THEORIES OF HYPNOSIS
Current Models and
Perspectives

THE GUILFORD CLINICAL AND EXPERIMENTAL HYPNOSIS SERIES

EDITORS
MICHAEL J. DIAMOND AND HELEN M. PETTINATI

THEORIES OF HYPNOSIS
Current Models and Perspectives

Edited by
Steven Jay Lynn
Judith W. Rhue

THE GUILFORD PRESS
New York   London

© 1991 The Guilford Press

Published in the United States of America by
The Guilford Press
A Division of Guilford Publications, Inc.
72 Spring Street, New York, N. Y. 10012

Printed in the United States of America

This book is printed on acid-free paper

Last digit is print number   9 8 7 6 5 4 3 2 1

Library of Congress Cataloging-in-Publication Data

Theories of hypnosis :   current models and perspectives   /   edited by
    Steven Jay Lynn and Judith W. Rhue.
        p.   cm. —(The Guilford clinical and experimental hypnosis
    series
        Includes bibliographical references and index.
        ISBN 0-89862-343-X
        1. Hypnotism.   2. Hypnotism—Therapeutic use.   I. Lynn, Steven J.
    II. Rhue, Judith, W.   III. Series.
        [DNLM: 1. Hypnosis.   2. Models, Psychological.   3. Psychological
    Theory.   WM 415 T385
    BF1141.T44   1991
    154.7—dc20
    DNLM/DLC
for Library of Congress   91-28531
                                                                     CIP

To my aunt, Harriette Lesser,
and my uncle, Rowen Glie,
with love, for being who and all that they are.
Steven Jay Lynn

To my mother, Raye Williams,
and my daughter, Martha Kate Rhue,
with much love.
Judith W. Rhue

Foreword

The distinction between the expansionist view of "something-more" and the reductionist view of "nothing-but" continues to lie at the center of theoretical diversity in the field of hypnosis. Some theorists and practitioners have interpreted the phenomena of hypnosis as revealing manifestations of basic mental processes and structures. Others have sought to explain the same phenomena as directly or indirectly suggested enactments and illusions.

However, some significant changes have taken place during the 30-odd years that I have followed developments in this area. Researchers and clinicians are now in closer agreement about what constitutes sound research methods and credible findings. There is a larger body of experimental and individual-difference data that a serious theory must explain. Today's major something-more models do not treat hypnotic phenomena as entirely singular, nor do the nothing-but competitors treat them as entirely ordinary. The former make systematic efforts to assimilate hypnotic phenomena into modern psychodynamic and psychostructural frameworks; the latter have enlarged their explanatory base to include subtle attributional and interpersonal processes. The field of hypnosis is becoming a testing ground for general psychological theories.

Theories of Hypnosis: Current Models and Perspectives offers neophytes and experts a scholarly and engaging overview of these contemporary developments and their historical background. The essays, written specifically for this volume by recognized experts, present and compare alternative views and provide vigorous and carefully argued critiques. Drs. Lynn and Rhue themselves have been active editors. Their personal contributions—the introductory and concluding chapters, and theoretical essay—are sure to mobilize the reader's integrative efforts. I expect this book to serve as a major reference for years to come.

Auke Tellegen
August 26, 1991

Acknowledgments

In editing and writing our chapters for this book, we have incurred many debts, both intellectual and personal. In addition to the students whose curiosity and questions provided the impetus for undertaking this project, we are particularly grateful to our family members, Jennifer and Jessica Lynn, and Raye Williams and Martha Kate Rhue, for their love, understanding, and support. Beyond that, we would like to thank James Council, Joseph Green, John Chaves, Irving Kirsch, Steven Kvall, David Sandberg, Harry Sivec, Nicholas Spanos, and Cheryl Yatsko for their comments on the manuscript, which helped to improve the book in many ways. We also would like to express our appreciation to our editor, Sharon Panulla, for her shrewd judgment and sound advice. Of course, this book would not have been possible without the interest, enthusiasm, and expertise of the contributors to this volume, and they deserve our special thanks and deep appreciation.

Preface

For the past 10 years, we have taught hypnosis to clinical psychology and medical students. Teaching hypnotic inductions, the administration of suggestions, and therapeutic applications of hypnosis is met with excitement and even awe when students first encounter a subject who exhibits such classical hypnotic responses as posthypnotic amnesia or age regression. Yet no hypnosis course is complete without exposing students to the fascinating history of hypnosis and the theoretical accounts that have been advanced to explain the dramatic phenomena that so intrigue the novice hypnotist. Teaching this aspect of the course is particularly challenging, because students often confront us with thoughtful questions about the opinions and viewpoints of historical and contemporary contributors to the hypnosis literature. Unfortunately, we have not always been able to answer our students' questions, at least to our satisfaction. Perhaps a little (student) knowledge is a dangerous thing, at least with respect to professors who fumble for answers to difficult questions.

We have heard it said, "If you do not know the answer to something, then write (or edit) a book." If the practicality of this advice is questionable, we nevertheless decided to heed it in this instance; there simply was no sourcebook available that provided a coherent picture of contemporary theoretical developments in the field of hypnosis. We therefore invited authors who had made substantial contributions to advancing the conceptual understanding of hypnosis to submit definitive statements of their current thinking about hypnosis.

Fortunately, it was not difficult to convince many eminent authorities that a resource book of contemporary theories, models, and perspectives would fill a void in the hypnosis literature. The list of authors who shared our enthusiasm and were able to participate is not exhaustive; however, their contributions represent important clinical and research traditions, which extend beyond the territory of hypnosis to mainstream psychology. These traditions include psychoanalysis, neodissociation theory, general systems theory, role theory and symbolic interactionism, social learning theory, communications theory, contextualism, and social and cognitive psychology.

We selected these theories not only because of their heuristic value and innovative insights, but also because they represent major hypnosis paradigms and schools of thought. One of our reasons for inviting contributors who are leading exponents of competing viewpoints was to share a sense of excitement about hypnosis with our readers. This excitement derives in large measure from the lively and at times acrimonious debates that have kindled the flame of discovery and expanded the borders of knowledge about hypnosis.

Controversies and disputes also extend to research findings and their interpretation. Vigorous debate often follows close on the heels of the publication of research in apparent support of a particular theory. A consideration of supportive research is necessary to evaluate the evidential basis of any theory. In Parts Two through Five of our book, research findings relevant to each perspective are summarized after the theory is introduced and the theoretical concepts and principles are set forth. This streamlined organization is intended to facilitate comparison of core concepts and research findings across theories. To lend a vital quality to the writing, we encouraged authors to write first-person accounts of their thinking that included statements of the intellectual lineage of their approach.

As a backdrop for contemporary hypnosis theories, the two chapters of Part One provide very different perspectives on the history of hypnosis. The decision to include two historical chapters is in keeping with our intention of providing readers with the broadest possible vista from which to view contemporary hypnosis. A brief introductory chapter preceding Part One, and a concluding section, complete the book's organizational scheme.

Our book is intended to appeal to students, instructors, researchers, and clinicians who desire an insider's view of major hypnosis theories, models, and perspectives. It goes beyond a straightforward rendering of theories to provide a thorough discussion of hypnotic phenomena, summaries of cutting-edge research programs, and a discussion of strengths and weaknesses of research strategies and methods used to address crucial theoretical questions. Many of the chapters tackle prickly questions, such as whether hypnosis evokes an altered state of consciousness; whether hypnotic behavior is involuntary; whether hypnotizability is stable, trait-like, and modifiable; and whether hypnotic and nonhypnotic behavior can be distinguished in meaningful ways. If the book does not contain *answers* to readers' questions about hypnosis, we hope that it will at least address them from multiple vantage points. More than that, we hope that our book stimulates critical thinking, research, and the sorts of questions that are at the leading edge of the theoretical and scientific advances described in the pages that follow.

S. J. L.
J. W. R.

Contributors

Éva Bányai, Ph.D., is the Head of the Department of Experimental Psychology, Eötvös Loránd University (ELTE), Budapest, Hungary. After earning her doctorate in psychology at ELTE in 1973, she spent a fellowship year with E. R. Hilgard at Stanford University where she developed active-alert hypnosis. For 15 years she was research associate at the Department of Comparative Physiology at ELTE, where her research focused mainly on the psychophysiological mechanisms of hypnosis. Since her research interests became extended to the subjective, behavioral, and interpersonal aspects of hypnosis, she moved to her present department in 1985, where she is heavily engaged in teaching and clinical activities. Dr. Banyai is a past president of the Hypnosis Section of the Hungarian Psychiatric Society, and is a member of several governing bodies of the Hungarian psychologists' community.

Joseph Barber, Ph.D., is Associate Clinical Professor in the Departments of Psychiatry and Pediatrics, UCLA School of Medicine, and received his doctorate at the University of Southern California, where Professor Perry London was his mentor. He is co-editor (with Cheri Adrian) of *Psychological Approaches to the Management of Pain*, which earned the Shapiro Award of the Society for Clinical and Experimental Hypnosis. He is a Diplomate of the American Board of Psychological Hypnosis and a Fellow of both the American Society of Clinical Hypnosis and The Society for Clinical and Experimental Hypnosis. He is President-Elect of The Society for Clinical and Experimental Hypnosis, and serves as Associate Editor and Book Review Editor for the *American Journal of Clinical Hypnosis*.

Kenneth S. Bowers, Ph.D., is a professor in the clinical psychology program at the University of Waterloo. He has participated, during sabbaticals, in Ernest Hilgard's hypnosis laboratory at Stanford University. During his most recent sabbatical, he served as Hilgard Visiting Professor of Psychology. While his primary committment is the study of hypnosis, he has also published work in the area of personality, unconscious processes, and intuition. He is a past president of the Society for Clinical and Experimental Hypnosis.

John F. Chaves, Ph.D., is Professor and Head of the Behavioral Sciences Section, School of Dental Medicine, Southern Illinois University at Edwardsville. He received his doctorate in psychology from Northeastern University, and has subsequently held positions at the Children's Hospital Medical Center in Boston and the Medfield Foundation. Dr. Chaves is Fellow of the American Psychological Association and past president of its Division of Psychological Hypnosis and of the Missouri Psychological Association. A recipient of the Milton H. Erickson Award, he is also a Fellow of the Society for Clinical and Experimental Hypnosis and the American Psychological Society. Dr. Chaves is the author of more than 30 chapters and articles, and co-authored, with T. X. Barber and N. P. Spanos, *Hypnosis, Imagination, and Human Potentialities,* and co-edited, with N. P. Spanos, *Hypnosis: The Cognitive-Behavioral Perspective.* He has authored an audiotape series, 'Tactics and Strategies of Clinical Hypnosis,' as well as clinical videotapes on pain management. He has presented more than 100 continuing education programs on clinical hypnosis in pain management for psychologists, dentists, and physicians throughout the United States and Canada.

William C. Coe, Ph.D., is a Professor of Medical Psychology at California State University at Fresno. After receiving his doctorate in clinical psychology at the University of California, Berkeley, he worked for three years at Langley-Porter Neuropsychiatric Institute in San Francisco. For 22 years, he maintained a private practice in clinical psychology. Dr. Coe co-authored, with Theodore Sarbin, *Hypnosis: A Social Psychological Analysis of Influence Communication,* and has written six chapters and published over 50 articles on hypnosis, in addition to presenting many papers at conventions and workshops. Past president of Division 30 of the American Psychological Association, Psychological Hypnosis, he also reviews for a number of journals. His other major interest is in behavioral and cognitive therapy.

Thomas M. Davidson, Ph.D., received his doctorate in clinical psychology from the University of Waterloo, where he cultivated his interest in social-cognitive and dissociative theories of hypnosis - particularly in relation to cognitive models of memory. He currently works as a forensic psychologist at the maximum security Mental Health Centre Penetanguishene, assessing men who have committed serious criminal offenses, and is an expert on the insanity defense, sexual offenders, and psychopathy. Dr. Davidson also has an active private practice where he continues to explore the clinical applications of hypnosis for habit control and self-management.

William E. Edmonston, Jr., Ph.D., is Professor of Psychology and Director of the Neuroscience Program at Colgate University and president of Edmonston Publishing. In 1988, he was a National Gold Medalist in the CASE Professor of the Year program and was named New York State Professor of the Year. He is the author of *Hypnosis and Relaxation: Modern Verification of an Old Equation* and *The Induction of Hypnosis* and editor of *Unfurl the Flags: Remembrances of the American Civil War.* The focus of his present research is the assessment of the protein composition of the CNS relative to CNS regeneration. A Fellow of the A.A.A.S., the American Psychological Association, the American Psychopathological Assocation, and the Society for Clinical and Experimental Hypnosis, Dr. Edmonston is a past president and founding member of the Division of Psychological Hypnosis (APA) and past president of the American Society of Clinical Hypnosis. From 1968 to 1976 he was editor of the *American Journal of Clinical Hypnosis.*

Frederick J. Evans, Ph.D., is Adjunct Professor in the Department of Psychiatry, UMDNJ-Robert Wood Johnson Medical School, Piscataway, NJ, and Vice-President, Texas Institute of Behavioral Medicine and Neuroscience, Houston. A licensed psychologist, Dr. Evans is the immediate past president of the International Society of Hypnosis, and has served as president of the Division of Psychological Hypnosis (APA) and the Society for Clinical and Experimental Hypnosis. He is also a Vice-President of the International Society for Mental Training and was a founding member of the Board of Directors of the American Pain Society. An Associate Editor of the *American Journal of Clinical Hypnosis*, he is on the editorial board of several journals. Much of the research summarized in his chapter was conducted when he was at the Insitute of the Pennsylvania Hospital and as Director of Research at the Carrier Foundation in Bell Mead, NJ.

David P. Fourie, Ph.D., is an Associate Professor in the Department of Psychology at the University of South Africa, Pretoria. He is involved in the training of psychologists in ecosystemic psychotherapy and also runs a part-time private practice. He is a member of the Psychological Association of South Africa, the South African Society of Clinical Hypnosis, the British Psychological Society, and the International Family Therapy Association.

Melvin A. Gravitz, Ph. D., received his doctorate in clinical psychology from Adelphi University. He is currently a Clinical Professor of Psychiatry and Behavioral Sciences at George Washington University, and has a private practice in Washington, D.C. A former president of the American Society of Clinical Hypnosis, the American Board of Psychological Hypnosis, and the American Board of Professional Psychology, and past editor of the *American Journal of Clinical Hypnosis*, Dr. Gravitz is a frequent contributor to the scientific literature, and has presented numerous workshops and seminars on hypnosis throughout the country.

Ernest R. Hilgard, Ph.D., received his doctorate in experimental psychology from Yale University. Currently Emeritus Professor of Psychology and Education at Stanford University, he has served that institution for over fifty years. Professor Hilgard is past president of the American Psychological Association and of Divisions 26 (History of Psychology) and 30 (Psychological Hypnosis), and of the International Society of Hypnosis and the Society for Clinical and Experimental Hypnosis. He was awarded the Franklin Gold Medal, International Society of Hypnosis, and has been the recipient of five other awards and medals. He has provided a broad range of public services to the U.S. government and private institutions, and has written, co-authored, and edited 10 books and numerous papers in scientific journals.

Irving Kirsch, Ph.D., is a Professor of Psychology at the University of Connecticut. A fellow of the American Psychological Association and the American Psychological Society, he is a North American Editor of *Contemporary Hypnosis*. Author of more than 60 journal articles, Dr. Kirsch is best known for his development of response expectancy theory, an extension of social learning theory. His book, *Changing Expectations: A Key to Effective Psychotherapy*, was published in 1990. Besides hypnosis, Dr. Kirsch has published research on anxiety disorders, depression, behavior therapy, and placebo effects.

Jean-Roch Laurence, Ph.D., is an Associate Professor of Psychology at Concordia University, Montréal, Québec, Canada. He is the founding president of la Société Québécoise de l'Hypnose and is a Fellow of the Society for Clinical and Experimental Hypnosis. He co-authored, with Campbell Perry, *Hypnosis, Will, and Memory: A Psycholegal History*.

Steven Jay Lynn, Ph.D., is a Professor of Psychology at Ohio University and has a private practice. He is a former president of the American Psychological Association, Division of Psychological Hypnosis, an American Psychological Association, American Psychological Society, and Society for Clinical and Experimental Hyposis Fellow, and a diplomate of the American Board of Psychological Hypnosis. He has received two SCEH awards for research excellence. An advisory editor of *Journal of Abnormal Psychology* and the *International Journal of Clinical and Experimental Hypnosis*, and a North American Editor of *Contemporay Hypnosis*, Dr. Lynn has written or edited textbooks on abnormal psychology and psychotherapy, and has published more than 80 articles on hypnosis, child abuse, psychotherapy, and behavioral medicine.

Kevin M. McConkey, Ph.D., received his doctorate in psychology from the University of Queensland, Australia, and is currently Associate Professor of Psychology at Macquarie University. A recipient of the Early

Career Award of the Australian Psychological Association, Dr. McConkey is a Fellow of that Society as well as of the American Psychological Association, the American Psychological Society, and the Society for Clinical and Experimental Hypnosis. His research interests include hypnosis and related phenomena, mood and emotion, and memory and amnesia.

Robert Nadon, Ph.D., is Assistant Professor and a Social Sciences and Humanities Research Council (SSHRC) Canada Fellow at Brock University, St. Catharines, Ontario, Canada. He is a Consulting Editor of *Contemporary Hypnosis*.

Michael R. Nash, Ph.D., is Associate Professor of Clinical Psychology at the University of Tennessee. He is a Fellow of the Society for Clinical and Experimental Hypnosis and is past president of Division 30 of the American Psychological Association. Dr. Nash's clinical and research interests include the assessment and treatment of sexually abused women, psychosocial intervention with cancer patients, and short-term psychoanalytic psychotherapy.

Campbell W. Perry, Ph.D., is Professor of Psychology at Concordia University, Montréal, Québec, Canada. A Fellow of both the Society for Clinical and Experimental Hypnosis and the American Psychological Society, he is also Book Review Editor for the *International Journal of Clinical and Experimental Hypnosis*. Dr. Perry has co-authored, with Jean-Roch Laurence, *Hypnosis, Will, and Memory: A Psycholegal History*, and with Peter Sheehan, *Methodologies of Hypnosis: A Critical Appraisal of Contemporary Paradigms of Hypnosis*.

Peter J. Rennick, M.S. (Counseling Psychology), has been a member of the clinical staff of the Milton H. Erickson Center for Hypnosis and Psychotherapy, Phoenix, Arizona, and teaches in training programs in Eriksonian approaches to hypnosis organized by the Milton H. Erickson Foundation. He is employed by the city of Tempe as a family therapist, involved with providing education programs for the city, and conducts a private practice there. During the past several years he has developed an expertise in working with anxiety disorders and is particularly interested in the use of metaphors and stories in therapy.

Judith W. Rhue, Ph.D., is an Associate Professor of Family Medicine at the Ohio University College of Osteopathic Medicine. She is actively involved in the Society for Clincial and Experimental Hypnosis and the American Psychological Association, Division of Psychological Hypnosis, and has received awards for excellence in research from both organizations. Dr. Rhue serves on the editorial board for *Contemporary Hypnosis*, and as a reviewer for four American journals. She is co-editor of two hypnosis books, and has written numerous articles and book chapters. Her research interests include hypnosis, fantasy, and child abuse.

Theodore R. Sarbin, Ph.D., received his doctorate in psychology from Ohio State University and is currently Professor Emeritus of Psychology and Criminology at the University of California, Santa Cruz. His bibliography includes over 200 titles on various topics in theoretical, social, and personality psychology. A recipient of the Morton Prince Award, he has been a long-time contributor to the scientific literature on hypnosis and related phenomena. The Society for Clinical and Experimental Hypnosis recognized him and his collaborator, William C. Coe, with its award for the Best Theoretical Paper of 1979: "Hypnosis and Psychopathology: Replacing Old Myths with Fresh Metaphors."

Peter W. Sheehan, Ph.D., is Professor of Psychology and Academic Director of Research at the University of Queensland, Brisbane, Australia. He has worked at the Unit of Experimental Psychiatry at the Institute of the Pennsylvania Hospital, University of Pennsylvania; the City College of the City of New York; and the The University of New England, Armidale, Australia. His special interests are the imagery and its relationship to hypnotic phenomena, and the role of memory in hypnosis. He co-authored with C. W. Perry *Methodologies of Hypnosis: A Critical Appraisal of Contemporary Paradigms of Hypnosis,* and with K. McConkey, *Hypnosis and Experience: The Exploration of Phenomena and Process.* Dr. Sheehan is currently President of the Academy of the Social Sciences in Australia.

Nicholas P. Spanos, Ph.D., is a Professor of Psychology and Director of the Laboratory for Experimental Hypnosis at Carleton University. He received his doctorate in sociology from Boston University, and subsequently worked at the Medfield Foundation and was Director of Clinical Services at Boston Psychological Associates. A fellow of the American Psychological Association, and member of Division 30, Psychological Hypnosis, Dr. Spanos has publishede over 200 papers and book chapters on hypnosis, multiple personality, the history of psychiatry, and psychology and the law.

Graham F. Wagstaff, Ph.D., is Senior Lecturer in Psychology in the Department of Psychology at the University of Liverpool, England. His main teaching area is social psychology, and his research interests are the social psychology of hypnosis, with special reference to compliance and belief processes, and forensic aspects of hypnosis. He also has interests in the psychology and philosophy of social and criminal justice.

Jeffrey K. Zeig, Ph.D., is the Director and Founder of The Milton H. Erickson Foundation in Phoenix, Arizona. He received his doctorate from

Georgia State University and currently maintains an active private practice. In addition, he regularly conducts teaching seminars on Ericksonian psychotherapy and hypnosis throughout the world. Dr. Zeig has organized all of the yearly Erickson Congresses and Seminars since 1980, including the landmark 1985 and 1990 Evolution of Psychotherapy Conferences. He serves on the editorial board of two foreign and three American journals, and has edited or co-edited eight books and three monographs. He authored *Experiencing Erickson*, and a book about his work has been published in Italy. His books have been translated into seven languages.

Contents

THEORIES OF HYPNOSIS
Current Models and
Perspectives

Theories of Hypnosis: An Introduction

STEVEN JAY LYNN and JUDITH W. RHUE
Ohio University

HYPNOSIS: INCREASING ACCEPTANCE, DIFFERING PERSPECTIVES

The hypnotist drones, "Your hand is getting lighter, lighter, it is rising, rising by itself, lifting off the resting surface." Slowly but perceptibly, the subject's hand lifts in herky-jerky movements, in synchronization with the suggestions. After hypnosis, she insists that the movements felt involuntary and automatic. The hypnotist then suggests that she will remember many events from her past that she has forgotten. When she hears the words "Now you can remember everything," she experiences a flood of vivid childhood impressions. Two more suggestions follow: one for numbness in her hand, after which the subject appears insensitive to painful levels of stimulation, and another for the unsightly warts on her arm to fade away and disappear. She reports a mild tingling in the area, which is now noticeably tinged with red.

For more than 200 years, these sorts of demonstrations have fired the curiosity of laypersons, researchers, and clinicians. The seemingly magical, dramatic changes in hypnotized subjects' appearance, experiences, and behaviors have no doubt been responsible for the widespread interest in hypnosis and the application of hypnotic techniques to treat an array of psychological and psychophysiological problems (Kraft & Rudolfa, 1982). As Graham (1991) observes, "Today hypnosis is a loved sibling within the family of therapeutic techniques, and signs of that love abound" (p. 79).

What are the signs? Not only is hypnosis becoming increasingly accepted in scientific and scholarly circles, but the 1980s have witnessed appreciable growth in the numbers of clinical colleagues who identify with hypnosis and are interested in learning about and applying hypnotic techniques in their practices (Baker, 1987). That many professionals identify with hypnosis is made plain by consideration of the fact that from 1980 to 1990, the membership of the American Psychological Association (APA) Division of Psychological Hypnosis more than doubled, to total nearly 1,500 members. In the United States alone, there are about 20 different hypnosis societies or associations, with a combined membership of more than 21,000 (Burek, Koek, & Novallo, 1989).

Applications of hypnotherapy are booming. According to a national sample of psychologists, substantial numbers use hypnosis regularly in treating problems from anxiety disorders to personality and schizophrenic disorders (Kraft & Rudolfa, 1982). Furthermore, nearly half of the sample, drawn from the general membership of the APA, had received hypnosis training.

Baker (1987) notes that this recent surge of interest in clinical applications of hypnosis stems in part from a more solid research base supporting the scientific status of hypnosis. Baker is joined by like-minded clinicians and investigators (Fromm, 1987; Fromm & Shor, 1979; Kraft & Rudolfa, 1982; Pulver & Pulver, 1975), who agree that the field of clinical hypnosis has become more scientifically oriented. Although well-controlled clinical studies are few in number, and it has not been documented that hypnotic techniques are superior to other treatment interventions (Spanos & Chaves, 1989), there is a growing appreciation of the need to conduct more rigorous investigations.

In addition to the popular trend toward integrating hypnotic techniques into clinical practice, recent years have witnessed an unprecedented interest in hypnosis as a scientific phenomenon (Rudolfa et al., 1988). Graham (1990) notes that 30 years ago the *Psychological Abstracts* contained only 56 citations under hypnosis and related headings. Yet by 1978 the number had increased to 124, and by 1989 the number had more than doubled to 271. Nash, Minton, and Baldridge (1988) categorized over 3,500 scientific articles on hypnosis that were published between 1966 and 1985. During the most recent 4-year period (1982–1985, inclusive), they found evidence of a sharp increase in articles, with more articles published in this period than any other. The authors conclude that there is a stable level of acceptance and interest in hypnosis across years and disciplines (dental, medical, and psychological journals; core hypnosis specialty journals; and interdisciplinary journals). They further conclude that this stability, along with the growth of hypnosis specialty journals, portends maturation of the field.

Yet, despite the undeniable signs of increasing interest in and popularity of hypnosis, voices can be heard that are critical of the lack of a commonly accepted definition or unifying theory of hypnosis. Baker (1987) believes that an increasing pragmatic and technological emphasis has supplanted the drive to understand hypnotic phenomena and the complexities of human behavior. Hall (1989) has commented that hypnosis is a "collection of techniques in need of a unifying theory" (p. 7). Rossi (1986) bemoans the fact that "Since the inception of hypnosis more than 200 years ago, it has been impossible to find general agreement among professionals on just exactly what hypnosis is" (p. 3). In this book, Nadon, Laurence, and Perry (Chapter 16) virtually echo Rossi's remark by noting that two centuries' worth of research has not resolved the question of what hypnosis is. Hilgard (Chapter 3), in turn, agrees that a universally accepted definition of what constitutes hypnosis is elusive.

There is no question that hypnosis has eluded a single, simple definition. This is not surprising; the field is far from reaching a consensus about how to explain hypnotic phenomena. What is the essence of hypnosis for one theorist is mere artifact for another. Whereas some theorists are credulous about the parallel between hypnotic effects and corresponding natural phenomena (e.g., blindness, hallucinations), other theorists assume a more skeptical stance about hypnotic phenomena. These latter theorists assume that subjects' actions simply reflect mundane responses to suggestion, rather than a special state of consciousness induced by hypnotic communications (Kihlstrom, 1991; Sutcliffe, 1960).

As Sutcliffe (1960) observed more than 30 years ago, different schools of thought about hypnosis make radically different assumptions, adopt different methodologies, and accept different data as admissible evidence (see McConkey, Chapter 18, this volume). The state of affairs is not much different today. It reflects a field of inquiry that has grown in its knowledge base but has not matured to the point that consensus exists regarding basic assumptions and methods of inquiry. We would argue that this reflects not so much a hiatus or impasse in the evolution of the scientific study of hypnosis, as a fertile yet prolonged period of consolidation of research findings around differing paradigms that continue to compete for scientific support and validation.

Even though disagreement about how to define and conceptualize hypnosis abounds, it is nevertheless possible to specify a "domain of hypnosis" (Hilgard, 1973) that characterizes the sorts of phenomena that are included and lie outside it. As Hilgard notes in Chapter 3 of this book, there is widespread agreement about what phenomena (e.g., muscular movements, sensory distortions, hallucinations, posthypnotic amnesia, and hypnotic dreams) are included within this domain. In fact, the items that comprise contemporary hypnosis scales reflect a consensus about what sorts of phenomena are considered "hypnotic," which can be traced back to the 19th century. This consensus makes it possible for disparate theorists to converge in terms of the phenomena that are the subjects of their theory-building efforts.

In addition to the fact that they address a circumscribed and relatively well-delineated set of phenomena, contemporary hypnosis theories converge in many of the observations and issues they address. For example, it is virtually incumbent on a hypnosis theory to account for the well-documented finding of individual differences in hypnotic responsiveness; for alterations in suggestion-related subjective experience; and for the fact that hypnotic performance is generally stable over time, barring interventions designed to enhance hypnotizability.

Views of hypnosis differ in terms of whether they are aptly characterized as theories, as models, or simply as approaches to understanding hypnosis. Many contributors to this book edge away from describing their views as formal theories; they recognize that their viewpoints are tentative and lacking in detail and specificity. The authors who seem the least reluctant to describe their approaches as theories derive their viewpoints from well-established theories (e.g., dissociation, social learning) originally tendered to account for events outside the arena of hypnosis. In each case, puzzling hypnotic events are explained in terms of more familiar or established concepts (see Hanson, 1965).

Many of the formulations presented herein have properties of models, and can be so described. That is, they rely in part on metaphors and analogies to select events as relevant for study, to represent aspects of hypnotic behavior and experience, and to hypothesize about how the events are organized (see Price & Lynn, 1986). For example, theorists draw attention to the parallels between the behavior or condition of the hypnotized subject and role playing, relaxation, dissociation, and psychological regression outside the hypnotic context.

We use the term "perspective" to capture the fact that by adopting a particular model, analogy, or conceptual scheme for representing hypnosis, a powerful effect is exerted on how we "see" or perceive the events in question (see Price & Lynn, 1986). We contend that at least two major perspectives can be identified—the neodissociation and the sociocognitive perspectives—that view the transactions constituting hypnosis in fundamentally different ways. The fact that puzzling hypnotic behaviors are viewed from divergent perspectives creates flashpoints of tension among conflicting perspectives that vie for empirical support. These tensions are well represented in this book, as are areas of agreement and accommodation among different models. In order to highlight major issues and important points of convergence and divergence among theories, we introduce the chapters in the section that follows.

OVERVIEW OF THE BOOK

Views of Hypnosis in History

The historical context of the major debates in the field is examined in Part One, which consists of two chapters on the history of hypnosis. The first chapter, by Gravitz, provides an overview of early clinical theories of hypnosis. The second chapter, by Spanos and Chaves, delineates a very different history of hypnosis, written from the perspective that hypnosis can be thought of as a cultural creation.

Single-Factor Theories

Part Two of the book is introduced by theorists who maintain that a single process, trait, or mechanism is at the heart of diverse hypnotic phenomena. The first three chapters in this section are contributed by theorists (Hilgard, Bowers & Davidson, and Evans) who attribute profound alterations in consciousness and behavior during hypnosis to dissociative processes and abilities. These neodissociation theories are followed by Nash's and Edmonston's theories, which replace dissociation with psychological regression and relaxation, respectively, as central explanatory constructs.

The Neodissociation Perspective: Hypnosis as Dissociation

The neodissociation perspective is one of the dominant contemporary hypnosis perspectives. Many hypnosis theorists either embrace dissociation or reject it outright as an explanatory mechanism. Whether investigators are hostile or friendly to the construct, hypotheses derived from neodissociation theory have served as a platform for a great deal of contemporary hypnosis research. Indeed, the conceptual borders of a number of theories, particularly the sociocognitive approaches described below, have been brought into relief by contrast with neodissociation theory. In short, the impact and the heuristic value of neodissociation theory are formidable.

In the first chapter in this section, Hilgard notes that neodissociation theory is based on the idea that there exist multiple cognitive systems or cognitive structures in hierarchical arrangement under some measure of control by an "executive ego." The executive ego, or "central control structure," is responsible for planning and monitoring functions of the personality. Under special circumstances, such as hypnosis, these systems may become independent of or dissociated from each other. During hypnosis, relevant subsystems of control are temporarily dissociated from conscious executive control and are instead directly activated by the hypnotist's suggestions.

According to neodissociation theory, both motoric and nonmotoric responses, such as analgesia and amnesia, are potentially mediated by dissociative processes. For example, in the case of analgesia, the activation of a subsystem of pain control during hypnosis is temporarily less guided by plans and intentions than would ordinarily be the case. This diminished conscious executive control is responsible for the subjective impression of nonvolition that typically accompanies hypnotic responses. The fact that neodissociation theorists acknowledge that hypnosis may involve a change in the subject's state or condition has earned them the appellation of "state theorists" (Fellows, 1990). Finally, dissociation theorists believe that hypnotizability is generally stable and has trait-like properties.

In Chapter 4, Bowers and Davidson provide a critique of Spanos's sociocognitive/social-psychological position, while they present an ardent defense of the neodissociation position that Spanos, in turn, has criticized over the years. Following Hilgard, Bowers and Davidson cast neodissociation theory in the light of a general model of cognitive functioning. They maintain that the essence of the concept of dissociation is a simple idea: Not all action is consciously intended, initiated, or controlled. Bowers and Davidson assert that hypnotically suggested behavior is purposeful, in the sense that it is goal-directed—that is, it achieves the suggested state of affairs. However, they also note that hypnotic behavior is nonvolitional, in the sense that it is not performed on purpose—that is, it does not flow from executive initiative and effort. Bowers and Davidson maintain that it is neither contradictory nor paradoxical to assert that goal-directed behavior can also be nonvolitional.

In Chapter 5, Evans elaborates the construct of dissociation by presenting converging evidence that individual differences exist in the degree of control with which it is possible to access different states of consciousness, psychological awareness, or cognitive functioning. According to Evans, this general ability is associated with hypnotic responsiveness, but is also related to a wide range of psychological and physiological phenomena, some of which have clinical significance concerning the development and alleviation of symptoms. Evans's wide-ranging research includes studies on sleep and hypnosis; interrelationships between and among hypnotizability, punctuality, and absorption; and the relevance of hypnotizability to psychiatric patient populations and treatment outcome.

Hypnosis as Psychological Regression

Nash, in Chapter 6, maintains that hypnosis represents an altered state or condition of the person. However, he contends that processes other than dissociation or relaxation are responsible for this altered state. From a psychoanalytic perspective, Nash argues that hypnosis is a special case of psychological regression. This regression is characterized by fundamental alterations in the experience of self, relationship, and the way information is processed. Phenomena such as transference, in which the hypnotist becomes the repository of the subject's archaic interpersonal schema, are actually products of a topographic regression attendant upon a shift from secondary process to more primary-process thinking. In its reference to a hierarchical model of the mind in which subsystems of the ego can act independently of the executive ego, and in the view that hypnosis involves a relaxation of executive ego functioning, Nash's theory resembles neodissociation theory.

Hypnosis as Relaxation: Anesis

According to Edmonston (Chapter 7), it is not dissociation or psychological regression but relaxation that precedes and "forms the fundamental basis of subsequent phenomena associated with the term 'hypnosis.'" After citing a large body of clinical and physiological evidence, which suggests that many parallels exist between the effects of a hypnotic induction and the effects of relaxation, Edmonston proposes to replace the term "hypnosis" with "anesis," the noun form of the Greek verb *aniesis*—"to relax, to let go." Edmonston contends that relaxation is so basic a process that other mechanisms, such as dissociation and psychological regression, are in fact secondary to it.

Clinical Perspectives

Many contributors to this book note that their theories are applicable to clinical as well as experimental populations and settings. However, the next two chapters present viewpoints with explicit relevance to the practice of psychotherapy. J. Barber (Chapter 8) tenders an eclectic model of hypnosis; in so doing, he invokes a variety of explanatory mechanisms to account for the curative properties of hypnosis. Zeig and Rennick (Chapter 9) set forth an Ericksonian model of hypnosis, which represents an increasingly popular and influential clinical tradition.

Barber attributes the therapeutic influence of hypnosis to the interaction between a hypnotically induced altered state of consciousness and an intense, even archaic therapeutic relationship with the patient. The patient's imaginative and dissociative capacities, which predict the likelihood of responding to hypnotic suggestions, can be accessed and exploited for therapeutic purposes. To maximize treatment gains, it is possible to vary the hypnotic proceedings and the relationship idiosyncratically to unlock the client's naturally occurring dissociative capacities and other beneficial unconscious processes— hence the name of Barber's approach, the "locksmith model."

Zeig and Rennick's approach is rooted in Milton Erickson's communications model of hypnosis. Along with Barber, they contend that hypnotic responsivity and treatment gains can be optimized by customizing techniques to fit the individual's needs, personality, and unique life circumstances. One of the therapist's most important tasks is to cultivate the patient's responsiveness to minimal cues. Zeig and Rennick's description of hypnosis, as responsive behavior elicited from one person by another, is so vast in scope that it places virtually no bounds on situations defined as "hypnotic." As in single-factor theories, the utility of positing a hypnotic state or condition is supported by Zeig and Rennick and by Barber as well, at least in terms of characterizing the subjects' phenomenology.

The Sociocognitive Perspective

The next six chapters are contributed by sociocognitive theorists (Coe & Sarbin, Spanos, Wagstaff, ourselves, Kirsch, and Fourie), who contend that social and situational aspects of the hypnotic context, along with subjects' attitudes, expectations, and beliefs about hypnosis, must be considered in any complete theory of hypnosis. Given this dual emphasis on the social and cognitive dimensions of hypnosis, the term "sociocognitive" (see Spanos & Chaves, Chapter 2) is apt.

According to sociocognitive theorists, hypnosis is so defined not because of the operation of a single process, ability, or condition of the person but because it occurs in the context of an interaction that is labeled by the participants as "hypnosis." In this interaction, one person typically assumes the role of hypnotist and the other assumes the role of the subject. Shaped by attitudes, beliefs, and features of the situational context, the unfolding hypnotic proceedings are mutually constructed by the participants. In this sense, hypnosis is defined in a subjective yet operational manner.

According to this line of thinking, there is nothing "special" or unusual about hypnotic behavior (e.g., arm lifting, eye closing, forgetting, visualizing objects), apart from the properties ascribed to it by participants or observers who categorize a particular behavior as "hypnotic." Sociocognitive theorists are skeptical of the ability of hypnosis to transcend normal waking capacities, and claim that behaviors traditionally associated with hypnosis (e.g., age regression) can be achieved by appropriately motivated or instructed subjets (Kihlstrom, 1991). Unlike theorists who hold that hypnotizability is trait-like and mutable only within narrow limits, sociocognitive theorists maintain that hypnotic responsiveness can be substantially modified.

The authors of the first four chapters (Coe & Sarbin, Spanos, Wagstaff, and ourselves) in this section have been identified with a social-psychological approach to hypnosis. One of the primary assumptions of the social-psychological approach is that hypnotic behavior is fundamentally mundane, role-governed social behavior. The general scheme of what constitutes the mutual roles of hypnotist and subject is culturally transmitted. However, hypnotic communications—the induction and suggestions—are also influential in scripting elements of the coparticipants' roles. Rather than being passive automata, hypnotized subjects retain control of their behavior. Even their reports of suggestion-related involuntariness and alterations in consciousness reflect their active and ongoing attempts to have suggested experiences and gear their responses to shifting contextual and role-related demands. Subjects' use of cognitive strategies, which involve imagery, fantasy, and the allocation of attention, are implicated in creating convincing subjective experiences, such as the experience of nonvolition or posthypnotic amnesia.

Coe and Sarbin's theory (Chapter 10) relies heavily on the metaphor of "role" to capture parallels between the hypnotic interaction and a theatrical performance in which both the hypnotist and the subject enact reciprocal roles. Six role theory variables are deemed important: role location ("what is expected of me"), self–role congruence (match of role requirements with self-perceptions), role expectations (expectations regarding appropriate conduct), role skills (e.g., imaginative skills), role demands (situational demand characteristics), and the reinforcing properties of the audience. The withholding of secrets, the practice of deception, and self-deception strategies are viewed as playing a part in the way subjects come to think of their hypnotic conduct.

From Spanos's sociocognitive perspective (Chapter 11), hypnotic behavior, like ordinary behavior, is directed by personal goals, perceptions, and attributions of contextual demands and private experiences. For instance, subjects' reports of suggestion-related nonvolition are related to their interpretations of their responses to suggestion. These perceptions are shaped in part by passively worded suggestions, which imply that responses are "happenings" rather than mundane actions. According to Spanos, stability of hypnotic responding across testings reflects stability in subjects' interpretations and understandings of hypnosis, rather than the trait-like nature of hypnotizability. Finally, positive attitudes and at least moderate levels of imaginal abilities (e.g., absorption) may boost hypnotic responsivity, but are not sufficient to generate high levels of hypnotic responding in the absence of an active interpretational set that enables subjects to translate imaginal abilities into subjectively compelling hypnotic enactments.

Wagstaff (Chapter 12) argues that the notion of hypnosis as a state has erroneously implied that there exists some common element binding hypnotic phenomena together. According to Wagstaff, different hypnotic phenomena (i.e., pain control, posthypnotic amnesia) require different explanations. Furthermore, several processes may interact to give rise to individual phenomena, and the interactions between and among these processes may differ from situation to situation, and even from person to person. To describe these processes, and to account for hypnotic phenomena, Wagstaff suggests replacing traditional state terminology with terms and concepts such as "conformity," "compliance," "belief," "attitudes," "expectations," "attention," "concentration," "relaxation," "distraction," "role enactment," and "imagination."

In Chapter 13, we describe hypnotic subjects as creative agents who shape their experience and direct their actions in terms of their agendas, performance standards (criteria for judging the adequacy of their behaviors and experiences), relationship with the hypnotist, and perceptions of contextual and interpersonal demands. Our "integrative" model is so termed because it integrates concepts from social-psychological and cognitive perspectives on hypnosis, and it views the talented hypnotic subject as a seeker and integrator of information from an array of situational, personal, and interpersonal sources. Imaginings, goal-directed strivings, and expectancies are viewed as interactive and inseparable facets of subjects' behavioral and experiential stream.

The next two theories rely less on social-psychological concepts and principles than the sociocognitive theories we have summarized. Kirsch's response expectancy theory (Chapter 14) is an extension of social learning theory, and is based on the premise that expectancies can generate nonvolitional responses, both within and apart from the hypnotic context. In fact, Kirsch contends that subjects' expectancies can account for the gamut of hypnotic phenomena and can play an important role in accounting for individual differences. Kirsch believes that response expectancies can be immediate causes of hypnotic responses. For example, rather than directly affecting hypnotic responsiveness, imagery may enhance responsiveness by virtue of its effects on expectancy. Nevertheless, Kirsch is open to the possibility that response determinants, such as fantasy proneness, may exert an influence on hypnotic conduct that is independent of expectancies.

Based on systems theory, Fourie's ecosystemic approach (Chapter 15) uses the metaphor of the ecology of ideas to describe a complex, unfolding network of opinions, expectations and attributions in which "certain classes of behavior come to be seen as of a type called 'hypnotic'." According to Fourie, "hypnosis" is regarded as a concept that denotes a situation in which behaviors are designated as "hypnotic" by a process of co-construction or "ongoing mutual qualification" of the participants. Fourie's ecosystemic approach to hypnosis represents a move away from the traditional Newtonian tenets of reductionism, linear causality, and objectivity of observation, which Fourie believes characterize both state and nonstate theories. The hypnotist and subject are thus interpenetrating aspects of the whole situation, which is not readily divisible into constituent parts.

The focal themes (e.g., expectancies, interpretations of suggestions, impact of context) of sociocognitive approaches have been acknowledged, if not adopted, by other hypnosis theories (e.g., psychoanalytic, synergistic, contextual, social-psychobiological). Whereas single-factor theories de-emphasize expectancies and social-psychological determinants, and do not regard hypnotic behavior as mundane, goal-directed social behavior, no hypnosis theory summarily rejects cognitive and social-psychological processes as potential response determinants. The influence of the sociocognitive perspective on other lines of inquiry is evident in the interactive–phenomenological theories that follow.

Interactive–Phenomenological Theories

Theories that place particular emphasis on the interaction of multiple variables during hypnosis, and on understanding the subjects' experience, are classified under the rubric of "interactive–phenomenological" theories. Parallels can be drawn between the final group of contributors (Nadon, Laurence, & Perry; McConkey; Sheehan; Bányai) and the sociocognitive theorists. Agreement exists about the need to recognize multiple and interactive cognitive and situational determinants of hypnosis, such as attitudes, beliefs, expectancies, and demand characteristics. Nevertheless, the final group of contributors places more explicit emphasis on the study of interactive processes and underscores differences between hypnotic and waking behavior and cognitive activity. In addition, subjects' personality traits, styles, and/or abilities are accorded a prominent role in shaping or facilitating hypnotic experiences.

We have positioned Nadon, Laurence and Perry 's synergistic model (Chapter 16) first in this section because it makes a strong argument for the advantages of examining the interrelationship of personality, cognitive, and social-psychological factors as a means of understanding the contingencies that are integral to hypnotic performance. By "synergy," the authors mean the effects of various influences on hypnotic response in combination. Accordingly, the study of combined or synergistic effects is necessary in order to avoid the pitfalls of explanations that emphasize either personality or situational factors without duly considering their interrelationship or the host of potential variables (e.g., affective, cognitive) that can affect hypnotic responding. By advocating the use of correlational and experimental methodologies within single research designs, the authors advance a spirit or strategy of inquiry that captures the multidimensional nature of hypnosis.

Sheehan's contextual model (Chapter 17) highlights the interactive reciprocal relations between an active organism and an active context; the "fine-grained variation" in responsiveness to suggestion that exists among very hypnotizable subjects; rapport with the hypnotist; and processes believed to be distinctive in the way they operate during hypnosis. More specifically, the study of hypnosis and waking behavior can be distinguished by the nature of the subjects' motivations and cognitions. The core of Sheehan's model is the construct of "motivated cognitive commitment." This concept is not to be equated with conformity, compliance, or simple cooperation. Rather, it expresses subjects' motivated cognitive effort, or problem-solving attempts to respond appropriately to suggestions as they are understood within a particular framework, defined by the hypnotist and by the evolving hypnotic relationship.

According to McConkey (Chapter 18), it is a priority to understand the essential variability that characterizes subjects' hypnotic responses. To do so, it is necessary to examine the meaning that subjects assign to the hypnotist's communications, the idiosyncratic ways in which they cognitively process suggestions, and intraindividual differences that can occur in responding across suggestions. High hypnotizability reflects the interplay of subjects' cognitive skills (e.g., attention) and personal traits (e.g., absorption), along with the ability to process information that is both consistent and inconsistent with a suggested event in such a way that it facilitates the belief in the virtual reality of the event.

McConkey's and Sheehan's models emphasize subjects' cognitive commitment or readiness to cooperate with the hypnotist and to resolve conflicting role demands in a focused, goal-directed manner akin to problem solving. These models are particularly concerned with exploring subjects' experience of hypnosis and understanding the phenomenal meaning of suggested events. Hence, Spanos and Chaves's (Chapter 2) labeling of these theories as "social-phenomenological" is apropos. Elements of McConkey's and Sheehan's viewpoints have penetrated the formulations of disparate theorists, including J. Barber, Nash, and ourselves, in particular.

Bányai's social-psychobiological model is a multidimensional approach that is unique insofar as it encompasses physiological processes and concomitants of hypnosis in its purview. This interactional framework accords equal importance to the behavioral, experiential, relational, and physiological dimensions of hypnosis. To fully appreciate the meaning of the transactions between the subject and hypnotist, it is necessary to understand the interactions among these dimensions and the reciprocal nature of the hypnotist–subject relationship. According to this model, a hypnotically altered state of consciousness may have a socially and biologically adaptive value by spurring meaningful cognitive and emotional experiences that enrich both the hypnotist and the subject.

CONCLUSIONS

Our overview of the book suggests that theoretical viewpoints differ from one another in many respects. Yet there is substantial overlap among certain theories, with facets of one theory subtly shading into facets of another theory. The reader may take thus exception with our classification scheme. Indeed, a case could be made for placing a number of theories under different rubrics.

For example, Kirsch's and Fourie's theories could perhaps be classified as social-psychological theories. We have resisted this temptation for two reasons. First, Kirsch and Fourie do not identify themselves as social-psychological theorists. Second, unlike many social-psychological theories, neither Kirsch's nor Fourie's theory relies on metaphors and concepts derived from social psychology or role theory (e.g., self-presentation, role enactment, compliance, conformity). Nevertheless, many aspects of Kirsch's and Fourie's theories are not readily distinguishable from social-psychological theories, rendering conceptual boundaries fuzzy. To be sure, sharp distinctions are not possible among social-psychological theories themselves, although they differ with respect to the emphasis placed on conformity and compliance, role enactment, imaginative skills, cognitive strategies, performance standards, and interpersonal factors. Social-psychological theories are thus not monolithic (Kihlstrom, 1991).

Our categorical scheme is perhaps best regarded as a heuristic framework for organizing theories of hypnosis. What we wish to avoid is a rigid "pigeonholing" of approaches that obscures points of confluence among theories. To facilitate comparisons of theories, we identify a number of points of overlap that exist among theories before concluding our introductory comments.

First, many theorists represented in this volume (e.g., Coe & Sarbin, Spanos, ourselves, Zeig & Rennick, J. Barber, Nash, Sheehan, McConkey, Bányai) acknowledge that hypnotic behavior is interpersonal in nature, and that subjects' sensitivity to the hypnotist, subtle cues, and the tacit implications of hypnotic communications have a bearing on how they respond.

Second, even those theorists (e.g., Coe & Sarbin, Spanos, ourselves, Wagstaff, Sheehan, McConkey) who emphasize the conscious, goal-directed nature of hypnotic responding are alert to the fact that subjects may engage in self-deception, may be unaware of the intrapsychic and contextual determinants of their actions, and may engage in behaviors that fulfill suggested demands with little awareness that they are doing so. The view that hypnotic behavior and its determinants are not necessarily consciously articulated is a prominent feature of the neodissociation, psychoanalytic, Ericksonian, and locksmith models.

Third, a number of theorists (i.e., Coe & Sarbin, Spanos, ourselves, Wagstaff, Sheehan, McConkey, J. Barber, Fourie, Kirsch) are impressed by the active, even creative ways that subjects devise to fulfill suggested demands and resolve conflict about how to respond appropriately to suggestions.

Fourth, in many quarters, there seems to be at least a skeptical "wait-and-see" attitude toward (e.g., Bányai, Hilgard, Bowers & Davidson, Nadon et al.), if not an outright endorsement of (e.g, Spanos, ourselves, Wagstaff, Zeig & Rennick, J. Barber, Kirsch, Fourie), the possibility that hypnotizability is plastic or modifiable—at least within certain limits.

Fifth, many theorists (e.g., Coe & Sarbin, Spanos, ourselves, Wagstaff, Nadon et al., Zeig & Rennick, Nash, J. Barber, Bányai, Sheehan, McConkey, Fourie) believe that no single determinant is necessarily sufficient to account for the complexities of hypnotic behavior, which are increasingly being explained in terms of multiple, interactive social and cognitive variables.

And finally, virtually all of the contributors to our book locate their theory of hypnotic behavior within the larger arena of contemporary psychology, and draw on concepts from this larger domain to buttress their arguments.

In the concluding chapter, we address points of convergence and divergence among hypnosis theories in greater detail. We do so by considering three broad questions that have captured the attention of theorists who represent different schools of thought: (1) Is hypnosis an altered state of consciousness? (2) Is hypnotic behavior involuntary? (3) How stable, trait-like, and modifiable is hypnotizability? Finally, we discuss a number of pertinent research issues and directions for future research, with the goal of maximizing the heuristic value of the theories presented in our book.

REFERENCES

Baker, E. L. (1987). The state of the art of clinical hypnosis. *International Journal of Clinical and Experimental Hypnosis, 35,* 203–214.

Burek, D. M., Koek, K. E., & Novalllo, A. (Eds.). (1989) *Encyclopedia of associations: 1990.* (24th ed.). Detroit: Gale Research.

Fellows, B. J. (1990). Current theories of hypnosis: A critical overview. *British Journal of Clinical Hypnosis, 7,* 81–92.

Fromm, E. (1987). Significant developments in clinical hypnosis during the past 25 years. *International Journal of Clinical and Experimental Hypnosis, 35,* 215–230.

Fromm, E., & Shor, R.E. (1979). Underlying theoretical issues: An introduction. In E. Fromm & R. E. Shor (Eds.), *Hypnosis: Developments in research and new perspectives* (2nd ed., pp. 3–13). Chicago: Aldine.

Graham, K. R. (1991). Hypnosis: A case study in science. *Hypnos, 17,* 78–84.

Hall, J. A. (1989). *Hypnosis: A Jungian perspective.* New York: Guilford Press.

Hanson, N. R. (1965). *Patterns of discovery.* New York: Cambridge University Press.

Hilgard, E. R. (1973). The domain of hypnosis, with some comments on alternative paradigms. *American Psychologist, 28,* 972–982.

Kihlstrom, J. F. (1991). [Review of *Hypnosis: The cognitive–behavioral perspective*]. *Contemporary Psychology, 36,* 11–12.

Kraft, W. A., & Rudolfa, E. R. (1982). The use of hypnosis among psychologists. *American Journal of Hypnosis, 24*(4), 249–257.

Nash, M. R., Minton, A., & Baldridge, J. (1988). Twenty years of scientific hypnosis in dentistry, medicine, and psychology: A brief communication. *International Journal of Clinical and Experimental Hypnosis, 36,* 198–205.

Price, R. H., & Lynn, S. J. (1986). *Abnormal psychology* (2nd. ed.). Homewood, IL: Dorsey Press.

Pulver, S. E., & Pulver, M.P. (1975). Hypnosis in medical and dental practice: A survey. *International Journal of Clinical and Experimental Hypnosis, 23,* 28–47.

Rossi, E. L. (1986). *The psychobiology of mind–body healing.* New York: Norton.

Spanos, N. P., & Chaves, J. F. (Eds.). (1989). *Hypnosis: The cognitive–behavioral perspective.* Buffalo, NY: Prometheus Books.

Sutcliffe, J. P. (1960). "Credulous" and "skeptical" views of hypnostic phenomena: A review of certain evidence and methodology. *International Journal of Clinical and Experimental Hypnosis, 8,* 73–101.

PART ONE

HISTORICAL
PERSPECTIVES

CHAPTER 1

Early Theories of Hypnosis: A Clinical Perspective

MELVIN A. GRAVITZ
George Washington University

The theories and phenomena of modern hypnosis are not entirely congruent with those observed in the past, although most of the behaviors that are today associated with hypnosis were known more than a century ago. Temple sleep, demoniacal possession, royal touch, planetary influence, and mineral and animal magnetism, among others, were all theoretical points on the historical path that has led to our present understanding. Necessarily considered within the context of the "science" of those times, these antecedents of theory and practice were associated with therapeutic changes based upon belief, imagination, and undoubtedly other healing mechanisms that are as yet unknown. These latter constructs are what constitute the link between antiquity and today. This chapter discusses the historical and theoretical development of hypnosis as it has evolved from quasi-science and controversy, and as it has in turn shaped the larger field of psychological understanding and treatment for several centuries.

HYPNOSIS FROM ANCIENT TIMES TO THE MID-1700s

Healing utilizing the medium of induced states of altered awareness (trances) was practiced by the ancient Chinese, Egyptians, Hebrews, Indians, Persians, Greeks, Romans, and others. More than 4,000 years ago, Wang Tai, the founder of Chinese medicine, taught a therapeutic technique that utilized incantations and manual passes over the body of the patient. The Hindu Veda, written about 1500 B.C., described similar

19

procedures, while the Egyptians more than three millenia ago described healing methods similar to modern-day hypnosis (Muses, 1972).

The interrelated influence of mental and physical forces in health and illness was known to the ancients. Hippocrates, for example, observed that the "soul sees quite well the affections suffered by the body" (Adams, 1886). The legendary Greek physician–god, Asclepiades, who was known to the Romans as Aesculapius, allayed pain and suffering by the stroking of his hands and the induction of lengthy sleep-like states. In the many temples dedicated to Asclepiades, proper thoughts of trust and faith were required and expected. Related to the "laying on of hands" described in the Bible, the "royal touch" of powerful figures came to be regarded as therapeutic. The Roman emperors, including Constantine, Vespasian, and Hadrian, used their touch to cure illness, and by the time of the Middle Ages this method had become widely used in Europe. Together with the even older uses of charms, amulets, and certain metals, suggestion, belief, and expectancy began to emerge as therapeutic agents, although their mechanisms were not then understood. At a time when it was widely believed that many physical ailments were caused by demoniacal possession (Diethelm, 1970), Hieronymous Nymann, who lived in the late 1500s, emphasized the power of the imagination on health; he also attributed the effects of certain drugs to the imagination. It was through bold conceptual insights such as this that the link between bodily function and mental influence began to be established.

The related use of mineral magnets in the treatment of illness can also be traced back to antiquity. In the late 15th century, Petrus Pomponatius (1462–1525) maintained that sickness and disease could be cured by magnetic emanations. "When those who are endowed with this faculty [of magnetism] operate by employing the force of the imagination and the will, this force affects their blood and their spirits" (cited in Vincent, 1893, p. 8). A century later, Philippus Aureolus Theophrastus Bombastus von Hohenheim (1493–1541), who was better known as Paracelsus, was an eminent (albeit controversial) Swiss-born physician and philosopher who challenged the contemporary medical establishment, which then used archaic forms of treatment based upon the centuries-old teachings of Galen and others. An important aspect of Paracelsus's theories was the belief that a subtle magnetic influence from the planets and stars affected the mind, while magnetic radiation from the earth affected the body. This potent magnetism, which he called the Monarch of Secrets, was considered to possess both positive and negative qualities. Since magnets could cure, and the dysfunction of the body's own magnetic properties caused illness, he logically applied mineral magnets directly to affected body areas in order to correct such imbalance. Yet he also sagely recognized, as had Hippocrates before him, that thought, belief, and will were significant influences upon human behavior.

During this period, a belief widely held by Paracelsus and others was that an invisible fluid pervaded the universe, including the heavenly bodies and all animate and inanimate objects. Good health required that there be an optimal balance of this fluid.

In the next century, Johann van Helmont (1577–1644) taught that people had a natural power based upon magnetism, which enabled them to influence each other and to promote health. A similar view was held by William Maxwell (1581–1641), a Scotsman who was the physician of King Charles I of England. In his monumental *De Medicina Magnetica*, which was published in 1679, he described a system of so-called "magnetic medicine" and claimed that human disease could be cured by magnetically transferring it to animals and plants. Maxwell believed that a "vital spirit" affected everyone; and by means of this spirit, all living things were related to each other. A contemporary, Kenelm Digby, developed his own theory of sympathetic medicine, which assumed that there was an imperceptible "powder of sympathy" by which wounds could be treated from a distance. Another important figure of the 1600s was Valentine Greatrakes (1628–1680), who treated hundreds by faith and by manually stroking the affected parts of the body. The underlying belief was that in so doing, the disease was driven first into the extremities and then entirely out of the body. Frequently his patients exhibited convulsive-like movements, which were similar to what Mesmer decades later termed the "crisis."

An English follower of Paracelsus, Robert Fludd (1547–1637), theorized that each person possessed the qualities of a magnet and that when two people met, an interactive magnetic field developed. He was another who claimed that the heavenly bodies influenced human behavior. Similar views were held during this time by Rudolf Goclenius, Agrippa von Nettesheim, J. E. Burgraav, Sebastian Wirdig, and Athanasius Kirchner, all of whom were eminent physicians who used magnets in their practice. Not all authorities of the time believed magnetism to be a positive force, however, and some attributed magnetic effects to satanic agency; consequently, magnetism as a therapeutic modality had both good and bad connotations.

A different kind of healer was Johann Joseph Gassner (1727–1779), a cleric who was a well-known authority on exorcism. He distinguished between two types of illness: the "natural," which was to be treated by physicians, and the "preternatural" or "spiritual," which belonged under the care of the clergy. The latter were diabolical in origin and could be managed only by faith and exorcism. As a result of his encounter with Franz Anton Mesmer in 1776, Gassner influenced the latter's theories and thereby helped prepare the way for a therapeutic method that was separate from religion and that satisfied the requirements of an enlightened age. What became evident was that curing the sick was in itself not enough: It had to be accomplished by methods that were acceptable to the community and to the times.

Richard Mead (1673–1754), a prominent English physician, was another important figure. In addition to voluminous contributions to the contemporary medical literature on a variety of topics, he wrote a treatise titled *De Imperio Solis ac Lunae in Corpora Humana et Morbis inde Oriundis* (Mead, 1704), in which he mathematically formulated the position that periodic atmospheric tides arising from planetary forces produced alterations of gravity, elasticity, and air pressure; in turn, these changes affected the human body in health and disease. Mead's book is important in the history of hypnosis theory because of its impact upon the later writings of Mesmer.

The theories and practices discussed above were developed over the course of centuries, and they anticipated the much later psychological views of interpersonal relationships and influence, including transference, in psychotherapy. They were also significant antecedents of Mesmer's theories of animal (i.e., biological) magnetism in the late 1700s. The period from the mid-1500s to the mid-1700s was one of rapid growth of scientific knowledge. New Cartesian thought, empirical observations, and doubts about the accepted teachings of the past replaced dogmatism, even though powerful vestiges of the old notions persisted for many years. In particular, knowledge of the relationship of body and mind and of the influence of emotions on health and illness began to emerge. Thus it was that the vague outlines of modern psychology and psychotherapy began to take further shape.

MESMER AND HIS FOLLOWERS

Against the background of the preceding developments, a 32-year-old medical student, Franz Anton Mesmer (1734–1815), presented a paper originally entitled *Dissertatio Physico-Medica de Planetarum Influxu* (*Physical–Medical Dissertation on the Influence of the Planets*) to the faculty of the University of Vienna on May 27, 1766. Although Mesmer's theories drew widely from other writers, including Paracelsus, Maxwell, Fludd, and van Helmont, his dissertation borrowed liberally and in places verbatim from Mead's (1704) *De Imperio Solis* (Pattie, 1956). In his highly technical thesis, Mesmer proposed the existence of tides on the earth and within the human body that responded to the movements of the moon and sun, which were classed as planets in those days. In addition to these physical forces upon human behavior, he emphasized another influence, which he first termed "animal gravitation" and which was considered to be the source of all bodily properties. He also held that planetary influence established an effect he termed "universal gravitation," which was caused by animal gravitation and was the force by which human bodies are brought into harmony with stellar configurations.

Several years after the completion of his dissertation, Mesmer advocated the use of mineral magnets in order to restructure the tide of artificial magnetism in his patients, and he enlarged on the earlier theory of animal gravitation. "I called this property of the animal body which makes it sensitive to universal gravitation 'gravity' or 'animal magnetism' " (Bloch, 1980, p. 25). Conceptualized as a fluid, "animal magnetism" was the term he ultimately adopted to describe the force.

In January 1768, Mesmer married the affluent widow of an Austrian cavalry officer. This union provided him with monetary security and entry into the high social position of fashionable Viennese society. At the same time, he continued his clinical practice. One of his patients in 1773 was a young woman, Francisca Oesterlin, who suffered from an intermittent illness with a variety of puzzling symptoms. Conventional remedies had proven ineffective, so on the historic date of July 28, 1774, Mesmer (1775), after first having her swallow a preparation containing iron filings, then applied custom-shaped magnetized steel plates to parts of her body in order to produce an artificial magnetic tide. This was intended to restore her health by an appropriate rebalance of fluidic harmony, in accord with the theory of magnetism outlined in his dissertation. Mesmer had obtained the plates from a friend, Maximillian Hell (1720–1792), who was the Royal Astronomer to the Austrian court and who was himself interested in magnetism. As was common with Mesmer's early patients, Oesterlin first entered a drowsy, semiconscious trance state, which was considered to be facilitative of the cure. Despite several relapses and episodes of convulsions that alarmed onlookers, Oesterlin subsequently was cured of all symptoms.

The official Viennese medical establishment was first indifferent and eventually hostile to Mesmer and his practice of animal magnetism. This antagonism peaked as the result of the outcome of the treatment of another of his young patients, Maria-Thérèse Paradis. The 18-year-old daughter of a prominent court official, she had suddenly become blind at the age of 3. Because of her precocious talent as a pianist and as compensation for her disability, she had become a protegé of her namesake, the Empress Maria-Thérèsa, who granted the Paradis family a generous pension. Although her parents had consulted the best medical experts, none had been able to restore her sight, and they eventually brought her to Mesmer in early 1777. Since she had been frightened by many years of bleeding, purging, blistering, and electric shocks, in accordance with the accepted methods of the day, Mesmer reasoned that rapport and confidence were first needed, and he undertook to build a bond of trust between them. This early recognition of the importance of a positive therapeutic relationship was facilitated by having the young patient move into his own home.

In this case, as previously, the patient's reaction to the magnetic therapy included the development of remarkable spasms throughout her body, including the eyes; this was another forerunner of the therapeutic "crisis" upon which Mesmer elaborated in later years. Although Paradis's parents were at first pleased with their daughter's progress in Mesmer's clinic, doubts began to surface as the reportedly beneficial treatment generated skepticism, resentment, and overt hostility from a group of influential members of the traditionally conservative Viennese medical community. It was not long before the parents became alarmed at the course of treatment, perhaps in part because they were threatened with the loss of the royal pension as their daughter began to change from a blind musical prodigy to merely another talented pianist. Eventually, the mother came to Mesmer's mansion, where she demanded that her daughter be delivered to her. When the physician demurred, she became loudly abusive and physically agitated. The spectacle caused the young patient to relapse to her former condition of blindness and convulsive behavior, at which point she was thrown against a wall by her mother. At that moment of turmoil, her father stormed into the clinic waving his sword. Eventually, the servants succeeded in expelling both parents from the house, but the harm had already been done. The Paradis matter quickly became a topic for scandal and malicious gossip based upon Mesmer's unorthodox methods and his alleged relationships with his young female patients. The unfortunate belief of some critics that animal magnetism was associated with unsavory conduct and eroticism remained part of the mythology of the modality long after Mesmer himself passed from the scene.

As a result of the Paradis debacle, Mesmer decided to leave Vienna. His professional reputation was besmirched, despite the undoubted successes in other cases; his marital life had deteriorated over a number of years; and there were no true ties to keep him there. Consequently, he moved to Paris in February 1778.

Upon arriving in the French capital, Mesmer opened a new practice based upon his continued strong conviction that he had discovered a revolutionary natural physical fluid that existed everywhere in nature and in all people, and that required no medications. Eager to disseminate his views, groups of devoted followers were soon organized into a number of so-called Societies of Harmony throughout France. His methods of treatment included touching, stroking, manual passes over the body, and some use of magnets. The magnets, however, had been largely discontinued before he left Vienna, because he had become convinced that the therapeutic power of animal magnetism existed within himself; that is, the magnetizer himself was the therapeutic instrument, although a relationship first had to be established with the patient before a cure could proceed. He also continued the use of a device called the *baquet*. Based upon a similar apparatus that he had first used in 1776 with a Hungarian patient, the *baquet* was a large oak vat that was placed on the floor in front of the patient or group of patients. It contained a slurry of "magnetized" water, glass fragments, and iron filings, while from its sides protruded magnetized iron rods that the patients touched to the afflicted parts of their bodies. Cords connected the patients to each other and to the *baquet*, in order to enhance the flow of the magnetic fluid. Musical instruments played soothing melodies in an anteroom; mirrors designed to reflect the magnetic fluid were everywhere; thick drapes allowed only dim light to enter; and temperature, humidity, sound, and air pressure were all regulated in accord with Mesmer's theories. Mesmer himself was attired in purple silk, and he carried a magnetized iron wand as he moved from patient to patient, touching them and staring into their eyes.

Mesmer wrote voluminously, and in particular published his celebrated *Mémoire* in 1779, the year following his arrival in Paris. In it he described 27 propositions to explain animal magnetism, which can be summarized in four basic principles:

> (1) A subtle fluid fills the universe and forms a connecting medium between man, the earth, and the heavenly bodies, and also between man and man. (2) Disease originates from the unequal distribution of this fluid in the human body; recovery is achieved when the equilibrium is restored. (3) With the help of certain techniques, this fluid can be channeled, stored, and conveyed to other persons. (4) In this manner, "crises" can be provoked in patients and disease cured. (Ellenberger, 1970, p. 62)

At the same time, Mesmer understood the importance of the interrelationship between the magnetizer and patient, which was known as "rapport." He emphasized that the emotional component of the rapport was crucial, for he held that animal magnetism "must in the first place be transmitted through feeling" (Mesmer, 1781). One of his close associates, Charles de Villers (Villers, 1787), noted that "for one soul to act upon another, the two souls must be in a measure united." Magnetic rapport also referred to the patient's special feelings toward the magnetizer and to the belief that the patient could sense the magnetizer's thoughts. The reverse was recognized, too, and the term "magnetic reciprocity" was used in 1784. These concepts were to lead a century later to the important psychotherapeutic findings of transference and countertransference, especially through the work of Sigmund Freud.

An essential goal of the treatment was that the patient experience the "crisis" while in trance. This was a series of typically prolonged and agonizing convulsive contortions that occurred at the height of the treatment session and that left the patient emotionally and physically drained—but frequently with remission of the presenting symptoms. That this was a precursor of catharsis and abreaction can be readily determined. Such crisis reactions, however therapeutic, were alarming to scientific observers, as was the fact that the majority of Mesmer's patients were young women. Once again, he became the object of innuendo, ridicule, satire, and malice. What is known today is that many of the patients seen at that time were hysterics who were hypersuggestive to the expectations of the mesmeric situation (demand characteristics) and who believed in the therapeutic value of the crises.

Working with male assistants, Mesmer treated many of his patients in groups because of the heavy demands on his time, and he set aside a day each week to treat the indigent without charge. He also traveled to outlying locales to provide magnetic care for those who could not otherwise obtain it. In those ways, Mesmer anticipated both group psychotherapy and community-based health outreach programs.

It may have been his narcissism that led Mesmer to expect that the French medical establishment would accept and even welcome a foreigner's radical theory, which could render invalid all that had been discovered over the previous centuries and which would cause their profession to become superfluous. Not surprisingly, and as had previously occurred in Vienna, there soon arose powerful opposition to mesmerism as treatment and to Mesmer as a person (e.g., Thouret, 1784). As a consequence of the controversy surrounding animal magnetism, but also at the request of Mesmer himself, Louis XVI appointed two investigative commissions of inquiry. One consisted of members of both the Academy of Sciences and the Faculty of Medicine. This was chaired by Benjamin Franklin, then the first American diplomatic minister to Paris. A second panel was comprised of noted members of the Royal Society of Medicine.

After a series of generally well-designed experiments and observations, which focused on the work of a disciple and of Mesmer himself, the commissions concluded that the theoretical fluid did not exist and that whatever salutary effects were produced by animal magnetism were solely the result of imagination (Commissaires de l'Académie de Sciences et la Faculté de Médecine, 1784; Commissaires de la Société Royale de Médecine, 1784). Furthermore, since imagination was then an unacceptable topic for enlightened scientific study, magnetism was considered at best unworthy of comment and at worst a fraud perpetrated by a charlatan upon a naive public. To his credit, one of the commissioners, Antoine-Laurent de Jussieu, an eminent botanist, dissented from the majority view. In his minority statement, Jussieu (1784) wrote that the positive effects of mesmerism had been overlooked by the investigation, and he raised the point that stimulation of the imagination might in itself be a therapeutic force. He realized that the body was influenced by both internal moral (i.e., mental) and external physical factors; however, he did not take the next step to conclude that animal magnetism was a new form of treatment based upon mental influence. One of Mesmer's colleagues, who ironically had been ostracized for his views, did come closer to that realization. Charles d'Eslon (Eslon, 1784), in his own reaction to the commission's reports, concluded that imagination played the greatest role in the effects of mesmerism, and that the extensive and powerful forces of imagination might be the real agent responsible for the undenied efficacy of animal magnetism. "If Mesmer had no secret than that he has been able to make the imagination exert an influence upon health, would he not still be a wonder doctor? If treatment by the use of the imagination is the best treatment, why do we not make use of it?" With that insight, Eslon laid another cornerstone of modern psychotherapy, and the idea that the mind influenced the body took another step forward.

Jean Sylvain Bailly, the reporter for the Franklin commission's public report, simultaneously penned a secret report that was "designed only for the eyes of the King" and which remained hidden for many years (see Bertrand, 1826). This communication alleged that a moral threat arose from the purported erotic attraction of the mesmerized female patient to her male magnetizer. The report overlooked the fact that some magnetizers were women and some patients were men; once again, mesmerism was tainted by undocumented charges of immorality and hints of sexual misconduct.

With the publication of these reports, mesmerism and Mesmer both went into eclipse for the most part. He left France soon after their publication and died in relative obscurity in 1815, not far from where he was born on the shores of Lake Constance.

However, certain of Mesmer's colleagues did not discontinue their work. One of the most renowned of these was Amand-Marie-Jacques de Chastenet, the Marquis de Puységur (1751–1825), a distinguished military officer and scion of a noted family. On his estate in Buzancy, he established a laboratory where he conducted experiments in the late 1700s and early 1800s on such matters as electricity and animal magnetism (Puységur, 1784). On one occasion, he observed that Victor Race, an employee, exhibited none of the expected convulsions or other signs of crisis. Instead, Race appeared to enter an unusual state in which he appeared to be more alert than usual: He spoke louder, with greater confidence, and seemed to possess more information than he ordinarily had. Once removed from this induced state, Race had no memory of what had transpired. Because this behavior resembled sleepwalking, Puységur called it "artificial somnambulism," and the relationship itself was termed "intimate rapport." He also made the important observation that somnambulists would often speak spontaneously of matters that concerned them, after which they would feel relieved. This was a precursor of the later emergence of catharsis as a therapeutic technique.

Realizing that erotic factors might enter into the relationship, Puységur sought to create a condition of virtually infantile dependence of the patient upon the magnetizer. This regressive approach was designed to provide therapeutic benefit similar to the mother–child interaction, although he recognized the necessity of eventually ending the patient's dependence on him. This was a conceptual forerunner of the present-day method of working through of transferential issues, and his views were also relevant to the much later development of object relations theory.

As had Mesmer before him, Puységur undertook to magnetize trees, which afflicted persons could touch and obtain therapeutic relief. Francois-Joseph Noizet, a contemporary magnetizer, insightfully noted, "To me it is obvious that the effect of the tree was non-existent, and that which occurred in its shade was entirely the result of the confidence that was placed in its magnetic virtues" (Noizet, 1854, p. 245). Noizet also emphasized the importance of suggestion, positive anticipation, and mutual feelings of trust between the magnetist and patient. These noteworthy conclusions were theoretical contributions that led to the rise of the Nancy school in the late 19th century, and were forerunners to what today is termed "expectancy set" in experimental psychology and "transference" in psychodynamic psychotherapy. Jules Charpignon, another mesmerist, later found that suggestions made to the magnetized subject could influence subsequent behavior, thereby anticipating the therapeutic technique of posthypnotic suggestion (Charpignon, 1841).

EUROPEAN DEVELOPMENTS IN THE 19TH CENTURY

The early 1800s continued to produce other important developments in France. José Custodio da Faria (1756–1819), a Goanese cleric who came to Paris in 1813, theorized that no special fluid was transmitted by the magnetizer; instead, the stimulus for what he termed "lucid sleep" came from the subject himself or herself, and therefore there were individual differences in response (Faria, 1819). He also introduced a new induction technique in which the subject was asked to fixate attention on a specific point or object, such as Faria's raised hand. This was accompanied by loud commands to sleep. While in the state of lucid sleep, the subject was given suggestions for beneficial change—precursors for what later came to be known as "posthypnotic suggestions." Together with Faria, Alexandre Bertrand (1795–1831) is considered to be an originator of the theory that the essential causes of somnambulistic behavior lay in the patient's own imagination and response to suggestion (Bertrand, 1826). These views were subsequently enlarged upon and made therapeutically relevant with considerable success by the Nancy school, and they form the basis of much of modern hypnotherapeutic theory.

Despite his new theory and methodology, Faria was unable to revive the course of magnetism in France following its post-Mesmer decline. That was accomplished instead by Joseph Philippe Francois Deleuze (1753–1835), who published an important text (Deleuze, 1810) and many other contributions. His *Instruction Practique sur le Magnétisme Animal* (Deleuze, 1825) was a classic manual that went through several French editions and was translated into a number of other languages, including English. Influenced by Puységur, Deleuze was an active and respected participant in the clinical practice and scientific study of animal magnetism.

In 1826, Simon Mialle (1790–?) published an impressive and valuable two-volume book, in which he outlined in alphabetical order numerous cases in which animal magnetism had been used successfully to treat a large variety of mental and physical disorders. The book also contained one of the earliest references to nomenclature based upon the "hypn-" prefix, as in the English-language cognates "hypnology" and "hypnologist" (Mialle, 1826, p. xxxix). He acquired this terminology from the earlier writings of Etienne Felix d'Henin de Cuvillers, a contemporary French mesmerist who in 1820 employed the words "hypnotist," "hypnotism," and so on, after the Greek god of sleep, Hypnos (Gravitz & Gerton, 1984). Indeed, similar terms had been used even earlier in several French dictionaries, as d'Henin de Cuvillers acknowledged. This was several decades before James Braid was to popularize that nomenclature in the English language.

Magnetic healing in France continued its activity as the modality recovered from the criticisms of mesmerism and Mesmer. Theoretical considerations and therapeutic practice proceeded in tandem, and a number of scientific journals dedicated exclusively or principally to the field were founded in a number of countries (Gravitz, 1981, 1987). The first such periodical was the *Annales de la Société Harmonique des Amis Réunis de Strasbourg*, which appeared in 1787. In the early 1800s, the modality began to be utilized for surgical anesthesia at a time when surgery, when it was undertaken at all, was a death warrant for more than half the patients who suffered through it (Gravitz, 1988). The first documented hypnoanesthesia was in 1829, when a Parisian surgeon performed a mastectomy. By the advent of chemical anesthetics in the 1840s, the use of magnetism for such purposes had become commonplace.

Mesmerism arrived in England in 1788 when J. B. de Mainauduc, a student of Eslon, came to present a series of lectures on the topic. He was followed by others who gave public displays of the phenomena throughout the country, and textbooks that described the theory and methodology began to be published. In 1829, Richard Chevenix, who had studied with Faria in Paris, published a number of scientific articles on animal magnetism that generated considerable comment in the British medical community. Among those who as a result became interested in the field was John Elliotson (1791–1862), a dedicated physician and noted educator who had introduced Laennec's wooden stethoscope to England. In 1837, the noted French magnetizer, Jules Denis du Potet de Sennevoy, came to London at Elliotson's request. Du Potet was well known for his work with animal magnetism in Paris, and his theories stressed the importance of the "soul," or mental influence, in treatment (Du Potet de Sennevoy, 1838). Elliotson's interest was enhanced by his work with Du Potet, and he began to treat his own patients in the 1830s. He was able to attract others, and his work on hypnotic anesthesia was known even in America (Elliotson, 1843). The British medical establishment was hostile to his efforts, however, and when he was unable to publish his research in traditional journals because of editorial bias, he founded a new periodical called the *Zoist* that became the most important mesmeric journal of the time. His harsh critics in the medical hierarchy were eventually able to provoke him to resign his academic honors and hospital appointments in 1839. With the professional demise of Elliotson, mesmerism in England became discredited as a legitimate practice area, as had previously occurred with Mesmer; however, as in those earlier times, animal magnetism survived—principally, in this case, through the work of James Braid and several others.

Braid (1795–1860), a surgeon, was introduced to mesmerism by Charles Lafontaine, a popular Swiss magnetizer who in late 1841 presented several public lectures and demonstrations of somnambulism in Manchester, where Braid resided. By his own account, Braid, a skeptic who originally considered mesmerism to be a "system of delusion and collusion," came to scoff at Lafontaine's presentations, but was sufficiently impressed by his observations that he became an instant advocate. He then quietly began his own experiments with magnetic treatment of his medical and "insane" patients.

At first, Braid theorized that the effects of animal magnetism were due to induced fatigue of the eye muscles, which in turn led to a brain-mediated physiological variant of natural sleep. After initially using the term "neuro-hypnology" in 1842, he then devised the word "neurypnology" the following year (Braid, 1843). That term, which served as the title of his principal work (Braid, 1843), was derived from the Greek *neuron* or "nerve," *hypnos* or "sleep," and *logos* or "discourse," the combination of which referred to the doctrine of "nervous sleep." This terminology was soon replaced by "hypnotism," but while Braid is generally given credit for originating that nomenclature, in actuality that was not so. As noted above, it was a Frenchman, Etienne Felix d'Henin de Cuvillers, who had applied the "hypn-" prefix in 1820 to a wide array of words descriptive of the mesmeric process (Gravitz & Gerton, 1984), and there had been even earlier uses of that terminology by others.

Braid subsequently discarded the mesmeric passes and scientifically untenable theory of a magnetic fluid. Instead, he proposed a new natural and nonmystical system based upon physiology, in which "physico-psychical" stimulation of the retina acting through brain mechanisms induced rapid fatigue of the nervous and sensory systems, which in turn resulted in nervous sleep or hypnotism (Braid, 1843). He also believed that it was the hypnotist who set these forces in motion within the patient; consequently, he stressed the importance of subjective elements, such as belief and suggestion, and he was a strong adherent of the view that the mind and body influence each other. After beginning with a theoretical model of hypnotism based upon sleep and physiology, he then came to believe that the essential action was as much psychological as physiological, and he emphasized that hypnotic phenomena were the result of mental concentration on a single idea. The latter theory was given the name of "monoideism" by him in 1847 (Braid, 1855).

Elliotson's contribution had been that he had lent his then considerable prestige in support of a new and at times controversial therapeutic methodology. Even though Braid began from a less prominent position, his contribution was more significant. He popularized a new name for the old "mesmerism," which made it more acceptable, and he formulated a physiologically based explanation that fit into the scientific frame of reference of his medical colleagues. Thus, Braid's theory of "hypnotism" meshed better than "animal magnetism" with the accepted thinking of the day and was therefore not as controversial. Once again, as with Gassner a century before, curing the sick was not enough in itself: It had to be done by theories and techniques that were acceptable at the time to the broader community.

Another landmark figure contemporary with Elliotson and Braid was James Esdaile (1808–1859), a Scottish surgeon under contract with the British East India Company. He was familiar with the work being done with hypnotism in England and elsewhere, and he also knew of the therapeutic trance states used by the local Indian healers. Although he was not a psychotherapist, Esdaile's (1846) major contribution was that he performed thousands of surgical operations, including over 300 major procedures, using hypnotism as the anesthetic agent. Because his mortality rate was about 5% compared to some 50% in surgery elsewhere, his work served to encourage the use of hypnotism in Europe and America. Despite its success, the modality was unacceptable to the medical community, and after the arrival of chemical anesthetics the use of hypnotism for such purposes faded. The inhalation agents were more acceptable to surgeons because they required little training; were more reliable; and perhaps most of all were part of the doctrinaire medical mainstream, which was based upon mechanistic formulations of diagnosis and treatment in terms of a disease model.

Another important reason for the decline of hypnotism in the third quarter of the 19th century was that the field was infiltrated and largely pre-empted by stage entertainers and outright charlatans, as well as spiritualists and other believers in extrasensory paranormal phenomena. Beginning with the notorious 1847 case of the Fox sisters of New York State (Podmore, 1902), who claimed to be able to communicate with the dead through the medium of ghostly rappings (and who were subsequently exposed as liars and manipulators), a wave of spiritualism swept the United States and then crossed the Atlantic several years later. Even before then, there had been some mesmerists who had blended animal magnetism with occult beliefs in table turning, phrenology, clairvoyance, telepathy, and the like. Given such taints, it is understandable that generally conservative practitioners and scientists had their traditional misgivings about hypnotism reinforced.

One cannot help comparing those years with the late 1980s, which have seen the emergence of certain hypnosis-related theories and methods that have proven on investigation to lack sufficient merit. These have tended to be promulgated and marketed by self-designated experts who have managed to convince some onlookers that their views represent the leading edge of the field. As history has demonstrated on any number of occasions, when science and respectable practice in hypnosis are in effect abandoned to fringe elements, then respectability and the field itself will inevitably decline (Gravitz, 1985).

Fortunately, the inherent merit of hypnosis as a therapeutic modality has resulted in responsible investigation and leadership. So it was in the late 1880s. Some 40 years after the publication of Braid's (1843) monumental *Neurypnology, or the Rationale of Nervous Sleep*, that work was translated into French by Jules Simon. Braid's theories, now called "braidism," then served to influence a generation of serious French theorists and practitioners, such as Etienne Eugene Azam, Paul Broca, Joseph Pierre Durand de Gros, Alfred Velpeau, Jean Martin Charcot, Charles Richet, Auguste Ambroise Liébeault, and Hippolyte Bernheim.

Azam (1822–1899), a physician and psychologist of Bordeaux, experimented with hypnotism and suggestion as anesthesia and psychotherapy. He was a friend of Braid and an exponent of his work. It was Azam's later investigations that eventually led to the establishment of the Nancy school of hypnosis, which was conceptually based on Braid's theories and which revolutionized the scientific understanding of hypnosis and hypnotherapy. Broca (1824–1860), in late 1859, and Velpeau (1795–1867), in early 1860, presented favorable reports on Braid's experiments to the French Academy of Sciences. The acceptance of these papers by the same esteemed learned body that had condemned mesmerism 75 years earlier gave a cachet of renewed respectability to the field, and thereby made it easier for others to acknowledge their interest and undertake research.

Richet (1850–1935) was a brilliant Nobel laureate in physiology who helped lead the way to dynamic psychology and psychotherapy through his work with hypnosis. His influence was such that, when he published an article on induced somnambulism in 1875, this helped greatly to legitimize the field (Richet, 1875). It was Richet's experimentation with hypnosis that introduced his colleague, Jean Martin Charcot, to his own use of the modality in 1878.

Charcot (1825–1893) was the most noted neurologist of his time. Director of the Salpêtrière, a large hospital for the neurologically and mentally disordered in Paris, he was a world-renowned teacher and researcher. Because he was seeking to differentiate between hysterical and organic convulsions, and because he was interested in all aspects of mental function, he turned to hypnosis when Richet discussed it with him. His work with hysterics brought him the title "Napoleon of Neuroses," but unfortunately several of his assistants misled him by demonstrations of increasingly extraordinary hysterical and hypnotic behaviors, which they had rehearsed with several of his patients. Charcot (1882) became the leader of the Paris school of hypnosis, and by defining the modality as somatically determined in a paper that he read before the Academy of Sciences (as Broca and Velpeau had done), he helped to reinstate the method as an acceptable area for study and application. Charcot was a mesmeric fluidist who held that magnets, auditory stimulation, tactile pressure, and certain metals could induce the trance state; he also believed that hypnosis was a pathological somatogenic condition virtually synonymous with hysteria. On the basis of research with a very few patients, he theorized three stages of hypnosis, each of which had its own characteristics: "lethargy," "catalepsy," and "somnambulism." He and his associates published many contributions in support of the theories of the Paris school, but other investigators did not agree with their views.

In 1860, the year of Braid's death, a modest rural physician from Pont Saint Vincent, a small village near the city of Nancy across the country from Paris, became familiar with Braid's teachings. After incorporating them into his own medical practice, Auguste Ambroise Liébeault (1823–1904) offered his patients the choice of traditional care at full fee or hypnotherapy at no charge. Not surprisingly, the number of those who opted for hypnosis grew each year, especially since the method proved to be effective in many cases. In 1866, exactly 100 years after Mesmer's dissertation was published, Liébeault wrote a book in which he theorized that hypnosis was similar to natural sleep, the essential differences being that the modality was produced by suggestion and concentration on the idea of sleep (i.e., braidism) and that the patient was "en rapport" with the hypnotist (Liébeault, 1866). In addition to emphasizing the interpersonal aspects of the treatment, he also utilized direct psychotherapeutic suggestions for symptom relief and remission. Interestingly, toward the end of his life, Liébeault reversed course and became a believer in the theory of a magnetic fluid (Ellenberger, 1970).

Although most of his colleagues treated him with neglect and even disdain, Liébeault gained respect in 1882 when he successfully treated a severely sciatic patient whom the noted Hippolyte Bernheim had been unable to help with traditional medical methods. Bernheim (1840–1919) was a professor at the University of Nancy, and he was discerning and honest enough to become Liébeault's student and eventual colleague. Bernheim wrote a number of important publications (e.g., Bernheim, 1884), many of which were translated into other languages. From the beginning, he theorized that suggestion was the key to hypnosis. Before long, a small group of dedicated like-minded scientists, including Henri Beaunis (1830–1921) and Jules Liégeois (1833–1908), joined the Nancy school as productive contributors to its theoretical and clinical views. They conceptualized hypnosis as a normal, nonpathological psychological state of mind, in which suggestion played a vital if not an essential role. As time went on, Bernheim especially employed hypnotic techniques less frequently, and he eventually concluded that suggestion without hypnotic ritual ("suggestive therapeutics") was equally effective (Bernheim, 1891). The Nancy school was bitterly opposed by the Paris school, and there ensued an intellectual struggle that lasted several years; eventually, however, the Nancy theorists prevailed, and their doctrines have remained primary to the present day.

Students from throughout Europe came to Paris to learn from Charcot. Among them in October 1885 was a young Viennese physician, Sigmund Freud (1856–1939). During his brief stay of several months in the French capital, Freud was exposed to Charcot's influential views on mental disorder and hypnosis, and as a result he changed his career choice from neurology to psychopathology. Freud was no stranger to hypnosis, however, for he had been interested in the field since his medical school days. In addition, he and his close colleague and friend, Josef Breuer (1842–1925), had earlier discussed the latter's puzzling patient named Bertha Pappenheim, who became known in the scientific literature as "Anna O" (Breuer & Freud, 1895). The unraveling of the hypnotically based transferential dynamics of this classic case was crucial in Freud's subsequent development of his psychoanalytic theories. But although he is a stellar figure in the evolution of the larger field of psychotherapy, Freud has been a relatively minor force in the history of hypnosis. His clinical techniques were basically limited to direct authoritarian commands for symptom remission, and his theoretical position was that hypnosis was essentially an eroticized dependent relationship. Furthermore, although he was an enthusiastic supporter of the modality while beginning his practice, he "abandoned" its use in 1896 for a number of reasons; these included countertransferential dynamics derived from his personal experiences with hypnotherapy and Breuer's traumatic reaction to the Anna O case. Perhaps his greatest impact on the field was that his rejection of hypnosis came at a time when his own prestige was rising as the result of the rapid growth and influence of his psychoanalytic views; consequently, his negative stance caused many professionals to consider the modality as unworthy of study and use, and when he left the field, others did the same.

Thus, by the end of the 19th century, hypnosis had once again faded in importance, even though new techniques of induction and treatment were beginning to be utilized (Gravitz, 1983). More than a few practitioners, however, continued to use the method in psychotherapy. Notably, these included Morton Prince, Boris Sidis, and John Duncan Quackenbos in the United States; Pierre Janet, Edgar Berillon, and Alfred Binet in France; C. Lloyd Tuckey, Ralph Henry Vincent, and R. W. Felkin in Great Britain; Ivan Pavlov in Russia; Paul Dubois and Charles Baudouin in Switzerland; and Oskar Vogt, Rudolf Heidenhain, and Albert Moll in Germany. But until World War I, hypnosis and its therapeutic applications were in another period of eclipse. During that conflict, there was a brief revival on both sides of the use of hypnotic anesthesia and psychotherapy in the trench-line warfare of the time, but with the conclusion of hostilities matters were once again quiet. The theories and methods of the Nancy school predominated tnroughout those years, however.

HYPNOSIS IN THE UNITED STATES

Reference should be made at this point to developments in the United States, because it is there that the principal theoretical, clinical, and experimental advances of the past 75 years have been made. Hypnosis had been known in America from its earliest years. News of animal magnetism had been brought to its shores by the Marquis Marie-Joseph de Lafayette, a fervent French disciple of Mesmer, who came to aid the colonists in their struggle for independence. In 1784, he wrote to George Washington of his strong belief in mesmerism (Deleuze, 1825). The American leader did not endorse the modality, however, probably because his esteemed friend and colleague Benjamin Franklin had chaired the French commission of inquiry during the same period of time that he had been the first ambassador to Paris. In the early 1820s, Charles Caldwell (1772–1853) of Louisville, Kentucky, developed a system of magnetic medicine based upon Puységur's theory of the existence of both physical and psychological factors. Caldwell had also observed Elliotson's work while on a trip to England, and he was well read and knowledgeable about mesmeric progress in Europe. He was especially impressed by "the entire prevention of pain in severe surgical operations by the mesmeric influence" (Caldwell, 1842, p. 128). In 1829, Joseph du Commun, an immigrant French mesmerist, was a frequent lecturer on the topic (Du Commun, 1829). He noted that the effective magnetizer possessed three qualities; belief, will, and benevolence; he also endorsed the role of women as magnetizers, a position that was radical in its day. Du Commun and several friends with similar interests formed a "society of magnetizers" in New York City. This was one of the earliest professional organizations of its kind in the United States, predating similar groups in Cincinnati (Wester, 1976) and New Orleans (Gravitz & Gerton, 1986), but preceded by even earlier magnetic societies in Philadelphia and Clinton, New York.

Another important influence on the rise of hypnosis in the United States was the translation into English of Deleuze's *Instruction Pratique sur le Magnétisme Animal* (Deleuze, 1825) and its publication in Rhode Island in 1837. An appendix written by the translator, Thomas Hartshorn, presented information on a number of American cases. Charles Poyen, another French immigrant, lectured widely and published an important account of mesmeric cases in New England in 1837. During the same year, the first American translation of the French commission's report was published in Philadelphia (Franklin, 1784/1837). Public interest in mesmerism was high in those days, and reports of its applications received wide circulation in the popular press (Gravitz, 1981, 1988) and in a number of scientific journals (Gravitz, 1981, 1987).

One of Poyen's students in 1838 was Phineas Parkhurst Quimby (1802–1866) of Maine, who had been influenced by the fluidic theory of John Bovee Dods (1795–1872). The latter had devised a variation of animal magnetism, which he called "electrical psychology" (Dods, 1843). Quimby was a successful and well-known mesmerist who had numerous patients from throughout New England, one of whom was Mary Baker Eddy, the later founder of Christian Science. Several decades before Freud's theories of the id, ego, and unconscious, Quimby held that the human mind had two levels—the upper, characterized by thought (i.e., rationality), and the lower, associated with belief (i.e., irrationality). Together with other prominent American mesmerists, he believed that the therapeutic process involved the patient's will, imagination, and faith (Dresser, 1895). These tenets led to the development of a school of treatment called "faith healing" or "mind cure," which attracted numerous adherents. This in turn evolved into the "New Thought" movement, which then blurred into spiritualism and other quasi-religious philosophies of treatment. Hypnosis suffered from the dilution of respectability that these fringe movements brought to the field, and from the consequent loss of approval and acceptability in the scientific community. Even so, mesmerism at that time had several important effects upon scientific thinking: It stimulated interest in psychology; it predisposed the general public to accept the view of unconsciously determined behavior; and it encouraged the blending of secular self-help psychological principles with spiritual thought. In general, American mesmerism in the middle to late 1800s focused much more upon the facilitation of philosophical and spiritual fulfillment than on the treatment of medical and psychological problems. Indeed, developments in therapeutic applications tended to limp along until the end of the century.

An important influence upon American clinical hypnosis at the turn of the century was Pierre Janet (1859–1947), a French medical psychologist who had been associated with Charcot in the study of hysteria and hypnosis. In 1904 and 1906, he lectured on his findings in the United States, and he was a prolific writer (Ellenberger, 1970). He claimed priority for the discovery of the cathartic cure, and he disagreed with Freud's theories of dreams and the sexual origin of neurosis. His classic work *Les Médications Psychologiques*, which was translated into English and widely read, contained a large section on hypnosis and hypnotherapy (Janet, 1919). He had a special interest in the phenomenon of psychological automatism, which implied that part of the personality could split off from conscious awareness and then follow an autonomous subconscious development. This evolved into the concept of "dissociation," as he termed it, which he believed could be facilitated and studied by hypnosis. Janet's work with hypnosis and dissociation became the stimuli for later studies of multiple personality by Morton Prince and Boris Sidis in Boston.

Prince (1854–1929), a psychologist with a medical degree, was the founder of both the Psychological Clinic at Harvard University and the *Journal of Abnormal Psychology*; the latter has ever since been especially hospitable to articles dealing with hypnosis and multiple personality. Prince was familiar with the work of the French hypnotists and, indeed, had visited both the Salpêtrière and the clinic at Nancy. His famous patient, "Miss Beauchamp," became the prototypical case of multiple personality, which he regarded as a dissociative disorder and which he treated with hypnosis for several years (Prince, 1905). A contemporary Harvard psychologist, Sidis (1867–1923) studied suggestion and its relation to hypnosis and hypnoid states by laboratory experimentation. He, too, was interested in the theory of mental dissociation and multiple personality. The public at large was intrigued by the work of Prince and Sidis, which served to popularize both hypnosis and psychopathology; however, the concept of dissociation faded together with overall interest in hypnosis and was not revived until the 1970s by Ernest R. Hilgard (1987).

Two important figures came on the American scene in the early 1920s. These were Clark L. Hull (1884–1952) and Milton H. Erickson

(1901–1980). Hull was an academic psychologist at the University of Wisconsin who designed a series of ingenious laboratory experiments to test some of the fundamental questions of hypnosis. He was not a clinician (although he did successfully use hypnosis in the treatment of phobia), but as a teacher he helped popularize hypnotic techniques at his university, and he published a classic discussion of controlled scientific research in hypnosis (Hull, 1933). Erickson was one of Hull's undergraduate students in 1923. The two initially collaborated, but eventually conflicted because Erickson disagreed with his professor's theoretical emphasis on the primary role of the hypnotist and the need for a standardized induction procedure for use in laboratory research; he himself stressed the individual subject's own dynamically complex inner processes as they operated in hypnosis. Erickson proceeded to develop an approach that was naturalistic, permissive, and indirect, while Hull was more traditional (Erickson, 1983). The career demands on Hull attenuated his interest in hypnosis, and he moved on to a distinguished career in other areas of psychology, notably learning theory. Erickson went on to become a prolific and innovative contributor to the therapeutic and experimental literature (Gravitz & Gravitz, 1977), as well as the best-known American practitioner of hypnosis in the 20th century.

Prior to Erickson's death in 1980, he received many honors, and his impact on the field has been impressive. In recent years, concern has arisen that certain of his followers who are uncritical in their enthusiasm for his memory have sought to establish a unique "Ericksonian hypnotherapy" based upon their own interpretations of his work. The claim has been made that these "Ericksonians" have dogmatically and overzealously polarized the field through a plethora of meetings, workshops, and publications (e.g., Hilgard, 1987).

Erickson's true contributions should not be overlooked, even though his theoretical conclusions have not all withstood the rigorous scrutiny of scientific investigation. By his key position and a half century of practice, training, and research, he revitalized hypnosis in the United States after its long period of dormancy. His work also inspired many professionals in other countries to undertake similar activities there. Although he never developed a comprehensive, synthesized system of hypnosis, his theoretical principles may be summarized as follows: (1) The unconscious need not be made conscious, and unconscious processes can be facilitated so that they can function autonomously to solve each patient's problems in an individual way. (2) Mental mechanisms and personality characteristics need not be analyzed for the patient: They can be utilized as processes, dynamisms, or pathways facilitating therapeutic goals. (3) Suggestion need not be direct, and indirect suggestions can frequently bypass a patient's learned limitations and thus can better facilitate unconscious processes. (4) Therapeutic suggestion is not a process of programming the patient with the therapist's point of view; rather, it involves an inner resynthesis of the patient's behavior achieved by the patient himself or herself (Rossi, 1980). It is evident that these principles are applicable to psychotherapy in general and not only to hypnosis.

A FINAL WORD

With the participation of many, hypnosis has developed significantly over the last four decades. Research is voluminous, and there are many modern applications in a variety of areas (see, e.g., Crasilneck & Hall, 1985; Udolf, 1987). It can truly be said that the current wave of worldwide scientific and clinical interest is the strongest and most enduring in the long history of this modality.

REFERENCES

Adams, F. (Ed.). (1886). *The genuine works of Hippocrates*. New York: William Wood.

Bernheim, H. (1884). *De la suggestion dans l'état hypnotique et dans l'état de veille* [*On suggestion in the hypnotic state and the state of will*]. Paris: Doin.

Bernheim, H. (1891). *Hypnotisme, suggestion, psychothérapie: Études nouvelles* [*Hypnotism, suggestion, psychotherapy: New studies*]. Paris: Doin.

Bertrand, A. J. F. (1826). *Du magnétisme animal en France* [*On animal magnetism in France*]. Paris: Baillière.

Bloch, G. J. (1980). *Mesmerism: A translation of the original medical and scientific writings of F. A. Mesmer, M.D.* Los Altos, CA: William Kaufmann.

Braid, J. (1843). *Neurypnology, or the rationale of nervous sleep considered in relation with animal magnetism*. London: Churchill.

Braid, J. (1855). *The physiology of fascination; and the critics criticized*. Manchester: Grant.

Caldwell, C. (1842). *Facts in mesmerism, and thoughts on its causes and uses*. Louisville, KY: Prentice & Weissinger.

Charcot, J. M. (1882). Sur les divers états nerveux déterminés par l'hypnotisation chez les hystériques [On the different nervous states determined by hypnotism in hysterics]. *Comptes Rendues de l'Academie des Sciences, 94*, 403–405.

Charpignon, J. (1841). *Physiologie, médecine, et metaphysique du magnétisme* (*Physiology, medicine, and metaphysics of magnetism*). Orleans, France: Pesty.

Commissaires de l'Académie de Sciences et la Faculté de Médecine. (1784). *Rapport des commissaires chargés par le Roi de l'examen du magnétisme animal* [*Report of the commissioners charged by the King with the examination of animal magnetism*]. Paris: Imprimerie Royale.

Commissaires de la Société Royale de Médecine. (1784). *Rapport des commissaires de la Société Royale de Médecine nommés par le Roi pour faire l'examen du magnétisme animal*

[*Report of the commissioners of the Royal Society of Medicine who were named by the King to conduct an investigation of animal magnetism*]. Paris: Imprimerie Royale.

Crasilneck, H. B., & Hall, J. A. (1985). *Clinical hypnosis: Principles and applications* (2nd ed.) Orlando, FL: Grune & Stratton.

Deleuze, J. P. F. (1810). *Histoire critique du magnétisme animal* [*Critical history of animal magnetism*]. Paris: Schoell.

Deleuze, J. P. F. (1825). *Instruction pratique sur le magnétisme animal* [*Practical instruction on animal magnetism*]. Paris: Dentu.

Diethelm, O. (1970). The medical teaching of demonology in the 17th and 18th centuries. *Journal of the History of the Behavioral Sciences, 6,* 3–15.

Dods, J. B. (1843). *Six lectures on the philosophy of mesmerism.* Boston: Hall.

Dresser, A. G. (1895). *The philosophy of P. P. Quimby.* Boston: Ellis.

Du Commun, J. (1829). *Three lectures on animal magnetism.* New York: Desnous.

Du Potet de Sennevoy, J. D. (1838). *An introduction to the study of animal magnetism.* London: Saunders & Otley.

Ellenberger, H. F. (1970). *The discovery of the unconscious.* New York: Basic Books.

Elliotson, J. (1843). *Numerous cases of surgical operations without pain in the mesmeric state.* Philadelphia: Lea & Blanchard.

Erickson, M. H. (1983). *Healing in hypnosis.* New York: Irvington.

Esdaile, J. (1846). *Mesmerism in India and its practical application in surgery and medicine.* London: Longmans, Brown, Green, & Longman.

Eslon, C. d'. (1784). *Observations sur les deux rapports de MM. les commissaires nommés par Sa Majeste pour l'examen du magnétisme animal* [*Observations on the two reports by the commissioners named by His Majesty to study animal magnetism*]. Paris: Clousier.

Faria, J. C. da. (1819). *De la cause du sommeil lucide* [*On the cause of lucid sleep*]. Paris: Horiac.

Franklin, B. (1837). *Report of Benjamin Franklin and other commissioners charged by the King of France with the examination of the animal magnetism as practiced at Paris.* Philadelphia: Perkins. (Original work published 1784)

Gravitz, M. A. (1981). Bibliographic sources of nineteenth century hypnosis literature. *American Journal of Clinical Hypnosis, 23,* 217–219.

Gravitz, M. A. (1983). Early uses of the telephone and recordings in hypnosis. *American Journal of Clinical Hypnosis. 25,* 280–282.

Gravitz, M. A. (1985). Scientific responsibility and hypnosis. *American Journal of Clinical Hypnosis, 28,* 90.

Gravitz, M. A. (1987). Two centuries of hypnosis specialty journals. *International Journal of Clinical and Experimental Hypnosis, 35,* 265–275.

Gravitz, M. A. (1988). Early uses of hypnosis as surgical anesthesia. *American Journal of Clinical Hypnosis. 30,* 201–208.

Gravitz, M. A., & Gerton, M. I. (1984). Origins of the term hypnotism prior to Braid. *American Journal of Clinical Hypnosis, 27,* 107–110.

Gravitz, M. A., & Gerton, M. I. (1986). The Société du Magnétisme de la Nouvelle-Orléans: Its place in the early history of hypnosis in America. *International Journal of Psychosomatics, 33,* 11–14.

Gravitz, M. A., & Gravitz, R. F. (1977). The collected writings of Milton H. Erickson: A complete bibliography 1929–1977. *American Journal of Clinical Hypnosis, 20,* 84–94.

Hilgard, E. R. (1987). *Psychology in America: A historical survey.* Orlando, FL: Harcourt Brace Jovanovich.

Hull, C. L. (1933). *Hypnosis and suggestibility.* New York: Appleton-Century.

Janet, P. (1919). *Les médications psychologiques [Psychological healinq].* Paris: Alcan.

Jussieu, A. L. de. (1784). *Rapport de l'un des commissaires chargés par le Roi de l'examen du magnétisme animal [Report by one of the commissioners charged by the King with the investigation of animal magnetism].* Paris: Veuve Herissant.

Liébeault, A. A. (1866). *Du sommeil et des états analogues considérés surtout au point de vue de l'action du moral sur le physique [On sleep and related states considered entirely from the viewpoint of the action of the mind on the body].* Paris: Masson.

Maxwell, W. (1679). *De medicina magnetica [On magnetic medicine].* Frankfurt: Zubrodt.

Mead, R. (1704). *De imperio solis ac lunae in corpora humana et morbis indeoriundis [On the influence of the sun and moon on the human body].* London: Raphaelis Smith.

Mesmer, F. A. (1766). *Dissertatio physico-medica de planetarum influxu [Physical–medical dissertation on planetary influence].* Vindobonae (Vienna): Ghelen.

Mesmer, F. A. (1775). *Schreiben über die magnetkur [Writings on the magnetic cure].* Vienna: Kurtzbock.

Mesmer, F. A. (1779). *Mémoire sur la découverte du magnétisme animal, par M. Mesmer, docteur en médecine de la faculté de Vienne [Memoir on the discovery of animal magnetism, by Mr. Mesmer, doctor of medicine from the faculty of Vienna].* Geneva and Paris: Didiot.

Mesmer, F. A. (1781). *Précis historique des faits relatifs au magnétisme animal jusques en Avril 1781 [Historical summary of facts relating to animal magnetism as of April 1781].* London: No publisher available.

Mialle, S. (1826). *Exposé par ordre alphabétique des cures opérées en France par le magnétisme animal depuis Mesmer jusqu'a nos jours [An exposé in alphabetical order of cures achieved by animal magnetism from Mesmer to our time].* Paris: Dentu.

Muses, C. (1972). *Consciousness and reality.* New York: Dutton.

Noizet, F. J. (1854). *Mémoire sur le somnambulisme et le magnétisme animal [A memoir on somnambulism and animal magnetism].* Paris: Plon.

Pattie, F. A. (1956). Mesmer's medical dissertation and its debt to Mead's *De imperio solis ac lunae. Journal of the History of Medicine and Allied Sciences, 11,* 275–287.

Podmore, F. (1902). *Modern spiritualism: A history and a criticism.* London: Methuen.

Poyen, C. (1837). *Progress of animal magnetism in New England.* Boston: Weeks & Jordan.

Prince, M. (1905). *The dissociation of a personality: A biographical study in abnormal psychology.* New York: Longmans, Green.

Puységur, A. M. J. de Chastenet, Marquis de. (1784). *Mémoires pour servir à l'histoire et à l'établissement du magnétisme animal [Memoirs on the history and establishment of animal magnetism].* Paris: Dentu.

Richet, C. R. (1875). Du somnambulisme provoqué [On induced somnambulism]. *Journal de l'Anatomie et de la Physiologie Normales et Pathologiques de l'Homme et des Animaux, 11,* 348–378.

Rossi, E. L. (Ed.). (1980). *The collected papers of Milton H. Erickson on hypnosis. Vol. IV. Innovative psychotherapy.* New York: Irvington.

Thouret, M. A. (1784). *Recherches et doutes sur le magnétisme animal [(Research and doubts about animal magnetism].* Paris: Prault.

Udolf, R. (1987). *Handbook of hypnosis for professionals* (2nd ed.) New York: Van Nostrand Reinhold.

Villers, C. de. (1787). *Le magnétiseur amoureux, par un membre de la Société Harmonique du Regiment de Metz* [*The amorous magnetizer, by a member of the Society of Harmony of the Metz Regiment*]. Geneva: No publisher available.

Vincent, R. H. (1893). *The elements of hypnotism*. London: Kegan Paul, Trench, Trubner.

Wester, W. C. (1976). The Phreno-Magnetic Society of Cincinnati—1842. *American Journal of Clinical Hypnosis, 18,* 277–281.

History and Historiography of Hypnosis

NICHOLAS P. SPANOS
Carleton University
JOHN F. CHAVES
Southern Illinois University

Histories are always written from a particular point of view. They reflect the assumptions, both tacit and explicit, that provide the framework around which historians develop their narratives and with which they "make sense" of the events under consideration (Carr, 1961). Histories of hypnosis have almost always taken each of the following notions to be axiomatic: (1) The term "hypnosis" refers to a denotable state or condition of the person (e.g., "trance state"). (2) This state can be induced (at least in susceptible individuals) by certain identifiable rituals labeled "hypnotic induction procedures." (3) The hypnotic state induced by these rituals possesses at least some invariant or essential properties, which are independent of the means by which the trance is induced or the persons in whom the state is induced. It is this pivotal assumption of the invariance of the hypnotic condition itself that enables historians to classify as examples of hypnosis historical phenomena as diverse as Asclepian dream healing in ancient Greece, early modern Catholic exorcisms, the dancing of 18th-century Indian dervishes, the convulsions associated with mesmeric healing, and high levels of responsiveness to modern tests of hypnotizability.

These assumptions have led historians of hypnosis to conceptualize their task as similar to that of medical historians who trace such physical diseases as bubonic plague, ergotism, and tuberculosis across historical eras. Like medical historians, historians of hypnosis have assumed that they are studying an objective entity that, despite some variation engendered by culture and habit, can be traced down through the ages on the basis of its invariant features.

Contemporary researchers in the field of hypnosis are acutely aware that the axioms concerning hypnosis taken for granted by historians are, in fact, highly controversial (Barber, 1969; Barber, Spanos, & Chaves, 1974; Fellows, 1986, 1990; Sarbin & Coe, 1972; Wagstaff, 1981). Despite more than a century of empirical research, there is no convincing evidence to support the contention that hypnotic subjects enact behaviors, process information, or develop experiences in ways different from those of nonhypnotic control subjects (Spanos & Chaves, 1989). On the contrary, subjects are capable of enacting all of the phenomena currently associated with the notion of "deep hypnosis" (e.g., suggested amnesia, analgesia, "trance logic" hallucinations) without first being administered rituals that even remotely resemble what have come to be labeled "hypnotic induction procedures" (e.g., interrelated suggestions for relaxation, sleep, and entering hypnosis). Moreover, subjects can display such phenomena while appearing to be alert and wide awake, and while defining themselves as not hypnotized (Barber, 1969; Radtke & Spanos, 1981).

One theoretical perspective that challenges traditional assumptions about hypnosis conceptualizes hypnotic responding as contextually supported, goal-directed action (Spanos & Chaves, 1989). According to this perspective, the term "hypnosis" does *not* refer to a state or condition of the person. Instead, it refers to a historically and culturally rooted social construction—an interrelated set of ideas that provide guidelines concerning how hypnotists and hypnotized subjects are supposed to act and feel while enacting their respective roles in those social situations defined as hypnotic.

The implications of the constructivist perspective for the historiography of hypnosis are profound. To begin with, this perspective suggests that the historical study of hypnosis as conventionally conducted should be abandoned. Historians can and should continue to study the idea of hypnosis, the manner in which that idea evolved, the practices and reciprocal role enactments associated with that idea, and the cultural and historical circumstances that gave rise to that idea and its attendant practices. However, from a contextualist perspective, it is misleading and counterproductive to view hypnosis as an entity or condition that can be traced from one historical era to another.

From a contextualist perspective, the historiography of hypnosis can be fruitfully viewed as more analogous to the historiography of, say, law, table manners, or military tactics, than to the historiography of physical diseases. For example, the historical study of the jury system in English and American law might examine the social and cultural matrix in which that system evolved, changes in the roles that developed among the principal actors in courtroom minidramas over long temporal intervals, the manner in which political and economic events influenced legal practice and theory, and so on (Rembar, 1980). However, no serious historian would attempt to trace the historical continuity of "justice" or "lawfulness" as entities or states of mind associated with one or more of the participants in courtroom dramas. A contextualist perspective suggests that historical attempts to study "hypnosis" as an entity or condition are equally misleading.

In the next section, we illustrate our position by examining two phenomena from antiquity: Asclepian dream healing and New Testament religious healing. Both phenomena are frequently described as examples of hypnosis in the ancient world. We criticize this conceptualization and briefly describe a contextualist alternative.

HYPNOSIS IN ANTIQUITY?

Traditional historians of hypnosis implicitly or explicitly endorse the notion that "hypnosis" was manifested during earlier historical periods. However, because of ignorance or superstition, hypnosis was not recognized as such until modern times; instead, hypnotic phenomena were incorrectly ascribed to various forms of supernatural intervention, or to magic. Thus, from this perspective, Asclepian dream healing, New Testament exorcisms, and numerous other phenomena of antiquity were "really" manifestations of hypnosis (Conn, 1957; Edmonston, 1986; Kroger & Fezler, 1976; LeCron & Bordeaux, 1947; Ludwig, 1964; MacHovec, 1975, 1979; Pulos, 1980).

As indicated earlier, one serious difficulty with such formulations is their grounding in a set of unsupported and misleading assumptions about the nature of hypnotic responding. A second difficulty arises because such formulations tend to de-emphasize the diversity of the historical phenomena they cite and the complex social contexts in which they were embedded, in order to make comparisons between isolated and sometimes superficial aspects of these phenomena and certain aspects of contemporary hypnotic phenomena (Stocking, 1965; Spanos, 1978; Stam & Spanos, 1982). We illustrate these and other difficulties by examining the purported role of hypnosis in Asclepian temple healing.

Asclepian Temple Healing and Hypnosis

From the Homeric period to the reign of Constantine in the 4th century A.D., the figure in the ancient world most prominently associated with healing was the god Asclepos (Edelstein, 1937; Kee, 1983; Kitto, 1951).

The Asclepian cult played a central role in the cultural and religious life of antiquity, and healing temples dedicated to Asclepos (i.e., Asclepia) were common features in the Greco-Roman world. However, the traditions associated with Asclepos were varied. For instance, one healing tradition emphasized divine intervention, while another emphasized more naturalistic medical and surgical intervention. Moreover, the psychosocial functions subserved by the cult changed rather dramatically from the Hellenistic period (5th century B.C.) to the period of the early Roman Empire (Kee, 1983). During the Hellenistic period, Asclepos was viewed in a straightforward manner as a god of healing. During this period there is no evidence of external ritual and no suggestion that the healings held transcendental meanings. The Asclepia of this period functioned somewhat like outpatient clinics. Suppliants with medical problems slept overnight in the *abeton* (the place in the temple where the god purportedly appeared during dreams).

By the time of the early Roman Empire, the figure of Asclepos had been transformed from a healer of specific ills to a cosmic savior who appeared in dreams in the form of a personal guide. The transformation of Asclepos occurred in conjunction with numerous other sociocultural and religious changes in the Greco-Roman world. In his role as savior, however, Asclepos provided meaning and purpose to life through the experience of salvation and personal transformation as well as, and often instead of, physical healing (Kee, 1983).

Historians who attempt to link Asclepian healing to hypnosis usually ignore the complex and diverse nature of the Asclepian cult and the social and cultural matrix in which it evolved. Instead, these historians usually limit their focus to only one aspect of the cult's practice, the so-called "dream healings." During the dream healings patients slept in the temple, where they were supposedly visited by the god Asclepos in a dream. During this visitation the god either cured the patients outright or provided prescriptions for a cure (Edlestein & Edelstein, 1945; Stam & Spanos, 1982).

During the 19th century, several investigators suggested somnambulism and animal magnetism as explanations for the dream healings (Edelstein & Edelstein, 1945). More recent authors have posited hypnosis as an explanation (Kroger & Fezler, 1976; Edmonston, 1986; Ludwig, 1964; MacHovec, 1975, 1979; Pulos, 1980). According to these hypotheses, the temple priests used hypnosis (probably unwittingly) to guide suppliants' experiences while they awaited the appearance of the god in a dream. For instance, MacHovec (1979) suggested that suppliants were made more susceptible to hypnosis through repetitive and relaxing activities such as massage, hymn singing, and chanting; he also hypothesized that the priests "maintained rapport, formulated the treatment plan, and reinforced it in the mind of the patient. . . . influencing the dreamwork, guiding the trance state or making posthypnotic suggestions for recovery" (p. 88). MacHovec (1979), Deutsch (1946), and others further suggested that the priests disguised themselves as the god and, accompanied by trained snakes, visited the supplicants at night in the temple and whispered therapeutic suggestions to them.

The evidence concerning a role for hypnosis in the dream healings consists almost entirely of selective citations from sources of dubious credibility, or confusion between what was required of members of the cult and what was required of the sick who underwent dream healings. For instance, for the sick, the evidence indicates that there was little ritual and no need for chanting, singing, fasting, or other solemn ceremonies (Behr, 1968; Kee, 1983; Kerenyi, 1947/1960). Furthermore, the evidence that the priests "influenced the dreamwork" or administered posthypnotic suggestions derives from a single questionable source, a description of the dream healings given in Aristophanes's (448–330 B.C.) comic play *Plutus*.

In the play, a witness to an incubation watches the god, accompanied by two enormous snakes, cure the blindness of his sleeping friend. Those who argue for a role of hypnosis in the dream healings assume that this scene from the play is veridical and that priests disguised as the god treated the sick. As pointed out by Edelstein and Edelstein (1945), however, the writings of Aristophanes should not be accepted at face value "without making allowance for poetic fantasy and comic license" (p. 145). The temple priests did not think of themselves as physicians, and there is no evidence that they suggested treatments or "formulated [a] treatment plan." Instead, their role was to help supplicants implement the procedures prescribed in their dreams. In addition, there is no evidence to suggest that the temple priests attempted to trick supplicants into believing that they (the priests) were gods. Even in the play, the cure was effected by the god and not by a disguised priest. The visions of the god reported by the sick were dream visions. The god was never seen by anyone while awake (Edelstein & Edelstein, 1945; Kerenyi, 1947/1960).

In summary, reconstructions of Asclepian dream healing in terms of hypnosis are based almost exclusively on selective citation from secondary sources of questionable validity. These accounts begin with the assumption that hypnosis is a state induced by special rituals and identifiable in terms of specifiable characteristics. Next, certain aspects of Asclepian temple healings are defined as hypnotic because, when separated from their own social and historical context, they appear to bear some superficial resemblance to modern hypnotic events. For instance, hypnotists are, and Asclepian priests were authority figures. Clinical hypnotic procedures are, and the rituals of Asclepian priests were associated somehow with psychological healing. Hypnosis has historically been associated with sleep, and Asclepian healing purportedly occurred in sleep. Therefore, Asclepian healing must have involved hypnosis. If such an argument is not sufficient, it can be buttressed by creating historical scenarios that are of questionable validity but that make intuitive sense, once the premise of hypnosis as transhistorical entity has been accepted (e.g., priests guiding the trance, influencing the dreamwork, administering posthypnotic suggestions).

Usually, attempts to equate dream healing with hypnosis are also based on the contention that symptomatic improvement was produced in at least some dream healing patients by contextual factors that operated to strengthen patients' beliefs and expectations in the efficacy of the treatment. This assertion is certainly reasonable. In fact, it is a truism that can be (and often is) stated about any psychological treatment procedure (Barber, 1981; Frank, 1973). However, the validity of this assertion does not constitute evidence that Asclepian priests employed hypnosis or that hypnosis was involved in the cure of patients who slept overnight in Asclepian temples.

New Testament Healing and Hypnosis

A number of investigators in both the 19th and 20th centuries interpreted diverse phenomena described in the Old and New Testaments as examples of mesmerism and later of hypnosis (Edmonston, 1986; Grimes, 1845; Glasner, 1955; Hockley, 1849; Paton, 1921; Williams, 1954; Smith, 1986). Because of space limitations, we confine the present discussion to the notion that evidence of hypnosis can be found in the New Testament healings attributed to Jesus.

The method used to demonstrate hypnosis in the New Testament healings is typified by Edmonston (1986), who quotes short passages from the synoptic Gospels (Matthew, Mark, and Luke) that depict Jesus healing the sick. On the basis of these quotes, Edmonston (1986) concludes that Jesus used eye fixation, soothing suggestions, a laying on of hands, and posthypnotic suggestions as hypnotic procedures for the cure of various disorders. However, the hypnotic account of these events runs into difficulties almost immediately, even if, for the moment, we assume the accuracy of the New Testament depictions.

For example, modern experimental work makes it clear that eye fixation and a laying on of hands have little to do with responsiveness to hypnotic suggestions (Barber, 1969). Moreover, suggestions given in a firm tone of voice are responded to as readily as those given in a soothing tone (Barber & Calverley, 1964). In short, if there is no evidence to suggest that eye fixation, a soothing tone, and the like facilitate hypnotic responding in modern settings, there is even less justification in assuming that they produced hypnosis in ancient settings. Moreover, the New Testament descriptions make it clear that Jesus could heal without ritual of any kind (as in the case of the woman who was healed when, unbeknownst to Jesus, she touched his robe; Mark 5:29), and without the knowledge or even the presence of the patient (as when Jesus healed at a distance the slave of a Roman centurion; Luke 7:10).

The New Testament Gospel writers made a clear distinction between the procedures used by Jesus to cure physical disorders (e.g., touching the patient, applying spittle to the diseased area) and the procedures he used to cure demonic possession (direct verbal commands addressed to the indwelling demon). There is little resemblance between the treatments applied to these different disorders, and the authors of the New Testament obviously conceptualized these treatments as distinct. On the other hand, historians of hypnosis often lump the exorcisms and the physical healings together as examples of hypnosis. There appears to be no justification for doing so, and no explanation in terms of hypnosis for why these two treatments should be so different.

There is nothing in the New Testament descriptions to suggest that the patients healed by Jesus were first placed into an altered state. In fact, the only thing these patients appear to have in common is their more or less instantaneous cure at the hands of Jesus. In short, the only way to find evidence of hypnosis in the New Testament is first to assume it is there, and then to interpret individual passages as evidence of hypnosis on the basis of some superficial similarity between a Biblical event (e.g., Jesus healing with a touch) and some practice associated with mesmerism or hypnosis at some time during the 19th or 20th centuries (e.g., the touching of afflicted areas, sometimes practiced by mesmerists).

The most serious criticism to be leveled against those who interpret New Testament stories in terms of hypnosis stems from the implicit assumption made by these investigators that the New Testament provides accurate descriptions of real healings and exorcisms that were actually performed by Jesus. Few modern Biblical historians are willing to make this assumption (Hoffman, 1986; Kee, 1986; Wells, 1982). The New Testament texts that provide information about the miracles, healings, and exorcisms of Jesus were all originally written between 40 and 120 years *after* the purported events occurred. None of these texts were written by eyewitnesses. In fact, the oldest Gospel (Mark) may well have been written by a Gentile rather than a Jew. This author appears to have possessed a very hazy conception of the geography of Palestine, and he placed in the mouth of Jesus expressions that a pious Jewish healer/prophet would have been very unlikely to utter (Helms, 1989; Kee, 1986). Most important, the primary purpose of the gospel authors was not to write history. All of the Gospels were written with particular audiences in mind, in an attempt to present God's plan, win converts, sustain the faith of believers, attack and denigrate competing beliefs, provide answers to critics, and so on (Kee, 1986; Wells, 1975, 1982).

Although the four Gospels contain numerous similarities and often retell the same specific stories, they cannot be used as independent sources of verification for the events depicted. Most Biblical historians believe that the oldest Gospel is that of Mark, and that this Gospel was known to the other three writers. According to this hypothesis, Matthew and Luke copied extensively from Mark; hence the similarities among these three texts, which led to their being labeled "synoptic." Furthermore, similarities between Matthew and Luke that are not also contained in Mark occurred because both Matthew and Luke also copied from a source not available to Mark (the so-called "Q" source; Kee, 1986; Koester, 1980). Where the Gospels do not derive from common sources, they often differ widely from one another in emphasis and historical detail. In many cases these differences appear to have arisen from theological differences among the authors, from the different audiences to which they aimed their work, and from the fact that these authors wrote at different times and therefore addressed issues created by different historical circumstances (Koester, 1980).

Differences among historians concerning the veracity of the Gospel accounts have led to widely different interpretations of the biblical material. For instance, some modern historians (J. M. Hull, 1974; Smith, 1978, 1986) argue that the Biblical material, coupled with information from non-biblical sources concerned with healing and magical rituals in the first few centuries A.D., make it plausible that Jesus was a 1st-century itinerant Jewish magician or holy man who engaged in what today would be called psychological healing. However, even these historians caution that the Gospel narratives cannot be taken at face value, and that the descriptions of the healings presented therein are most likely inaccurate. According to Smith (1978), for example, the healings and exorcisms of Jesus were purposely described inaccurately by the Gospel writers in order to forestall the charge that Jesus healed by magic. The notion of Jesus as a 1st-century magician has been criticized on numerous grounds (Kee, 1986; Wells, 1982). The most important of these criticisms holds that those who adopt this position have made inappropriate inferences about events in the time of Jesus on the basis of magical texts and stories written primarily in the 2nd and 3rd centuries.

More common among contemporary Biblical historians is the position that the Gospels should not be treated as early attempts at history writing, but as religious tracts that attempted to convey their message by using a narrative, historical format. One version of this approach holds that the development of the Gospel narratives can be best understood by assuming that there never was a historical Jesus (Allegro, 1984, 1986; Leach &

Aycock, 1983; Wells, 1975, 1982, 1986). According to this hypothesis, Jesus and his disciples, as well as such events as the trial of Jesus, his healings; his miracles; the crucifixion, and so on, are mythological constructions. These stories were invented, elaborated upon, placed within an actual historical context, and finally committed to writing (somewhat like a modern historical novel) in order to serve the needs of a proselytizing new sect that required a savior/hero with a concrete history, miraculous abilities, and certain specific characteristics (e.g., a Davidic lineage).

Even modern historians who do not reject Jesus as a historical figure usually acknowledge that the New Testament writings cannot be used to reconstruct accurately the events of his life (Helms, 1989; Hoffman, 1986; Kee, 1986). Instead, these writers suggest that the Gospel stories must be understood in terms of the context and motives of the Gospel writers, and the religious messages they were attempting to convey. The basic Gospel message was that the death and resurrection of Jesus heralded a new age. The postresurrection world was in its final days, and only those who believed in Jesus would be saved (Kee, 1986). From this perspective, the events of Jesus's life—healings, exorcisms, miracles—foretold a new situation where Satan would be banished, the people of God vindicated, and the purpose of God accomplished.

Christianity began as a sect within Judaism. Consequently, legitimation for the Christian message was sought in the Old Testament. The Gospel writers created such legitimation by shaping their stories about Jesus to conform to (and confirm) Old Testament prophecies and views concerning the characteristics of the Jewish Messiah (Helms, 1986). For example, the Messiah was to be of Davidic lineage and come out of Egypt (Wells, 1975). Thus, both Matthew and Luke provide Jesus with Davidic ancestors. Matthew and Luke also have Jesus born in Bethlehem (David's birthplace), and Matthew has him taken to Egypt by his parents so that he can later return out of Egypt (Helms, 1989).

The healing stories of Jesus can be viewed in a similar light. For instance, the healing miracles of Jesus include curing the blind, deaf, and lame, and the raising of the dead. Why do the Gospel writers make a point of depicting Jesus as healing these particular disorders? Because the Old Testament prophet Isaiah had predicted just these events as signs heralding the new age: "The eyes of the blind shall be opened, and the ears of the deaf shall hear. Then shall the lame man leap as an hart" (Isaiah 35:5); "The dead shall rise, and they that are in the tombs shall be raised" (Isaiah 26:19).

The Gospel miracles are sometimes modeled so closely on Old Testament stories that their literary origins are obvious. For example, Helms (1986) points out the following similarities between Luke's account of Jesus raising the son of the widow of Nain from the dead, and the Old Testament prophet Elijah's raising of the dead son of the widow of

Sarepta as given in the Septuagent (i.e., the Greek translation of the Old Testament used by the Gospel writers) version of the book of Kings:

> Both stories begin with the Septuagent's favorite formula "And it came to pass" . . . Both stories concern the dead son of a widow. In both stories the prophet "went" to town, where he met the widow at the "gate of the city," even though archeological study has shown that the village of Nain in Galilee never had a wall, Nain's fictional gate is there for literary reasons, Sarepta's gate is transferred. In both stories, the prophets speak and touch the dead son, who then rises and speaks. Then in both stories it is exclaimed that the miracle certifies the prophet. . . . And both stories conclude with precisely the same words, "and he gave him to his mother." (Helms, 1986, pp. 137–138).

The Gospel writers were intent not only to present the activities of Jesus as fulfilling Old Testament prophecies, but also to present the Christian message as relevant to people outside the traditional Jewish community. Consequently, Jesus is depicted as healing people who, according to the rules of Jewish piety, were taboo by reason of their ritual condition (e.g., a menstruating woman, a leper), their occupation (e.g., a tax collector), their non-Jewish ethnicity (e.g., the slave of a Roman centurion), and so on (Kee, 1986).

The Gospels present Jesus as an exorcist of demons as well as a healer of physical maladies. Like the healing stories, the exorcisms are presented by the Gospel writers as confirming the Christian message that the new age had dawned, and the powers of evil (i.e., Satan) were defeated (Kee, 1968, 1986). Demons were believed to have powers of speech and supernatural knowledge. The Gospel writers use these characteristics to portray the demons in a manner that legitimated Jesus and his message. Thus, the demons are depicted as recognizing the divinity of Jesus, quaking before his power, and obeying his commands (Kee, 1968). The eschatological message to be conveyed by these stories is made explicit in Luke 11:20: "If it is by the finger of God that I cast out demons, then the kingdom of God has come upon you."

In summary, the assumption made by historians of hypnosis that New Testament stories can be read as history, and thereby scrutinized for evidence of hypnotic practice, is most certainly false. Instead, these stories constitute a kind of mythohistory (Leach & Aycock, 1983); they are fables that depict mythological events and personages in the form of historical narrative for the purpose of conveying a transcendental religious message. Some of the characters depicted were most assuredly real (e.g., Herod, Pontius Pilate); others, like Jesus, may or may not have had some connection to actual historical personages. Furthermore, some of the healing practices referred to may have been based on local custom and tradition (e.g., the application of clay made from spittle to the eyes as a magical cure for blindness; Smith, 1978). Nevertheless, these stories cannot be used as accurate descriptions of real events. Moreover, they cannot be understood if they are examined outside of the social and historical context in which they were written, and without reference to the motives and purposes of the authors. Because traditional histories of hypnosis consist of just such presentist accounts of New Testament healing narratives, they provide neither an understanding of the Biblical stories nor accurate information about the history of hypnosis.

MESMERISM, DEMONISM, MEDICINE AND HYPNOSIS

Modern ideas concerning hypnosis grew out of the 18th-century work of Franz Anton Mesmer (1781/1980) on animal magnetism. According to Mesmer, a "subtle fluid" permeated the universe, including the human body. An imbalance of this fluid within the body produced disease, and cure of disease was accomplished by redistributing and harmonizing the flow of fluid. Redistribution of the fluid in the sick was effected by transmitting magnetic fluid from certain healthy individuals ("magnetizers") to the sick (Ellenberger, 1970).

Mesmer's theorizing was embedded in the scientific *Zeitgeist* of his day. For instance, Mesmer's notion of an all-pervasive fluid has been related by historians to earlier scientific ideas concerning universal fluids propagated by Paracelsus, Von Hartman, Mead, and others, as well as to other aspects of the intellectual climate that pervaded 18th-century science (Darnton, 1970; Ellenberger, 1970; Pattie, 1956; Podmore, 1909; Sarbin, 1962; Spanos & Gottlieb, 1979).

The social role of the magnetized or mesmerized subject was multifaceted and evolved in a number of different directions throughout the 19th century. Nevertheless, by the early 19th century, the major components of that role were established. Enactment of the role consisted of a set of rather unusual behaviors that occurred within the confines of a mesmeric relationship. Among the most important of these behaviors were convulsions, amnesia, clairvoyance, augmented or diminished sensory and/or motor abilities (e.g., analgesia, increased strength), and the subjective experience of these behaviors as occurring without volition.

The procedures used by magnetizers to cure their patients also became standardized. These came to include not only specific curative procedures ("passes" made with the hands along the patient's body), but, equally important, the development by magnetists of a particular moral stance toward themselves and their patients (Spanos & Gottlieb, 1979). The personal characteristics of magnetizers, their faith in their procedures, and their belief in the moral purity of their undertaking became conceptualized as crucial to the success of their treatment (Deleuze, 1825/1879). The psychological characteristics of successful magnetizers came to be seen as opposite to the psychological characteristics of the patients they treated. Patients (who were frequently women) were seen as passive, fragile, and weak in both mind and body, whereas magnetizers (who were almost always men) came to be seen as strong, powerful, and intelligent (A Practical Magnetizer, 1843). This dominant–subservient aspect of the magnetic relationship reflected the way in which 19th-century physicians conceptualized the doctor–female patient relationship. These (male) physicians conceptualized themselves as strong, competent and intelligent, but viewed their "nervous" female patients as innately weak and relatively unintelligent and incompetent (Smith-Rosenberg, 1972; Wood, 1974).

Magnetists soon came to construe their healing activities in moral terms. Disease became a moral evil and health a moral good. Virtue became necessary for the maintenance of health, and vice could produce disharmony and disease. Magnetists pledged not only to cure sickness, but also to prevent injustice and to promote honesty and correct conduct (Bergasse, 1785/1970; Rostan, 1825). Magnetists were engaged in a moral confrontation with the evil of disease and would be victorious only if they first girded themselves with the appropriate moral stance (Darnton, 1970; Deleuze, 1825/1879; Dupeau, 1826). For instance, magnetizers who used incorrect techniques or who were morally or physically unfit to magnetize might develop symptoms of their patients' disorder (Deleuze, 1825/1879; Newman, 1847; Pearson, 1790). In short, the patterns of interaction between magnetizers and patients, and the manner in which both magnetizers and patients came to view themselves as well as each other, quickly became standardized.

Attempts to account for the standardization of roles seen in the magnetic interaction have usually focused on the patient and ignored the magnetizer. The most common historical account held that the behavior of magnetized patients flowed automatically from underlying physiological changes. Thus, from the perspective of the early magnetists (and later from that of hypnotists as well), behaviors such as convulsions, alterations in sensory acuity, intellectual enhancements, and spontaneous amnesia tended to occur together because of intrinsic changes in the nervous system that came about when patients entered magnetic or hypnotic sleep (Braid, 1843/1960; Charcot, 1889). The major difficulty with this hypothesis was pointed out by Bernheim when he criticized Charcot's (1889) three stages of *grand hypnotisme*. In essence, Bernheim pointed out that the "symptoms" of hypnosis or magnetism did not necessarily intercorrelate. Instead, behaviors such as lethargy, paralysis, and convulsions clustered together only when expectations for their occurrence were implicitly or explicitly suggested to subjects.

Nevertheless, the components of the magnetized role cannot be adequately explained in terms of suggestions emanating from the magnetizer. This hypothesis does not account for why magnetizers would choose to suggest such an odd array of behaviors to their patients. More important, this hypothesis also fails to explain why the behaviors in question were occurring together before the advent of magnetism. Mesmer's early patients often convulsed and exhibited catalepsy, paralysis, and various sensory dysfunctions before he met them. During the 18th century, many of these behaviors— especially when they occurred in women—were considered symptomatic of hysteria (Spanos & Gottlieb, 1979; Veith, 1965). Neither Mesmer nor other early magnetizers suggested the initial occurrence of these behaviors to their patients. Instead, they attempted to regulate the timing of their occurrence and their eventual disappearance.

Following Spanos and Gottlieb (1979), we suggest that the reciprocal social roles of magnetizer and magnetized patient evolved out of and were patterned to a large extent after an earlier form of social interaction: the interaction of exorcist and possessed person (demoniac).

From Exorcism to Magnetism

The phenomena of demonic possession and exorcism, and the dualistic religious cosmology in which they were embedded, emerged from Near Eastern religious beliefs and practices into Western history during the period between the Old and New Testaments (Russell, 1972). These phenomena then spread throughout the Western world as accompaniments to Christianity (Oesterreich, 1966). The history of possession and exorcism are described in detail elsewhere (Oesterreich, 1966; Kelly, 1974; Spanos, 1983). Suffice it to say here that from the earliest Christian centuries through the 17th and 18th centuries, the role behaviors enacted by demoniacs (despite local variations) remained relatively consistent. Among the most important behaviors displayed by demoniacs were those that later became associated with magnetism. These included convulsions, analgesia, sensory and motor deficits, heightened intelligence, sensory functioning and clairvoyance, spontaneous amnesia for the period in which the demon controlled the body, and the experience of role behaviors as occurring involuntarily (Spanos & Gottlieb, 1979).

Importantly, in the case of both possession and magnetism, role behaviors were contextually cued. The initiation and termination of these behaviors were influenced by the exorcist or magnetizer. For instance, in cases of possession exorcists often initiated and terminated convulsions, displays of analgesia, sensory and motor dysfunctions, and so on by issuing the appropriate verbal or nonverbal cues (e.g., sprinkling the possessed with holy water might elicit convulsions; Spanos, 1983). Similarly, magnetists often reported producing comparable behavioral displays in their patients by varying the direction of their "passes," the manner or location in which they touched patients, or the like (Deleuze, 1825/1879; Ellenberger, 1970). Moreover, during both exorcism and magnetism, symptoms tended to exacerbate as the treatment progressed; they reached a peak accompanied by dramatic displays of convulsions, which ultimately resolved with resulting symptom attenuation. As was later the case with magnetism, exorcism was construed not merely as a curative procedure, but as a moral confrontation between good and evil. Successful exorcism provided a legitimating function by illustrating the power of the church and affirming its values. The most obvious, and certainly the most frequently cited, similarity between exorcising and magnetizing was the use of "laying on of hands" by exorcists and the passes and touches employed by magnetists (Edmonston, 1986; Owen, 1971; Rose, 1971).

In addition to such behavioral similarities, the exorcist role, like the magnetist role, also involved the development of appropriate attitudes toward oneself and one's procedures. Exorcists, like magnetists, viewed their healing powers as emanating from a source other than themselves (God in the case of exorcism, magnetic fluid in the case of magnetism). Nevertheless, both exorcists and magnetists conceptualized their attitudes and beliefs as crucial in effecting cures (Spanos & Gottlieb, 1979; Spanos, 1983). Descriptions of the attitudes appropriate to exorcism sound very similar to the descriptions given earlier of the attitudes and beliefs thought to be appropriate for successful magnetism. Exorcists, like magnetists, viewed their activity as a moral confrontation between good and evil. In order to prevail against demonic forces, exorcists were required to lead a moral life, have a strong faith in God, and cleanse themselves spiritually before exorcising (Spanos & Gottlieb, 1979). Failure to meet these requirements might not only prevent a cure; it could also leave the exorcist vulnerable to demonic attack.

In summary, the relationship between exorcists and demoniacs resembled that between magnetizers and patients in a number of important respects. The interactions in both cases were construed as moral confrontations. Evil could be conquered in these confrontations only if the representatives of good (exorcists or magnetists) were morally purified, possessed abundant faith in their procedures, and maintained firm control over themselves and the situation. Moral failing in exorcists or magnetizers could lead to their developing the symptoms of their patients.

Similarities in the roles of exorcist–demoniac and magnetizer– patient are not the only evidence that the magnetized role was modeled on earlier demonic enactments. Evidence for such a modeling effect also comes from the fact that cases of demonic possession were still relatively common occurrences in the 18th century. Such cases were well known to early magnetizers, who themselves often noted similarities between their procedures and those carried out by exorcists (Ellenberger, 1970; Spanos & Gottlieb, 1979). For example, in the middle of the 18th century, Johann Joseph Gassner conducted well-attended public exorcisms in Swabia, Switzerland, and Tyrol. The behavior of Gassner's demonically possessed patients strongly resembled that of magnetized subjects, and Gassner's exorcism procedures closely resembled the procedures used by magnetists. Mesmer, in fact, observed some of Gassner's demonstrations and concluded that the results were due to Gassner's inadvertent use of animal magnetism (Ellenberger, 1970). Similar reinterpretations of possession as magnetism were made by many mesmerists and later by hypnotists as well (Dods, 1865; Haddock, 1849; Mahan, 1855; Sextus, 1893/1968). In fact, as indicated earlier, it even became common to reinterpret Biblical references to exorcism and healing as examples of the inadvertent use of magnetism and hypnosis.

The similarities of possession and magnetism were noted by many others than the magnetizers. For instance, many clergy and laypeople in the 18th and 19th centuries defined magnetism as a species of demonic possession (Spanos & Gottlieb, 1979). The transition from demonic to magnetic interpretations also involved various attempts to combine and integrate these perspectives. For example, notions of magnetism and somnambulism, which were initially described in naturalistic terms, quickly became integrated into supernaturalistic frames of reference. Magnetism began to be employed as a technique for divination and spirit communication. Somnambules became professionalized as spirit mediums; before the end of the 18th century, this spiritualist form of mesmerism had spread throughout Europe (Ellenberger, 1970; Darnton, 1970).

In the early 19th century, the notion of "demonico-magnetic affections" was developed by Justin Kerner, a German physician and Romantic poet (Spanos & Gottlieb, 1979). Kerner believed that people could become possessed by demons, and that they could be successfully treated by a combination of exorcism and magnetism.

In summary, the hypothesis that the magnetic relationship was to a large extent modeled after the exorcist–demoniac relationship is supported not only by the fact that both activities involved highly similar phenomena and overlapped during the 18th and 19th centuries, but also by the fact that both magnetists and proponents of the possession doctrine quickly and easily reinterpreted the phenomena of the other system within their own frames of reference, or sometimes developed hybrid practices that involved attempts at integrating the two theoretical systems.

From Mesmerism to Hypnosis

By the middle of the 19th century, both possession and magnetism were frequently interpreted by the medical community in terms of hysteria (Drinka, 1984; Ellenberger, 1970). With increases in scientific knowledge, explanations of physiological functioning or of behavior in terms of universal fluids fell into disfavor. Scientific and medical thinking during this period were influenced by a rise in the popularity and status of neurology. One important consequence of this change in scientific *Zeitgeist* was the replacement of both spiritual and "fluidist" hypotheses of magnetic phenomena with hypotheses based on contemporary notions of neurological functioning. The best-known neurological alternative to the fluidist hypothesis was Braid's (1843/1960) notion of "neurypnology." Misled by the lethargic appearance of his patients, Braid initially accounted for magnetic phenomena in terms of spreading neural inhibition induced by sustained visual attention and eye muscle fatigue. Purportedly, the spreading of this neural inhibition backward from the optic nerves to the brain produced a state akin to sleep, in which the phenomena of magnetism (now relabeled "hypnosis") became manifest.

A second consequence of adopting neurological accounts for hysteria and hypnosis was the placing of these phenomena under the rubric of medical disease. Perhaps the strongest reflection of this viewpoint was found in the work of Charcot, who contended that hysteria was a disease and that only hysterics could manifest the signs of *grand hypnotisme*. Charcot frequently drew attention to similarities between symptoms of hysterics and the behavior of the demonically possessed of previous centuries as evidence that the possessed had, in reality, been suffering from the disease of hysteria (Charcot & Marie, 1892; Charcot & Richet, 1887/1972).

Charcot's identification of hypnosis with nervous disease was undoubtedly facilitated by the fact that many of the most salient "symptoms" of hypnosis (when divorced from the social context in which they occurred) lent themselves easily to neuropathological interpretation (e.g., convulsions, analgesia). Thus, many of the odd behaviors that have remained a part of the modern hypnotic role probably received initial legitimation in 19th-century medical circles because their superficial resemblance to the symptoms of neurological disease encouraged their conceptualizations in medical terms (Wagstaff, 1981). These behaviors continue to be conceptualized as "symptoms" of hypnosis and have become enshrined as such on modern hypnotizability scales. The misleading medical names that, even today, continue to be applied to these behaviors clearly reflect their historical origins in medicine (e.g., "amnesia" as opposed to attempted forgetting; "hallucination" as opposed to imagining). The

19th-century medical accounts of these behaviors, like earlier accounts in terms of demonic possession, reinforced the notion that these behaviors were involuntary occurrences and, like the symptoms of other diseases, were not under the patient's control (Drinka, 1984; Spanos & Gottlieb, 1979).

Charcot's specific ideas about hypnosis were discarded before the end of the 19th century. Nevertheless, a number of implicit conceptions of the hypnotic subject propagated by him, as well as by most other 19th-century investigators, persisted as part of the general mythology of hypnosis well into the 20th century (e.g., the hypnotic subject as an automaton, hypnotic responsiveness as symptomatic of mental weakness). Historically, these notions derived in part from earlier conceptions of the exorcist–demoniac relationship, became an integral part of 18th- and 19th-century conceptions of the magnetic relationship, and have persisted down to the present day as part of the popular public image of hypnosis.

Hysteria, Hypnosis, and History

Using the notion of hysterical disease as an explanation for possession, mesmerism, and hypnosis did little to promote an understanding of the behaviors associated with this notion. Although the term "hysteria" can be traced to antiquity (Veith, 1965), there is little evidence to suggest that this term refers to a unitary disease process that can be traced down through the centuries. During the 19th and 20th centuries, the referents for this term have been highly ambiguous and changeable. The term has, in fact, referred to a wide range of relatively unusual and dramatic but often unrelated behaviors (Chordoff, 1974; Chordoff & Lyons, 1958; Janet, 1925; Szasz, 1961). In the 19th and early 20th centuries, this array of behaviors included spontaneous amnesia; fugue states; convulsions; sensory and motor disturbances occurring in the absence of demonstrable organic pathology; multiple personality; heightened suggestibility; hallucinations; anorexia; a host of sexual disturbances; and a personality configuration variously described as vain, coquettish, frigid, and so on (Spanos & Gottlieb, 1979). There is no evidence to support the contention that the various behaviors subsumed under the rubric "hysteria" reflect a unitary disease process or have a common etiology (Slater, 1965). Moreover, there is little evidence to suggest that the behavioral referents for the term "hysteria" in ancient times were similar to the constellation of behaviors labeled as "hysteria" in the 19th and 20th centuries. On the other hand, a growing body of historical evidence suggests that many of the behaviors that came to be classified in the 18th and 19th centuries as "hysteria" (or earlier as "possession") reflected the coping strategies of unhappy women who adopted the sick (or possessed) role as a means of both adapting to and rebelling against restrictive, harsh, or demeaning social conditions (Smith-Rosenberg, 1972; Drinka, 1984; Spanos, 1983).

The popularity of the diagnosis "hysteria" in the 19th century cannot be understood in terms of its medical utility. The diagnosis did not identify a unitary disorder, pinpoint a valid etiology, or lead to successful treatment. On the other hand, the popularity of this diagnosis can be explained in terms of the concurrent rise in the status of psychiatry as a medical discipline. Medical specialties, of course, require diseases that the specialists can diagnose and treat. In the 19th and early 20th centuries, the budding specialty of psychiatry required "diseases of the mind" that could be differentiated from the diseases of the nervous system, which were already the province of neurology. The reinterpretation of hysteria as a psychological rather than a neurological disease served such a function. The popularity of the hysteria diagnosis in the 18th and 19th centuries may be viewed as an example of the medicalization of deviant and disturbing behavior. The troubling and unusual behavior of some unhappy women, which had previously been viewed in terms of moral or religious concerns, was now viewed as symptomatic of disease. Even though hysteria was often employed as a catch-all diagnosis that covered a wide variety of unrelated behaviors, the medicalization of these behaviors reified hysteria as a mental disease, and supported the emergence of psychiatry as a legitimate medical discipline with its own distinct diseases (Szasz, 1961).

It should be kept in mind, that the 19th-century practitioners of psychiatry were also the discipline's first historians. These investigators were intent on legitimizing the notion that certain behavioral deviances were really diseases. The reification of hysteria as a disease entity was facilitated by demonstrating that the disorder had an ancient history. The symptoms of this "disease" could now be traced from Asclepian temples through 16th-century possessed nuns and Mesmer's 18th-century magnetized patients to 19th-century hysterics. In short, psychiatric histories legitimated the medical mythologies that provided the underpinnings for the emergence of psychiatry as a medical discipline (Drinka, 1984; Spanos, 1989b).

As pointed out by Spanos and Gottlieb (1979), a contextualist perspective applied to the history of possession, hysteria, mesmerism, and hypnosis acknowledges that disease theorists have been correct in pointing to behavioral similarities associated with these phenomena. However, the disease perspective lacks theoretical viability in conceptualizing these behavioral commonalities as deriving from a unitary process that produces invariant symptoms. A contextualist perspective suggests instead that the manifestations of possessed behavior were maintained for centuries as a coherent social role because the status of the demoniac became associated with a number of important social functions. For instance, in conjunction with exorcism procedures, the role of demoniac provided an avenue for reintegrating deviants into the social community; it also served as an important device for proselytizing, in addition to supporting the religious and moral values of the church and state (Spanos, 1983).

The gradual shift from possession to hysteria that occurred from the 16th through the 19th centuries was associated with changes in the behavior of the patients to whom those labels were applied. As behavioral deviance increasingly became defined in medical terms, patient behaviors that were not amenable to mechanistic explanations based on organic pathology gradually became less frequent (e.g., vomiting pins that the possessing demon purportedly brought with him when he entered the demoniac). On the other hand, behaviors that could be easily subsumed under a medical rubric remained (e.g., sensory–motor disturbances, convulsions; Spanos & Gottlieb, 1979).

In the late 18th and 19th centuries, many patients treated with magnetism and later hypnotism were diagnosed as hysterics (Drinka, 1984; Ellenberger, 1970). In other words, many patients (usually female), who in various respects behaved like earlier demoniacs, now defined themselves and were defined by their physicians as sick rather than as possessed. It was patients of this ilk—unhappy women who complained of vague aches and pains, reported sensory and motor deficits with little evidence of organic dysfunction, convulsed, and appeared highly anxious and overly "sensitive"—who were treated by the early magnetizers (Binet & Fere, 1888, Janet, 1925; Podmore, 1902, 1909). It was these behavioral enactments— previously defined as demonic, now defined as sick—that the magnetizers brought under "control" and shaped into the role of the magnetic and later the hypnotic subject.

In summary, a contextualist approach to the history of possession, hysteria, mesmerism, and hypnosis rejects the traditional view that hysteria and hypnosis are invariant phenomena that have been discovered by modern science and can now be used to explain the historical occurrences of possession, exorcism, and religious healing. The contextualist approach, on the other hand, transposes the traditional view by suggesting that ancient notions of possession, exorcism, and religious healing created the groundwork from which the hysterical, magnetizer, and magnetized subject roles eventually emerged. From this perspective, the social roles of demoniac and exorcist acted as social templates that influenced the structure of the hysteric, magnetic, and magnetizer roles, which emerged as the magical/religious *Zeitgeist* of the 16th and 17th centuries was gradually transformed into the mechanistic/scientific *Zeitgeist* of the 18th and 19th centuries.

PSYCHOLOGICAL THEORIES OF HYPNOSIS

After the middle of the 19th century, psychological theories of hypnosis became increasingly prominent and increasingly differentiated from neurological theorizing. Nevertheless, these psychological theories, like their neurological predecessors, remained rooted in a mechanistic/positivist *Zeitgeist* and took for granted the proposition that hypnotic responses were automatic occurrences rather than goal-directed activities. Despite the assumption of automaticity, it became increasingly apparent that hypnotic subjects modified their behavior in terms of the wishes, commands, and expectations of the hypnotist (Sarbin, 1962). From time to time, this recognition led to the criticism that hypnotic responses were simply faked by wily patients in order to gain the approval and attention of credulous hypnotists (e.g., Hart, 1898). However, accusations of faking were typically employed not as serious scientific hypotheses aimed at explaining hypnotic behavior, but instead as moral condemnation aimed at discrediting the work of particular investigators. Moreover, it was commonly believed in the 19th and early 20th centuries that hypnotic subjects could perform at least some behaviors that transcended the capabilities of nonhypnotized individuals. By definition, of course, faking could not account for transcendent behavior.

Ideomotor Responding

One of the earliest psychological theories, aimed at accounting both for the apparent automaticity of hypnotic responding and for the influence of the hypnotist's expectations, was formulated by Braid (1855/1970). By 1847, Braid had become dissatisfied with his own earlier quasi-physiological speculations concerning "neurypnology," and, as an alternative, developed the concept of "monoideism." Monoideism was based on the notion of "ideomotor action"—the hypothesis that ideas that remain uncontradicted by other ideas lead automatically to the corresponding action. According to this formulation, the hypnotist communicates a particular idea to the subject— say, the idea that the subject's arm is becoming stiff and rigid. Supposedly, the focusing of attention by the subject exclusively on the idea of arm stiffness leads automatically to a stiffening of the arm.

Although Braid's notion of monoideism had no influence on Charcot, it strongly influenced the work of Liébeault, Bernheim, and other members of the so-called Nancy school, who made ideomotor action the central tenet in their theory of "suggestion" (Sarbin & Coe, 1972). Thus, for Bernheim, the suggestions of the hypnotist were translated by the patient into representations or ideas. These ideas then led automatically to corresponding behaviors. Because the elicitation of the behaviors was automatic, the behaviors were experienced as "unwilled."

Bernheim's notion of suggestion as ideomotor action became the cornerstone of much hypnotic theorizing throughout the early 20th century. For example, this notion, although formulated in somewhat different language and elaborated upon in somewhat different ways by each investigator, was central to the theories of hypnosis and/or suggestion posited by Coue (1922), Wundt (1892), C. L. Hull (1933), and Arnold (1946).

Dissociation

Charcot's notion of hypnosis as a neuropathological state that could be produced in full only in hysterics was modified and expanded upon in Janet's (1925) concept of "dissociation." According to the dissociation hypothesis, ideas or behavioral patterns that normally occurred together or in sequence could become separated or dissociated from one another. Purportedly, such dissociation was most likely to occur when individuals who were constitutionally predisposed by a "weak" nervous system were exposed to psychological stress or trauma. In such predisposed subjects, however, dissociations could also be produced by the suggestions or commands of the hypnotist. The dissociation hypothesis appeared to explain not only such relatively simple "automatisms" as limb catalepsy, but also complex behaviors such as automatic writing and multiple personality, which seemed to imply the existence of intelligent but unconscious selves or personalities that appeared to be isolated from the person's "normal" or "conscious" self. Although dissociation theory initially gained numerous influential adherents in both Europe and America, by the middle of the 20th century it had been largely displaced in theories of hypnosis by variants of Bernheim's theory of suggestibility. Some of the reasons for the decline of the dissociation hypothesis were outlined by White and Shevach (1942):

> Dissociative boundaries, we have noticed, by no means necessarily follow natural lines of cleavage; they do not have to surround innate biological systems nor are they required to enclose systems built up in the person's experience. Instead, the pattern of dissociative barriers is in a great many cases directly dependent on what is suggested, following in minute detail even the most bizarre conceits of the operator. Thus, post-hypnotic amnesia may be established for a single arbitrarily chosen event within the hypnotic trance . . . In short, the operator

can impose a dissociative barrier almost wherever he chooses. This fact tends to shift our interest from dissociation to suggestion . . . (p. 327)

R. W. White and the Rejection
of Mechanism

R. W. White was the first modern investigator to explicitly reject mechanistic approaches to hypnotic behavior. In a seminal paper, White (1941) underscored the limitations of both the concept of ideomotor action and dissociation theory. Some of White's criticisms of dissociation theory have been cited above. With respect to ideomotor action, he pointed out that the responses of hypnotic subjects are too complex to be understood as flowing automatically from ideas "implanted" by the hypnotist. On the contrary, once the demands of a suggestion are clear, subjects often creatively improvise and elaborate a performance that goes well beyond the explicit ideas suggested. For example, in order to give a convincing performance of age regression, subjects must draw on their abstract knowledge of childhood as well as personal remembrances of their own childhood, and then weave this information into a coherent, childlike performance (which includes interacting with the experimenter in a childlike manner, answering questions in a childlike manner, etc.). The creative and goal-directed aspects of such a performance, White pointed out, cannot be accounted for adequately by the notion of ideomotor action.

White's (1941) own views of hypnosis were influenced on the one hand by pre-World War II academic social psychology, and on the other by psychoanalytic theorizing. He proposed that

> hypnotic behavior be regarded as meaningful goal-directed striving, its most general goal being to behave like a hypnotized person as this is continuously defined by the operator and understood by the subject . . . The subject, it is held, is ruled by a wish to behave like a hypnotized person, his regnant motive is submission to the operator's demands, he understands at all times what the operator intends, and his behavior is striving to put these intentions into execution. (p. 483)

Despite his emphasis on goal-directed strivings and subjects' expectations, White (1941) retained the notion of an altered state of the person. In part, this reflected White's belief (common at the time but now known to be mistaken) that hypnotic procedures produced enhancements in performance that transcended the enhancements produced by nonhypnotic procedures. White further believed that the relaxation component of hypnotic procedures could induce a "restriction of consciousness" that facilitated the experience of responding involuntarily, and that perhaps led to subtle alterations in the cognitive functioning of hypnotized subjects.

The Methodological Tradition

The manner in which all modern psychological theories of hypnosis are presented and tested has been shaped by the pervasive experimental–behavioral tradition that has formed the methodological underpinning of most modern approaches to experimental social psychology, as well as to psychological research more generally. This methodological tradition, with its emphasis on operationalization of concepts, quantification, the use of controlled experiments, and the statistical treatment of data, was introduced into hypnosis research during the 1930s by C. L. Hull (1933). However, the systematic application of this tradition to hypnotic phenomena only began in earnest in the late 1950s and early 1960s with the empirical work of Sutcliffe (1960, 1961), Barber (1969), Orne (1959), and Hilgard (1965).

The importance of this methodological tradition to contemporary theorizing about hypnosis would be difficult to overemphasize. For example, the implicit mistrust of verbal report and the emphasis on objective and quantifiable response indices inherent in this tradition were important supports for the development of empirically based research programs, which have largely laid to rest the notion that hypnotic subjects enter an unusual state enabling them to transcend the behavioral capabilities of nonhypnotic subjects. At an even more fundamental level, the implicit acceptance of the assumptions that underlie this methodological tradition provides modern investigators with a common language and a shared set of empirical standards with which to anchor theoretical ideas and with which to test their own and competing theoretical formulations (e.g., the common methodologies that underlie the controversy over "hidden-observer" responding; Hilgard, 1979; Spanos, 1986).

Modern Approaches in Historical Perspective

Despite their grounding in a common methodological tradition, modern theories of hypnosis differ from one another in the extent to which they attempt to account for hypnotic responding by positing the operation of unusual, unique, or essential cognitive activities. It is important to keep in mind, however, that these approaches share numerous similarities as well as differences (Spanos & Barber, 1974; Sheehan & Perry, 1976); that differences in the variables chosen for investigation often reflect differences in relative emphasis, rather than fundamental disagreements; and that methodologies and research instruments developed by those who favor one approach are frequently incorporated into the research studies of those who favor different approaches.

Sociocognitive Perspectives

The most explicit rejection of the notion of a hypnotic or trance state is found in the work of investigators broadly identified with what is variously labeled as the "social-psychological," "sociocognitive," "cognitive–behavioral," or simply the "nonstate" approach toward hypnosis (Barber, 1969; Sarbin & Coe, 1972; Spanos, 1986; Wagstaff, 1981). The earliest definitive statement on this perspective was formulated by Sarbin (1950). Sarbin was heavily influenced by White's (1941) notion of hypnotic responding as goal-directed action. Unlike White (1941), however, Sarbin (1950) rejected both the notion that hypnotic responding was facilitated by an altered state of consciousness and the related notion that hypnotic responding was associated with subtle cognitive transformations. Instead, Sarbin accounted for both the behavioral and subjective report aspects of hypnotic responding in terms of the concept of "role enactment." Sarbin's (1950) role theory perspective emphasized the importance of contextual variables in communicating the social demands that shaped subjects' expectations of the hypnotic role. This formulation also emphasized that subjects were actively involved in generating the behaviors and subjective experiences that constituted hypnotic role enactments. In short, Sarbin's (1950) approach involved an explicit rejection of the mechanistic assumption that hypnotic responding was caused by an antecedent "trance state." Instead of viewing hypnosis as a state or condition that "happened to" (i.e., was induced in) subjects, Sarbin viewed hypnotic responding as actively generated by subjects who used contextual information to create the experiences and behaviors that constituted the hypnotic role.

Despite his seminal theorizing, Sarbin conducted relatively little empirical research. Throughout the 1960s, however, his ideas, along with those of White, strongly influenced the experimental work conducted by Barber (1969, 1979). In an extensive series of studies, Barber and his associates (Barber, 1969) empirically demonstrated the important roles played by subjects' attitudes, expectations, and motivations in hypnotic responding. Importantly, Barber's empirical work also provided repeated demonstration of the fact that nonhypnotic subjects, given brief instructions to perform maximally, showed increments in responsiveness to suggestions that were as large as the increments produced by hypnotic procedures. This finding supported the contention that despite external appearances, hypnotic responses were not particularly unusual, and therefore did not require the positing of unusual states of consciousness.

More recently, investigators within the sociocognitive tradition have focused on the detailed examination of individual hypnotic phenomena, and the ways in which subtle and sometimes ambiguous social demands influence subjects' cognitive appraisals of and response to suggestions for amnesia, analgesia, limb catalepsy, and the like (for reviews, see Coe, 1989;

Lynn, Rhue, & Weekes, 1989; Spanos, 1989a). These investigators have also conducted a good deal of research that examines the assumptions underlying competing formulations and emphasizes the role of contextual variables in hypnotic responding.

Sociophenomenological Perspectives

An influential alternative to sociocognitive formulations that retains White's emphasis both on the goal-directed nature of hypnotic responding and on the notion of altered cognitive functioning during hypnotic responding is, for lack of a better term, labeled the "sociophenomenological" perspective here. This perspective is most closely identified with the work of Orne (1959, 1979), but also influenced the work of Shor (1959, 1962) and continues to influence the search for experiential and cognitive style correlates of hypnotic responding that characterizes the work of Tellegen (Tellegen & Atkinson, 1974), Sheehan and McConkey (1982), Laurence and Perry (1983), and others.

Like White and Sarbin, Orne emphasized the goal-directed nature of hypnotic responding and viewed the subject as actively involved in interpreting and responding to the social demands of the experimental situation. Unlike Sarbin, however, Orne did not reject the concept of a hypnotic state. Instead, Orne (1959) retained White's belief that hypnotic responding was characterized by relatively subtle changes in cognitive functioning. Orne developed a simulator control methodology that he initially believed would enable the separation of those subtle cognitive characteristics that constituted the "essence" of hypnosis from what he considered to be behavioral artifacts produced in response to social demands. The experimental work generated by the use of Orne's simulator control design, like the experimental work conducted by Barber (1969), was important in demonstrating that a wide range of hypnotic responding that had been assumed to reflect a hypnotic state could instead be explained more parsimoniously in terms of the expectations transmitted to subjects by the social demands of the experimental situation. On the other hand, experimental designs employed by both Orne and Barber have been criticized by those approaching hypnosis from alternative perspectives. These controversies are explored in detail elsewhere (e.g., de Groot & Gwynn, 1989; Spanos, 1986) and in some of the chapters that follow.

Regardless of the limitations of the simulator control design, the tradition represented by the work of Orne, Shor, Sheehan, and others continues to focus research attention on the diverse subjective experiences reported by hypnotic subjects and on the development of methodologies for the assessment and classification of such experiences (Sheehan & McConkey, 1982). Investigators within this tradition have also been instrumental in developing questionnaires for the assessment of stable experiential or phenomenological styles that might be correlated with hypnotizability (Shor, Orne, & O'Connell, 1962; Tellegen & Atkinson, 1974).

The major difference between the sociocognitive and sociophenom-enological perspectives stems from the explicit rejection of the hypnotic state construct by the former, and its at least tacit acceptance in the work of Orne, Shor, and others. For instance, in Orne's (1959) early work, genuine hypnotic experiences were implicitly conceptualized as events that happened to subjects, rather than as experiences generated by subjects in response to the contextual cues present in the experimental situation. "Hypnotized" subjects were seen as being in a state or condition in which the usual rules of logic no longer applied, and in which at least some complex behaviors (e.g., posthypnotic responding) could be elicited automatically and independently of contextual demands and conscious control (Orne, Sheehan, & Evans, 1968).

More recently, at least some investigators identified with this perspective have conceptualized both hypnotic experiences and hypnotic behavior as actively created by subjects, and as a function of subjects' varied cognitive styles in interplay with the communications of the hypnotist (Sheehan & McConkey, 1982). In short, at least some of the investigators that we have identified with the sociophenomenological perspective and those identified with the sociocognitive perspective appear to be converging on a common theoretical perspective. The differences between the proponents of these two perspectives may, to an increasing degree, reflect differences in research emphasis more than fundamental differences in the conceptualization of hypnotic responding as passive happening rather than context supported action.

The Neodissociation Perspective

In the mid-1970s, E. R. Hilgard (1977) reintroduced Janet's notion of dissociation into theories of hypnosis. Hilgard (1977) postulated that dissociations between cognitive systems were often partial rather than complete, and contended that this postulate differentiated his notion of dissociation from that of Janet. By maintaining that dissociations were often incomplete, Hilgard was able to make his version of this concept congruent with the common observation that the memories purportedly forgotten by subjects during hypnotic amnesia continue to influence performance in a variety of subtle ways.

Dissociation regained substantial influence as a perspective toward hypnosis within a relatively short period of time. In part, the ready acceptance of this notion reflected Hilgard's stature as a well-known pioneer in the field of psychology. In addition, such acceptance probably also reflected the deeply ingrained and long-standing belief that hypnotic behavior really does differ in some fundamental way from nonhypnotic behavior. Finally, the notion of dissociation both supported and gained support from the recent renewed popularity of multiple personality as a psychiatric diagnosis. Most of the clinical investigators who deal with multiple-personality patients consider the phenomenon to result from dissociation and to be intimately connected with hypnotic responsivity (e.g., Bliss, 1986).

Unlike sociocognitive and sociophenomenological formulations, the neodissociation perspective de-emphasizes the role of contextual factors in hypnotic responding, and denies (or at least greatly de-emphasizes) the view that hypnotic responding reflects goal-directed activity. Instead, the neodissociation perspective conceptualizes hypnotic behavior and hypnotic experiences as events that happen to subjects. Thus, hypnotic subjects do not create their experiences of amnesia or pain reduction. Instead, these experiences happen to them when certain cognitive subsystems somehow become separated (dissociated) from one another. In short, according to neodissociation theory, subjects are by and large the passive observers rather than the active initiators of their hypnotic experiences.

As we have pointed out earlier, one of White and Shevach's (1942) most important criticisms of Janet's notion of dissociation was that the concept explained nothing and was therefore unnecessary. According to those investigators, the experiences and behaviors that appeared to be dissociated were those for which dissociation had been implicitly or explicitly suggested by the hypnotist. In other words, dissociation could be reduced to suggestion and therefore was not required as a separate concept.

In contrast to White and Shevach (1942), Hilgard (1977, 1979) has argued that dissociations are *not* the direct result of suggestion. Instead, dissociations of cognitive functioning are supposedly present during hypnotic responding even when the dissociations have not been directly suggested and when neither the hypnotist nor the subjects are aware of their presence. Hilgard (1977) supported his hypothesis by presenting data that he interpreted as indicating that hypnotic subjects simultaneously process sensory information at two levels of consciousness, while remaining consciously aware of only the information at one level. For example, in several studies (reviewed by Hilgard, 1979), subjects who reported little pain during hypnotic analgesia also reported feeling high levels of pain at the same time. These reports of high pain were supposedly obtained directly from a dissociated part of the hypnotic subject. This dissociated part of the person was labeled the "hidden observer," and Hilgard argued that during hypnotic analgesia a hidden part of the person continues to feel high levels of pain. Normally, however, this hidden part of the person is never contacted by the hypnotist; as a consequence, neither the hypnotist nor the subject is aware that a dissociated part of the subject feels high levels of pain. It is important to keep in mind that subjects do not spontaneously report hidden experiences. Such reports have been observed only when the hypnotist has informed subjects that they possess a hidden part that experiences events differently than does their "normal" self (Hilgard, 1979).

The obvious criticism of the hidden-observer studies conducted by Hilgard and by others (e.g., Zamansky & Bartis, 1985) is the same criticism leveled by Bernheim against Charcot's idea that *grande hypnotisme* involved three stages, with each stage characterized by invariant and unsuggested symptoms. Bernheim's point was that the symptoms Charcot took to be invariant and unsuggested were, in fact, the result of implicit and explicit suggestions of which Charcot was unaware. Along similar lines, a good deal of experimental work (reviewed by Spanos, 1986) now indicates that hidden-observer reports, rather than reflecting unconscious dissociations, reflect role enactments carried out by subjects who develop expectations concerning the characteristics of hidden-observer responding from the social demands inherent in their experimental test situation. Thus, rather than unambiguously reflecting unconscious dissociations, the findings of hidden-observer studies can also be interpreted as providing more support for a view of hypnotic responding as context-supported, goal-directed action.

Several experimental strategies that do not depend on the "hidden-observer" methodology have been employed in an attempt to garner support for the dissociation concept. In some cases these studies have yielded data that appear to contradict predictions derived from neodissociation theory (Stava & Jaffa, 1988). Although other studies (e.g., Kihlstrom, 1980; Miller & Bowers, 1986) have yielded more positive findings, they do not unambiguously support the notion of dissociation, or yield results that cannot also be easily and parsimoniously interpreted within a sociocognitive framework (Spanos & Katsanis, 1989; Spanos, Radtke, & Dubreuil, 1982).

It is now generally accepted by investigators in cognitive and social psychology that a great deal of information processing occurs outside of awareness; that people are often unable to specify the most important variables that determine their behavior; and that the causal attributions people do develop to explain behavior are often inaccurate and reflect cultural convention rather than accurate introspection (Gilbert & Cooper, 1985; Nisbett & Wilson, 1977; Wilson, 1985). Perhaps the most valuable contribution of neodissociation theorists to the study of hypnotic behavior stems from their insistence that unconscious processing of this kind is likely to be important in explaining at least some aspects of hypnotic responding. However, notions of unconscious processing and misattribution are not inconsistent with the concept of goal-directed action. White (1941), for example, despite rejecting the concept of dissociation, argued that goal-directed activities could occur outside of awareness. More recently, a number of investigators within the sociocognitive tradition (Diamond, 1989; Lynn et al., 1989; Sarbin, 1989; Spanos, Salas, Bertrand, & Johnston, 1989) have suggested that some hypnotic phenomena (e.g., reports that responses to suggestion occurred involuntarily) involve misattributions, self-deception, cue-induced shifts in attention to or reflection on the wrong stimulus features when generating causal attributions, or other factors that clearly imply the processing of information outside of awareness. Perhaps the continued development of these notions within theoretical frameworks that also emphasize the goal-directed nature of hypnotic responding will allow for some rap-prochement between neodissociation and sociocognitive theorists.

CONCLUSIONS

The constellation of unusual behaviors that evolved into the hypnotic role was well established by the beginning of the 19th century. By the middle of that century, enactments of the hypnotic role were firmly associated with pathology, and the most common explanations given for those enactments were couched in terms of altered neurological functioning that gave rise to an altered or trance state of consciousness. Most of the 19th-century investigators who wrote about hypnotic behavior were trained as physicians. Consequently, the reification of the hypnotic state with its implications of automatism, the explanation of that "state" in terms of physiological alteration, and the relative lack of attention paid to contextual antecedents or to the motives and intentions of subjects, fit comfortably within the positivist/mechanistic framework that these physician/investigators took for granted. The concept of the hypnotic state was given further legitimacy by providing it with an ancient history. This process was accomplished by singling out various historical phenomena that bore some superficial resemblance to hypnotic events, wrenching those phenomena from the social and historical context that made them understandable in their own terms, and then labeling those phenomena as hypnotic events that went unrecognized as such by contemporaries. In this manner, hypnosis could be traced back through the ages and supported as a condition that transcended time and historical circumstance.

The fact that mesmeric and later hypnotic responding was related to the motivations and intentions of subjects and to expectations transmitted by hypnotists was noted repeatedly, from at least the time of the French royal commission that investigated mesmerism during the late 18th century. Nevertheless, a morally neutral theoretical language for describing interpersonal behavior in terms of the expectations, motivations, and intentions of the participants did not develop until the 20th century (Sarbin, 1962). When such a language evolved during the development of modern social psychology, faking and fraud were no longer the only means of describing the goal-directed nature of hypnotic responding; more generally, mechanistic views of human functioning began to be replaced with scientifically legitimate theoretical frameworks that viewed people as "intentional doers," rather than as organisms who simply reacted mechanically to stimuli.

White's (1941) work constituted a watershed in theorizing about hypnosis. White clearly recognized the goal-directed nature of hypnotic responding and the limitations of the mechanistic notions of ideomotor action and dissociation. Nevertheless, White remained unable to free himself entirely from mechanism, and retained that notion of a hypnotic state associated with subtle cognitive alterations.

Modern perspectives on hypnosis differ with respect to their treatment of White's compromise position. Sociocognitive theorists have built on the notion of goal-directed action while rejecting such mechanistic notions as the "trance state." Neodissociation theorists, on the other hand, have re-embraced mechanism while de-emphasizing the goal-directed nature of hypnotic responding, and sociophenomenological theorists have attempted to maintain White's compromise position and develop its empirical implications. The success of these alternative perspectives in providing a useful account of hypnotic responding should be judged by the readers who compare and contrast the chapters of the present volume.

REFERENCES

Allegro, J. M. (1984). *The Dead Sea Scrolls and the Christian myth*. Buffalo, NY: Prometheus Books.

Allegro, J. M. (1986). Jesus and Qumran: The Dead Sea Scrolls. In R. J. Hoffman & G. A. Larue (Eds.), *Jesus in myth and history* (pp. 89–96). Buffalo, NY: Prometheus Books.

Arnold, M. B. (1946). On the mechanism of suggestion and hypnosis. *Journal of Abnormal and Social Psychology, 41*, 107–128.

Barber, T. X. (1969). *Hypnosis: A scientific approach*. New York: Van Nostrand Reinhold.

Barber, T. X. (1979). Suggested ("hypnotic") behavior: The trance paradigm versus an alternative paradigm. In E. Fromm & R. E. Shor (Eds.), *Hypnosis: Developments in research and new perspectives* (2nd ed., pp. 217–271). Chicago: Aldine.

Barber, T. X. (1981). Medicine, suggestive therapy and healing. In R. J. Kastenbaum, T. X. Barber, S. C. Wilson, B. L. Ryder, & L. B. Hathaway. *Old, sick and helpless: Where therapy begins*. Cambridge, MA: Ballinger.

Barber, T. X., & Calverley, D. C. (1964). Effect of experimenter's tone of voice on "hypnotic-like" suggestibility. *Journal of Clinical Psychology, 20*, 438–440.

Barber, T. X., Spanos, N. P., & Chaves, J. F. (1974). *Hypnosis, imagination and human potentialities*. Elmsford, NY: Pergamon Press.

Behr, C. A. (Trans.). (1968). *Aelilus Aristides and the sacred tales*. Amsterdam: Hakkert.

Bergasse, N. (1970). Ideés generales sur le système du monde et l'accord des lois physiques et morales dans la nature. In R. Darnton (Ed.), *Mesmerism* (pp. 183–185). New York: Schocken Books. (Original work published 1785)

Bernheim, H. (1900). *Suggestive theraputics*. New York: Putnam.

Binet, A., & Fere, C. (1888). *Animal magnetism*. New York: Appleton.

Bliss, E. L. (1986). *Multiple personality, allied disorders and hypnosis*. New York: Oxford University Press.

Braid, J. (1960). *Braid on hypnotism* (reprint of *Neurhypnology*, with an introduction by A. E. Waite). New York: Julian. (Original work published 1843)

Braid, J. (1970). The physiology of fascination and the critics criticized. In M. M. Tinterow (Ed.), *Foundations of hypnosis* (pp. 365–389). Springfield, IL: Charles Thomas. (Original work published 1855)

Carr, E. H. (1961). *What is history?* New York: Random House.

Charcot, J. M. (1889). *Clinical lectures on the diseases of the nervous system* (Vol. 3). London: New Sydenham Society.

Charcot, J. M., & Marie, P. (1892). Hysteria. In D. Hack Tuke (Ed.), *Dictionary of psychological medicine* (p. 69). London: Churchill.

Charcot, J. M., & Richet, C. (1972). *Les doemoniaques dans l'art*. Amsterdam: B. M. Israel. (Original work published 1887)

Chordoff, P. (1974). The diagnosis of hysteria: An overview. *American Journal of Psychiatry, 131*, 1073–1087.

Chordoff, P., & Lyons, H. (1958). Hysteria, the hysterical personality and "hysterical" conversion. *American Journal of Psychiatry, 114*, 734–740.

Coe, W. C. (1989). Posthypnotic amnesia: Theory and research. In N. P. Spanos & J. F. Chaves (Eds.), *Hypnosis: The cognitive–behavioral perspective* (pp. 110–148). Buffalo, NY: Prometheus Books.

Conn, J. H. (1957). Historical aspects of scientific hypnosis. *International Journal of Clinical and Experimental Hypnosis, 5*, 17–24.

Coue, E. (1922). *Self mastery through conscious autosuggestion* (A. S. Van Orden, Trans.). New York: Malkan.

Darnton, R. (Ed.). (1970). *Mesmerism*. New York: Schocken Books.

de Groot, H. P. & Gwynn, M. I. (1989). Trance logic, duality, and hidden observer responding. In N. P. Spanos & J. F. Chaves (Eds.), *Hypnosis: The cognitive–behavioral perspective* (pp. 206–240). Buffalo, NY: Prometheus Books.

Deleuze, J. P. F. (1879). *Practical instruction on animal magnetism* (T. Hartshorn, Trans., with an appendix of notes and letters added). New York: Wells.

Deutsch, A. (1946). *The mentally ill in America: A history of their care and treatment from Colonial times*. New York: Columbia University Press.

Diamond, M. J. (1989). The cognitive skills model: An emerging paradigm for investigating hypnotic phenomena. In N. P. Spanos & J. F. Chaves (Eds.), *Hypnosis: The cognitive–behavioral perspective* (pp. 380–399). Buffalo, NY: Prometheus Books.

Dods, J. B. (1865). *Philosophy of mesmerism*. New York: Fowler & Wells.

Drinka, G. F. (1984). *The birth of neurosis*. New York: Simon & Schuster.

Dupeau, J. A. (1826). *Lettres physiologiques et morales sur le magnétisme animal*. Paris:

Edelstein, L. (1937). Greek medicine in its relation to religion and magic. *Bulletin of the Institute of the History of Medicine*, 5, 201–246.

Edelstein, E. J., & Edelstein, L. (1945). *Asclepius: A collection and interpretation of the testimonies* (2 vols.). Baltimore: John Hopkins University Press.

Edmonston, W. E., Jr. (1986). *The induction of hypnosis*. New York: Wiley.

Ellenberger, H. (1970). *The discovery of the unconscious*. New York: Basic Books.

Fellows, B. J. (1986). The concept of trance. In P. L. N. Naish (Ed.), *What is hypnosis?* (pp. 37–58). Philadelphia: Open University Press.

Fellows, B. J. (1990). Current theories of hypnosis: A critical overview. *British Journal of Experimental and Clinical Psychology*, 7, 81–92.

Frank, J. D. (1973). *Persuasion and healing: A comparative study of psychotherapy*. Baltimore: John Hopkins University Press.

Gilbert, D. T., & Cooper, J. (1985). Social psychological strategies of self-deception. In M. W. Martin (Ed), *Self-deception and self-understanding* (pp. 75–94). Lawrence: University of Kansas Press.

Glasner, S. (1955). A note on allusions to hypnosis in the Bible and Talmud. *International Journal of Clinical and Experimental Hypnosis*, 3, 34–39.

Grimes, S. J. (1845). *Etherology: Or the philosophy of mesmerism and phrenology*. New York: Saxton & Miles.

Haddock, J. (1849). *Psychology: Or the science of the soul*. New York: Fowler & Wells.

Hart, E. (1898). *Hypnotism, mesmerism and the new witchcraft*. New York: Appleton.

Helms, R. (1986). Fiction in the Gospels. In R. J. Hoffman & G. A. Larue (Eds.), *Jesus in myth and history* (pp. 135–142). Buffalo, NY: Prometheus Books.

Helms, R. (1989). *Gospel fictions*. Buffalo, NY: Prometheus Books.

Hilgard, E. R. (1965). *Hypnotic susceptibility*. New York: Harcourt, Brace & World.

Hilgard, E. R. (1977). *Divided consciousness*. New York: Wiley.

Hilgard, E. R. (1979). Divided consciousness in hypnosis: The implications of the hidden observer. In E. Fromm & R. E. Shor (Eds.), *Hypnosis: Developments in research and new perspectives* (2nd ed., pp. 45–79). Chicago: Aldine.

Hockley, M. (1849). On the ancient magic crystal and its connection with mesmerism. *The Zoist*, 7, 251–266.

Hoffman, R. J. (1986). The life of Jesus in research. In R. J. Hoffman & G. A. Larue (Eds.), *Jesus in myth and history* (pp. 89–96). Buffalo, NY: Prometheus Books.

Hull, C. L. (1933). *Hypnosis and suggestibility: An experimental approach*. New York: Appleton-Century-Crofts.

Hull, J. M. (1974). *Hellenistic magic and the synoptic tradition*. London: SCM Press.

Janet, P. (1925). *Psychological healing*. New York: Crowell-Collier & Macmillan.

Kee, H. C. (1968). The terminology of Mark's exorcism stories. *New Testament Studies*, 14, 232–246.

Kee, H. C. (1983). *Miracle in the early Christian world*. New Haven, CT: Yale University Press.

Kee, H. C. (1986). *Medicine, miracle and magic in New Testament times*. New York: Cambridge University Press.

Kelly, H. A. (1974). *The devil, demonology and witchcraft*. Garden City, NY: Doubleday.

Kerenyi, C. (1960). *Asklepios: Archetypical image of the physician's existence* (R. Manheim, Trans.). London: Thames & Hudson. (Original work published 1947)

Kihlstrom, J. F. (1980). Posthypnotic amnesia for recently learned material: Interactions with "episodic" and "semantic" memory. *Cognitive Psychology, 12,* 227–251.

Kitto, H. D. F. (1951). *The Greeks.* Chicago: Aldine.

Koester, H. (1980). *Introduction to the New Testament: History and literature of early Christianity.* New York: Walter De Gruyter.

Kroger, W. S., & Fezler, W. D. (1976). *Hypnosis and behavior modification: Imagery conditioning.* Philadelphia: J. B. Lippincott.

Laurence J.-R. & Perry, C. (1983). Hypnotically created pseudomemories among highly hypnotizable subjects. *Science, 222,* 523–524.

Leach, E., & Aycock, D. A. (1983). *Structuralist interpretations of Biblical myth.* New York: Cambridge University Press.

LeCron, L. M., & Bordeaux, J. (1947). *Hypnotism today.* New York: Grune & Stratton.

Lynn, S. J., Rhue, J. W., & Weekes, J. R. (1989). Hypnosis and experienced nonvolition: A sociocognitive integrative model. In N. P. Spanos & J. F. Chaves (Eds.), *Hypnosis: The cognitive–behavioral perspective* (pp. 78–109). Buffalo, NY: Prometheus Books.

Ludwig, A. M. (1964). A historical survey of the early roots of mesmerism. *International Journal of Clinical and Experimental Hypnosis, 12,* 205–217.

MacHovec, F. J. (1975). Hypnosis before Mesmer. *American Journal of Clinical Hypnosis, 17,* 215–220.

MacHovec, F. J. (1979). The cult of Asklipios. *American Journal of Clinical Hypnosis, 22,* 85–90.

Mahan, A. (1855). *Modern mysteries explained and exposed.* Boston: Jewitt.

Mesmer, F. A. (1980). *Mesmerism* (G. Bloch, Ed. and Trans.). Los Altos, CA: Kaufman. (Original work published 1781)

Miller, M. E., & Bowers, K. W. (1986). Hypnotic analgesia and stress inoculation in the reduction of pain. *Journal of Abnormal Psychology, 95,* 6–14.

Newman, J. B. (1847). *Fascination.* New York: Fowler.

Nisbett, R. E., & Wilson, T. D. (1977). Telling more than we can know: Verbal reports on mental processes. *Psychological Review, 84,* 231–259.

Oesterreich, T. K. (1966). *Possession: Demoniacal and others.* Secaucus, NJ: Citadel.

Orne, M. T. (1959). The nature of hypnosis: Artifact and essence. *Journal of Abnormal and Social Psychology, 58,* 277–299.

Orne, M. T. (1979). On the simulating subject as a quasi-control group in hypnosis research: What, why and how. In E. Fromm & R. E. Shor (Eds.), *Hypnosis: Developments in research and new perspectives* (2nd ed., pp. 519–565). Chicago: Aldine.

Orne, M. T., Sheehan, P. W., & Evans, F. J. (1968). The occurrence of posthypnotic behavior outside the experimental setting. *Journal of Personality and Social Psychology, 26,* 217–221.

Owen, A. R. G. (1971). *Hysteria, hypnosis and healing.* London: Dobson.

Paton, L. B. (1921). *Spiritism and the cult of the dead in antiquity.* New York: Macmillan.

Pattie, F. A. (1956). Mesmer's medical dissertation and its debt to Mead's *De imperio solis ac lunae. Journal of the History of Medicine and Allied Sciences, 11,* 275–287.

Pearson, J. A. (1790). *A plain and rational account of the nature and effects of animal magnetism.* London: W. & J. Stratford.

Podmore, F. (1902). *Modern spiritualism: A history and a criticism.* London: Methuen.

Podmore, F. (1909). *From mesmerism to Christian Science: A short history of mental healing.* London: Methuen.

A Practical Magnetizer. (1843). *The history and philosophy of animal magnetism.* Boston: Bradley.

Pulos, L. (1980). Mesmerism revisited: The effectiveness of Esdaile's technique in the production of deep hypnosis and total body hypnoanaesthesia. *American Journal of Clinical Hypnosis, 22,* 206–211.

Radtke, H. L., & Spanos, N. P. (1981). Was I hypnotized? A social psychological analysis of hypnotic depth reports. *Psychiatry, 44,* 359–376.

Rembar, C. (1980). *The law of the land.* New York: Simon & Schuster.

Rose, L. (1971). *Faith healing.* Harmondsworth, England: Penguin Books.

Rostan, L. (1825). *Magnetisme dictionaire de médecine par MM. Adelon.* Paris.

Russell, J. B. (1972). *Witchcraft in the Middle Ages.* Ithaca, NY: Cornell University Press.

Sarbin, T. R. (1950). Contributions to role-taking theory: I. Hypnotic behavior. *Psychological Review, 57,* 255–270.

Sarbin, T. R. (1962). Attempts to understand hypnotic phenomena. In L. Postman (Ed.), *Psychology in the making* (pp. 745–785). New York: Knopf.

Sarbin, T. R. (1989). The construction and reconstruction of hypnosis. In N. P. Spanos & J. F. Chaves (Eds.), *Hypnosis: The cognitive–behavioral perspective* (pp. 400–416). Buffalo, NY: Prometheus Books.

Sarbin, T. R., & Coe, W. C. (1972). *Hypnosis: A social psychological analysis of influence communication.* New York: Holt, Rinehart & Winston.

Sextus, C. (1968). *Hypnotism.* Hollywood, CA: Wilshire. (Original work published 1893)

Sheehan, P. W., & McConkey, K. (1982). *Hypnosis and experience.* Hillsdale, NJ: Erlbaum.

Sheehan, P. W., & Perry, C. W. (1976). *Methodologies of hypnosis.* Hillsdale, NJ: Erlbaum.

Shor, R. E. (1959). Hypnosis and the concept of the generalized reality orientation. *American Journal of Psychotherapy, 13,* 582–602.

Shor, R. E. (1962). Three dimensions of hypnotic depth. *International Journal of Clinical and Experimental Hypnosis, 10,* 23–28.

Shor, R. E., Orne, M. T., & O'Connell, D. N. (1962). Validation and cross-validation of a scale of self-reported personal experiences which predict hypnotizability. *Journal of Psychology, 53,* 55–75.

Slater, E. (1965). Diagnosis of "hysteria." *British Medical Journal, 29,* 1395–1399.

Smith, M. (1978). *Jesus the magician.* New York: Harper & Row.

Smith, M. (1986). The historical Jesus. In R. J. Hoffman & G. A. Larue (Eds.), *Jesus in myth and history* (pp. 47–54). Buffalo, NY: Prometheus Books.

Smith-Rosenberg, C. (1972). The hysterical woman: Some reflections on sex roles and role conflict in 19th century America. *Social Research, 39,* 652–678.

Spanos, N. P. (1978). Witchcraft in histories of psychiatry: A critique and an alternate conceptualization. *Psychological Bulletin, 85,* 419–439.

Spanos, N. P. (1983). Demonic possession: A social psychological analysis. In M. Rosenbaum (Ed.), *Compliance behavior* (pp. 149–189). New York: Free Press.

Spanos, N. P. (1986). Hypnotic behavior: A social psychological interpretation of amnesia, analgesia and trance logic. *Behavioral and Brain Sciences, 9*, 449–467.

Spanos, N. P. (1989a). Experimental research on hypnotic analgesia. In N. P. Spanos & J. F. Chaves (Eds.), *Hypnosis: The cognitive–behavioral perspective* (pp. 206–241). Buffalo, NY: Prometheus Books.

Spanos, N. P. (1989b). Hypnosis, demon possession and multiple personality: Strategic enactments and disavowals of responsibility for actions. In C. A. Ward (Ed.), *Altered states of consciousness and mental health: A cross cultural perspective* (pp. 96–124). Newbury Park, CA: Sage.

Spanos, N. P., & Barber, T. X. (1974). Toward a convergence in hypnosis research. *American Psychologist, 29*, 500–511.

Spanos, N. P., & Chaves, J. F. (Eds.). (1989). *Hypnosis: The cognitive–behavioral perspective.* Buffalo, NY: Prometheus Books.

Spanos, N. P., & Gottlieb, J. (1979). Demonic possession, mesmerism and hysteria: A social psychological perspective on their historical interrelations. *Journal of Abnormal Psychology, 88*, 527–546.

Spanos, N. P., & Katsanis, J. (1989). Effects of instructional set on attributions of nonvolition during hypnotic and nonhypnotic analgesia. *Journal of Personality and Social Psychology, 56*, 182–188.

Spanos, N. P., Radtke, H. L., & Dubreuil, D. L. (1982). Episodic and semantic memory in posthypnotic amnesia: A reevaluation. *Journal of Personality and Social Psychology, 43*, 565–573.

Spanos, N. P., Salas, J., Bertrand, L. D., & Johnston, J. (1989). Occurrence schemas, context ambiguity and hypnotic responding. *Imagination, Cognition and Personality, 8*, 235–247.

Stam, H. J., & Spanos, N. P. (1982). The Asclepian dream healings and hypnosis: A critique. *International Journal of Clinical and Experimental Hypnosis, 30*, 9–22.

Stava, L. J., & Jaffa, M. (1988). Some operationalizations of the neodissociation concept and their relationship to hypnotic susceptibility. *Journal of Personality and Social Psychology, 54*, 898–996.

Stocking, G. W. (1965). On the limits of "presentism" and "historicism" in the historiography of the behavioral sciences. *Journal of the History of the Behavioral Sciences, 1*, 211–218.

Sutcliffe, J. P. (1960). "Credulous" and "skeptical" views of hypnotic phenomena: A review of certain evidence and methodology. *International Journal of Clinical and Experimental Hypnosis, 8*, 73–101.

Sutcliffe, J. P. (1961). "Credulous" and "skeptical" views of hypnotic phenomena: Experiments on esthesia, hallucination and delusion. *Journal of Abnormal and Social Psychology, 62*, 189–200.

Szasz, T. (1961). *The myth of mental illness.* New York: Hoeber-Harper.

Tellegen, A., & Atkinson, G. A. (1974). Openness to absorbing and self-altering experiences ("absorption"), a trait related to hypnotic susceptibility. *Journal of Abnormal Psychology, 83*, 268–277.

Veith, I. (1965). *Hysteria.* Chicago: University of Chicago Press.

Wagstaff, G. F. (1981). *Hypnosis, compliance and belief.* New York: St. Martin's Press.

Wells, G. A. (1975). *Did Jesus exist?* London: Pemberton.

Wells, G. A. (1982). *The historical evidence for Jesus.* Buffalo, NY: Prometheus Books.

Wells, G. A. (1986). The historicity of Jesus. In R. J. Hoffman & G. A. Larue (Eds.), *Jesus in myth and history* (pp. 27–46). Buffalo, NY: Prometheus Books.

White, R. W. (1941). A preface to a theory of hypnotism. *Journal of Abnormal and Social Psychology, 36,* 477–505.

White, R. W., & Shevach, B. J. (1942). Hypnosis and the concept of dissociation. *Journal of Abnormal and Social Psychology, 37,* 309–328.

Williams, G. W. (1954). Hypnosis in perspective. In L. M. LeCron (Ed.), *Experimental hypnosis* (pp. 4–21). New York: Macmillan.

Wilson, T. D. (1985). Self-deception without repression: Limits on access to mental states. In M. W. Martin (Ed.), *Self-deception and self-understanding* (pp. 95–116). Lawrence: University of Kansas Press.

Wood, A. D. (1974). "The fashionable diseases": Women's complaints and their treatment in 19th century America. In M. Hartman & L. W. Banner (Eds.), *Clio's consciousness raised* (pp. 1–22). New York: Harper & Row.

Wundt, W. M. (1892). *Hypnotismus und suggestion.* Leipzig: Engelman.

Zamansky, H. S., & Bartis, S. P. (1985). The dissociation of an experience: The hidden observer observed. *Journal of Abnormal Psychology, 94,* 243–248.

PART TWO

SINGLE FACTOR
THEORIES

THE NEODISSOCIATION
PERSPECTIVE

C H A P T E R   3

A Neodissociation Interpretation of Hypnosis

ERNEST R. HILGARD
Stanford University

INTRODUCTION

Neodissociation theory may be considered a contemporary endeavor to deal with the kinds of problems that gave rise to classical theories of dissociation in the later 19th century and the early 20th century by theorists such as Pierre Janet in France and Morton Prince in the United States. The plausible aspects of dissociation became neglected in the early half of this century, in part because Freud's theory of repression to the unconscious appeared to cover much of the same ground (E. R. Hilgard, 1973a). However, in the latter half of the century new interest in dissociation has asserted itself, partly through a revived interest in multiple personalities and related phenomena. An International Society for the Study of Multiple Personality and Dissociation was established, and it sponsored a new journal called *Dissociation*, the first issue of which appeared in March 1988. The new interest also led to an extensive treatment of dissociative disorders in the revised third edition of the Diagnostic and Statistical Manual for Mental Disorders (DSM-III-R; American Psychiatric Association, 1987).

Neodissociation Theory Briefly Characterized

Classical dissociation theory, as well as the dissociations presented in DSM-III-R, tied the dissociations to psychopathological conditions. The neodissociation theory presented here arose through hypnotic experimentation, chiefly on university students who were not patients but "subjects" in the kinds of experiments with unselected students familiar in experimental psychology; thus it is not limited to those who show symptoms of pathological dissociations. The use of the term "neodissociation theory" has been selected to indicate that although the historical background is pathological dissociation, the modern theory does not rest on the same assumptions as the older theory and is in that sense new, or "neo" (E. R. Hilgard, 1986).

The phenomena that gave rise to dissociation theory in the first place included hysterical symptoms of functional paralyses and anesthesias (now referred to as "conversion symptoms"), but more particularly somnambulisms, amnesias, fugues, and multiple personalities. These states, although not always encountered frequently, occur spontaneously as natural experiments, and they are instructive as to manifestations of human personality and consciousness. The revived interest in these states is interesting, but does not require that the theoretical treatment of dissociation should follow the old lines. Were the older theories to be taken literally and revived in their original form (e.g., as proposed by Janet), it would imply belief that these and related states are found only among hysterical personalities, and one would find it necessary to support many observations of doubtful value. Using the concept of "neodissociation" makes it possible to take a fresh start, with no obligation to remain loyal to the views of those who founded the classical dissociation doctrines.

The nature of the hypnotic phenomena leading to the dissociation theory is discussed in greater detail later, but at this point it may suffice to say that if dissociation is conceived broadly to imply an interference with or a loss of familiar associative processes, most phenomena of hypnosis can be conceived as dissociative. One or two illustrations should make this clear. Consider, for example, the shifts in control of motor functions so familiar in hypnotic demonstrations: the suggested inability to bend a stiff arm, with the stiffness itself produced by hypnotic suggestion; or the loss of ability to say one's own name when such loss of normal control of the speech apparatus is suggested. These are illustrative of the loss of voluntary control under hypnosis.

A second illustration is posthypnotic amnesia. The typical demonstration is that after the hypnotized person has responded to a series of suggested acts or experiences while hypnotized, and told that he or she will forget what was done during hypnosis after hypnosis is terminated (until the memory is restored by an implanted signal), the experience is commonly that a few (or occasionally all) of the happenings within hypnosis will be forgotten until the release signal is given, when much of the forgotten material is restored. This qualifies as dissociation, if the loss and recovery of memories are evident. It then shows that the material has been "stored" in memory, but is not subject to the usual associative recall because of something that happened during hypnosis to interfere with the recovery of the memory before the amnesia was reversed.

In addition to the dissociations found in the familiar demonstrations of the responses of the hypnotized person, a further set of evidence that provides support to the neodissociation theory is derived from research on what I have characterized as a "hidden observer," detected through the use of automatic writing and related methods. These studies have shown, in subjects highly responsive to hypnosis, that when pain or hearing have been reduced by hypnotic procedures, the hypnotically analgesic or deaf persons are at some level aware of the intensity of the pain or the loudness of the tone that was not experienced at the time. Evidence of this kind is generalized into a theory of alternative cognitive control structures in hierarchical arrangement under some measure of control by an "executive ego." It is the elucidation of this neodissociation theory to which the bulk of this chapter is devoted.

The Background of Functional Psychology

When a psychological theory is proposed, it is desirable to know something of the orientation of the author of the theory. Although I grew up in an era of behaviorism, I have never called myself a behaviorist. Instead I have taken the somewhat eclectic position, common among American experimental psychologists, known as "functionalism." This tradition began with William James, and was then developed at the University of Chicago by Dewey, Angell, and Carr, and at Columbia by Cattell, Woodworth, and Thorndike; however, it has been adopted as an orientation by many others, so that Boring (1950) could write, "Functional psychology *is* American psychology" (p. 559).

In writing about functionalism in relation to learning theory, I have stated what I liked about the functionalist position as follows (these points are summarized from E. R. Hilgard, 1956, pp. 333–336):

1. Functionalists are tolerant but critical. This means that functionalists are free from self-imposed constraints that sometimes shackle other systematists. They can use psychological concepts such as "behavior," "consciousness," "unconscious processes," "states of awareness," and "physiological substrata" without taboos against them if they appear relevant. At the same time, functionalists seek to be as clear as circumstances allow.

2. Functionalists prefer continuities over discontinuities or typologies. This sometimes leads to a dimensional analysis, because there are changes along a continuum, rather than sharp breaks.

3. Functionalists are experimentalists, so that they like to drive issues back to specifics in order to settle controversies through experimental demonstration.

These statements reflect my general orientation.

Basic Assumptions about Hypnosis

What I have said about my functionalist orientation I now apply to my assumptions about hypnosis.

The Domain of Hypnosis Can be Delineated

It would appear to be unwise to devise a theory about phenomena that are not well enough recognized to fit into a common category with some recognizable boundaries to exclude phenomena that do not fit. Hence, a theory should be clear about what it is a theory of. Because a universally accepted definition of what constitutes hypnosis is elusive, I prefer to begin by specifying what I have called "the domain of hypnosis"—that is, a characterization of what sorts of phenomena are included and what lie outside it (E. R. Hilgard, 1973c). That also is not an easy task, and arguments about what to include and what to exclude continue to this day.

I first met the issue clearly when André Weitzenhoffer and I undertook to construct the Stanford Hypnotic Susceptibility Scales. A summary of the Stanford scales, up to that date, can be found in E. R. Hilgard (1965). Such scales are constructed according to the methods of other empirically derived and standardized psychological tests. In hypnosis there are enough familiar behaviors and experiences in demonstrations of hypnosis, or in its use by practicing hypnotists, that finding appropriate topics is generally not too difficult. Included are such phenomena as muscular movements or inhibitions, sensory distortions, positive and negative hallucinations, posthypnotic amnesia, and dreams within hypnosis. We had the advantage of an earlier scale devised by Friedlander and Sarbin (1938), with which Dr. Weitzenhoffer had had considerable experience while working on his doctoral dissertation at the University of Michigan.

Apart from familiarity with the substance of the test items in other demonstrations of hypnosis, how did we know that our new items fell within the domain of hypnosis? Because of the "face validity" of most items, the test of internal consistency was satisfactory when applied to the new items. If an item correlated with the whole (with that item omitted), it was identified as belonging to the common domain. This criterion— that scores on an item can be considered representative of hypnosis only if these scores correlate with the scores of a number of other items known to represent hypnosis—is easy to understand and is coherent with what we have long known about hypnosis.

This is not, of course, the only way to proceed to define the domain of hypnosis. For example, Weitzenhoffer (1980) argued that the scales do not measure the classical conception of hypnosis, which is *an increase in suggestibility* following hypnotic induction. I replied to his arguments by pointing out the many problems that would arise in constructing scales based on the changes in scores from tests in waking suggestion to tests following attempted hypnotic induction (E. R. Hilgard, 1981).

The Problems Created by Resistance and Simulation

A clever actor (and even a not-so-clever one) can resist hypnosis and then score too low on a hypnotic scale, or can act like a hypnotized person and then score too high. It is easy to jump to the conclusion that these difficulties must be a major obstacle to the experimenter on hypnosis. These possibilities have to be recognized, noted, and guarded against, but experience with thousands of students tested in the Stanford Laboratory of Hypnosis Research indicates that the problem is not nearly as severe as it conceivably might be. There are various checks on this, which are somewhat difficult to state simply. On the matter of resistance, the genuine disappointment often shown by the low scorer is partial evidence that any "resistance" is not deliberate. Repeated tests with a variety of scales may, in fact, show the kind of improvement expected of a hypnotizable subject who was originally resistant. The subject himself or herself may report that in the first session he or she "held back" in order to see what it was like, and, when convinced that there was nothing threatening about it, cooperated fully in the next session.

Simulation is somewhat harder to deal with, although there is a tendency for simulators to overreact by giving maximum conventional hypnotic responses to all of the demands. By so doing, they may give themselves away. The use of instructed simulators, according to a procedure devised by Orne (1971), helps in this respect. In this procedure, a confederate of the experimenting hypnotist assigns two groups of subjects, the "reals" and the instructed "simulators." These are selected from a larger sample of subjects whose hypnotic responsiveness is known from prior hypnotic testing, but the subjects are unknown individually to the hypnotist. Each subject, although assigned to one of the two groups, is tested individually in a randomized order. The reals are all highly responsive, and the simulators all score low on the scales. The confederate instructs the reals to participate in the usual way in hypnosis: "Let things happen" rather than "Make things happen," and "Do nothing to deceive the hypnotist." The other half are told to act "as if" they are hypnotizable, doing what the hypnotist appears to be expecting. "This is part of the experiment, and there should be no guilt about deceiving the hypnotist."

Following the completion of the experiment, the confederate, who instructed the simulators as well as the reals, conducts a careful interrogation, insisting on absolute honesty. If some of the reals were deliberately "helping out," the confederate wants to know; so, too, if some of the simulators felt that they actually became responsive to hypnosis, he or she wants to know that. As mentioned above, when the data are all in, it is common to find that on many items the simulators report responses at a higher level than do the reals, but in their "honesty" reports the reals report a genuine hypnotic experience, and the simulators almost never do.

The design does not call into question the "proper" demand characteristics in the hypnotic setting ("proper," because any explicit suggestion has within it a specified demand). Clearly, the hypnotist, in suggesting "Now your arm is getting stiff," implies that if a subject is hypnotizable his or her arm will get stiff. This is inherent in the nature of hypnotic suggestion, but there are often subtle suggestions that contain implicit demands rather than explicit ones, and it is for them that the real–simulator arrangement is planned.

It should perhaps be noted that the issues of resistance and of simulation are not limited to scores on hypnosis scales, but may be found in other test situations as well. Some of the draftees who did not wish to go to officer candidate school in World War II deliberately made lower scores on the Army tests. On the Strong Vocational Interest Blank, it is possible for a person to "fake good" by answering as he or she believes a doctor would or a lawyer would, instead of honestly reporting his or her own interests. This does not happen when the test is used for guidance purposes, because then the person is trying to find out how he or she compares with others. Perhaps if a test were used for selection purposes, the temptation to deception would be greater.

The Problem of Experimenter Bias

The problem of experimenter bias is a serious one in hypnosis experimenta- tion, as it is in many other forms of psychological experimentation. This was brought to the fore some years ago when "task motivation" was offered as a substitute for hypnotic induction, particularly by T. X. Barber and his associates (e.g., Barber & Calverley, 1962). The "task motivation" instructions were actually deceptive in implying that everyone could have visual hallucinations (and other hypnotic experiences) if they wished to, and the pressure for acquiescence was very great, as the following quotations from the instructions indicate:

> Everyone passed these tests when they tried. . . . Yet when these people [who felt that imagining a movie so vividly that they felt as if they were actually looking at the picture was awkward or silly] later realized that it wasn't hard to imagine, they were able to visualize the movie and they felt the imagined movie was as vivid and real as an actual movie . . . if you try to imagine to the best of your ability, you can easily imagine and do the interesting things that I tell you and you will be helping this experiment and not wasting any time. (Barber & Calverley, 1962, p. 366)

Of five antecedent conditions that might have achieved hypnosis without induction, this was the only one that approached the success following a usual induction.

Although the pressure for conformity was evidently strong, Bowers (1967) subsequently made a convincing test through the use of honesty instructions following the hypnotic performances of those given such "task motivation" instructions. He showed that results such as those reported by Barber and Calverley could be obtained by using their "task motivation" instructions, but when the successful subjects were questioned after the experiment by someone other than the hypnotist, with the instruction to be altogether honest, they readily reported that the experiences were not as real as they reported them to be under the conformity pressure.

There are other types of task motivation instructions that do not include any deceptive phrases, such as "Everyone can do it" or "By responding like others, you will be helping the experiment." In addition, there are "exhortation" instructions and "involving" instructions— motivating suggestions that supplement rather than displace hypnotic induction, with control subjects used to determine what occurs without induction. Results from such experiments have been reported in E. R. Hilgard (1965, pp. 114–118) and are not to be confused with the "task motivation" experiments described above. The issue, from a functionalist standpoint, is what combination of circumstances will produce the highest asymptote, if the criterion is something as objective as the ability to enhance motor performance. No experimenter bias need enter.

This completes the introductory remarks that give a preliminary sketch of the neodissociation standpoint, and the basic orientation toward hypnotic experimentation.

THEORETICAL CONCEPTS AND PRINCIPLES

With this much background, the neodissociation theory itself can take central stage, on the assumption that the basics of hypnotic interaction as

I perceive them provide a data base to serve as a test of theoretical propositions.

I have already stated in general terms how the point of view of neodissociation is differentiated from classical dissociation, and how much of it depends upon an interpretation of familiar hypnotic phenomena, such as alteration of controls over motor functions and postyhypnotic amnesia. The second consideration, briefly introduced, is the kind of response within hypnosis that I have described as a "hidden observer," but this needs much further elucidation in order for readers to understand its central role in the development of the neodissociation theory. However, it is worth noting that my interest in dissociation in relation to hypnosis antedated any hint about the hidden observer. My own interest in dissociated experiences began with my reading of William James and William McDougall as a graduate student, but it was only after I began experimenting with hypnosis that I took dissociation more seriously.

The Developmental–Interactive Standpoint

Our first attempts at theorizing were attempts to account for individual differences in hypnotic responsiveness. We offered the framework for such a theory, called a "developmental–interactive theory" (J. R. Hilgard & Hilgard, 1962: E. R. Hilgard, 1965). The emphasis was on how individual differences could come about. The "developmental" part of the proposed theory was that whatever innate propensities there were would be modified by early social interactions with parents and other persons, thus affecting the hypnotic responsiveness at a later time. The "interactive" portion of the theory proposed that the propensities for hypnosis, acquired in the interaction between nature and nurture, still had to be capitalized upon through appropriate current interventions if the hypnotic potential were to be realized. A third category of propositions was then called "hypnotic state propositions," intended to deal with some of the phenomenology of the hypnotic condition.

Developmental Aspects

The developmental portion of the theory was soon buttressed by an interview program undertaken by Josephine Hilgard, in which students to become subjects in tests of hypnotic performance and experience were interviewed before and after experiencing hypnosis, partly in the search for childhood antecedents associated with measured susceptibility (e.g., J. R. Hilgard, 1965, 1979). She later, in collaboration with Samuel LeBaron, studied further aspects of the development of hypnotic ability in childhood through such protohypnotic experiences as pretend play. This theorizing was a significant by-product of an investigation of hypnotherapy of children with cancer (J. R. Hilgard & LeBaron, 1984). These supplements to the early developmental–interactive theory have not been formalized, but provide the kinds of raw material not available when the theory was first outlined.

The developmental discussion allowed for the possibility that there might be some native characteristics bearing upon later hypnotizability, but the evidence did not become available until Arlene Morgan published her dissertation (done in our laboratory) on the possible heritability of hypnotizability, based on a study of twins and their families (Morgan, 1973). All members of twin pairs were tested individually and separately, each of a set of twins at the same time but in separate rooms, so that there could be no communication between them about the hypnotizabilty scales. She found that hypnotizability might have a hereditary component because of the higher correlations found between identical twins than between fraternal twins. There are always some qualifications to be made in such studies, many of which have been done with intelligence tests. However, a distinguished geneticist who advised Morgan on the study said she could safely conclude that there was a high likelihood of genetic contribution to the similarities and differences found between the members of different kinds of twin pairs. Hence, the nature–nurture problem persists here as in other studies employing twins; the suggestion is that the changes as a consequence of home environment and special circumstances during development may be changes from a hereditary baseline.

Interactive Aspects

The interactive aspects were intended to deal with the here-and-now changes taking place in a successful induction of hypnosis, explicit or implicit, whether the agent be a hypnotist or the person's own self. Much of the experimentation on hypnosis to be discussed has to do with what happens in the present.

Two statements about dissociation were made in the early account of the developmental–interactive theory. The first statement asserted that the specific dissociations developed in hypnosis might be correlated with developmental experiences, and illustrations of possibilities followed (E. R. Hilgard, 1965, pp. 388–390). The second statement asserted that hypnosis is characterized by *partial* dissociations, to avoid a rejection of the concept of dissociation if complete functional independence of the dissociated material from other aspects of consciousness is not found.

Hypnosis as State, Trait, or Neither

There are conceptual problems in defining hypnosis as an altered state, and these have been a source of controversy. From the point of view both of the subject experiencing hypnosis and of the experimenter (or any other unbiased observer), the indications are of alterations that at a phenomenal level are most readily described as changes in the total condition or state, just as drunkenness and sleep are described as altered states, subject to differences in the profundity of the change at any given time.

There is no reason for a taboo against the word "state." I prefer to speak of the "hypnotic condition," however, rather than to enter the controversy over "state" or "trance," partly because I accept the gradualism of the neodissociation position. It allows for partial dissociations, so that the "hypnotic condition" or "state" is not an all-or-nothing change from the normal waking condition.

The issue of whether to consider hypnotizability as a "trait" (i.e., a more or less enduring ability or skill) is also controversial, partly because of the critique of personality traits in general by social psychologists, but also because of the controversy over the extent to which individual differences in measured hypnotizability can be modified.

My own belief in hypnotic ability as a relatively stable trait is supported by our 25-year follow-up of the same subjects tested first in college, then 10 years later, and again 15 years beyond that or 25 years after the initial testing (Piccione, Hilgard, & Zimbardo, 1989). The stability coefficients, expressed as significant coefficients of correlation between scores on the Stanford Hypnotic Susceptibility Scales, Forms A or B, were .64 for the 10-year retest, .82 for the subsequent 15-year retest, and .71 for the total 25-year retest. The means were highly stable also. This relative stability over time compares favorably with other measures of enduring individual differences. These results were obtained without efforts to modify hypnotizability, but were found despite the great changes in personal and socioeconomic circumstances over these many years since college. Most efforts to modify hypnotizability have shown slight changes, often statistically significant but of little consequence for changing nonhypnotizable subjects into highly hypnotizables ones.

A more recent study has challenged these findings by reporting massive changes through training in "sociocognitive skills" (Gorassini & Spanos, 1986). The findings are somewhat debatable, however, because the training methods blurred the distinction between "letting things happen" and "making things happen" by using assurances that "everybody can succeed by trying"—reminiscent of the earlier "task motivation" instructions. The final position on the degree of modifiability of hypnotizability will be determined by additional empirical studies.

The "Hidden Observer" Phenomenon

Despite my friendliness to the dissociation concept, I did little with it until the early 1970s, when some experiments on automatic writing were

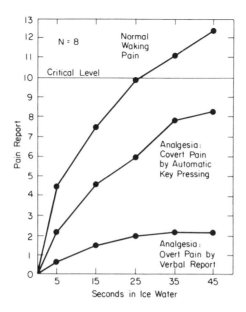

FIGURE 3.1. Normal waking pain, overt pain, and covert pain in hypnotic analgesia. Results for the 8 most successful subjects of 20 subjects selected for high hypnotizability. The data were originally from E. R. Hilgard, Morgan, and Macdonald (1975). From *Hypnosis in the Relief of Pain* (rev. ed., p. 172) by E. R. Hilgard & J. R. Hilgard, 1983, Los Altos, CA: William Kaufmann. Copyright 1983 by William Kaufman, Inc. Reprinted by permission.

undertaken in the laboratory, and the so-called "hidden-observer" phenomena began to be explored. By using techniques such as automatic writing in the context of hypnosis, or its equivalent technique that we have by analogy called "automatic talking," we have been able to demonstrate that a highly responsive hypnotic subject may report considerable pain (or memory for it) from information previously at a covert level—that is, from pain that the subject had not consciously felt or reported (E. R. Hilgard, Morgan, & Macdonald, 1975). We have designated such reports as coming from a "hidden observer." An illustration of these findings is given in Figure 3.1.

When hypnotic analgesias had been suggested prior to the insertion of the hand and forearm into circulating ice water, these highly responsive subjects reported no pain or very little pain at the overt level: They gave an average report of pain as a level of 2, on a scale in which 10 was defined as a critical level at which they would very much wish to remove the hand from the water. However, they simultaneously reported by automatic key pressing (an equivalent to automatic writing) that the revealed pain was rising to a mean of 8 on the same scale that yielded a mean of 2 as overtly reported. This was slightly below the mean of normal waking pain they reported without analgesic suggestions. Perhaps the lesser reported pain was in part due to the general relaxation of hypnosis, as well as the lack of feedback from the grimacing, squirming, and other signs usually associated with felt pain in this setting. Why some highly responsive subjects, capable of reducing pain under hypnosis, do not yield the hidden-observer reports remains to be explained. For those who do report differences of the type shown in Figure 3.1, it is appropriate to consider the two different reports as evidence of a split in consciousness between the overt (conscious) level and the covert (subconscious) level, and hence as evidence of dissociative processes.

Although this kind of dissociation is dramatic in experiments on pain, it is by no means limited to pain. It has been known informally for a long time that some cognitive system within the hypnotized person processes information beyond that available to that person while hypnotized and under the influence of suggestions that counter the awareness of that information. William James devoted several pages in his *Principles of Psychology* to an account of gaps in consciousness, with evidence that the mind is active even when the person ignores the fact (James, 1890, Vol. 1, pp. 201–213). James recorded his own experiment:

> In a perfectly healthy young man who can write with a planchette, [a device like the pointer on a Ouija board] I lately found the hand to be entirely anesthetic during the writing act. I could prick it severely without the subject knowing the fact. The writing on the planchette, however, accused me in strong terms of hurting the hand. (James, 1890, Vol. 1, p. 208)

We have been able to demonstrate in our own laboratory that hypnotic blindness, hypnotic deafness, and positive hallucinations can all be penetrated by automatic responses. That is, at the level of the concealed cognitive processing (the "hidden observer") the subjects who had distorted normal reality in the context of hypnosis were able to report the actual physical situation: numbers not seen, sentences not heard, and "nothing" (which was perceived as a playful dog).

Assumptions in the Elaboration of the Neodissociation Theory

Three assumptions have been proposed in taking the next steps toward a neodissociation theory that goes beyond the mere fact that dissociations occur. The first assumption is that that there are subordinate cognitive systems, each of which has some degree of unity, persistence, and autonomy of function. These systems are interactive, but occasionally, under special circumstances, may become somewhat isolated from each other. The concept of the unity of the total consciousness is an attractive one, but it does not hold up under examination. There are too many shifts in the ordinary course of the day, such as those between waking and night dreaming, or as the lapses of consciousness in the control of well-learned habits (e.g., driving a car, playing a musical instrument, or reciting the alphabet). Such activities, having been overlearned in the past, can proceed with a minimum of conscious control once the activity is underway.

The second assumption is that there is some sort of hierarchical control that manages the interaction or competition between and among these structures. If there were no process of selective dominance, there would be a veritable deluge of thoughts and actions trying to go on at once.

A third assumption is that there must be some sort of monitoring and controlling structure. The alternative, without this assumption, is that the hierarchy is determined by some sort of relative strength (as in the pecking orders of barnyard fowl); however, I have rejected this as inappropriate from what we know about human decision making and planned action toward distant goals.

The Evolved Theory in Greater Detail

On the basis of the assumptions just mentioned, the evolved theory can be given in diagrammatic form (Figure 3.2). This highly generalized diagram is designed to convey the idea of multiple cognitive processing systems or structures (of which only three of the many possible ones are shown). They are arranged in hierarchical order as suggested by their positions on the chart, but each is equally independent with its own appropriate inputs and outputs, and with multiple feedback relations between them. At the top is an "executive ego" or "central control structure," which has the planning, monitoring, and managing functions that are required for appropriate thoughts and actions involving the whole person.

We may now turn to a fuller characterization of the individual cognitive structures, their hierarchical arrangement, and the role of the central control structure or executive ego.

Separate Cognitive Structures

The expression "cognitive structure" was an older term revived by Tolman (1932) and taken over by Lewin (1935), who acknowledged his debt to Tolman. A related concept, called "schema," was used by Bartlett (1932). Meichenbaum and Gilmore (1984), in their discussion of cognitive structures, found at least nine different terms used to express the same idea.

From a different starting point, Chomsky (1957) implied that there exist innate cognitive structures in the brain that permit the child to learn language. Hence there is nothing alien to familiar theories when I include cognitive structures in neodissociation theory.

The Concept of Hierarchy

The concept of hierarchy has been added to indicate that one structure can be dominant at a given time, to be succeeded by the activation of another when the first recedes. Consider the bilingual person who has decided to speak in one of his or her familiar languages, perhaps in reply to a question phrased in that language. Then the appropriate vocabulary and grammatical forms of that language become dominant and the other language is inhibited, although still available in latent form.

One of Clark Hull's central concepts was a habit-family hierarchy, including a number of habits (each of which may be thought of as a small substructure). As the organism seeks to achieve its goals in a given situation, if the habit highest in the hierarchy cannot function, the one next below in the hierarchy is activated (Hull, 1934).

The Executive Ego

The nature of the executive ego as a central control structure is an important but troublesome problem. The extreme possibilities are that there is a powerful central control, equivalent to the old idea of a strong will, or that there is really none at all. If there is none, the hierarchy is determined by a competition among the parts for the control of a final common path. The one that is strongest at any given moment will win over those that are weaker. For many years psychologists evaded the problem of a planning self, so that, in essence, the second of these alternatives was implicitly accepted. To the extent that the person is controlled by past conditionings and present stimuli, what the person does will be a compromise that adapts to the total forces operating.

The importance of planning was brought to attention in a book titled *Plans and the Structure of Behavior* (Miller, Galanter, & Pribram, 1960). If one examines the concept of planning, it appears that a planner must be inferred. Even such a simple matter as making an appointment for a luncheon next week is written down or otherwise remembered and acted upon at a later date. The person as planner controls the behavior for fulfilling the plan quite effectively, by rejecting other invitations and setting aside competing interests in order to give priority to the plan adopted during the prior week. Appointments of this kind are kept with a high probability—perhaps over 90% of the time—so that the planning function must be taken seriously. It appears to control the hierarchical

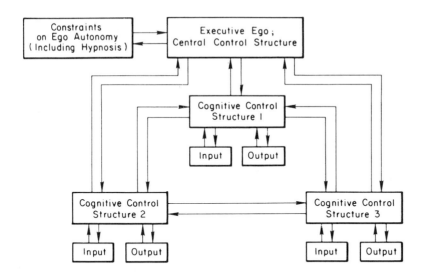

FIGURE 3.2. Subordinate cognitive control structures in a hierarchical order. Hierarchical positions are subject to change under control of the executive ego. From "Neodissociation Interpretation of Pain Reduction in Hypnosis" (p. 405) by E. R. Hilgard, 1973, *Psychological Review*, 80, 396–411. Reprinted by permission of American Psychological Association.

determinants of specific behavior far in advance. The illustration is trivial, but the implications for central control are not.

Support for an executive function has come from an unlikely source: the computer. Heuristic computer programs commonly have an executive program that monitors the computer's attempt to solve problems (e.g., Newell & Simon, 1972). If the program sets out in one direction and goes on too long without reaching a solution, the executive calls a halt, and a new direction of attack on the problem is entered upon. This close analogy to what a thinker does makes the idea of an executive ego a plausible one.

The Role of Hypnosis

Neodissociation theory is intended to be more general than a theory of hypnosis, but its origin has been within hypnosis experimentation, and its relevance can be demonstrated by calling attention to both the prominence of dissociations within hypnosis and the control that hypnosis exerts over cognitive control systems.

The major bearing upon hypnosis of the hierarchical structure shown in Figure 3.2 rests in the cell labeled "constraints on Ego Autonomy."

Hypnosis enters because effective suggestions from the hypnotist take much of the normal control away from the subject. That is, the hypnotist may influence the executive functions themselves and change the hierarchical arrangements of the substructures. This is what takes place when, in the hypnotic context, motor controls are altered, perception and memory are distorted, and hallucinations may be perceived as external reality.

A fuller exposition of the interrelationships shown in a general way in Figure 3.2 would provide the essence of the neodissociation theory. I regret to leave the theory in this incomplete form, so that it is more of a promise than a finished theory. The line of experimental investigation that it has supported may, in the hands of others, provide more elegant versions of the kind of theory intended.

RESEARCH AND APPRAISAL

The neodissociation theory arose primarily out of findings in our experiments. Hence the appraisal of the theory by others has depended to a large extent on how persuasive they found the experimental evidence.

Divided Control Processes in Automatic Writing

A dissertation by James Stevenson on automatic writing marked the beginning of special studies of dissociation in our laboratory, beyond the dissociations found in usual hypnotic behavior and experience. Although the dissertation was completed in 1972, the published version came out after some other reports had appeared (Stevenson, 1976).

In brief, using a variety of control conditions (including Orne's real–simulator design) Stevenson studied the interference between two tasks. One was performed consciously; the other, as a consequence of hypnotic suggestion, was performed subconsciously—that is, without awareness. The subjects were necessarily previously tested to demonstrate that they were highly responsive to hypnosis. One of the tasks was color naming of colored patches mounted in rows on a gray background. The task could be varied so that the colors could be presented in varied order. The same patches were always used, so that color discrimination was not a difficulty. The alternative task was either of two arithmetic tasks, of two levels of difficulty. The easier task required the subject to write the numbers from 1 to 10 in repeated cycles. The more difficult arithmetic task was serial addition—that is, starting with a two-digit seed number to add 7 to it successively.

In a later experiment along the same lines (although it appeared earlier), we (Knox, Crutchfield, & Hilgard, 1975), used color naming competing with rhythmic pressing of two keys in a cycle: three times for the left key, followed by three times for the right key. In both of these experiments, although the subjects were successful in dissociating the "subconscious" task, the individual differences were striking.

In the Stevenson experiment, the amount of interference was much greater with the more difficult arithmetic task. In both experiments, the actual performances of the subjects deteriorated under the subconscious condition, as though maintaining the dissociation was using cognitive effort. Curiously, the simulators were more successful than the reals, possibly because the demand on their cognitive processing did not carry the burden of keeping the task out of awareness.

A related experiment from another laboratory was more successful in yielding the normally expected results. Bowers and Brenneman (1981) used shadowing of a verbal message to one ear (repeating it word for word while listening to it), along with an occasional signal to the other ear, to which the subjects were to respond by touching their noses. They found less interference with nose touching when the nose touching was subconscious, but there was still some interference. It is quite possible that nose touching is a much easier task to perform out of awareness than the more structured tasks used in the other experiments, and the result follows from Stevenson's finding that the less difficult the subconscious task, the less interference. However, all three of the experiments confirmed the general finding that a task can be dissociated and still interfere with concurrent tasks.

The results of these experiments were not dramatic enough to arouse controversy.

Reactions to the Hidden Observer in Hypnotic Analgesia

The early experimental evidence on the hidden observer was based primarily on experiments with the reduction of pain in hypnosis in experiments using the so-called "cold-pressor" test, in which the pain is produced by inserting the hand and forearm in circulating ice water (e.g., E. R. Hilgard, 1973b, 1974; E. R. Hilgard et al., 1975). Later experiments, using the real–simulator design, validated the earlier findings (E. R. Hilgard, Hilgard, Macdonald, Morgan, & Johnson, 1978).

Additional experiments were done with pain obtained by a tourniquet to the upper arm, followed by exercise of the occluded arm. Careful earlier experiments by Smith, Egbert, Markowitz, Mosteller, and Beecher (1966) had shown that this was the preferred method for simulating surgical pain in the laboratory, validated by the fact that it showed a dose sensitivity reaction to morphine. The major publication was that by Knox, Morgan, and Hilgard (1974). The results were essentially those found with the cold-pressor response, in that the hidden-observer responses following hypnotic analgesia closely paralleled the responses when the pain was felt in the nonhypnotic condition.

Unlike the experiments on automatic writing, these somewhat more dramatic experiments invited more attention—favorable or unfavorable. The most favorable initial attention came from Donald Hebb, whose own theory of cell assemblies he viewed as a physiological basis for cognitive structures. In a talk before the Canadian Psychological Association in 1974, he noted a possible coordination between his proposals and the existence of the "hidden observer" as I described it (Hebb, 1975). He repeated his support in an article in *Psychology Today* entitled "Hilgard's Discovery Brings Hypnosis Closer to Everyday Experience" (Hebb, 1982).

At the other extreme were those who totally rejected the theory (Spanos & Hewitt, 1980; Spanos, 1983). The main possibility was that the findings might have resulted from the demand characteristics in the instructions given to the subjects. Recognizing this as a charge to be corrected, investigators at Concordia University in Montreal (Nogrady, McConkey, Laurence, & Perry, 1983), having earlier done experiments replicating and extending the Stanford findings, designed an experiment specifically to test the influence of possible demand characteristics. Their meticulous experiment supported the original findings, and satisfactorily answered the charge of undue pressure for compliance.

The Concordia group's earlier findings had added to an understanding of some concomitants of the hidden-observer experience. I had already noted that even among very highly responsive subjects, who could reduce their pain extensively through suggested hypnotic analgesia, those who showed hidden observers constituted only about half of these highly selected subjects. I could find no reason for this, and conjectured that it might have something to do with amnesia, but there was no evidence for such differences in their prior performances.

Laurence and Perry (1981) found an interesting correlate that distinguished between those highly responsive subjects with and without a hidden observer. In the course of hypnosis, they included age regression as one of the test items: Subjects were to experience themselves again as children of 5 years of age. For successful subjects, such an experience may take one of two forms. In one form the subject becomes completely absorbed in the experience of being a child again; in the second form the subject is convinced of being a child again, but in addition retains the presence of an adult observer. This observer has some of the properties of the hidden observer in pain, in that it knows all that is going on in the inward experience as well as in the contexts of the experience. Sometimes the regressed subject reports this in statements that are variants of this one: "I felt sorry for that child who was lost and frightened lest her mother would not find her, because I knew all along that she would return soon." Laurence and Perry proposed to call this an experience of duality—at once a child and an adult. Although regression had been tested in advance of the hidden observer in pain, they found that the subjects with the duality experience were the ones who later reported a hidden observer. The result was confirmed in the previously mentioned study by Nogrady et al. (1983), and adds a great deal to the knowledge of differences in information processing by the two groups of highly hypnotizable subjects, one with and one without a reported hidden observer.

Support and Elaboration of the Neodissociation Theory

The unfinished theory represented in Figure 3.2 was carried further by Kihlstrom (1984) in a book chapter entitled "Conscious, Subconscious, Unconscious: A Cognitive Approach," in which he tied the neodissociation theory more closely than I had done to modern cognitive psychology, including the interpretations of models of memory and the distinctions between procedural and declarative knowledge. While elaborating the neodissociation theory, he gave it strong support, and indicated regret that many cognitive theorists had failed to take the implications of dissociation into account. The book in which Kihlstrom's chapter appears has many other chapters bearing on cognitive conceptions of unconscious processes (Bowers & Meichenbaum, 1984).

CONCLUDING REMARKS

This chapter is designed primarily to present a theory of hypnosis. The theory is built upon evidence from hypnosis, and may be undertstood as one among other theories. The phenomena of the human mind are not divided into natural categories to serve our convenience, however, and any satisfactory theory of hypnosis should also be a theory bearing on psychology at large. It is my hope that neodissociation theory, as it develops, will serve this larger purpose.

Acknowledgments. The neodissociation theory of hypnosis described in this chapter is based primarily on investigations of hypnosis that were carried on for over 20 years (primarily from 1957 to 1979) in the Stanford Laboratory of Hypnosis Research, within the Department of Psychology of Stanford University. The generosity of funding agencies was important for this program of research. Although some other agencies gave periodic support, in the initial period the laboratory was established by a grant from the Ford Foundation. From 1961 on, the primary sustaining grant was that from the National Institute of Mental Health (Grant No. MH-03859). This support permitted the maintenance of a well-equipped laboratory, as well as financial assistance to a substantial number of research assistants and associates (not only graduate students but some full-time staff members, postdoctoral fellows, and visiting scholars from other universities located in many parts of the world).

REFERENCES

American Psychiatric Association. (1987). *Diagnostic and statistical manual of mental disorders* (3rd ed., rev.). Washington, DC: Author.

Barber, T. X., & Calverley, D. S. (1962). "Hypnotic behavior" as a function of task motivation. *Journal of Psychology, 54,* 363–389.

Bartlett, F. C. (1932). *Remembering.* Cambridge, England: Cambridge University Press.

Boring, E. G. (1950). *A history of experimental psychology.* (2nd ed.). New York: Appleton-Century-Crofts.

Bowers, K. S. (1967). The effects of demands for honesty upon reports of visual and auditory hallucinations. *International Journal of Clinical and Experimental Hypnosis, 15,* 31–36.

Bowers, K. S., & Brenneman, H. A. (1981). Hypnotic dissociation, dichotic listening, and active versus passive modes of attention. *Journal of Abnormal Psychology, 90,* 55–67.

Bowers, K. S., & Meichenbaum, D. (Eds.). (1984). *The unconscious reconsidered.* New York: Wiley.

Chomsky, N. (1957). *Syntactic structures.* The Hague: Mouton.

Friedlander, J. W., & Sarbin, T. R. (1938). The depth of hypnosis. *Journal of Abnormal and Social Psychology, 33,* 473–475.

Gorassini, D. R., & Spanos, N. P. (1986). A sociocognitive skills approach to the successful modification of hypnotic susceptibility. *Journal of Personality and Social Psychology, 50,* 1004–1012.

Hebb, D. O. (1975). Science and the world of imagination. *Canadian Psychological Review, 16,* 4–11.

Hebb, D. O. (1982, May). Hilgard's discovery brings hypnosis closer to everyday experience. *Psychology Today,* pp. 52–54.

Hilgard, E. R. (1956). *Theories of learning* (2nd ed.). New York: Appleton-Century-Crofts.

Hilgard, E. R. (1965). *Hypnotic susceptibility.* New York: Harcourt, Brace & World.

Hilgard, E. R. (1973a). Dissociation revisited. In M. Henle, J. Jaynes, & J. Sullivan (Eds.), *Historical conceptions of psychology* (pp. 205–219). New York: Springer.

Hilgard, E. R. (1973b). A neodissociation interpretation of pain reduction in hypnosis. *Psychological Review, 80,* 396–411.

Hilgard, E. R. (1973c). The domain of hypnosis, with some comments on alternative paradigms. *American Psychologist, 28,* 972–982.

Hilgard, E. R. (1974). Toward a neodissociation theory: Multiple cognitive controls in human functioning. *Perspectives in Biology and Medicine, 17*, 301–316.

Hilgard, E. R. (1981). Hypnotic susceptibility scales under attack: An examination of Weitzenhoffer's criticism. *International Journal of Clinical and Experimental Hypnosis, 29*, 24–41.

Hilgard, E. R. (1986). *Divided consciousness: Multiple controls in human thought and action* (expanded ed.). New York: Wiley.

Hilgard, E. R., & Hilgard, J. R. (1983). *Hypnosis in the relief of pain* (rev. ed.). Los Altos, CA: William Kaufmann.

Hilgard, E. R., Hilgard, J. R., Macdonald, H., Morgan, A. H., & Johnson, L. S. (1978). The reality of hypnotic analgesia: A comparison of highly hypnotizables with simulators. *Journal of Abnormal Psychology, 87*, 239–246.

Hilgard, E. R., Morgan, A. H., & Macdonald, H. (1975). Pain and dissociation in the cold pressor test: A study of hypnotic analgesia with "hidden reports" through automatic key-pressing and automatic talking. *Journal of Abnormal Psychology, 84*, 280–289.

Hilgard, J. R. (1965). Personality and hypnotizability: Inferences from case studies. In E. R. Hilgard, *Hypnotic susceptibility* (pp. 343–374). New York: Harcourt, Brace & World.

Hilgard, J. R. (1979). *Personality and hypnosis: A study of imaginative involvements* (2nd ed.). Chicago: University of Chicago Press.

Hilgard, J. R., & Hilgard, E. R. (1962). Developmental–interactive aspects of hypnosis: Some illustrative cases. *Genetic Psychology Monographs, 66*, 143–178.

Hilgard, J. R., & LeBaron, S. (1984). *Hypnotherapy of pain in children with cancer.* Los Altos, CA: William Kaufmann.

Hull, C. L. (1934). The concept of habit-family hierarchy and maze learning. *Psychological Review, 41*, 33–54, 134–152.

James, W. (1890). *Principles of psychology* (2 vols.). New York: Henry Holt.

Kihlstrom, J. F. (1984). Conscious, subconscious, unconscious: A cognitive approach. In K. S. Bowers & D. Meichenbaum (Eds.), *The unconscious reconsidered* (pp. 149–211). New York: Wiley.

Knox, V. J., Crutchfield, L., & Hilgard, E. R. (1975). The nature of task interference in hypnotic dissociation: An investigation of hypnotic behavior. *International Journal of Clinical and Experimental Hypnosis, 23*, 305–323.

Knox, V. J., Morgan, A. H., & Hilgard, E. R. (1974). Pain and suffering in ishemia: The paradox of hypnotically suggested anesthesia as contradicted by reports from the "hidden observer." *Archives of General Psychiatry, 39*, 1201–1214.

Laurence, J.-R., & Perry, C. (1981). The "hidden observer" phenomenon in hypnosis: Some additional findings. *Journal of Abnormal Psychology, 90*, 334–344.

Lewin, K. (1935). *A dynamic theory of personality.* New York: McGraw-Hill.

Meichenbaum, D., & Gilmore, J. B. (1984). The nature of unconscious processes: A cognitive–behavioral perspective. In K. S. Bowers & D. Meichenbaum (Eds.), *The unconscious reconsidered* (pp. 273–298). New York: Wiley.

Miller, G. A., Galanter, E., & Pribram, K. H. (1960). *Plans and the structure of behavior.* New York: Holt.

Morgan, A. H. (1973). The heritability of hypnotic susceptibility in twins. *Journal of Abnormal Psychology, 82*, 55–61.

Newell, A., & Simon, H. A. (1972). *Human problem solving.* Englewood Cliffs, NJ: Prentice-Hall.

Nogrady, H., McConkey, K. M., Laurence, J.-R., & Perry, C. (1983). Dissociation, duality, and demand characteristics in hypnosis. *Journal of Abnormal Psychology, 90,* 334–344.

Orne, M. T. (1971). The simulation of hypnosis: Why, how, and what it means. *International Journal of Clinical and Experimental Hypnosis, 19,* 183–210.

Piccione, C., Hilgard, E. R., & Zimbardo, P. G. (1989). On the stability of measured hypnotizability over a 25-year period. *Journal of Personality and Social Psychology, 56,* 289–295.

Smith, G. M., Egbert, L. D., Markowitz, P. A., Mosteller, F., & Beecher, H. K. (1966). An experimental pain method sensitive to morphine in man: The submaximum effort tourniquet technique. *Journal of Pharmacological and Experimental Therapeutics, 154,* 324–332.

Spanos, N. P., & Hewitt, E. C. (1980). The hidden observer in hypnotic analgesia: Discovery or experimental creation? *Journal of Personality and Social Psychology, 39,* 1201–1214.

Stevenson, J. H. (1976). The effect of posthypnotic dissociation on the performance of interfering tasks. *Journal of Abnormal Psychology, 85,* 398–407.

Tolman, E. C. (1932). *Purposive behavior in animals and men.* New York: Appleton-Century.

Weitzenhoffer, A. M. (1980). Hypnotic susceptibility revisited. *American Journal of Clinical Hypnosis, 22,* 130–146.

A Neodissociative Critique of Spanos's Social-Psychological Model of Hypnosis

KENNETH S. BOWERS
University of Waterloo

THOMAS M. DAVIDSON
Mental Health Centre, Penetanguishene

INTRODUCTION

Current thinking in hypnosis research is dominated by two schools of thought—E. R. Hilgard's (1973a; 1977a) neodissociation model of hypnosis, and the social-psychological model of hypnosis. Although the two schools agree about some fundamental facts and observations that delineate the domain of hypnosis (E. R. Hilgard, 1973b; Spanos & Barber, 1974), there is continuing disagreement about how best to understand the phenomena.

In this chapter, we present a neodissociative account of hypnosis, but do so in the context of an analysis and a critique of the social-psychological view of the phenomenon. The main investigators identified with this latter view are Theodore Sarbin and his former student William Coe, and Theodore Barber and his former student Nicholas Spanos. Although these investigators differ from each other in some aspects of their approach to hypnotic phenomena, the similarities are by and large more conspicuous than the differences. Accordingly, we focus on the contributions of Nicholas Spanos as representative of the social-psychological model of hypnosis. We have done so because Spanos is currently the most prolific investigator of hypnosis, and the most vocal critic of the neodissociation model. By providing an extended critique of Spanos's social-psychological position, and by contrasting it with the neodissociation model of hypnosis, we hope to bring the advantages of the latter into sharp relief.

THEORETICAL CONCEPTS AND PRINCIPLES

Classical dissociation theory, as formulated by Pierre Janet (1901, 1907/ 1965; see also Ellenberger, 1970; Perry & Laurence, 1984) and Morton Prince (1915), maintained that certain aspects of human mental functioning could be "split off" (dissociated) from consciousness. Hypnosis, according to this classical formulation, was a quintessentially dissociative phenomenon. Thus, hypnotized subjects could perform suggested activities without any awareness that they had been told to perform them—as in posthypnotic suggestion with amnesia for the suggestion. Or subjects could allegedly perform two tasks simultaneously without being aware of the secondary (hypnotically suggested) performance, and without the cognitive demands of the two tasks interfering with each other.

There were difficulties with this classical view of dissociation (White & Shevach, 1942). For example, it turned out that the hypnotically suggested performance of a secondary task by no means ensured its functional independence from a primary, consciously performed task (Hull, 1933). Hilgard's neodissociation model acknowledges these problems (Knox, Crutchfield, & Hilgard, 1975; Stevenson, 1976), and reformulates classical dissociation theory in terms of contemporary cognitive psychology (E. R. Hilgard, 1973a, 1977a). According to Hilgard's model, executive control of thought and behavior is at the top of a control hierarchy, with various subsystems of control ordinarily being subject to executive initiative and monitoring. When the control hierarchy is operating in an integrated, seamless manner, a person's goals, intentions, and purposes are realized in action. Typically, action that flows from such an integrated network of control is experienced as conscious and volitional.

However, Hilgard's neodissociation model also proposes that under certain circumstances, lower levels of control can function in a manner that is dissociated from higher, executive levels of control. To illustrate, when people sleep, executive functions are in abeyance; nevertheless, subsystems of control remain responsive to locally significant information. People typically do not fall out of bed, they can awaken to the cry of a distressed newborn, and they typically respond to bladder pressure by waking up and going to the bathroom. They may even wake up at an appropriate time in the morning if the the alarm clock fails to go off. Note that each of these sleep-enacted behaviors serves an important purpose; however, it stretches a point to argue that they are enacted on purpose. Performing a behavior on purpose implies a conscious intention to perform it, something that a sleeping subject cannot readily achieve. Accordingly, *actions that serve a purpose are not always performed on purpose.*

Hilgard's neodissociation model constitutes a general model of cognitive functioning. It was not developed, as some have supposed (e.g., Spanos, 1982), solely to account for hypnotic phenomena. Indeed, Hilgard (1977a) draws upon a variety of everyday occurrences, such as dreams and tip-of-the-tongue phenomena (Brown & McNeill, 1966), as well as minor and major psychopathological disorders (e.g., fugue states and multiple personality), to illustrate and support the model.

It is nevertheless true that the neodissociation model has been applied primarily to an understanding of hypnosis. With respect to hypnotic phenomena, Hilgard's neodissociation model proposes that hypnotic responsiveness involves a somewhat reduced influence of executive control over hypnotically enacted behavior (Shor, 1959, 1970; Gill & Brenman, 1959; G. A. Miller, Galanter, & Pribram, 1960). "The planning function is inhibited, and the hypnotized person does not independently undertake new lines of thought or action" (E. R. Hilgard, 1979, p. 50). In addition, lower systems of control are more responsive to the suggested state of affairs, and less responsive to the reality (stimulus) state of affairs, than would ordinarily be the case. In other words, suggestions administered to a hypnotized person can more or less directly activate subsystems of control, which are partially and temporarily dissociated from executive (intentional, conscious) control.

The neodissociation model also provides an account of the so-called "classic suggestion effect" (Weitzenhoffer, 1978, 1980)—the experience of nonvolition that frequently accompanies hypnotically suggested behavior. The experience of volition or intention ordinarily reflects executive control over behavior. However, it is precisely such executive control that is minimized or bypassed when a hypnotized subject enacts the suggested state of affairs. Consequently, hypnotically suggested behaviors are typically experienced as nonvolitional.

An important implication of the considerations described above is this: The neodissociation model proposes that hypnotically suggested behavior is purposeful, in the sense that it is goal-directed—that is, it achieves the suggested state of affairs. However, it also implies that the behavior can be nonvolitional, in the sense that it is not performed on purpose—that is, it does not flow from executive initiative and effort. Thus, from the point of view of the neodissociation model of hypnosis, it is neither contradictory nor paradoxical to assert that goal-directed behavior can also be nonvolitional.

In effect, Hilgard's neo-dissociation model recognizes that not everything people do is achieved consciously, intentionally, or on purpose (cf. Uleman & Bargh, 1989). However, when behavior is not consciously controlled, it does *not* mean that people exercise no control at all over their behavior; rather, the control being exercised is dissociated from high-level, executive plans, intentions, and effort. Such "dissociated control" (Bowers, in press; M. E. Miller & Bowers, 1990) is particularly (but not exclusively) evident in various action slips (Norman, 1981; Reason, 1979; Heckhausen & Beckmann, 1990). For example, when a person dials a more familiar telephone number rather than the intended one, a subsystem of control has been activated—more, perhaps, by vagrant thoughts of a close friend than by conscious plans and intentions.

By way of contrast, Spanos often describes hypnotic behavior as "purposeful"—a word that does not capture the distinction between goal-directed behavior and behavior that is enacted volitionally (i.e., on purpose). Indeed, Spanos strongly implies that hypnotic behavior is goal-oriented and *therefore* volitional. From our point of view, this conflation of purpose and volition is one of the most important ways in which the social-psychological model of hypnosis differs from its neodissociative counterpart. As well, this conflation has helped fuel his skepticism about the dissociative basis of hypnosis, which, as we have seen, permits hypnotic behavior to be both purposeful and nonvolitional.

To be sure, skepticism is not new to hypnosis. Historically, it has taken the form of denying the very reality or genuineness of hypnotically suggested effects (e.g., Rosen, 1946; Bowers, 1983). For example, Barber (1970) stated:

> The motivation for denial of pain is present in the clinical hypnotic situation. The physician who has invested time and energy hypnotizing the patient and suggesting that pain will be relieved, expects and desires that his efforts will be successful, and by his words and manner communicates his desires and expectations to the patient. The patient in turn has often formed a close relationship with the physician–hypnotist and would like to please him or at least not to disappoint him. Furthermore, the patient is aware that even though the patient may have suffered, it may be difficult or disturbing for him to state directly to the physician–hypnotist that he experienced pain and it may be less anxiety-provoking to say that he did not suffer. (pp. 211–212)

Similar sentiments have more recently been expressed by Wagstaff (1986).

Spanos's skepticism has taken a different tack, however. He acknowledges that various hypnotically suggested effects, such as hypnotic analgesia (e.g., Spanos, Brown, Jones, & Horner, 1981) and hypnotic amnesia (Spanos, Radtke, Bertrand, Addie, & Drummond, 1982), are genuine— though, as Kihlstrom (1986) and others (Orne, Dinges, & Orne, 1986) have noted, he sometimes gives the contrary impression. For the most part, however, skepticism in the last 10 or 15 years has evolved from questioning whether the hypnotically suggested state of affairs represents a genuine alteration in experience (Bowers, 1983) to question-ing the traditional view about how these suggested alterations are achieved. In particular, Spanos believes that hypnotic analgesia, say, is achieved by the purposeful use of cognitive strategies. And, as we have seen, Spanos seems to mean by "purposeful" that reductions in pain are achieved by the conscious and intentional use of various cognitive strategies.

Unfortunately, the experience of nonvolition that ordinarily accom-panies hypnotic enactments appears to contradict such a view. In an attempt to address this apparent contradiction, Spanos has reconceptual-ized subjects' reports of nonvolition as "contextually cued interpretations made by subjects about behaviors that are, in fact, purposeful, goal-directed actions. . . . [Moreover], suggestion-related imaginings are seen as facilitating and legitimating the attributions of involuntariness that are demanded by the structure of the typical hypnotic test situation" (Spanos, Cobb, & Gorassini, 1985, p. 283). In effect, then, the experience of nonvolition is not part and parcel of hypnotic responding; rather, it is an attritutional error made by a person who remains unaware of the blunder (Spanos, 1986a).

Spanos's attempt to explain away reports of nonvolitional experience as attributional errors is one indication that he regards hypnotically suggested behavior as thoroughly volitional (i.e., as performed "on purpose"). In addition, Spanos's concerted efforts to discredit dissociation as a "special process" is directed against an important premise made by a neodissociative account of hypnosis—namely, that cognitive controls can be altered by hypnotic suggestion in a way that makes behavior less volitional (which is to say, less dependent on conscious plans and intentions). Indeed, a good deal of Spanos's published research is organized around demonstrating the alleged bankruptcy of dissociation as a viable explanation of hypnotic behavior.

The most impressive result of this mission is the sheer number of papers he has published in the area of hypnosis. For example, in the 10 years beginning in 1979 and ending in 1988, Spanos has authored or coauthored 89 papers on hypnosis, which is 7% of the 1,267 papers written on this topic during this time.[1] For the interested reader, the most accessible summary of his work was recently published in *Behavioral and Brain Sciences* (*BBS*) (Spanos, 1986a).

Despite Spanos's voluminous contributions to the literature, his own research has for the most part escaped the systematic and extended scrutiny he has visited on the work of others (though see the commentaries to his *BBS* paper). One purpose of this chapter is to redress this imbalance. Given the sheer number of papers he has published, it is not feasible to consider them one by one. However, there is a thematic and stylistic continuity that runs throughout most of Spanos's contributions to the hypnosis literature, so we proceed by highlighting problematic features of his position, citing particular papers to document our concerns.

We proceed by first critically reviewing some of Spanos's research in three representative domains: hypnotic analgesia, hypnotic amnesia, and the modifiability of hypnotic ability. His research in each of these areas has been quite critical of a more traditional account of hypnosis, with particular emphasis on its alleged methodological weaknesses. We examine these claims carefully in light of methodological concerns we have about his own research. Later in the chapter, we present some research recently conducted at the University of Waterloo that highlights the advantages of the neodissociative model of hypnosis, while exposing the weaknesses of a social-psychological model.

RESEARCH AND APPRAISAL

Hypnotic Analgesia

In his 1986 *BBS* article, Spanos states:

> According to Hilgard, . . . subjects low in hypnotic suggestibility are unable to experience dissociation; hence, conscious attention diversion and relaxation are the only psychological strategies open to them for reducing pain. Attention diversion and relaxation, however, are much less effective pain reducers than dissociation. *Consequently, low suggestibles can achieve only relatively small reductions in pain.* (1986a, p. 458; italics added)

This quotation is true only insofar as it refers to reductions in pain that are achieved by *hypnotic* suggestions for pain analgesia. When subjects low in hypnotizability are explicitly trained in the use of strategies to counter pain (e.g., distraction, relaxation, imaginative transformation of pain), they seem to do much better. It should be emphasized, however, that Hilgard nowhere states or implies that low-hypnotizability subjects are unable to reduce pain substantially as a result of such nonhypnotic interventions; he was interested in pain analgesia produced by specifically hypnotic procedures, not in pain reduction regardless of how it was produced. Nevertheless, Spanos argues that Hilgard's neodissociation position is disconfirmed when low-hypnotizability subjects achieve substantial pain reductions as a result of nonhypnotic treatment interventions. A recent publication illustrates our point.

Spanos and Katsanis (1989) assert that recent research from their laboratory "contradicts Hilgard's . . . hypothesis that low hypnotizable subjects are unable to experience large suggestion-induced reductions in pain" (p. 183). This quotation occurs in a context indicating clearly that the term "suggestion-induced" refers to a particular kind of *nonhypnotic* suggestion—namely, suggestions delivered to waking subjects that encourage them in the conscious use of cognitive coping strategies (e.g., distraction, imagining events inconsistent with pain). These are the kind of interventions that Meichenbaum and his associates (Turk, Meichenbaum, & Genest, 1983) have used so successfully in their program of research on the cognitive control of acute pain. However, their work has been conducted without any reference to hypnosis or individual differences in hypnotic ability. Nevertheless, when Spanos (1986a) reviews these and related (Neufeld & Thomas, 1977) findings, he argues that "hypnotic analgesia and waking [i.e., nonhypnotic] analgesia appear to be basically similar; in both cases, pain is reduced by motivated subjects actively coping with the noxious stimulation" (p. 458). The clear implication is that hypnotic analgesia results from a conscious and intentional use of various cognitive strategies, which counter both the pain experience and associated stress reactions.

In order to address these concerns empirically, M. E. Miller and Bowers (1986) recently conducted a study in which the similarities and differences between hypnotic and nonhypnotic analgesia were examined. The investigators analyzed the pre- and posttreatment pain reports of carefully selected low- and high-hypnotizability subjects (hereafter referred to as "lows" and "highs," for the sake of brevity) in each of three treatment conditions. One treatment involved hypnotizing subjects and administering suggestions for hypnotic analgesia. A second treatment involved stress inoculation (Turk et al., 1983), which Spanos has likened to hypnotic analgesia (see above). A third treatment was identical to the second treatment, except that subjects were told at the last moment that the cognitive strategies they had been taught were, in essence, hypnotic techniques for controlling pain. Subjects in all three groups were naive about the investigative relevance of hypnosis during the pretreatment baseline trial, and subjects in the second group remained so for the posttreatment assessment as well. Submersion of the forearm in circulating ice water (cold pressor) served as the pain stimulus in this experiment.

The rationale of this study was based on the fact that straightforward suggestions for hypnotic analgesia reduce pain more for highs than for lows (E. R. Hilgard & J. R. Hilgard, 1975). If, as Spanos argues, active cognitive strategies are the basis for hypnotic analgesia, then highs and lows in the two stress inoculation conditions should have differed from each other as much as highs and lows in the hypnotic analgesia condition. However, this did not occur. In correlational terms, hypnotic ability correlated .48 ($p < .02$) with the amount of pain reduction in the hypnotic analgesia condition, but only .04 (n.s.) in the stress inoculation condition, and .18 (n.s.) in the stress inoculation condition defined as hypnosis. In addition, Miller and Bowers (1986) demonstrated that 33 out of 36 subjects in the two stress inoculation groups retrospectively reported using the various cognitive strategies they had been taught as a means of reducing cold-pressor pain; only 3 of 18 subjects in the hypnotic analgesia condition did so. Apparently, hypnotic ability mediated the effect of hypnotic analgesia, but not the analgesia produced by stress inoculation; on the other hand, stress inoculation training reduced pain, but not differentially for high and low subjects. It is difficult to reconcile this pattern of data with Spanos's assertion that hypnotic analgesia and cognitive strategies both reduce pain in pretty much the same way.

Spanos (Nolan & Spanos, 1987) vigorously objected to the M. E. Miller and Bowers (1986) investigation. We have some sympathy with one of his objections: Unaccountably, neither the published article nor the original dissertation (M. E. Miller, 1986) reported a direct 2×2 comparison of high and low subjects exposed to stress inoculation and hypnotic analgesia. In raising the question of this missing analysis, Nolan and Spanos (1987) are quite clear about what the social-psychological prediction would be: "[T]he high and low scorers in the stress-inoculation condition [should] report as little posttest pain as the highly hypnotizable hypnotic subjects" (p. 97). As it turns out, however, this was not the case. In fact, the pain reduction achieved by the highs in the hypnotic analgesia condition was 23% greater than the mean reduction across the other three cells, which were virtually identical to one another.[2] Both the main effect of hypnotic ability and the condition $\times$ hypnotic ability interaction were significant ($p < .01$). (Incidentally, this outcome will come as no surprise to anyone who examines the graphic presentation of the posttreatment results, which *were* presented in both the published paper and Miller's dissertation.) Thus, contrary to recent reports from Spanos's laboratory (e.g., Spanos, Kennedy, & Gwynn, 1984), highs in receipt of suggestions for hypnotic analgesia showed considerably more pain reduction than did highs or lows who were administered nonhypnotic interventions for pain analgesia. All in all, there is little comfort in these findings for Spanos's view that lows are disadvantaged by suggestions for hypnotic analgesia, and that when they receive appropriately motivating instructions to cope actively with pain, "both low and high scorers in nonhypnotic treatments can achieve as much pain reduction as highly hypnotizable hypnotic subjects" (Nolan & Spanos, 1987, p. 96).

Spanos and Katsanis (1989) have recently published an extended empirical rebuttal to the M. E. Miller and Bowers (1986) investigation. They employed a nonhypnotic condition in which analgesic suggestions were identical to those administered in the hypnotic condition. Moreover, subjects in the nonhypnotic condition were "informed . . . that they were selected for participation because they were highly responsive to suggestion . . . [and] that because of their natural abilities in this regard they would be very responsive to suggestion even though they were not first hypnotized" (p. 184). In contrast to his earlier nonhypnotic interventions (see above), the nonhypnotic condition employed by Spanos and Katsanis (1989) is quite different from the interventions used in the literature on the cognitive control of pain. Indeed, it closely resembles what has traditionally been called "waking suggestion"—that is, *hypnotic-like* suggestions administered in the absence of a prior hypnotic induction. Waking and hypnotic suggestibility correlate about .60 (e.g., E. R. Hilgard, 1965; E. R. Hilgard & Tart, 1966), so high subjects exposed to Spanos and Katsanis's version of nonhypnotic suggestions would doubtless be far more analgesic than their low counterparts. Such an outcome would of course be problematic for the social-psychological position, because it contends that low and high subjects exposed to *non*hypnotic suggestions for analgesia reduce pain as much as do highs administered hypnotic suggestions for analgesia.

Unfortunately, Spanos and Katsanis (1989) ran only highly hypnotizable subjects in their investigation. Consequently, the study could not reveal the superior pain reduction of highs relative to lows in response to *both* hypnotic and nonhypnotic (but hypnotic-like) suggestions for analgesia. In effect, the omission of lows from this investigation creates ambiguity regarding the impact of "nonhypnotic suggestions" for analgesia. Earlier, "nonhypnotic suggestions" referred to interventions bearing no resemblance to hypnotic analgesia (e.g., stress inoculation techniques of pain control). We henceforth refer to this kind of intervention as a "Type I" nonhypnotic suggestion. In response to such Type I interventions, lows might conceivably perform as well as highs do in response to hypnotic suggestions (though it will be recalled that this was not the case in the M. E. Miller & Bowers [1986] investigation).

However, after Miller and Bowers (1986) demonstrated that suggestions for hypnotic analgesia and Type I nonhypnotic suggestions reduce pain in different ways, Spanos and Katsanis (1989) shifted to a second meaning of nonhypnotic suggestion—namely, suggestions that are distinctly hypnotic-like, though presented in the absence of a formal hypnotic induction. We henceforth refer to this kind of intervention as a "Type II" nonhypnotic suggestion. Type II nonhypnotic suggestions are very likely to produce higher levels of responsiveness in high than in low subjects—simply because on the average, highs demonstrate more waking suggestibility than do lows.

Spanos is thus faced with a conundrum. On the one hand, he can hope to demonstrate that lows are as responsive to Type I nonhypnotic suggestions as highs are to hypnotic suggestions; however, as M. E. Miller and Bowers (1986) demonstrated, even if that were true, different mechanisms seem to mediate the analgesic effects produced by these two different treatments (see also M. E. Miller & Bowers, 1990, summarized below). On the other hand, Spanos can use Type II nonhypnotic suggestions for both highs and lows; however, doing so would surely lead highs to outperform lows—an outcome that is at odds with Spanos's social-psychological views.

In effect, Spanos and Katsanis's (1989) omission of low subjects from a study employing Type II nonhypnotic suggestions for analgesia means that the superior responsiveness of high subjects to nonhypnotic (but hypnotic-like) suggestions remains empirically invisible. But the entire point of the Miller and Bowers (1986) investigation, to which Spanos and Katsanis (1989) have taken such exception, was to see how individual differences in hypnotic ability are expressed in different treatment conditions. The Spanos and Katsanis paper thus distracts attention from issues raised by the Miller and Bowers paper, rather than addressing them.[3]

To summarize, Spanos has attempted to discredit the neodissociative account of hypnosis on the grounds that low subjects can substantially reduce pain by means other than hypnotic analgesia—a claim that is both irrelevant and misleading. It is irrelevant because Hilgard's account of hypnosis never made any prediction about the analgesic impact of nonhypnotic interventions with either high or low subjects. It is misleading because Miller and Bowers (1986) have shown that the mechanism by which Type I nonhypnotic suggestions (e.g., stress inoculation) produces analgesia is different from the mechanism underlying hypnotic analgesia. Spanos's own work in response to these findings also perpetrates a misleading picture by omitting low subjects from a follow-up experiment. Their inclusion would surely have demonstrated that Type II nonhypnotic suggestions engender more pain reduction in highs than in lows.

Hypnotic Amnesia

In a series of studies designed to clarify the cognitive process underlying hypnotic amnesia (Radtke-Bodorik, Planas, & Spanos, 1980; Radtke-Bodorik, Spanos, & Haddad, 1979; Spanos & Bodorik, 1977; Spanos & D'Eon, 1980; Spanos, Radtke, Bertrand, et al., 1982; Spanos, Radtke-Bodorik, & Shabinsky, 1980; Spanos, Stam, D'Eon, Pawlak, & Radtke, 1980), Spanos and his colleagues concluded that hypnotic amnesia is accomplished when subjects "attend away" from those normally relevant retrieval cues that would otherwise oblige recall. These investigations utilized a recall organization paradigm to investigate amnesia for a list of words. In this paradigm, (1) subjects learn a categorized word list to criterion over a series of free-recall trials; (2) they are given an amnesia suggestion to forget the word list; (3) they are asked to recall the words again (amnesia trial); (4) the amnesia suggestion is canceled, and (5) the subjects are asked to recall the words a final time (recovery trial).

Spanos's investigations on amnesia revealed several consistent findings. First, amnesia is associated with recall disorganization: Relative to the last learning and the recovery trial, recall is less organized on the amnesia trial. In other words, during the amnesia trial, remembered items are less likely to be recalled in an orderly, category-by-category fashion. (Note that this paradigm requires some items to be remembered, so that recall disorganization can be assessed. Thus, people who are amnesic for all the words cannot be included in the analysis of the data; instead, the paradigm focuses on subjects who are partially amnesic.) Second, the relationship between recall disorganization and partial amnesia is mediated by hypnotic ability. Third, the disorganization effect is not a product of demand characteristics.

The principle of "encoding specificity" (Tulving & Thomson, 1973) was invoked as a cognitive mechanism to account for these effects. This principle states that the efficiency of recall is determined by the degree of similarity between the specific retrieval cues present at the time of attempted recall, and those present at the time of initial learning (encoding) of the target material. In short, if the subject attends to the same retrieval cues during attempted recall that were employed to learn the material in the first place, recall is efficient; on the other hand, to the extent that the subject does not attend to the same retrieval cues during attempted recall that were also present during learning, then recall is inefficient. According to Spanos, the recall of amnesic subjects is inefficient precisely because they do not attend to relevant retrieval cues.

To review, there are four essential points to Spanos's inattention hypothesis as it applies to amnesia for an entire list of words:

1. Successful recall is a function of the match between retrieval cues present at the time of both learning and attempted recall (encoding specificity).
2. The organizational features of the word list (i.e., the category membership of words on the list) are the most salient retrieval cues present when the words are memorized to criterion.
3. Therefore, successful amnesia (unsuccessful recall) depends upon diverting attention from the organizational features of the list.
4. By not attending to the organizational features of the list, the word categories cannot serve as the basis for attempted recall, and the words that are remembered by partial amnesics are therefore disorganized.

In the University of Waterloo hypnosis laboratory, we conducted two studies (Davidson, 1986; Davidson & Bowers, 1991) that evaluated the inattention hypothesis in the context of *selective* amnesia. Rather than administering suggestions to forget an entire list of categorized words, we administered suggestions to forget 4 of the 16 words subjects had just learned to criterion. The 4 words to be forgotten were all in one category (e.g., birds), and the remaining 12 words not targeted for amnesia belonged to one of three other categories. (Note that in this selective amnesia paradigm, people who forget all four target words can still be included in the analysis, because the organization of their recall can be based on the 12 remaining words not targeted for amnesia. Consequently, subjects most responsive to suggestions for hypnotic amnesia can be retained for analysis.) Recalling these 12 words in an orderly fashion during the amnesia trial should considerably increase the probability of recalling the remaining 4 words. This prediction follows from the principle of encoding specificity, endorsed by Spanos as follows:

> When hypnotic subjects shift their attentional focus away from the task of list recall, the content of the information to which they are now attending is unlikely to match the information contained in the memory traces of the target events. Retrieval is therefore inefficient. When presented with the cancellation cue, *subjects simply refocus attention to the retrieval cues that were present during encoding and the target material immediately comes to mind.* (Spanos, Radtke, & Dubreuil, 1982, p. 565; italics added)

However, results from our first study of selective amnesia disconfirmed this prediction (Davidson & Bowers, 1991). In the first experiment, subjects high, medium, and low in hypnotizability who totally or partially forgot the words targeted for amnesia nevertheless recalled most of the remaining 12 words category by category—that is, in a manner that was highly organized. In other words, attending to the relevant retrieval (organizational) cues did *not* engender recall of the four words targeted for amnesia, as the principle of encoding specificity would predict.

A second study, also reported in Davidson and Bowers (1991), replicated these findings. In addition, it controlled for some possibly extraneous factors—such as the length of time between receiving the suggestion for posthypnotic amnesia and the test for it, and whether the test for amnesia took place within hypnosis or posthypnotically. Regardless of condition, subjects who were selectively amnesic for the words in the targeted category nevertheless recalled all or most of the remaining words in a highly organized fashion. Interestingly, some of the subjects in this study testified that they were aware, during the amnesia trial, of the *category of words* targeted for amnesia, but were nevertheless unable to recall the particular words in the category. In other words, these subjects reported attending to the main retrieval cues, but nevertheless evidenced amnesia.

After preliminary presentations of these experiments (Davidson & Bowers, 1982, 1983), Spanos also reported two studies that attempted to evaluate the cognitive processes underlying selective amnesia (Bertrand & Spanos, 1985; Spanos & de Groh, 1984). Instead of detailing the particulars of these experiments, it is sufficient to spell out their rationale and findings. Spanos begins by acknowledging:

> Subjects instructed to forget only a specific portion of a categorized word list while recalling the remainder cannot meet task demands by simply disattending from the recall task. Instead, they must employ a strategy that will segregate the material to be forgotten from the material to be recalled. Any such segregative strategy is likely to be associated with a high level of organization in the material recalled during amnesia testing. (Bertrand & Spanos, 1985, p. 250)

For example, subjects asked to forget words in one category while recalling the words in the remaining categories can "cluster items perfectly and then rehearse the items in two of the clusters as a means of disattending the items in a third cluster" (Bertrand & Spanos, 1985, p. 251). On the other hand, subjects asked to forget one item from each category can most easily accomplish this by "clustering the items in memory, 'mentally removing' one item from each category, and then rehearsing the to-be-recalled items" (Bertrand & Spanos, 1985, p. 251). It should be noted that differential rehearsal of the to-be-remembered words did not occur during the learning of the words; rather, it took place *after* the learning criterion had been met. There was, however, no apparent impact of this differential rehearsal on the recall of the word list during the recovery trial.

One of us (Davidson, 1986) has provided a detailed criticism of both the Bertrand and Spanos (1985) investigation, and a companion report by Spanos and de Groh (1984). We confine ourselves here to a couple of comments. Conceptually, there is the awkward fact that subjects must recall precisely what words to forget in order to avoid rehearsing them. Methodologically, one problematic feature of the investigations concerns the fact that the amnesic suggestions did not specify which category of words (or which word from each category) was to be forgotten; the decision in this regard was left to the subject. However, leaving the category or word unspecified means that we can readily discern only whether the subjects were *partially* amnesic; whether they were *selectively* amnesic is not as clear. In other words, it is more difficult by this procedure to distinguish between forgotten words that had been self-selected for amnesia, and forgotten words that had not been. Since the main purpose of the investigations was to examine the selectivity of amnesia, the use of a procedure that renders it difficult to do so must be viewed as problematic.

Finally, Bertrand and Spanos (1985) and Spanos and de Groh (1984), in assessing their results, quietly abandon the principle of encoding specificity that had been so central to Spanos's thinking and theorizing *vis à vis* his investigations of entire-list amnesia. According to Spanos, subjects in the selective amnesia paradigm rehearse the words *not* targeted for amnesia in an organized, category-by-category fashion. By doing so, they obviously attend to the specific retrieval cues used during encoding of the words during the learning trials. Therefore, according to the principle of encoding specificity espoused by Spanos and his colleagues, the target material should immediately come to mind (Spanos, Radtke, & Dubreuil, 1982, p. 565). Such recall should have been particularly evident for those subjects who were given a suggestion to forget only one word from each of the three categories. Not only did the words forgotten by these subjects have the organizational features of the list as an important retrieval cue, but their association with other words in the same category should also have acted as an important retrieval cue. Nevertheless, these subjects were able to maintain organized recall of words *not* targeted for amnesia without cueing the recall of words that were.

In sum, the question Spanos never addresses is this: Why is the principle of encoding specificity—so central to his understanding of entire-list amnesia—repealed by him without comment or qualification in the context of selective amnesia? Whatever the reason for his silence on this issue, the results of recent investigations on selective amnesia by Spanos and his colleagues confirm our own similar findings: Despite the principle of encoding specificity, attention to relevant retrieval cues does not ensure successful recall of words selectively targeted for amnesia.

Before we leave this topic, it is important to compare a neodissociative and a social-psychological view of hypnotic amnesia. As we have seen, Spanos emphasizes "purposeful strategies" (Bertrand & Spanos, 1985, p. 258) as the basis for suggested forgetting. In other words, his social-psychological model proposes that hypnotic amnesia involves a successful attempt to forget something; in contrast, the neodissociation model of hypnosis implies that suggested amnesia represents a failed attempt to remember something.

Ironically, Spanos's position on hypnotic amnesia is reminiscent of Freud's early view of repression: In both cases, a person tries not to recall something. In his earliest writing on repression, Freud stated that a patient "wished to forget, and therefore intentionally repressed" (Breuer & Freud, 1893–1895/1974, p. 61). The source of the patient's wish to forget was the anxiety associated with remembering a painful memory. For Spanos, the motivation to forget flows from the wish to self-present as a deeply hypnotized person (Spanos & Radtke, 1982). In both cases, forgetting is, at least at the outset, a voluntary act. (Freud later altered this early notion of repression so that not only the the repressed material, but the act of repression itself became unconscious; see Erdelyi, 1985, pp. 218–222.)

We do not deny the possibility that hypnotic amnesia may sometimes be due to motivated forgetting, but it does not seem to capture the core of the phenomenon (cf. Kihlstrom, 1983)—*particularly when cues for recall are quite salient*, as they are with selective forgetting of organized word lists. To illustrate what we mean, consider an embarassing social situation familiar to many of us, in which the name of a friend one is trying to introduce remains inaccessible. The cue value of the friend's physical presence does not jiggle the name free from the recesses of one's mind; nor is the high social motivation to recall it enough to muscle the mind into revealing the recalcitrant name. It would surely be bizarre to view this temporary inability to recall a friend's name as a successful attempt to forget it; rather, despite highly motivated efforts to remember the name, and despite the cue value of the friend's presence, his or her name fails to come to mind. We propose that in its most fully realized form, posthypnotic amnesia resembles the situation of trying to recall a friend's name and failing. This kind of "unmotivated" forgetting occurs all the time in everyday life: We forget where we put the car keys just moments ago; we forget to turn off the exit ramp that would get us to our destination; we temporarily forget what we went upstairs to get; and so on. This kind of forgetting seems to involve a temporary inaccessibility of a memory representation, rather than a motivated attempt to forget.

The question that makes hypnotic amnesia so perplexing is this: How can hypnotic suggestions for amnesia activate the kind of forgetting that occurs spontaneously all the time? For example, how can a posthypnotic suggestion to forget a friend's name engender amnesia for it later on when introductions are attempted? Some hints toward an answer have been provided by Kihlstrom (1980, Kihlstrom & Evans, 1979), but we are partial to the possibilities inherent in a recent proposal of Schacter (1989). He argues that the output of an activated memory does not necessarily activate consciousness of the memory. If activating information and activating consciousness of it are separate and distinct cognitive processes, the apparent paradox of selective amnesia is averted: A person forgets material targeted for amnesia because a suggestion-activated memory is temporarily unable to activate consciousness of the memory. Just how or why an activated memory can be temporarily unable to activate consciousness of it is not entirely clear—just as it is not clear why the name of a friend can become temporarily inaccessible just as one is about to introduce him or her, and despite the fact that memory of the name is at least partially activated by the friend's physical presence.

In the long run, we do not think that Spanos's attempt to account for hypnotic amnesia solely as a strategic and motivated enactment will succeed; rather, we think the most satisfying explanation of it will also involve a temporary breakdown of specific *mnemonic* mechanisms that ordinarily generate access to memories and represent them in conscious experience.

Hypnotic Responsiveness: Stable or Changeable?

Individual differences in hypnotic ability are critical factors in defining the domain of hypnosis (E. R. Hilgard, 1973b). The reliability and stability of hypnotic ability as assessed on standardized scales are quite extraordinary, especially considering the fact that it is typically measured by scales consisting of no more than 12 items. Even when investigators of different persuasions employ different scales consisting of different items and different scoring formats, the correlations between the scales is seldom lower than about .60 (Bowers, 1976/1983). When parallel forms of the same scales are employed, the correlation is about .90 (see, e.g., E. R. Hilgard, 1965).

Furthermore, longitudinal testing of hypnotic ability establishes its stability with some authority. In a 1974 study, Morgan, Johnson, and Hilgard reported a correlation of .60 ($n=85$) between the hypnotic ability measured first in Stanford undergraduates, and then 10 years later when the former students were adults. A more recent report assessed 50 of the original 85 subjects for the third time, 25 years after their initial test of hypnotic ability (Piccione, Hilgard, & Zimbardo, 1989). From the first to the third testing, $r=.71$; from the second to the third testing (representing a 15-year intertest interval), $r=.82$. Clearly, measured hypnotic ability is unusually stable over extended periods of time, especially considering that the period between late adolescence and middle adulthood is so beset with important life changes.

On the face of it, such trait-like stability is somewhat problematic for a social-psychological view of hypnosis, which is conceptually predisposed to see situational or treatment factors as being more important than person factors in accounting for hypnotic responsiveness. Nevertheless, Barber (1969) and Spanos (Spanos, Radtke, Hodgins, Stam, & Bertrand, 1983) have both devised their own measures of hypnotic ability, and both of them have found the same kind of high test–retest correlations as have advocates of a more traditional view. However, Barber (1969) did not systematically incorporate these individual differences into his understanding of hypnosis, and Spanos has lately been arguing that individual differences in hypnotic ability provide an illusion of stability, but that systematic efforts to improve hypnotic responsiveness are increasingly showing it to be a highly modifiable characteristic (e.g., Gorassini & Spanos, 1986; Spanos, Robertson, Menary, & Brett, 1986; Gfeller, Lynn,

& Pribble, 1987). The question thus comes down to how the evidence for stability and change in hypnotic ability should be understood. On the one hand, the stability of hypnotic ability may be merely apparent—a function of the fact that the circumstances surrounding the assessment of hypnotic ability are pretty much the same from one occasion to another, even when the assessments are years apart. On the other hand, treatment-induced increases in scores achieved on standardized scales of hypnotic susceptibility may reflect hypnotic ability less than they do compliance to unambiguous demands for hypnotic responsiveness to increase.

Although there have been many reported attempts to show treatment-induced increases in hypnotic responsiveness (for earlier reviews of the stability and change in hypnotic ability, see Perry, 1977; Diamond, 1977; Bowers, 1983, Ch. 5), the recent reports from Spanos's laboratory have clearly sparked renewed interest in the possibility of turning hypnotic duffers into virtuosos. For example, in one such study (Spanos, Robertson, Menary, Brett, & Smith, 1987) it was reported that 80% of low hypnotizability subjects were reclassified as highs after being subjected to a treatment program designed to increase hypnotic responsiveness. Across several such studies, Spanos has never reported fewer than 50% of low subjects scoring as highs after being administered his program (see Bates, Miller, Cross, & Brigham, 1988, Table 6, for a summary account of Spanos's findings).

These improvements are quite astonishing, given the relatively modest increases that have been reported prior to Spanos's development of the Carleton Skills Training Program for the enhancement of hypnotic responsiveness, and they provoke two contrary impulses. On the one hand, it raises the hope that the benefits of high hypnotic responsiveness (e.g., analgesia for surgical-level pain—Perry & Laurence, 1983; J. R. Hilgard & LeBaron, 1984) are not as limited as has been generally assumed, and that Spanos and other like-minded investigators will soon be documenting their claims with evidence for the clinical utility of hypnosis in people initially having very low hypnotic responsiveness. On the other hand, the claim that low subjects can be transformed into highs by a 75-minute treatment program rather flies in the face of our emerging understanding of hypnotic ability as a developmentally based characteristic (J. R. Hilgard, 1979; J. R. Hilgard & LeBaron, 1984, especially Ch. 9) that is no more subject to dramatic change than intelligence, say. Clearly, a critical appraisal of Spanos's claims for dramatic increases in hypnotic ability, in light of the procedures and methods for producing them, is in order.

The Carleton Skill Training Program for Modifying Hypnotic Ability

The training program that Spanos has developed for enhancing hypnotic responsiveness consists of three component parts: (1) presentation of positive information and elimination of misconceptions about hypnosis; (2) emphasis on becoming imaginatively absorbed in the suggested state of affairs; and (3) "detailed information concerning how to interpret specific types of suggestions coupled with practicing responses to such suggestions" (Gorassini & Spanos, 1986, p. 1005). Despite the fact that the three components are presented as if they were equally important, Spanos's investigations have clarified that it is the third, "detailed information" component that is critical to treatment-enhanced hypnotic responsiveness (see, e.g., Spanos et al., 1986, Table 1). So, we can focus on this component to examine why it so powerfully alters subjects' hypnotic responsiveness.

This third component (see Spanos et al., 1986, p. 351, for a complete description of it) was developed from a simple premise: Hypnotic suggestions are typically ambiguous because they often convey that a suggested response will simply happen, and that a hypnotized subject should await its occurrence without doing anything to make it happen. According to Spanos, "high-susceptible subjects tend to treat [such] suggestions as tacit requests to bring about suggested responses [which they then interpret] as events happening to them rather than as actions that they carry out" (Spanos et al., 1986, p. 350). Low subjects, on the other hand, interpret a suggestion to mean that they should await its occurrence rather than enacting it. In other words, the main difference between high and low subjects is how they interpret hypnotic suggestions. By this understanding, the way to transform lows into highs is straightforward: Make it unambiguously clear to lows during the course of their training that they should first enact the suggested response rather than await its occurrence, and then interpret this enactment as subjectively real and involuntary.

To implement this strategy, Spanos provides low subjects with four practice suggestions. Prior to receiving each such suggestion, subjects are given explicit instructions about how to understand and respond to it. For example:

> [The suggestion] will specifically tell you that your arm is like a hollow balloon being pumped up with helium . . . and that it's rising into the air by itself . . . you must do everythng that is required of someone making believe such a thing. *You must lift your arm up* and you must imagine that the arm is really a hollow balloon that is being pumped full of helium, rising by itself. You must . . . actually make it seem real. . . . Rivet your attention on the hollow arm, the lightness, the fact it's going up by itself and so on. Don't imagine anything or pay attention to anything that is unrelated to the make-believe situation. (Spanos et al., 1986, p. 351; italics added)

Subjects are then exposed to a tape-recorded model of a young woman who is described as someone "who [was] initially unresponsive to test suggestions, but who [has] learned the cognitive skills required to respond successfully" (Gorassini & Spanos, 1986, p. 1006). In the first part of the tape, the model simply enacts the suggestion a subject is about to receive, and expresses appropriate accompanying sensations and experiences. In a second portion of the tape, the model is interviewed and reinforced for interpreting the suggested effects appropriately. After receiving the "informational component" for each of four practice suggestions, and practicing the four suggestions accordingly, subjects are submitted to a posttraining assessment of their hypnotic ability.

Critique of the Carleton Skills Training Program

We would like our readers to imagine being subjects in this experiment. How would this "detailed information" intervention be received? What does it seem to communicate about appropriate behavior on the practice suggestions, and on the subsequent tests of hypnotic ability?

We submit that one very likely reading of the "detailed information" component of the treatment package is this: "When I later receive a suggestion (say, for my arm to rise), I should treat it as a simple request to behave accordingly (in much the same way as I would pass the salt when asked to do so at the dinner table). So, *first of all*, I should simply lift my arm (thereby satisfying the italicized portion of the training instructions, and also mimicking the model's behavior). *Then* comes the interesting part—namely, seeing whether I experience the arm as hollow, light, going up by itself, and so on."

Depending on a variety of personal and contextual factors, one may actually experience the arm in the manner suggested; on the other hand, the alteration in experience may not occur. In the latter event, one may admit the absence of the suggested experience; alternatively, one can merely acquiesce to the suggestion—less to express one's actual subjective experience than to satsify unambiguous external demands and expectancies for the raised arm to be experienced in this way. However, alterations in subjective experience are really the critical features of hypnotic responsiveness (Orne, 1966; Bowers, 1983); thus, misrepresenting one's arm as feeling hollow, feeling light, and rising by itself are uninteresting from the point of view of hypnosis. Hence, the obvious question we need to ask of Spanos's training program is this: To what extent does this program genuinely enhance hypnotic responsiveness, and to what extent does it provoke outward compliance in the absence of altered experience?

To address this question, it is first of all necessary to examine the way in which Spanos assesses hypnotic responsiveness before and after administering his treatment package. One measure employed is the Carleton University Responsiveness to Suggestion Scale (CURSS; Spanos et al.,

1983), which is scored in three separate ways. The CURSS:O index simply measures the number of passed responses to the seven separate suggestions that comprise the scale (maximum score, 7); the CURSS:S measures on a rating scale of 0–3 the extent of subjective experience associated with each suggestion (maximum score, 21); finally, the CURSS:O-I measures the degree of involuntariness associated with each overt response (maximum score, 7). (Spanos also uses a 10-item group adaptation of the Stanford Hypnotic Susceptibility Scale, Form C [SHSS:C]—scored in an analogous three-way fashion—as a supplementary, posttraining index of hypnotic responsiveness.)

Recall that Spanos's summary claim is that his treatment program transforms 50–80% of initially low subjects into high subjects. This claim is based on increases in subjects' CURSS:O index. In other words, the very high rate of success Spanos reports in tranforming low into high hypnotic responders is based on an index of overt behavior that in many people is likely to be received as a simple request (e.g., to raise one's arm). After going along with the request, the issue of whether it is experienced as subjectively real and involuntary can be tapped by the CURSS:S and CURSS:O-I, respectively. In the event, these indices both increase considerably. For example, in the first article in the series (Gorassini & Spanos, 1986), low subjects went from a mean of 6.17 to 11.20 on the CURSS:S index, and from 0.90 to 3.20 on the CURSS:O-I index ($p < .001$ for both comparisons). Although these latter findings are impressive, it is clearly important to determine how much these increases are artifactual (i.e., constitute increased compliance to the suggestions fostered by the treatment program), and how much they reflect genuine increases in hypnotic responsiveness.

One way in which Spanos et al. (1986) attempt to address this question is by including a simulator control group in the design. These subjects are initially selected for their low hypnotic ability; they are not exposed to the training program, but are instead told to fake being deeply hypnotized throughout the upcoming (i.e., second) assessment of hypnotic ability. These subjects demonstrate gains on all three CURSS indices even greater than those achieved by their counterparts in the complete training program condition. Spanos et al. (1986) view this outcome as indicating that simulators overplay the role of hypnotized subjects. Although this interpretation of their behavior may well be true, it does not really help us assess how much the posttraining increases in hypnotic responsiveness are due to compliance factors on the one hand, and to genuine increases in hypnotic ability on the other. In effect, the simulator control group does not really serve its intended function in this experiment.[4]

Another recent report addresses the compliance issue in a more focused and compelling fashion (Bates et al., 1988). The authors of this investigation reasoned that if subjects initially selected for their low hypnotizability were provided a phony rationale for receiving Spanos's skills training program, they would be less disposed to see posttraining increases in hypnotic ability as the *raison d'être* of the investigation. Consequently, one group of people receiving this training program was told that the purpose of the study "was to increase hypnotic suggestibility to see whether imaging ability increased along with it" (Bates et al., 1988, p. 122). The assumption was that if these subjects were persuaded by this rationale for the training program, they would be less pressured to respond positively to a second, posttraining assessment of hypnotic ability, introduced as part of a completely independent experiment. This "experimental condition" could then be compared on the second test of hypnotic responsiveness to two other conditions. In one of these other conditions, subjects were treated like those receiving the complete training package in the initial (Gorassini & Spanos, 1986) study (the "replication condition"); in the other condition, subjects were simply hypnotized a second time (the "practice condition"). All three CURSS indices (i.e., O, S, and O-I) and analogous indices on the Harvard Group Scale of Hypnotic Susceptibility (HGSHS; Shor & Orne, 1962), were employed as dependent variables for both initial screening and subsequent testing for treatment effects.

The findings of this experiment indicated that the replication condition showed a significant increase from initial to test assessment of hypnotic responsiveness on four of the six indices of hypnotic responsiveness (all three CURSS indices and the HGSHS:O), whereas in the experimental condition (i.e., the one presented with a phony rationale), only one of the six indices, the CURSS:O, increased significantly. As mentioned previously, this particular index may well reflect a subject's understanding that subsequent suggestions should be regarded as a simple request for overt compliance.

Evidently, providing a false rationale for the training program lessens the need to comply with the demand for increased hypnotic responsiveness when it is subsequently assessed—particularly on those indices that tap subjective experience rather than overt behavior. In addition, the data reported by Bates et al. (1988) indicate that the mean number of created highs in their replication group (the one comparable to those run by Spanos and his associates) was only about 26%, rather than the 50–80% reported by Spanos and his colleagues. A similarly modest increase was also found in another replication attempt by Gfeller et al. (1987). In sum, demands for compliance considerably influence subjects' hypnotic responsiveness after receiving Spanos's cognitive skills training program; what is more, such demands seem to be an even greater factor in Spanos's laboratory than in those of other sympathetic investigators attempting to replicate his work.

Finally, Bates et al. (1988) conducted a 4-month follow-up of some of the subjects who had been run in either the replication or the experimental condition. They were administered only the CURSS on this occasion. None of the three CURSS indices differed from one condition to the other, nor did any of the follow-up means differ from those achieved at initial (baseline) assessment. So the gains that had been demonstrated immediately after training were not maintained 4 month's later—an outcome that is inconsistent with an earlier longitudinal report from Spanos's lab (Spanos, Cross, Menary, & Smith, 1987). Given the previously mentioned stability of hypnotic ability over a 25-year period (Piccione et al., 1989), the return to pretraining baseline after 4 months should perhaps not be surprising. Maybe the explicit demands for low subjects to respond hypnotically were simply neutralized by time; alternatively, any genuine gains in hypnotic responsiveness occurring as a result of exposure to the training package may be relatively unstable, compared to naturally occurring high levels of hypnotic responsiveness. In either case, any claim for the long-term effectiveness of the Carleton Skills Training Program is compromised by the Bates et al. (1988) investigation. So too is Spanos's argument that the traditional claims for the stability of hypnotic ability are illusory.

This is not to say that genuine increases in hypnotic responsiveness are impossible to achieve with time and practice. Clinicians have long argued that even subjects who initially appear to be low in hypnotizability may in fact prove to be far more responsive to hypnotic interventions than first impressions would indicate. Even advocates of a trait view acknowledge the possibility that low hypnotic responsiveness may be due to defensiveness and concern over loss of control, and that practice and increased familiarity with the hypnotist and the hypnotic proceedings may help to overcome these initial apprehensions. The report by Gfeller et al. (1987) is a particularly persuasive account of how special training may in fact increase hypnotic responsiveness, and may generalize to hypnotic suggestions never before encountered. However, these latter investigators especially emphasize the role of rapport in effecting substantial increases in hypnotic ability. It will be interesting to see whether future research assigns as much importance (or more) to subtle interpersonal factors as to specific training regimens in the enhancement of hypnotic responsiveness.

Finally, it should be noted that a trait of hypnotic ability does not imply that hypnotic responsiveness is competely fixed. Rather, it implies constraints on the degree to which hypnotic responsiveness will vary as a function of experience. An analogy to music may be helpful here. A person with marginal musical talent will never be converted into a Mozart, no matter how much he or she practices; nevertheless, such a person will learn to play the piano much better with practice. This improvement does not mean that musical ability *qua* trait does not exist. Similarly, improvement in hypnotic responsiveness as a result of practice does not tell against the existence of hypnotic ability, which constrains the extent to which such change is likely to occur. Thus we can almost agree with Gfeller et al. (1987) when they assert that "there is no intrinsic conflict between the contention that hypnotizability can be modified and enhanced and the notion that certain personal attributes and abilities exist that are stable, enduring, and perhaps resistant to modification" (p. 594). We would only change the word "hypnotizability" in this quotation to "hypnotic responsiveness," and reserve the word "hypnotizability" for those "personal attributes and abilities . . . that are stable, enduring, and perhaps resistant to modification."

Is Hypnotic Behavior Purposeful or Nonvolitional? Some Empirical Findings

When hypnotized subjects are asked about their hypnotic experience, they are likely to say that suggested behaviors "happened by themselves," or that they "did nothing to achieve the suggested state of affairs." According to the social-psychological position of hypnosis, however, these reports of nonvolitional experience should not be taken at face value. However fascinating and compelling this experience may seem, the hypnotic subject is *mistaken* in interpreting his or her behavior as nonvolitional. The subject is simply not viewed as competent to judge whether or not behavior is purposefully achieved. Instead, the social-psychological position asserts that when hypnotic behavior is consistent with the wording of suggestions, and when the subject reports any imagery or other cognitions consistent with the suggested state of affairs, the behavior is regarded as actively, purposefully, and volitionally achieved, regardless of how the subject experiences it. To quote Spanos (1986b) directly,

> Hypnotic subjects often report that their suggested responses occurred involuntarily. According to social-role interpretation, subjects who make such reports retain control over their behavior. Nevertheless, the wording of suggestions and other cues in the test situation leads these subjects to interpret their actions as involuntary. . . . Subjects who interpret their responses as involuntary experience them as such and report accordingly. However, the fact that subjects may be sincere in stating that their statements occurred involuntarily does not mean that their statements are correct. Sincere reports of having lost control over suggested responses can simply be mistaken. (p. 490)

In general, it is quite clear from Spanos's writings that he considers it virtually impossible for purposeful, goal-directed behavior to be involuntary (Spanos, 1982). By contrast, our position is that the experience of nonvolition, which so frequently accompanies a hypnotic response, results from the fact that executive initiative and effort are minimally involved in its production. Instead, subsystems of control are more or less directly activated by hypnotic suggestions. The behavior that results is purposeful, in the sense that it is goal-oriented and achieves the purposes described by the suggestions; but the behavior is also involuntary, in the sense that it is not performed *on purpose* (i.e., it does not flow from executive initiative and effort).

Perhaps an analogy to physical theories of motion usefully highlights the difference between a social-psychological and a neodissociative account of hypnotic responsiveness in general, and of nonvolition in particular. Aristotle proposed that a constant force was necessary to keep an object moving at a constant rate. Newton, on the other hand, proposed that an object in motion stayed in motion until opposed by a countervailing force—friction, for example. There is a sense in which the social-psychological theory of hypnosis has an Aristotelian flavor. Spanos, for example, proposes that an ongoing cognitive "force" (read "strategic enactment") is required to achieve a hypnotic response such as suggested analgesia. The neodissociative view, on the other hand, is more Newtonian, since it implies that analgesia to cold pressor is not something that requires ongoing executive effort, but is set into motion by suggestions that activate subsystems of pain control. Once activated, hypnotic analgesia has a momentum that does not require a constant cognitive (i.e., executive) "force" to maintain it.

Analogies can themselves be more forceful than reality warrants, so the question remains whether the distinction highlighted in this analogy can be sustained by productive research. Below are summaries of two studies recently completed at the University of Waterloo hypnosis laboratory. Each study in its own way addresses the issue of whether or not high-level cognitive work is required to achieve a hypnotically suggested state of affairs.

Is High-Level Cognitive Work Required to Produce Hypnotic Analgesia?

The second half of M. E. Miller's (1986) doctoral dissertation begins with the premise that if executive initiative and ongoing cognitive work are necessary to maintain effective strategies to counter pain, this process should involve considerable allocation of attention and effort (cf. Kahneman, 1973). Such an ongoing allocation of high-level cognitive work to reduce pain should in turn diminish the available resources for performing a concurrent, cognitively demanding task. The diminished capacity to perform this secondary task should occur even if the cognitive effort required to produce analgesia is hidden from consciousness by an amnesia-like barrier, as Hilgard has sometimes proposed (E. R. Hilgard, 1977b). Indeed, the effort involved in erecting such an amnesic barrier should further tax a person's cognitive resources (Stevenson, 1976; Knox et al., 1975), thereby impairing a concurrent task even more. However, suppose that hypnotic analgesia is achieved, not by an ongoing allocation of high-level cognitive resources, but by a suggestion-activated subsytem of pain control. If this were true, a highly hypnotizable person administered suggestions for hypnotic analgesia could perhaps show reduced pain without impairing performance on a concurrent, cognitively demanding task.

To examine this possibility, Miller (1986) selected 36 subjects who were first screened for their low and high hypnotizability on the HGSHS, and then scored less than 4 or more than 8 on a group adaptation of the SHSS:C (Weitzenhoffer & Hilgard, 1962). The 18 high and 18 low subjects remained unaware that the research had anything to do with hypnosis unless and until they were actually hypnotized. The experimenter was blind regarding the subjects' hypnotic ability throughout the entire experiment.

Each subject was administered three successive subtests of the Nelson Denny Reading Test (Brown, Bennett, & Hanna, 1973). This test adopts a multiple-choice format, in which the subject is given a word to define and five single-word definitions to choose from, only one of which is correct. After an initial baseline assessment of vocabulary, the subject was assessed again, this time while the subject's forearm was submerged in circulating ice water. It was assumed that pain caused by this pretreatment immersion in the cold pressor would impair a person's ability to perform well on the reading test.

Before a second immersion in the cold pressor took place, subjects were either hypnotized and administered suggestions for hypnotic analgesia, or told to use various cognitive strategies they had just learned in order to cope with cold-pressor pain. Then, during a posttreatment immersion in cold pressor, subjects took yet a third form of the reading test. The design of this study permitted Miller to answer the following question: Assuming that the two treatments were about equally effective in reducing pain, does hypnotic analgesia interfere less with performance on the reading test than a treatment requiring the purposeful marshaling of cognitive strategies?

Let us look first at the pain data. Subjects gave retrospective pain ratings from 1 to 10 concerning the level of pain experienced at the beginning, middle, and end of the cold-pressor immersion. There was no difference in the effectiveness of hypnotic analgesia and cognitive strategies, and both interventions were more effective for high than for low subjects. Since the two treatments were equally effective in reducing the pain of the cold pressor, it is legitimate to ask whether, as predicted, the cognitive cost of reducing pain was greater for subjects in the cognitive strategy condition than it was for subjects in the hypnotic analgesia condition.

From its baseline assessment, performance on the reading test declined by about 35% during the first (pretreatment) immersion in the cold pressor. Clearly, the pain of the cold pressor adversely affected subjects' ability to perform a cognitively demanding task. What, then, was the effect of the two different treatment interventions on the reading test during the last cold-pressor immersion?

For both high and low subjects in the cognitive strategy condition, there was an additional drop of about 30% in their vocabulary performance from pre- to posttreatment immersion in the cold-pressor. This reduction in the subjects' reading test scores occurred despite the fact that they successfully reduced pain—presumably through the use of cognitive strategies that further interfered with their ability to deal with the reading test. The situation in the hypnotic analgesia condition was quite different. The low subjects showed only a slight additional decrease (8%) in their reading test performance from the pre- to posttreatment immersion in the cold pressor; the high subjects, on the other hand, showed a slight (10%) *increase* in their vocabulary performance from the pre- to posttreatment immersion. In other words, despite the fact that hypnotic analgesia was quite effective in reducing the highs' pain, it permitted some recovery of the cognitive functioning that was badly impaired by the pain of the cold pressor. Presumably, this modest recovery was due to the fact that hypnotic analgesia made the cold pressor less painful, and did so in a manner that did not require diverting conscious attention from the reading test.

Miller's study demonstrates (as do many others) that cognitive strategies are effective in reducing pain, but in addition, her study shows that such strategies impair performance on a competing task in a manner that is not true of hypnotic analgesia. The fact that hypnotic analgesia does not impair performance on the competing task strongly suggests that its effectiveness does not depend on the subject's utilization of high-level cognitive resources. Rather, hypnotic analgesia seems to involve the dissociated control of pain—in other words, control that is relatively free of the need for high-level, executive effort. This pattern of findings is difficult to explain by a social-psychological model.

Moreover, Miller's findings give striking support to the notion that the suggested state of affairs can serve a purpose without any implication that it is enacted on purpose. Hypnotic analgesia reduces pain and is therefore beneficial to the hypnotized person; in this sense, it clearly serves or achieves an important purpose. However, because executive initiative and ongoing effort are apparently not required to produce hypnotic analgesia, it seems inappropriate to view the reduction in pain as something achieved on purpose. Unfortunately, by referring to the suggested state of affairs as "purposefully" achieved, Spanos and his colleagues do not make the distinction between "achieving a purpose" and "behaving *on purpose*." However, as the Miller investigation clarifies, this distinction may be critical to an understanding of how hypnotic responsiveness can be both purposeful and nonvolitional—a state of affairs that seems contradictory to advocates of a social-psychological model of hypnosis.

The next investigation further documents the point that hypnotic suggestions can engender behavior that is both purposeful (in the sense of achieving the suggested state of affairs) and nonvolitional (in the sense that executive initiative and ongoing effort do not seem required to achieve this purpose).

Wherefore Nonvolition? The Heart of the Matter

As already indicated, one of the most striking features of hypnotically suggested behavior is that its enactment is typically experienced as nonvolitional or effortless—as something that happens to the person, rather than something actively achieved (the so-called "classic suggestion effect"). From the neodissociative point of view, the experience of nonvolition means one of two things: Either a subsystem of control has been activated by the hypnotic suggestions in a manner that does not require executive initiative and effort, or the executive effort required to achieve the hypnotically suggested state of affairs is hidden behind an amnesic barrier. Both of these possibilities have been proposed by E. R. Hilgard (1977b). However, if the M. E. Miller (1986) findings just reported are at all representative, the experience of nonvolition is due more to the relative absence of executive control in producing a hypnotic response than it is to amnesia for it. Note that for amnesia to account for nonvolitional experience, it would in most cases have to be spontaneous rather than suggested amnesia. Given the rarity of spontaneous amnesia (Cooper, 1966), it is just as well that the neodissociation model of hypnosis has an alternative way of accounting for nonvolitional experience.

In a recent dissertation completed in the University of Waterloo laboratory, Hughes (1988) examined the experience of nonvolition in a novel way—via heart rate indices of cognitive effort. She employed heart rate as a dependent measure because past research (Lacey, 1967; Kahneman, Tursky, Shapiro, & Crider, 1969) had demonstrated that cognitive effort involved in generating imagery and other internal information is accompanied by heart rate increase: The more effort, the greater the heart rate increase. Thus, heart rate has some claim to being a reasonable index of cognitive work.

However, heart rate does not singularly reflect just one aspect of psychological functioning. For example, heart rate increases have also been successfully used to index emotionality, especially fear (e.g., Bauer & Craighead, 1979). Whether heart rate increases reflect cognitive effort or emotional arousal presumably depends on the specific experimental conditions. In particular, under conditions of neutral imagery, an increase in heart rate should reflect primarily the cognitive effort required to maintain a suggested image. Under conditions of fear imagery, however, past research indicates that an increase in heart rate registers emotional arousal. Since highly hypnotizable subjects become more emotionally involved in their imaginings than lows (J. R. Hilgard, 1979; Tellegen & Atkinson, 1974), imagining fearful scenes should increase heart rate more for high than for low subjects.

However, the main point of Hughes's research was to investigate whether heart rate changes to neutral and fear imagery would correlate with subjects' retrospective ratings of the effort involved in generating imagery, and of the fear accompanying it. The hope was that if heart rate changes did correlate with effort and fear ratings, they would do so differentially for highs and lows, and in a manner that would help clarify the relative merits of the neodissociative and social-psychological accounts of hypnotically suggested behavior.

Hughes first selected 30 low and 30 high male subjects, each of whom scored between 0–4 or 8–12, first on the HGSHS, and then on a group adaptation of the SHSS:C. Following earlier work conducted in our laboratory by Rothmar (1986), subjects were then administered three trials of neutral and three trials of fearful images in counterbalanced order. After each imagery trial, subjects were asked to rate on separate 7-point scales both the effort required to produce the imagery, and the amount of associated fear. Heart rate was continuously monitored throughout by electrodes attached to the sternum and ribs, and recorded on a Beckman RP dynagraph. For each subject, the mean amount of heart rate change from a pretrial baseline was calculated for the three fearful and the three neutral imagery trials. Mean heart rate change and ratings of fear and effort served as the main dependent variables.

The main analysis of Hughes's investigation concerned the pattern of correlations between the three dependent variables. Since she ran 30 high and 30 low subjects, Hughes could examine the relatively stable relationships that emerged *within* each level of hypnotic ability. The hope was that, despite the range restriction imposed by examining only highs and lows, reliable and meaningful differences in the two groups would emerge in how heart rate change correlated with the two rating variables.

For low subjects, the correlation between heart rate change and ratings of effortfulness was about .50 for both neutral and fearful imagery; evidently, the more effort required to "build" an image, the more the heart rate increased. This positive relationship between effort ratings and cardiac indices of cognitive effort is precisely what a social-psychological model would predict. Moreover, when lows engaged in fearful imagery, the correlation between effort and fear ratings was .66, indicating that the more cognitive work they expended to create a fearful image, the more frightened they became. This outcome also makes good sense from a Spanosian perspective. However, fear ratings and heart rate increase for these subjects correlated only .16, suggesting that for low subjects in this experiment, heart rate did not register fear very well.

For high subjects, the pattern of findings was very different. Effort ratings and heart rate correlated $-.05$ under conditions of neutral imagery. Evidently, for the highs, an increase in heart rate did *not* index the cognitive effort involved in producing suggested imagery. Moreover, for fear imagery, the correlation of $-.52$ between heart rate and effort ratings suggests that within high subjects, the *less* cognitive effort involved in imagining a fearful scene, the *more* heart rate increased. Furthermore, a correlation of .59 between heart rate increase and fear ratings suggests that for highs, unlike lows, cardiac responding registered emotionality (rather than cognitive effort). Finally, for the highs, the lower the ratings of cognitive effort, the *higher* the ratings of fear ($r = -.68$)—implying that fear was potentiated by experiencing it as nonvolitional.

Subsequent partial correlation analyses substantiate the impression that heart rate increase reflected cognitive effort for low subjects, and fear for highs. Thus, for lows in the fearful imagery condition, when ratings of fear were partialed out of the (.49) correlation between effort ratings and heart rate increase, the relationship remained virtually unchanged ($r = .52$)—implying that for them, the relationship between cognitive effort and increased heart rate was not mediated by fear. In highs, on the other hand, partialing out the impact of fear on the sizeable negative correlation between effort ratings and heart rate increase substantially reduced the relationship (from $-.52$ to $-.20$). So, for high subjects, fear seems to have been largely responsible for the substantial negative relationship between effort ratings and heart rate increase.

In sum, for low subjects, the more cognitive effort they expended to produce hypnotically suggested imagery, the more their heart rate increased, and the higher they rated their fear (to fearful imagery). This "Aristotelian" pattern of data accords quite well with the predictions of a social-psychological theory of hypnosis, which argues that active and purposeful (i.e., intentional) deployment of high-level cognitive strategies is required to achieve the hypnotically suggested state of affairs. However, the "Newtonian" pattern of data from the high subjects does not fulfill the social-psychological model at all. When highs engaged in neutral imagery, they demonstrated no correlation between ratings of cognitive effort on the one hand, and heart rate increase on the other. The implication is that ongoing cognitive effort was not involved in maintaining neutral imagery. Once this imagery was set in motion, it had its own psychological momentum. And when highs engaged in fear imagery, *less* rated effort was associated with *more* fear and heart rate increase. Perhaps experiencing fear imagery as effortless and nonvolitional—that is, as not being under conscious control—was alarming in its own right, and contributed to the emotional arousal of the high subjects.

This possibility may help account for the fact that heart rate increases associated with fear imagery were significantly greater for high than for low subjects. Analysis revealed that in response to fear imagery, highs demonstrated 1.8 times more heart rate increase than lows, whereas such increases for both highs and lows were relatively small and about equal *vis à vis* neutral imagery. Average effort and fear ratings for both levels of hypnotizability and imagery were also examined. Highs showed a significantly lower average effort rating for neutral imagery than did lows— implying that the classic suggestion effect was more evident in highs than in lows. Fearful imagery also generated lower effort ratings in highs than in lows, but the difference did not quite reach significance. As far as fear ratings are concerned, there was, unsurprisingly, no difference between lows and highs in the neutral imagery condition. However, in the fear imagery condition, highs, as predicted, rated themselves as significantly more fearful than did lows.

All in all, the findings from the high subjects fit a neodissociation model of hypnosis quite well. This model predicts that hypnotically suggested behavior is not necessarily due to high-level, executive effort, but instead occurs when a dissociated subsystem of control is more or less directly activated by suggestions. That is what Hughes's study seems to have demonstrated. The findings imply that a suggested state of affairs can be achieved nonvolitionally while nevertheless achieving the purposes set out by the suggestions. In other words, hypnotic responses can be purposeful without being enacted on purpose.

SUMMARY AND CONCLUSIONS

Spanos has occasionally demonstrated a real appreciation of work in cognitive psychology as a point of entry into understanding hypnotic phenomena. This appreciation was particularly evident in his earlier work on hypnotic amnesia, where encoding specificity, for example, played a major role in his thinking (Spanos & Bodorik, 1977). However, with time, he seems more and more committed to a social-psychological account of hypnosis (Spanos, 1986a, 1986b). The careful reader will discern three main aspects to this account.

First of all, the concept of strategic enactment emerges over and over again in his writings. Strategic enactment involves goal-oriented, purposeful behavior in accordance with the suggested state of affairs. Second, these strategic enactments are motivated, and the source of the motivation is the desire to self-present as a deeply hypnotized subject. Thus, at least part of the reason for individual differences in hypnotic responsiveness resides in differential levels of motivation rather than of hypnotic ability per se. Finally, there is an idea, increasingly evident in Spanos's recent writings, of a final common pathway for hypnotic responsiveness. This pathway consists of the way in which subjects typically interpret hypnotic suggestions. Highly hypnotizable subjects tend to interpret suggestions as something they must actively achieve; low subjects, on the other hand, typically interpret the suggested state of affairs as something that will simply happen to them. This difference in the typical interpretation of hypnotic suggestions is another (and modifiable) basis for individual differences in hypnotic responsiveness. The essence of hypnotic responsiveness for Spanos thus involves motivated, contextually guided strategic enactments in accordance with hypnotic suggestions that are interpreted as something to achieve actively and purposefully. In effect, hypnotic behaviors are consciously intended, initiated, and controlled, even though they may be mistakenly interpreted by the subject as nonvolitional visitations.

What is most definitely *not* required for a proper understanding of hypnosis, according to Spanos, is any "special process" of dissociation. To be sure, the concept of dissociation as it has emerged in the hypnosis literature is imprecise around the edges, and it is sometimes invoked in sloppy and ill-defined ways. But the center of the idea is not at all mysterious: As indicated earlier, it simply points to the fact that not everything people do or achieve is consciously intended, initiated, or controlled (Kihlstrom, 1984, 1987). The possibility for such "dissociated control" (Bowers, 1990; M. E. Miller & Bowers, 1990) in everyday life is particularly well revealed in various mental lapses, but is the basis for hypnotic responsiveness as well. Such dissociated control of thought and behavior depends on a hierarchical model of mind, which assumes—quite reasonably, we think—that different cognitive control systems can operate in relative independence of each other.

Such functional independence is well illustrated by the fact that "forgotten memories" can nevertheless affect thought and behavior (e.g., Jacoby & Witherspoon, 1982). Schacter (1987) has been particularly vigorous in espousing the view that so-called "implicit memories" demonstrably influence thought and behavior, even though they are not explicitly (consciously) recalled. In other words, implicit memories are dissociated from the conscious experience of them. Such dissociations are most clearly seen in neurologically damaged patients (Squire, 1986), but are by no means confined to them. Indeed, many of the contributors to a recent volume honoring Endel Tulving (Roediger & Craik, 1989) speak quite respectfully of mental dissociations of one kind or another. Thus, Spanos's evident disdain for dissociation is more and more a rearguard action that is unresponsive to current developments in cognitive psychology.

In many respects, Spanos's treatment of hypnosis participates in a long tradition of rationalism, in which autonomy and control are identified with the *conscious* control of thought and behavior. The possibility that thought and behavior might have unconscious influences is repugnant to devotees of rationalism, which is one reason why Freud has had such a difficult reception in some quarters. However, Freud's emphasis on unconscious motivation as an important influence on thought and behavior, although doubtless of considerable importance in everyday life, has relatively little bearing on "garden variety" hypnosis as ordinarily seen in the research laboratory. Rather, specific cognitive mechanisms are implicated, including dissociation of various cognitive control systems from each other. Ordinarily, the integration of these systems under executive guidance and monitoring provides the basis for everyday, goal-oriented thought and behavior. However, the fact that subsystems of control can operate in relative independence of each other, and of high-level, executive control, means that purposeful behavior need not always flow from conscious intentions and purposes; it can also be directly and discriminatively responsive to meaningful stimulation (as when a sleeping mother awakens to the cry of her baby, but not to the much louder sounds of a passing truck). In addition, the multiple and independent controls that influence thought and behavior permit subsystems of control to be more or less directly activated by hypnotic suggestions. This relatively direct activation of the suggested state of affairs circumvents executive initiative and effort; consequently, hypnotic responses are typically experienced as nonvolitional.

By way of contrast, Spanos places all his eggs in the basket of conscious control and purposes; in doing so, he does not acknowledge the multiple and independent controls that engender thought and behavior. His recalcitrance in this regard makes Spanos's social-psychological theory of hypnosis as single-minded as his defense of it.

Acknowledgments. We would like to thank Jeffrey S. Bowers for his comments on an earlier draft of this chapter. Research conducted at the University of Waterloo that is reported in this chapter was supported by the Social Sciences and Humanities Research Council of Canada, and by the Spencer Foundation of Chicago.

NOTES

1. These data were derived from a computer search of *Psychological Abstracts*, using the descriptors "hypnosis" and "hypnotic susceptibility" as the search terms.
2. The means for the four conditions, averaged across the five report intervals are as follows: In the stress inoculation condition, the lows scored .73 and the highs .72; in the hypnotic analgesia condition, the lows scored .76 and the highs scored .57. The data is presented as the log of pain ratings from 1 to 10, with some subjects

reporting even higher pain ratings if they could tolerate remaining in the cold-pressor stimulus beyond the point at which they very much wanted to remove their arms. There were no significant interactions involving report interval.

3. Rather than comparing high and low subjects, Spanos and Katsanis (1989) exposed highs to active or passive suggestions for analgesia, administered with or without a prior hypnotic induction. They did so under the expectation that "both hypnotic and nonhypnotic subjects can be led to define their pain reduction as either passive occurrences or active achievements, depending on the interpretive set fostered by the wording of the instructions they are administered" (p. 183). And indeed, subjects exposed to active suggestions later rated their analgesia as achieved volitionally, whereas subjects exposed to the passive suggestions rated the analgesia as nonvolitionally achieved. However, the fact that only high subjects were run means that all the subjects in the experiment were highly responsive to suggestion—not only for analgesia, but for experiencing their achievement of it in a particular way (whether actively, passively, or as a result of tapping their feet in waltz time). Consequently, the differences Spanos and Katsanis obtained in the experiential reports of subjects exposed to active or passive suggestions simply means that highly hypnotizable subjects are very responsive to suggestions. But everyone already knew and agreed to that, so this outcome does not distinguish the neodissociative from the social-psychological model of hypnosis—claims to the contrary notwithstanding.

4. The simulator control is used to assess the existence of task demands that inform hypnotized subjects how to behave (Orne, 1979). Obviously, hypnotic suggestions are themselves demand characteristics, and they therefore inform subjects how to comply if that is what they want to do. So when simulator controls are used, there is typically an expectation for hypnotic suggestions to be realized in a somewhat counterintuitive way that will not be fully anticipated by simulator subjects. This simulator design has been used very effectively on occasion (e.g., Evans & Orne, 1971; Gray, Bowers, & Fenz, 1970), but it is a logistically difficult and conceptually subtle design that cannot be recommended as a matter of course. When simulators overplay the role of hypnotized subjects, it simply means that the task demands are very easy to read and comply with. Such an outcome does *not* imply that genuinely hypnotized subjects are merely complying with the hypnotic suggestions. Consequently, in the Spanos et al. (1986) investigation, the use of simulators tells us nothing about why the genuinely hypnotized subjects behaved the way they did.

REFERENCES

Barber, T. X. (1969). *Hypnosis: A scientific approach.* New York: Van Nostrand Reinhold.
Barber, T. X. (1970). *LSD, marihuana, yoga, and hypnosis.* New York: Aldine.

Bates, B. L., Miller, R. J., Cross, H. J., & Brigham, T. A. (1988). Modifying hypnotic suggestibility with the Carleton Skills Training Program. *Journal of Personality and Social Psychology, 55,* 120–127.

Bauer, R. M., & Craighead, W. E. (1979). Psychological responses to the imagination of fearful and neutral situations: The effects of imagery instructions. *Behavior Therapy, 10,* 389–403.

Bertrand, L. D., & Spanos, N. P. (1985). The organization of recall during hypnotic suggestions for complete and selective amnesia. *Imagination, Cognition and Personality, 4,* 249–261.

Bowers, K. S. (1983). *Hypnosis for the seriously curious.* New York: Norton. (Originally published in 1976)

Bowers, K. S. (1990). Unconscious influences and hypnosis. In J.L. Singer (Ed.), *Repression and dissociation: Defense mechanisms and personality styles,* (pp. 143–179). Chicago: University of Chicago Press.

Breuer, J., & Freud, S. (1974). *Studies on hysteria* (J. Strachey, Trans.). Harmondsworth, England: Pelican. (Original work published 1893–1895)

Brown, J. I., Bennett, J. M., & Hanna, G. (1973). *Nelson-Denny reading test.* Boston: Houghton-Mifflin.

Brown, R. W., & McNeill, D. (1966). The "tip-of-the-tongue" phenomenon. *Journal of Verbal Learning and Verbal Behavior, 79,* 325–337.

Cooper, L. (1966). Spontaneous and suggested posthypnotic source amnesia. *International Journal of Clinical and Experimental Hypnosis, 14,* 180–193.

Davidson, T. M. (1986). *Recall organization and volitional/nonvolitional experiencing in posthypnotic and intrahypnotic amnesia: Inattention versus dissociation hypothesis.* Unpublished doctoral dissertation, University of Waterloo, Waterloo, Ontario, Canada.

Davidson, T. M., & Bowers, K. S. (1982). *Recall disorganization, volitional/ nonvolitional experiencing, and posthypnotic amnesia: Inattention versus dissociation paradigms.* Paper presented at the annual convention of the Society for Clinical and Experimental Hypnosis, Indianapolis.

Davidson, T. M., & Bowers, K. S. (1983). *Controls without awareness: Dissociative strategies of hypnotic amnesia.* Paper presented at the annual convention of the Society for Clinical and Experimental Hypnosis, Boston.

Davidson, T. M., & Bowers, K. S. (1991). Selective hypnotic amnesia: Is it a successful attempt to forget or an unsuccessful attempt to remember? *Journal of Abnormal Psychology, 100,* 133–143.

Diamond, M. J. (1977). Hypnotizability is modifiable: An alternative approach. *International Journal of Clinical and Experimental Hypnosis, 25,* 147–166.

Ellenberger, H. (1970). *The discovery of the unconscious: The history and evolution of dynamic psychology.* New York: Basic Books.

Erdelyi, M. (1985). *Psychoanalysis: Freud's cognitive psychology.* New York: W. H. Freeman.

Evans, F. J., & Orne, M. T. (1971). The disappearing hypnotist: The use of simulating subjects to evaluate how subjects perceive experimental procedures. *International Journal of Clinical and Experimental Hypnosis, 19,* 277–296.

Gfeller, J. D., Lynn, S. J., & Pribble, W. E. (1987). Enhancing hypnotic susceptibility: Interpersonal and rapport factors. *Journal of Personality and Social Psychology, 52,* 586–595.

Gill, M. M., & Brenman, M. (1959). *Hypnosis and related states.* New York: International Universities Press.

Gorassini, D. R., & Spanos, N. P. (1986). A social-cognitive skills approach to the successful modification of hypnotic susceptibility. *Journal of Personality and Social Psychology, 50*, 1004–1012.

Gray, A. L., Bowers, K. S., & Fenz, W. D. (1970). Heart rate in anticipation of and during a negative visual hallucination. *International Journal of Clinical and Experimental Hypnosis, 18*, 41–51.

Heckhausen, H., & Beckmann, J. (1990). Intentional action and action slips. *Psychological Review, 97*, 36–48.

Hilgard, E. R. (1965). *Hypnotic susceptibility.* New York: Harcourt, Brace & World.

Hilgard, E. R. (1973a). A neodissociation theory of pain reduction in hypnosis. *Psychological Review, 80*, 396–411.

Hilgard, E. R. (1973b). The domain of hypnosis: With some comments on alternative paradigms. *American Psychologist, 28*, 972–982.

Hilgard, E. R. (1977a). The problem of divided consciousness: A neodissociation interpretation. *Annals of the New York Academy of Sciences, 296*, 48–59.

Hilgard, E. R. (1977b). *Divided consciousness: Multiple controls in human thought and action.* New York: Wiley.

Hilgard, E. R. (1979). Divided consciousness in hypnosis: The implications of the hidden observer. In E. Fromm, & R. E. Shor (Eds.), *Hypnosis: Developments in research and new perspectives* (2nd ed., pp. 45–79). Hawthorne, NY: Aldine.

Hilgard, E. R., & Hilgard, J. R. (1975). *Hypnosis in the relief of pain.* Los Altos, CA: William Kaufmann.

Hilgard, E. R., & Tart, C. T. (1966). Responsiveness to suggestions following waking and imagination instructions and following induction of hypnosis. *Journal of Abnormal Psychology, 71*, 196–208.

Hilgard, J.R. (1979). *Personality and hypnosis: A study of imaginative involvement* (2nd ed.). Chicago: University of Chicago Press.

Hilgard, J. R., & LeBaron, S. (1984). *Hypnotherapy of pain in children with cancer.* Los Altos, CA: William Kaufmann.

Hughes, D. (1988). *Factors related to heart rate change for high and low hypnotizables during imagery.* Unpublished doctoral dissertation, University of Waterloo, Waterloo, Ontario, Canada.

Hull, C.L. (1933). *Hypnosis and suggestibility.* New York: Appleton-Century.

Jacoby, L. L., & Witherspoon, D. (1982). Remembering without awareness. *Canadian Journal of Psychology, 36*, 300–324.

Janet, P. (1901). *The mental state of hystericals* (E. Paul and C. Paul Trans.). New York: G. P. Putnam.

Janet, P. (1965). *The major symptoms of hysteria* (E. Paul and C. Paul Trans.). New York: Hafner. (Original work published 1907)

Kahneman, D. (1973). *Attention and effort.* Englewood Cliffs, NJ: Prentice-Hall.

Kahneman, D., Tursky, B., Shapiro, D., & Crider, A. (1969). Pupillary, heart rate, and skin resistance changes during a mental task. *Journal of Experimental Psychology, 79*, 164–167.

Kihlstrom, J. F. (1980). Posthypnotic amnesia for recently learned material: Interactions with "episodic" and "semantic" memory. *Cognitive Psychology, 12*, 227–251.

Kihlstrom, J. F. (1983). Instructed forgetting: hypnotic and nonhypnotic. *Journal of Experimental Psychology: General, 112,* 73–79.

Kihlstrom, J. F. (1984). Conscious, subconscious, unconscious: A cognitive perspective. In K. S. Bowers & D. Meichenbaum (Eds.), *The unconscious reconsidered* (pp. 149–211). New York: Wiley.

Kihlstrom, J. F. (1986). Strong inferences about hypnosis. *Behavioral and Brain Sciences, 9,* 474–475.

Kihlstrom, J. F. (1987). The cognitive unconscious. *Science, 237,* 1445–1452.

Kihlstrom, J. F., & Evans, F. J. (1979). Memory retrieval processes during posthypnotic amnesia. In J. F. Kihlstrom & F. J. Evans (Eds.), *Functional disorders of memory* (pp. 179–218). Hillsdale, NJ: Erlbaum.

Knox, J., Crutchfield, L., & Hilgard, E. R. (1975). The nature of task interference in hypnotic dissociation: An investigation of hypnotic behavior. *International Journal of Clinical and Experimental Hypnosis, 23,* 305–323.

Lacey, J. (1967). Somatic response patterning and stress: Some revisions of activation theory. In M. H. Appley & R. Trumbell (Eds.), *Psychological stress* (pp. 14–37). New York: Appleton-Century-Crofts.

Miller, G. A., Galanter, E., & Pribram, K. H. (1960). *Plans and the structure of behavior.* New York: Holt.

Miller, M. E. (1986). *Hypnotic analgesia and stress inoculation in the reduction of cold-pressor pain.* Unpublished doctoral dissertation, University of Waterloo, Waterloo, Ontario, Canada.

Miller, M. E., & Bowers, K. S. (1986). Hypnotic analgesia and stress inoculation in the reduction of pain. *Journal of Abnormal Psychology, 95,* 6–14.

Miller, M. E., & Bowers, K. S. (1990). *Hypnotic analgesia: Dissociated experience or dissociated control?* Unpublished manuscript.

Morgan, A. H., Johnson, D. L., & Hilgard, E. R. (1974). The stability of hypnotic susceptibilty: A longitudinal study. *International Journal of Clinical and Experimental Hypnosis, 22,* 249–257.

Neufeld, W. J., & Thomas, P. (1977). Effects of perceived efficacy of a prophylactic controlling mechanism on self-control under pain stimulation. *Canadian Journal of Behavioral Science, 9,* 224–232.

Nolan, R. P., & Spanos, N. P. (1987). Hypnotic analgesia and stess inoculation: A critical reexamination of Miller and Bowers. *Psychological Reports, 61,* 95–102.

Norman, D. (1981). Categorization of action slips. *Psychological Review, 88,* 1–15.

Orne, M. T. (1966). Hypnosis, motivation, and compliance. *American Journal of Psychiatry, 122,* 721–726.

Orne, M. T. (1979). On the simulating subject as a quasi-control group in hypnosis research: What, why and how. In E. Fromm & R. E. Shor (Eds.), *Hypnosis: Developments in research and new perspectives* (2nd ed., pp. 519–565). Hawthorne, NY: Aldine.

Orne, M. T., Dinges, D. F., & Orne, E. C. (1986). Hypnotic experience: A cognitive social-psychological reality. *Behavioral and Brain Sciences, 9,* 477–478.

Perry, C. (1977). Is hypnotizability modifiable? *International Journal of Clinical and Experimental Hypnosis, 25,* 125–146.

Perry, C., & Laurence, J.-R. (1983). Hypnosis, surgery, and mind–body interaction: An historical evaluation. *Canadian Journal of Behavioral Science, 15,* 351–372.

Perry, C., & Laurence, J.-R. (1984). Mental processing outside of awareness: The contributions of Freud and Janet. In K. Bowers & D. Meichenbaum (Eds.), *The unconscious reconsidered* (pp. 9–48). New York: Wiley.

Piccione, C., Hilgard, E.R., & Zimbardo, P.G. (1989). On the degree of stability of measured hypnotizability over a 25-year period. *Journal of Personality and Social Psychology, 56,* 289–295.

Prince, M. (1915). *The unconscious.* New York: Macmillan.

Radtke-Bodorik, H. L., Planas, M., & Spanos, N. P. (1980). Suggested amnesia, verbal inhibition, and disorganized recall for a long word list. *Canadian Journal of Behavioral Science, 12,* 78–97.

Radtke-Bodorik, H. L., Spanos, N. P., & Haddad, M. G. (1979). The effects of spoken versus written recall on suggested amnesia in hypnotic and task-motivated subjects. *American Journal of Clinical Hypnosis, 22,* 8–16.

Reason, J. T. (1979). Actions not as planned. In G. Underwood & R. Stevens (Eds.), *Aspects of consciousness* (pp. 67–89). London: Academic Press.

Roediger, H. L., & Craik, F. I. M. (Eds.). (1989). *Varieties of memory and consciousness.* Hillsdale, NJ: Erlbaum.

Rosen, G. (1946). Mesmerism and surgery: A strange chapter in the history of anesthesia. *Journal of the History of Medicine,* 527–551.

Rothmar, E. E. (1986). *The relationship between hypnotic ability and heart rate responsiveness to imagery.* Unpublished doctoral dissertation, University of Waterloo, Waterloo, Ontario, Canada.

Schacter, D. L. (1987). Implicit memory: History and current status. *Journal of Experimental Psychology: Learning, Memory, and Cognition, 13,* 501–518.

Schacter, D. L. (1989). On the relation between memory and consciousness: Dissociable interactions and conscious experience. In H. L. Roediger & F. I. M. Craik (Eds.), *Varieties of memory and consciousness* (pp. 355–389). Hillsdale, NJ: Erlbaum.

Shor, R. E. (1959). Hypnosis and the concept of the generalized reality orientation. *American Journal of Psychotherapy, 13,* 582–602.

Shor, R. E. (1970). The three-factor theory of hypnosis as applied to the book-reading fantasy and to the concept of suggestion. *International Journal of Clinical and Experimental Hypnosis, 28,* 89–98.

Shor, R. E., & Orne, E. C. (1962). *Harvard Group Scale of Hypnotic Susceptibility.* Palo Alto, CA: Consulting Psychologists Press.

Spanos, N. P. (1982). Hypnotic behavior: A cognitive, social-psychological perspective. *Research Communications in Psychology, Psychiatry, and Behavior, 7,* 199–213.

Spanos, N. P. (1986a). Hypnotic behavior: A social-psychological interpretation of amnesia, analgesia, and "trance logic." *Behavioral and Brain Sciences, 9,* 449–467.

Spanos, N. P. (1986b). Hypnotic behavior: Special process accounts are still not required. *Behavioral and Brain Sciences, 9,* 776–781.

Spanos, N. P., & Barber, T. X. (1974). Toward a convergence in hypnosis research. *American Psychologist, 29,* 500–511.

Spanos, N. P., & Bodorik, H. L. (1977). Suggested amnesia and disorganized recall in hypnotic and task-motivated subjects. *Journal of Abnormal Psychology, 86,* 295–305.

Spanos, N. P., Brown, J. M., Jones, B., & Horner, D. (1981). Cognitive activity and suggestions for analgesia in the reduction of reported pain. *Journal of Abnormal Psychology, 90,* 554–561.

Spanos, N. P., Cobb, P. C., & Gorassini, D. R. (1985). Failing to resist hypnotic test suggestions: A strategy for self-presenting as deeply hypnotized. *Psychiatry, 48,* 282–292.

Spanos, N. P., Cross, W. F., Menary, E., & Smith, J. (1987). Long term effects of cognitive-skill training for the enhancement of hypnotic susceptibility. *British Journal of Experimental and Clinical Hypnosis, 5,* 73–78.

Spanos, N. P., & de Groh, M. (1984). *Effects of active and passive wording on response to hypnotic and nonhypnotic instructions for complete and selective forgetting.* Paper presented at the annual convention of the American Psychological Association, Toronto.

Spanos, N. P., & D'Eon, J. (1980). Hypnotic amnesia, disorganized recall and inattention. *Journal of Abnormal Psychology, 89,* 744–750.

Spanos, N. P., & Katsanis, J. (1989). Effects of instructional sets on attributions of nonvolition during hypnotic and nonhypnotic analgesia. *Journal of Personality and Social Psychology, 56,* 182–188.

Spanos, N. P., Kennedy, S. K., & Gywnn, M. I. (1984). Moderating effects of contextual variables on the relationship between hypnotic suceptibility and suggested analgesia. *Journal of Abnormal Psychology, 93,* 285–294.

Spanos, N. P., & Radtke, H. L. (1982). Hypnotic amnesia as strategic enactment: A cognitive, social-psychological perspective. *Research Communications in Psychology, Psychiatry, and Behavior, 7,* 215–231.

Spanos, N. P., Radtke, H. L., Hodgins, D. C., Stam, H. J., & Bertrand, L. D. (1983). The Carleton University Responsiveness to Suggestion Scale: Normative data and psychometric properties. *Psychological Reports, 53,* 523–535.

Spanos, N. P., Radtke, H. L., Bertrand, L. D., Addie, D. L., & Drummond, J. (1982). Disorganized recall, hypnotic amnesia and subjects' faking: More disconfirming evidence. *Psychological Reports, 50,* 383–389.

Spanos, N. P., Radtke, H. L., & Dubreuil, D. L. (1982). Episodic and semantic memory in posthypnotic amnesia: A reevaluation. *Journal of Personality and Social Psychology, 43,* 565–573.

Spanos, N. P., Radtke-Bodorik, H. L., & Shabinsky, M. A. (1980). Amnesia, subjective organization and learning of a list of unrelated words in hypnotic and task-motivated subjects. *International Journal of Clinical and Experimental Hypnosis, 28,* 126–139.

Spanos, N. P., Robertson, L. A., Menary, E. P., & Brett, P. J. (1986). Component analysis of cognitive skill training for the enhancement of hypnotic susceptibility. *Journal of Abnormal Psychology, 95,* 350–357.

Spanos, N. P., Robertson, L. A., Menary, E. P., Brett, P. J., & Smith, J. (1987). Effects of repeated baseline testing on cognitive-skill-training-induced increments in hypnotic susceptibility. *Journal of Personality and Social Psychology, 52,* 1230–1235.

Spanos, N. P., Stam, H. J., D'Eon, J. L., Pawlak, A. E., & Radtke-Bodorik, H. L. (1980). The effects of social-psychological variables in hypnotic amnesia. *Journal of Personality and Social Psychology, 39,* 737–750.

Squire, L. R. (1986). Mechanisms of memory. *Science, 232,* 1612–1619.

Stevenson, J. (1976). Effect of posthypnotic dissociation on the performance of interfering tasks. *Journal of Abnormal Psychology, 85,* 398–407.

Tellegen, A., & Atkinson, G. (1974). Openness to absorbing and self-altering experiences ("absorption"), a trait related to hypnotic susceptibility. *Journal of Abnormal Psychology, 83,* 268–277.

Tulving, E., & Thomson, D. M. (1973). Encoding specificity and retrieval processes in episodic memory. *Psychological Review, 80,* 352–373.

Turk, D., Meichenbaum, D. H., & Genest, M. (1983). *Pain and behavioral medicine: A cognitive–behavioral perspective.* New York: Guilford Press.

Uleman, J. S., & Bargh, J. A. (Eds.). (1989). *Unintended thought.* New York: Guilford Press.

Wagstaff, G. F. (1986). Hypnosis as compliance and belief: A sociocognitive view. In P.L.N. Naish (Ed.), *What is hypnosis? Current theories and research* (pp. 59–84). Philadelphia: Open University Press.

Weitzenhoffer, A. M. (1978). Hypnotism and altered states of consciousness. In A. A. Sugarman & R. E. Tarter (Eds.), *Expanding dimensions of consciousness* (pp. 183–225). New York: Springer.

Weitzenhoffer, A. M. (1980). Hypnotic susceptibility revisited. *American Journal of Clinical Hypnosis, 22,* 130–146.

Weitzenhoffer, A. M., & Hilgard, E. R. (1962). *Stanford Hypnotic Susceptibility Scale, Form C.* Palo Alto, CA: Consulting Psychologists Press.

White, R. W., & Shevach, B.J. (1942). Hypnosis and the concept of dissociation. *Journal of Abnormal and Social Psychology, 37,* 309–328.

Hypnotizability: Individual Differences in Dissociation and the Flexible Control of Psychological Processes

FREDERICK J. EVANS
UMDNJ-Robert Wood Johnson Medical School

INTRODUCTION

The aim of this speculative review is to present selected evidence supporting the hypothesis that there is a dimension of individual differences involving dissociation, or a cognitive flexibility in accessing multiple cognitive and/or psychodynamic pathways, or the ability to switch easily between different psychological states. Hypnosis is one special manifestation of this dimension of flexible control. As I indulgently engage in a somewhat speculative 35-year progress report on my understanding of the hypnotic phenomenon, I would like to set the stage much as it was set for me as an undergraduate in 1954 at the University of Sydney, by a case vignette (Bagby, 1928).

Bagby relates the case of a teenage girl he was unsuccessfully treating for phobia of running water. One day the girl reported that an aunt, whom she had not seen since she was 4 years old, had come to town and had greeted her with this statement: "I have never told, have you?" The aunt subsequently confirmed that when she was babysitting for the 4-year-old girl, she had fallen asleep in the park. The little girl had wandered off to play in a waterfall. Her screams of terror awakened the aunt, who, because of her own guilt, threatened the girl to secrecy. Not surprisingly, hypnotic regression and abreaction techniques, in which the girl was placed back under the waterfall so she could discover that she was removed safely, led to a dramatic cure.

Such case reports involving the acquisition of symptoms under stress-induced dissociative experiences are common, although it is rare that there is documentation of the occurrence of the stressful circumstances. My tutor, Professor Gordon Hammer, was fond of this case because he was fascinated by hypnosis and its potential for understanding psychopathology. He lectured and wrote extensively about the concept of "dissociation" when that term was at the height of its unpopularity. Gordon Hammer would probably say that he is not sure whether he was 25 years behind his time (Prince, 1929) or 20 years ahead of it (E. R. Hilgard, 1977). Nevertheless, the possibility that dissociative experiences occur within the realm of the normal personality intrigued me as much then as it does now.

THEORETICAL CONCEPTS AND PRINCIPLES

My hypothesis is that there are significant individual differences in a dimension of personality and/or cognitive functioning that has something to do with the degree of control with which people can access different states of consciousness, psychological awareness, or cognitive functioning. Recognizing that there are many different usages of the term, I choose to label this individual-difference dimension "dissociation." Several converging lines of evidence suggest that the individual differences in the ability to experience hypnosis may reflect one aspect of a more general ability to access, regulate, and alter states of consciousness.

In the water phobia case described above, running water served as a "trigger," which stimulated some form of reverbatory neural circuit in the part of the little girl's psyche that was still panicking under the waterfall. This memory trace was dissociated, however, so that she was unaware that she was safe because of the aroused state she was experiencing and re-experiencing when triggered. The ability to experience hypnosis may involve an important psychological dimension concerned with the control of consciousness. This dimension of labile accessibility to multiple levels of awareness has significant implications for understanding a wide range of psychological and physiological phenomena, some of which may have clinical significance concerning the development and alleviation of symptoms.

It is hypothesized that this mechanism involves individual differences in the ability to maintain labile control over the level of functioning or state of consciousness that is appropriate for the person at the time. This control mechanism apparently involves the ability to change readily from one kind of psychological state or activity to another, or to maintain a nonvolitional flexibility over psychological sets and cognitive focusing.

My goal is not to develop a theoretical account of "dissociation," but instead to delineate some of its attributes, as well as to describe the kind of data that when taken together help to establish the convergent validity of the construct. Thus, I give no formal definition of what I mean by "dissociation." Indeed, my views would not depart in major ways from E. R. Hilgard's (1977) neodissociation theory. However, I would expand his views by focusing on individual differences in accessing multiple cognitive pathways, and by focusing on what I would view as a broad dimension of personality structure.

RESEARCH AND APPRAISAL

I summarize several seemingly unrelated sets of data from my own research program, conducted with many colleagues, that are consistent with the existence of an ability or skill that allows some individuals to gain functional access to different cognitive, psychological, and physiological states, as needed. This includes some work on sleep and hypnosis; on the interrelationship between and among hypnotizability, punctuality, and absorption; and on the relevance of hypnotizability to psychiatric patient populations and treatment outcome. Little attempt is made to integrate this research with the hypnotic literature. This task, left to the reader, should stimulate new ideas and empirical data that will lend credence or disconfirmation of the general approach.

However, it should be noted that, following from the initial data reviewed on the multidimensionality of hypnotic behavior, this review is only related to one component of the hypnotic experience (albeit perhaps the central one). For example, I have discussed elsewhere the clinical implications of a segment of hypnotic behavior, uncorrelated with the dissociative dimension, that is analogous to the placebo component of drug therapy (Evans, 1985).

Hypnosis and Suggestibility: Factor-Analytic Evidence

At the time of my graduate student days in the late 1950s, the theory that hypnosis was a form of suggestibility was almost universally accepted, even though it was recognized that there was circularity in a definition in which one term was being explained by another undefined term. My colleagues and I were initially uneasy about the alleged close link between hypnosis and suggestibility. Influenced by the research of Hull (1933) and Eysenck (1955) hypnosis was mostly measured by simple motor suggestions such as the postural sway test, involving motor versus indirection paradigms. The existing scales did not seem to reflect the full range of psychodynamic and dissociative experiences that occurred during hypnosis. It seemed to us that the statement that waking suggestibility and hypnotic suggestibility were correlated had no more significance than the observation that a red-headed person in his or her normal waking state would still be red-headed if he or she became hypnotized! This led us to conduct factor-analytic studies (Evans, 1965; Hammer, Evans, & Bartlett, 1963) of a battery including tests of suggestion and traditional hypnotic phenomena, and, as E. R. Hilgard (1965) and his colleagues were simultaneously doing, to explore the relationships between these suggestions when given with or without standardized induction procedures. It became clear that a single general factor of hypnotizability or suggestibility could *not* adequately account for enough of the common covariance among these measures of the domain of hypnosis (E. R. Hilgard, 1973); therefore, several alternative factor solutions were statistically valid (although many others could be ruled out statistically). The solution we favored indicated that at least four separate dimensions could be isolated in both waking and hypnotic performance. Three involved passive and challenge suggestions and imagery. A fourth involved a cluster of tests, including posthypnotic suggestion, amnesia, and age regression, and we labeled this a "dissociation" factor.

From a current perspective, this research is now mostly of historical interest, although its implication for the measurement of hypnosis still needs to be worked out more carefully. These factors can be recognized in scales such as the Stanford Hypnotic Susceptibilty Scales, Forms A, B, and C (SHSS:A, SHSS:B, SHSS:C; Weitzenhoffer & Hilgard, 1959, 1962); however, SHSS:A and SHSS:B, and several other published hypnosis scales, do not have many (sometimes any) items sampled from the imager and/or dissociative domains. The important point to be drawn from this early work is that the dissociative experiences normally associated with hypnotic behavior could be isolated both following a hypnotic induction and in normal waking conditions. Although the tendency to view hypnosis as multidimensional has been downplayed in subsequent years, these early studies from several sources helped stimulate the intensive study of specific hypnotic phenomena, such as the program initiated by Hilgard on pain and hypnotic analgesia (E. R. Hilgard, 1977); my work with Kihlstrom on posthypnotic amnesia (Evans, 1980, 1988; Kihlstrom & Evans, 1979; Kihlstrom & Evans, 1979); Josephine R. Hilgard's (1970) now classic interview studies of imaginative involvement; and Spiegel's work on the so-called "grade 5 syndrome" (H. Spiegel, 1974).

Hypnosis as a Dissociative Process: Posthypnotic Amnesia

Our research program on posthypnotic amnesia provides a strong line of evidence about the dissociative mechanisms involved in hypnosis. These studies have been reviewed elsewhere, and only some key studies are summarized here (Evans, 1980, 1988; Kihlstrom & Evans, 1979).

The phenomenon of "source amnesia" (Evans, 1979), in which hypnotized subjects can recall information learned only a few minutes before in hypnosis, but fail to recall that they have just learned it (often rationalizing their sudden awareness of the trivia), represents a dissociation of the content of the recalled material from the context in which the material was acquired. We have shown that hypnotized subjects, unlike simulators, use different problem-solving strategies when confronted with the task of counting their fingers when they cannot use the number 6 (Evans, 1974, 1980). Over the years, Kihlstrom and I (Evans, 1980, 1989; Evans & Kihlstrom, 1979; Kihlstrom & Evans, 1979) have shown that posthypnotic amnesia represents a temporary failure to use those normal retrieval strategies that usually lead to efficient recall. Such data provide compelling evidence that the cognitive processes during hypnosis are not fully integrated with normal conscious experience. A subject may be able to vaguely recall two suggestions, but may not be able to recall which one he or she completed first; nor can he or she really be sure of which arm became stiff and rigid, except for the feeling in one arm that is apparently due to the heroic efforts made to bend it.

Studies outside of our group were simultaneously leading to similar conclusions. These particularly include E. R. Hilgard's (1977) work on the hidden observer in hypnotic analgesia, extended by Laurence and Perry (1981) into other hypnotic phenomena such as age regression. These and other studies provide compelling evidence of the descriptive utility, if not the explanatory power, of the dissociation concept.

Most of these exciting studies refer to events that occur *within* the hypnotic context. I would like to focus attention not so much on the hypnotic process itself as on the underlying ability or capacity to experience hypnosis. In short, the focus of the material I present here is on individual differences in the underlying skill subsuming hypnotic susceptibility. There are, of course, many good reviews of the frustrating attempts to find standard "personality" correlates of hypnotic susceptibility (e.g., E. R. Hilgard, 1965), and this approach has pretty much been abandoned. Part of the reason for this history of failure is that investigators have focused on extrinsic characteristics of the person, rather than the characteristics of the dissociative dimension in its own right.

Hypnosis and the Control of Sleep

Sleep Responding and Dissociative Control

It may seem momentarily unusual to consider sleep as paradigmatic of a dissociated state. Subjectively, sleep is mostly recognized *after* the event by the temporal discontinuity experienced on awakening. The phenomena of sleep walking and sleep talking, as well as the very active process of dreaming, provide compelling documentation of the occurrence of dissociative cognitive activity outside of normal awareness. Even more compelling is the surprise typically registered when I ask audiences in a lecture, "When was the last time you fell out of bed?" This is an extremely rare event for adults, though children have to learn the skill. Yet the sleep laboratory has shown us that we make gross bodily movements many times a night, and it is indeed a wonder that we do not fall out of bed regularly. We even have clearly defined territoriality agreements with our sleeping partners, which are reacted to strongly when violated. Yet this detailed monitoring of the bed-defined (and partner-defined) limits occurs while we are asleep, totally outside awareness.

We (Evans, Gustafson, O'Connell, Orne, & Shor, 1966, 1969; Perry, Evans, O'Connell, Orne, & Orne, 1978) were able to show that during sleep we could administer suggestions such as "Whenever I say the word 'itch,' your nose will feel itchy until you scratch it," without arousing many of our subjects. For those subjects who showed no electroencephalographic (EEG) signs of arousal during the suggestion, the mere repetition of the cue word "itch" was sometimes sufficient to elicit the targeted response of nose scratching. This occurred almost exclusively in the rapid eye movement (REM) sleep state. The response could be obtained when the suggestion was tested by giving the cue word in the same REM state, or when it was tested in a later REM period (without repeating the suggestion), 24 hours later, or even 6 months later—in spite of intervening unbreachable waking amnesia for the sleep-administered suggestion itself (Evans, 1990).

The ability to produce meaningful sleep-induced behavioral responses while asleep was significantly correlated with hypnotizability in three of the four studies we completed. The rate of successful response during sleep (see Table 5.1) was particularly correlated with the dissociative rather than the motor and imagery clusters of hypnotic behavior (Evans et al., 1969). Less hypnotizable subjects did not respond as frequently because they tended to wake up every time we tried to administer the test cue words and suggestions. The data implied that some subjects can process significant information even while maintaining control over their own sleep process. Other subjects must momentarily awaken in order to process novel events occurring in their environment.

TABLE 5.1. Correlations between Behavioral Response to Sleep-Induced Suggestion and Susceptibility to Hypnosis

Hypnosis	Sleep response (frequency)	Immediate	Delayed	Carryover
		Delay between suggestion cue and response[b]		
HGSHS:A	−.48*	.23	.32	.64*
SHSS:C	−.56	.38	.43	.60**
Suggestion[a]				
Waking	−.15	.11	−.42	.06
Passive	.32	.05	.40	.41
Challenge	.26	.33	.08	.44
Hallucinatory–reverie[a]	.54**	.35	.42	.52**
Posthypnotic–dissociative[a]	.46*	.23	.30	.58**

Note. From "Sleep-Induced Behavioral Response: Relationship to Susceptibility to Hypnosis and Laboratory Sleep Patterns" by F. J. Evans, L. A. Gustafson, D. N. O'Connell, M. T. Orne, and R. E. Shor, 1969, *Journal of Nervous and Mental Disease, 148*, 467–476. Copyright 1969 by The Williams & Wilkins Co. Reprinted by permission.
[a]The clusters of hypnotic items are derived from the SHSS:C.
[b]Refers to the interval between sleep induced suggestion administration, and response during sleep to the cue word related to the suggestion: "Immediate," tested in the same REM period as suggestion administered; "delayed," tested same night, but later REM period; "carryover," tested on a different night, with intervening waking amnesia.
*p < .05 (two-tailed). **p < .01 (two-tailed).

The fact that some hypnotizable subjects were able to control cognitive processes during sleep was all the more striking because of the related finding that these same subjects fell asleep much faster at night than unresponsive subjects, in terms both of laboratory EEG criteria and of their own self-reported sleep patterns (Evans et al., 1969). Thus, a subgroup of subjects was isolated in whom three characteristics were noteworthy (Evans, 1977a, 1990): (1) dissociative control of behavioral response during sleep; (2) ability to fall asleep quickly; and (3) hypnotizability. It is especially noteworthy, however, that the cognitive control observed in our sleeping and hypnotizable subjects is a control that does not imply volition. The "control" here is outside the domain of awareness (as in much of cognition).

Control-of-Sleep Dimension

In a second phase of this research (Evans, 1977b), factor-analytic studies of subjective sleep patterns demonstrated that sleep efficiency could be con-

TABLE 5.2. HGSHS:A Scores of Subjects with High and Low Control of Sleep (CS)

	Sample 1		Sample 2	
	n	$\overline{X}$	*n*	$\overline{X}$
High CS	17	7.9	124	6.7
Low CS	13	4.6	89	6.0
t (*p* <)	3.16 (.005)		2.03 (.05)	

Note. From "Hypnosis and Sleep: The Control of Altered States of Awareness" by F. J. Evans, 1977, *Annals of the New York Academy of Sciences, 296,* 162–175. Copyright 1977 by the New York Academy of Sciences. Reprinted by permission.

ceptualized along at least three different uncorrelated dimensions: difficulty in falling asleep; difficulty in staying asleep; and, uncorrelated with both of these insomnia factors, the ability to maintain control over sleep processes. The control-of-sleep dimension was indicated by the speed with which the subjects could fall asleep at night, and the flexibility of nighttime sleep patterns. For example, in two samples involving 640 subjects, the persons who scored highly on this control-of-sleep cluster reported that they fell asleep easily at night; fell asleep easily in a variety of unusual surroundings, such as during a movie or concert or in a plane or car; catnapped regularly; and slept even when not tired in anticipation of future sleep loss. Thus, high-scoring individuals reported being ready, willing, and able to fall asleep at almost any time and in any place. It was as though the individuals had a switch or trigger mechanism readily available to turn the sleep process on and off. The lability of the switch mechanism, not any volitional intent, is the important conceptual point. Not surprisingly, habitual nappers scored high on this dimension (Evans, 1977a).

Subjects who scored high on the control-of-sleep dimension were also more hypnotizable. The relationship between hypnotizability and the control of sleep is shown in Tables 5.2, 5.3, and 5.4 (Evans, 1977a). In Table 5.2, hypnotizability scores in two student samples of 30 and 213 are dichotomized at the mean on the control-of-sleep dimension. In both samples, those with high control-of-sleep scores had significantly higher HGSHS:A (Shor & Orne, 1962) scores than those with low control-of-sleep scores. Table 5.3 shows differences between extremely high- and extremely low-hypnotizability subjects on four of the criterion measures on the Control of Sleep Questionnaire (a 30-item questionnaire in which each item is scored from 1 to 5).

Table 5.4 shows the relationship between hypnotizability and habitual napping in college student samples. This table presents scores on the

TABLE 5.3. Hypnotizability (HGSHS:A) and Subjective Sleep Patterns Defining the Control-of-Sleep Dimension

Item	High ($n = 28$)	Low ($n = 12$)	$p <$	r ($n = 60$)
Fall asleep easily	3.7	3.1	.01	.30
Go to sleep at will	3.4	2.2	.001	.51
Sleep in theater, concert	1.8	1.3	.02	.25
Dream at night	3.9	3.1	.001	.45

Note. Subjects responded on a 5-point scale (5 = "always," 1 = "never"). From "Hypnosis and Sleep: The Control of Altered States of Awareness" by F. J. Evans, 1977, *Annals of the New York Academy of Sciences, 296*, 162–175. Copyright 1977 by the New York Academy of Sciences. Reprinted by permission.

key defining item in the Control of Sleep Questionnaire ("Do you fall asleep readily?"), cross-classified by hypnotizability (HGSHS:A) and control of sleep. High-hypnotizability subjects fell asleep more readily than low-hypnotizability subjects, and nappers fell asleep more readily than non-nappers. The interaction between hypnotizability and napping was insignificant. This implies that the dimension of labile control may manifest itself differently in different people. A variety of altered states of consciousness (napping, trance or absorption states, meditation, etc.) may be functionally equivalent in terms of the way in which they can be used by responsive people in problem solving or stress reduction. It appears that the ability to achieve deep hypnosis and the ability to fall asleep easily share some common mechanisms.

Flexible Control of Cognitive Processes

The hypothesized ease of accessibility of dissociative states suggests a cognitive flexibility that should be identifiable in hypnotizable individuals. Hypnotizable subjects should possess attributes of maintaining strong, automatized cognitive control in the face of distraction, as well as a facility in shifting cognitive control when it is deemed appropriate. Our work has supported this hypothesis in several areas. (1) The correlation between sleep control and hypnotizability has already been summarized. (2) Correlations have been reported (Graham & Evans, 1977) between hypnotizability and a brief objective measure of cognitive flexibility: random number generation (RNG). (3) Two other correlates of hypnotizability fit well within this conceptual framework: absorption and punctuality.

TABLE 5.4. Hypnotizability, Napping, and Control of Sleep

| | HGSHS:A | | |
	High (n = 152)	Low (n = 67)	All (n = 219)
Napper (n = 121)	3.81	3.64	3.76
Non-napper (n = 98)	3.64	3.13	3.48
All subjects	3.74	3.40	3.63

F (HGSHS:A) = 7.55 ($p < .005$)
F (Napper, non-napper) = 7.68 (p .005)
F (Interaction) = 1.87 (n.s.)

Note. Control of sleep here was defined by the item "Do you fall asleep readily?" From "Hypnosis and Sleep: The Control of Altered States of Awakeness" by F. J. Evans, 1977, *Annals of the New York Academy of Sciences, 296*, 162–175. Copyright 1977 by the New York Academy of Sciences. Reprinted by permission.

Randomization and Hypnotizability

We have been developing a brief, objective, practice-free measure of cognitive flexibility and attentive effort. Subjects are asked to free-associate numbers. Specifically, they are asked to produce aloud at the pace of one per second, random digits between 0 and 9. A chi-square-like index (RNG) provides a sensitive and reliable measure of sequential response bias in these randomized procedures (Evans, 1978). In other studies, we have shown that randomization varies according to the degree of learning and overlearning of a complex motor task (Evans & Graham, 1980). Randomization is better in children, but significantly poorer in patients with diagnoses of psychosis and organic brain involvement. These and other studies suggest that the RNG task is a measure of cognitive flexibility. It shows changes in clinical improvement for patients with attentional deficits such as schizophrenia (Horne, Evans, & Orne, 1982) and for emotionally disturbed adolescents (Salierno, F. J. Evans, & B. J. M. Evans, 1984). In several samples, we (Evans & Graham, 1980) were able to show that highly hypnotizable subjects performed better on this task than relatively unhypnotizable subjects. This finding has been replicated by R. A. Karlin (personal communication, 1982), by C. McL. Morgan (personal communication, 1983) and by Suita (1982), in samples in the United States, Australia, and Poland, respectively. Although we have not continued to use this particular measure of cognitive flexibility in our subsequent work, these studies are significant in providing documentation that dissociative processes are related to cognitive and attentional functioning.

Controlled Absorption

Although the work on absorption of Shor (1980), Aas (1963), and Tellegen and Atkinson (1974) has been of great conceptual importance, the correlations between these scales and single measures of hypnotizability have generally tended to be quite modest or even insignificant in studies where the HGSHS:A has been used as a single criterion measure. The items in such scales show considerable diversity, even in scales refined by factor-analytic techniques (Tellegen & Atkinson, 1974). It is apparent, for example, that only some items included under the general rubric of "absorption" relate to the accessibility of altered states. Absorption scale items differ according to whether there is implied control over the subjective experience.

On a purely *a priori* basis, an expanded 60-item Absorption Questionnaire was broken into several subscales, including two that appeared to differ in the kind of control maintained by the subject in the absorption process. The first subscale, which we labeled Controlled Absorption, pertains to the degree to which one allows absorption to happen. This scale includes questions such as "Have you ever been so lost in thought (or involved in reading a good book) that you did not understand what people said to you even though you nodded token agreement?" On the other hand, items in the Involuntary Absorption subscale include those in which the individual is almost a bystander and becomes overwhelmed by the involvement. Two items in this scale are "Have you ever been caught up and overwhelmed by a beautiful sunset?" and "Have you ever almost fallen asleep while driving a car?"

In one college student sample of 82 subjects, the Controlled Absorption and Involuntary Absorption subscales correlated highly with the remaining items of the 60-item test (.81 and .72, respectively); however, as expected, the two scales correlated only moderately (.35). As predicted, there was a significant correlation of .37 ($p < .01, n = 82$; Evans, unpublished data) between scores on Controlled Absorption subscale and the Control of Sleep Questionnaire. It will be seen in Table 5.5 below that controlled absorption, but not involuntary absorption, correlates with hypnotizability.

Some construct validity for the subset of absorption experiences hypothesized to be under an important voluntary control mechanism comes from our recent work demonstrating a relationship between hypnotizability and punctuality.

TABLE 5.5. Arrival Time Means and Hypnotizability

		Session		
HGSHS:A	*n*	1	2	Combined
High	18	−3.4	−4.8	−4.1
Low	18	+3.9	+3.9	+3.9
p (one-tailed)		< .10	< .05	< .025

Note. +, minutes early; −, minutes late.

Punctuality, Hypnotizability, and Absorption

On the basis of original observation by Emily C. Orne (personal communication, 1968), we have been able to show that more hypnotizable subjects sometimes arrive late for their experimental appointments (Markowsky & Evans, 1978). Typical results from two of several replicated samples are presented in Tables 5.5 and 5.6, in which it is clear that some highly hypnotizable subjects are late at least some of the time. It should be emphasized, however, that the relationship between punctuality and hypnotizability may not be observed in a single session; variability in arrival time over several sessions is the important characteristic of the hypnotizable subject.

There are, of course, many reasons why a person is occasionally late. One hypothesis is that the hypnotized subject's facility at gaining entry into a preferred altered state (e.g., absorption) may in another sense become a social encumbrance. To the extent that such a person can become intensively absorbed in one activity, such as reading a book, occasional

TABLE 5.6. Hypnosis, Punctuality, and Variability (*n* = 24)

	Mean Hypnosis Score (SHSS:C)		
Variability	Early[a]	Late[a]	Combined
Most consistent third	2.6[*]	7.3	4.4 (*n*=8)
Least consistent third	4.7	9.0[b]	7.4 (*n* = 8)

[a]Refers to arrival time over eight sessions
[*]*p* < .02.

TABLE 5.7 Hypnotizability Related to Control of Sleep and to Controlled versus Involuntary Absorption: Students (*n* = 56)

HGSHS:A	*n*	Control of Sleep Questionaire	Controlled Absorption subscale	Involuntary Absorption subscale
High	23	16.4	6.6	5.7
Medium	20	15.4	6.3	5.5
Low	13	14.7	5.0	5.4
p <		.15	.005	n.s.

lateness may be due to a partial failure of whatever trigger mechanism is necessary for the person to integrate a sense of time into his or her ongoing reality orientation or book-based fantasy. Lateness may be due not to the inability to process time, but to a failure to terminate an all too seductively achieved absorbed state. The subject will arrive on time for an appointment only at the cost of being able to enjoy temporary escapes into alternative psychological states.

Support for the hypothesis that occasional lateness is mediated by the control mechanism we postulate as central to hypnosis was observed from two student samples (*n*'s = 34 and 48). Students with high scores on the controlled absorption subscale items arrived significantly later, on the average, for the four experimental sessions for which ranked punctuality data were available, compared to those subjects with lower scores (*t* = 3.34, *p* < .001, *n* = 82). The other measures derived from the absorption scales were not related to punctuality (Makowsky & Evans, 1978).

Hypnotizability, Sleep, and Absorption: Normal Subjects

So far, in replicated studies, we have been able to relate hypnotizability to control of sleep and to controlled absorption, separately. Although the correlations are modest, we have confidence that they will recur in most future samples. The obvious question is this: Are the three measures interrelated? A sample of 58 paid volunteers tested at Rutgers University were administered the HGSHS:A and the Control of Sleep and Absorption Questionnaire.

Table 5.7 summarizes scores on the Control of Sleep Questionnaire as well as the Controlled and Involuntary Absorption subscales for subjects of high (8–12), medium (5–7), and low (0–4) hypnotizability on the HGSHS:A. Unfortunately, the significant relationship found in several previous samples between hypnotizability and control of sleep was only

TABLE 5.8. Hypnotizability Related to Control of Sleep and Controlled Absorption: Psychiatric Inpatients ($n = 45$)

SHSS:C[a]	n	Control of Sleep Question- naire	n	Controlled Absorption subscale
High	27	13.2	18	6.2
Medium	25	13.3	22	6.0
Low	12	10.4	5	3.2
$p <$		.05		.05

[a]Multiple r (predicting SHSS:C) = .45, $p < .001$.

marginally supported in this sample ($p < .15$). The progression of the means was in the predicted direction. Controlled Absorption scores were related to hypnotizability: The correlation between hypnotizability (as measured by the HGSHS:A) and the Controlled Absorption scores was .45 ($p < .005$, $n = 58$). However the correlation between scores on the Involuntary Absorption subscale and the HGSHS:A (.04) was insignificant.

When subjects were dichotomized into extremely high and extremely low scores on the Control of Sleep Questionnaire, the respective HGSHS:A scores of 7.2 versus 5.5 approached significance ($p < .10$, $n = 32$). If the subjects were dichotomized into high and low scores on the Controlled Absorption subscale, the mean hypnosis scores were 7.9 and 5.5, respectively ($p < .03$, $n = 45$).

We would predict that individuals with the underlying labile control capacity might well score high on only one of the two predictors, moderator variable style. If subjects were classified as scoring high on either of the control dimensions (i.e., high control of sleep and/or high controlled absorption), the mean HGSHS:A score of 7.5 was significantly ($p < .05$) higher than for those subjects who did not have high scores on either control dimension ($\overline{X} = 6.0$).

Hypnotizability, Sleep, and Absorption: Patients

We have replicated this finding in a sample of psychiatric inpatients. Table 5.8 shows a similar relationship among hypnotizability, control of sleep, and controlled absorption. The resulting multiple correlation predicting SHSS:C scores from the two variables was significant ($r = .45$, $p < .001$).

Summary

It seems that a number of mechanisms tend to cluster together, though not all combinations of these have been interrelated, and some aspects await replication. The ability to be hypnotized, conceived of as a trait; the ability to control sleep processes; production of random sequences as a measure of flexibility of attentional focus; punctuality; and type of absorption all cluster together to help define the limits of a broad individual-difference dimension involving ready accessibility of different psychological and/or physiological states. Presumably, this dimension will relate to other evidence of hypnotically induced memory change and pain control. Such a dimension should have significant clinical implications.

Clinical Relevance of the Accessibility Dimension

Control of Sleep, Insomnia, and Smoking

Before saying much about the hypnotizable patient, I present some evidence indicating that a key index of the postulated dissociative or flexibility dimension, control of sleep, is related to treatment outcome. I then turn briefly to the controversial questions: Are psychiatric patients hypnotizable? Does hypnotizability predict symptom alleviation?

Insomnia. Individual differences in a mechanism of flexible cognitive control have clear implications for the development, maintenance, and control of symptoms. For example, it suggests that most patients with insomnia are probably relatively unresponsive to hypnosis. If, however, some people with sleep-onset insomnia can experience hypnosis, then this implies that these individuals have the necessary control mechanism, and therefore it should be possible to *teach* such persons to fall asleep easily. A study by Graham, Wright, Toman, and Mark (1975) provides some support for this possibility. The response of 20 insomniac patients with sleep-onset insomnia on the Control of Sleep Questionnaire differed significantly from those of 20 control subjects ($p < .01$ for five of the subscale-defining items). Six months after the self-hypnosis/relaxation treatment procedure, the insomniac students had improved on the Control of Sleep Questionnaire ($p < .0001$), as manifest on all the criterion questions. The change was accompanied by reports of significantly improved daily sleep patterns. Unfortunately, the relationship between the amount of improvement and the level of hypnotic responsivity was not reported.

Smoking. In another study, we explored retrospectively some correlates of success versus lack of success at quitting smoking. On the basis of the controversial work by Eysenck (1981), we predicted that those who were successful in quitting smoking after several years of indulgence

TABLE 5.9. Control of Sleep and Smoking History

Subgroup	n	Control of Sleep Questionnaire X̄	SD
Current smokers	147	11.5	4.1
Unsuccessful quitters	169	11.5	4.2
Successful quitters	162	12.2*	3.9
Nonsmokers	198	12.3	3.9

*$p < .05$.

would have higher control-of-sleep scores than either those who tried hard to quit but failed, or those who never tried to quit (Evans, unpublished data). In a national random probability survey of 676 U. S. adults, the results in Table 5.9 were obtained.

Though the differences were small, successful quitters scored higher on the Control of Sleep Questionnaire than unsuccessful quitters ($p < .05$). For some people, smoking may be an attempt to change arousal/ cognitive state by artificial means because the psychological control mechanism is too weak. Of course, hypnotic techniques are at least as adequate as other methods in helping patients stop smoking (see Holroyd, 1980; Perry & Mullen, 1975; H. Spiegel, 1970). We predict that this occurs in those with high state flexibility (in the sense in which we use the term), rather than those with high hypnotizability per se.

Hypnotizability, Flexible Control, and Treatment Outcome in Hospitalized Psychiatric Patients

The relationship between hypnotizability and therapeutic outcome in psychiatric patients has not been studied extensively. Four different questions can be raised concerning the relationship between hypnosis and treatment outcome.

1. Does hypnosis facilitate the therapeutic improvement of patients with specific symptoms or diagnoses? This refers to the efficacy of hypnotic intervention as it relates to recovery and long-term outcome.
2. Can obtained treatment changes be specifically attributed to hypnosis rather than to the nonspecific aspects of the hypnotic relationship? Such an attribution can be made only if individual differences in hypnotizability correlate with the extent of treatment success.

TABLE 5.10. Hypnotizability in DSM-III Diagnostic Subgroups

Scale		Depres- sion (*n* = 18)	Alcohol Abuse (*n* = 12)	Schizo- phrenia (*n* = 25)	Anorexia (*n* = 60)	*F*	*p*
HGSHS:A	$\overline{X}$	8.00	8.25	7.32	7.35	0.65	*n.s.*
	SD	3.1	2.7	2.3	2.6		
SHSS:C	$\overline{X}$	6.94	8.00	5.76	6.32	3.07	< .05
	SD	2.4	2.0	1.9	2.4		
HIP	$\overline{X}$	5.35	6.73	4.81	5.52	1.29	*n.s.*
INDUCTION	SD	2.6	2.1	2.9	3.0		

Adapted from Pettinati, Kogan, Evans, Wade, & Horne (1989). Copyright 1989 by American Psychiatric Assication. Reprinted by permission.

(Both the first and second questions address issues relating to the therapeutic applications of hypnosis; these issues are not being addressed in this chapter.)

3. Do patients of different diagnoses have experiences with hypnosis that are comparable to those of normal controls? That is, are patients as hypnotizable as nonpatient populations?

4. To what extent are individual differences in hypnotizability (as a hypothesized marker for the more general accessibility or control dimension) related to the therapeutic success and treatment outcome, independently of the specific method of treatment adopted?

Hypnotizability in Psychiatric Patients. There has been a good deal of controversy in the literature as to whether or not schizophrenic patients are capable of experiencing hypnosis. This material has been reviewed by Lavoie and Sabourin (1980), Pettinati (1982), H. Spiegel and D. Spiegel (1978), and Murray-Jobsis (1983). Table 5.10 summarizes data (Pettinati, Wade, Horne, & Staats, 1990) showing that for the most part subjects with varying *Diagnostic and Statistical Manual of Mental Disorders*, third edition (DSM-III) psychiatric diagnoses demonstrated normal ranges of hypnotic susceptibility, at least on the HGSHS:A and SHSS:C. Pettinati et al. (1990) found that schizophrenic patients did show a lower score than other patients in the sample (*n* = 60) on the Hypnotic Induction Profile (HIP; H. Spiegel & D. Spiegel, 1978), though not significantly so on the SHSS:C or the HGSHS:A.

Thus, we are satisfied that, in spite of small differences between the various scales, there are relatively few differences in hypnotizability across schizophrenic, depressed, alcohol-abusing, and anorexic patients. Except perhaps at moments of acute psychotic/hallucinatory episodes, psychotic and depressed patients appear to have the same range of capacity to experience hypnosis as do other patients and normal subjects.

There are, however, two clinical groups that seem to have *higher* levels of hypnotic capacity than normals and other patient populations. Starting with the initial work by Frankel and Orne (1976), three out of four studies have now shown that phobic patients have higher scores on hypnotizability scales than others (Frischholz, D. Spiegel, H. Spiegel, Balma, & Markell, 1982; Gerschman, Burrows, Reade, & Foenander, 1979; John, Hollander, & Perry, 1983). The only exception is a study that used the HIP (Frischolz et al., 1982).

In a reanalysis of the data on anorexic patients, Pettinati, Horne, and Staats (1983) were able to show that bulimic patients who purged and vomited, as well as anorexics who used vomiting to control weight, had significantly higher hypnotizability scores than normal subjects, other patients, and particularly those anorexic patients who used abstaining rather than vomiting to control weight. Interestingly enough, Apfel, Kelly, and Frankel (1983) showed that women with excessive morning sickness during pregnancy were also highly hypnotizable, while Margolis (1983) and Zeltzer and LeBaron (1983) demonstrated the value of hypnosis in treating vomiting as a side effect of medication in cancer patients (both adults and children).

I hardly need to point out that phobias are often considered as paradigmatic for dissociative processes. It is not difficult to hypothesize that anorexia (particularly the vomiting/purging behavior), along with similar uses of vomiting mechanisms in these other patients, might have dissociative roots (Pettinati et al., 1986), in much the same way that hysterical fainting was a prominent symptom in a similar group of young women many years ago.

Hypnotizability and Treatment Outcome. Data obtained both in medical and in psychiatric settings have indicated that hypnotizability is directly correlated with treatment outcome when the treatment involves hypnotic intervention. Most of these studies are poorly controlled, and have been reviewed by Bowers and Kelly (1979), Perry, Gelfand, and Marcovitch (1979), Holroyd (1980), and H. Spiegel and D. Spiegel (1978). There are still a number of unanswered questions regarding the relation of hypnotizability to treatment outcome.

The therapeutic advantage of hypnosis when used with highly hypnotizable subjects may be relatively short-lived: Differences between subjects high and low in hypnotizability may not occur after a more extensive follow-up period of 6 months or more. Failure to find such differences in the long term may be due to a relapse by hypnotizable subjects or to slower

TABLE 5.11. Correlations (Pearson r) between Hypnotizability (SHSS:A) and Therapeutic Outcome (Change Scores)

	All patients ($n = 32$)		Followup patients ($n = 22$)			
	Pre- to Post-therapy		Pre- to Post-therapy		Pretherapy to followup	
	r	$p<$	r	$p<$	r	$p<$
SCL = 90						
Number of Complaints	.15	n.s.	.22	n.s.	.23	n.s.
Weighted score	.27	.10	.38	.05	.26	n.s.
Intensity score	.38	.025	.40	.05	.18	n.s.
Target symptom						
Primary	.35	.025	.36	.005	.02	n.s.
Total	.48	.005	.56	.005	.20	n.s.
Therapist change report	.27	.10	.41	.025	—	—

Note. One-tailed probabilites. From "Hypnotizability and Outcome in Brief Psychotherapy" by E. P. Nace, A. M. Warwick, R. L. Kelley, and F. J. Evans, 1982, *Journal of Clinical Psychiatry, 43*, 129–133. Copyright 1982 by Raven Press. Reprinted by permission.

but continued recovery by less hypnotizable patients. Both possibilities are consistent with individual differences in control flexibility.

I have been involved in three studies that have examined the relationship between hypnotizability and the outcome of treatment *not* involving hypnosis. In one of these (Nace, Warwick, Kelley, & Evans, 1982), we studied 32 soldiers with a mixture of nonpsychotic psychiatric diagnoses. The more highly hypnotizable patients showed significantly greater therapeutic change during a 10-session treatment program than the relatively unhypnotizable patients. At a 6-month follow-up, however, there was no significant difference between the two groups of patients. There was a tendency indicating that low-hypnotizability subjects improved more slowly, but no evidence of relapse in the highly hypnotizable. The correlations between hypnotizablity and measures of change were consistently significant. These data are presented in Table 5.11.

A study (Horne, Evans, & Orne, 1983) was conducted at the Hospital of the University of Pennsylvania ($n = 57$ inpatients with a variety of psychiatric diagnoses). Follow-up data were obtained on 54 patients at 6 months and 49 patients at 2 years. Patients' hypnotizability could only be classified using the HGSHS:A. Highly hypnotizable patients had greater symptom severity at admission than the less hypnotizable patients, but

TABLE 5.12. Hypnotizability and Rehospitalization Frequency: Psychiatric Inpatients (n = 54)

Rehospitalized	Hypnotizability		
	High (9–12)	Medium (6–8)	Low (0–5)
6 months: Yes	5[a]	3	1
6 months: No	13	18	14
2 years: Yes	12[b]	5	5
2 years: No	6	16	10

[a]χ^2 = 2.77, n.s.
[b]χ^2 = 7.85, p < .02.

improved more at discharge and at a 6-month follow-up on several measures, including the Symptom Checklist—90 (SCL-90; Derogatis, Lipman, Rickels, Uhlenhuth, & Covi, 1974). However, there was no significant difference between the high and low groups at a 2-year follow-up. Surprisingly, a more frequent rate of rehospitalization was found among the highly hypnotizable patients (χ^2 = 6.16, df = 2, p < .025 at 6 months; χ^2 = 5.28, df = 2, p < .05 at 2 years).

The provocative findings indicate an urgent need for replication before conclusions can be drawn about the prognostic significance of hypnotizability in the nonhypnotic treatment of psychiatric patients. The study was replicated by Evans, Horne, and Pettinati at the Carrier Foundation, New Jersey, involving 55 randomly selected hospitalized patients; the results are summarized in Table 5.12. (Evans, 1989). A close replication of the University of Pennsylvania data was obtained, including the surprising higher rehospitalization rate at 2-year follow-up of its highly hypnotizable patients (p < .01). Dissociative skills (indicated by hypnosis score) may be a double-edged gift: They may facilitate symptom removal, but may well lead to the (re-)establishment of symptomatic behavior. The Bagby (1928) case study presented earlier illustrates both aspects of the dissociative spectrum.

Treatment Outcome, Hypnotizability, and Control of Sleep. Pilot data are available from a study of the relationship among the control-of-sleep dimension, hypnotizability, and treatment outcome. The sample consisted of 64 anorexic and bulimic patients. Data are only available for admission and discharge status. The SCL-90 change between admission and discharge is presented in Table 5.13.

TABLE 5.13. Hypnotizability, Control of Sleep, and Therapeutic Change (SCL90): Patients with Anorexia/Bulimia ($n = 57$)

SHSS:C	Control of Sleep Questionnaire	SCL90 decrease
High	14.0	79.5
Medium	13.3	67.7
Low	7.3	44.6

The results show that both hypnotizability as measured on SHSS:C and the control of sleep were significantly related to changes in SCL-90 at discharge for these anorexic/bulimic patients. This not only confirms the earlier results (Nace et al., 1982; Horne et al., 1983) discussed above, but also shows that hypnotizability and the control of sleep are significantly related to these treatment changes. Thus, clinically relevant information about the dimension of labile accessibility can be obtained from measures of the control of sleep as well as of hypnotizability.

CONCLUSIONS

In summary, some of our recent data suggest that there are a number of interacting reliable correlates of hypnotizability, both in normal populations and in patient groups. None relate to suggestibility in the traditional sense. Although not all combinations of the variables measured have yet been intercorrelated, and some of the key correlations require additional replication, a pattern is emerging that is consistent with the hypothesized individual-difference dimension of the control of dissociative states or lability of psychological processes. Hypnotizability is related to the ability to process cognitive information during sleep, to the physiological ease of falling asleep, and to a dimension of subjective sleep characteristics we have labeled the "control of sleep" (involving, among other things, the ability to fall asleep easily and readily at will, and the tendency to take naps). Additional data have suggested that the concept of absorption can be meaningfully divided into subfactors that reflect the volitional control over the absorption process that correlates with hypnotizability in both normal and patient populations.

The usefulness of the concept of controlled versus involuntary absorption has been shown in its ability to mediate appointment arrival times—a variable that has already been shown to relate to hypnotizability. A study requiring replication has not only marginally confirmed the relationship between the control of sleep and hypnotizability, but has shown that controlled absorption correlates significantly with hypnotizability in both normal and patient populations—a result that might be predicted from the concept of multiple pathways as correlates of hypnotizability (J. R. Hilgard, 1970). Subjects who score high on either of these dimensions are more hypnotizable than subjects who do not score high on either of these dimensions. The multiple correlation of the SHSS:C and the Control of Sleep Questionnaire with hospital discharge treatment outcome was .45 (*n* = 62) in psychiatric patients (Evans, 1989). Finally, both the control-of-sleep dimension and hypnotizability relate to the reductions of symptoms and psychopathology even when psychiatric patients are not treated with hypnotic techniques.

It appears, therefore, that an individual-difference dimension reflecting the ability to control altered or dissociative states has heuristic value in understanding those abilities involved in the hypnosis experience, as well as in clinical applications.

REFERENCES

Aas, A. (1963). Hypnotizability as a function of nonhypnotic experience. *Journal of Abnormal and Social Psychology, 66,* 142–150.

Apfel, R., Kelly, S., & Frankel, F. H. (1983, May). *Hypnotizability and nausea and vomiting of pregnancy.* Paper presented at the annual meeting of the American Psychiatric Association, New York.

Bagby, E. (1928). *The psychology of personality.* New York: Holt.

Bowers, D. S., & Kelly, P. (1979). Stress, disease, psychotherapy, and hypnosis. *Journal of Abnormal Psychology, 88,* 490–505.

Derogatis, L. R., Lipman, R. S., Rickels, K., Uhlenhuth, E. H., & Covi, L. (1974). The Hopkins Symptom Checklist: A measure of primary symptom dimensions. In P. Pichot (Ed.), *Psychological measurements in psychopharmacology: Modern problems in pharmapsychiatry* (Vol. 7). Basel, Switzerland: S. Karger.

Evans, F. J. (1965). *The structure of hypnosis; A factor analytic investigation.* Unpublished doctoral dissertation, University of Sydney, Sydney, New South Wales, Australia.

Evans, F. J. (1974, October). Sixes on the tip-of-the-tongue: Problem solving during specific hypnotic amnesia. In A. M. Weitzenhoffer (Chair), *Suggested inability to recall.* Symposium presented at the 26th Annual Meeting of the Society of Clinical and Experimenal Hypnosis, Montreal.

Evans, F. J. (1977a). Hypnosis and sleep: The control of altered states of awareness. *Annals of the New York Academy of Sciences, 296,* 162–175.

Evans, F. J. (1977b). The subjective characteristics of sleep efficiency. *Journal of Abnormal Psychology, 86,* 561–564.

Evans, F. J. (1978). Monitoring attention deployment by random number generation: An index to measure subjective randomness. *Bulletin of the Psychonomic Society, 12,* 35–38.

Evans, F. J. (1979). Contextual forgetting: Posthypnotic source amnesia. *Journal of Abnormal Psychology, 88,* 556–563.

Evans, F. J. (1980). Posthypnotic amnesia. In G. D. Burrows & L. Dennerstein (Eds.), *Handbook of hypnosis and psychosomatic medicine* (pp. 85–103). Amsterdam: Elsevier/ North-Holland.

Evans, F. J. (1985). Expectancy, therapeutic instructions, and the placebo response. In L. White, B. Tursky, & G. E. Schwartz (Eds.), *Placebo: Theory, research, and mechanisms* (pp.215–288). New York: Guilford.

Evans, F. J. (1988). Posthypnotic amnesia: Dissociation of content and context. In H. M. Pettinati (Ed.), *Hypnosis and memory* (pp. 157–192). New York: Guilford.

Evans, F. J. (1989). The hypnotizable patient. In D. Waxman, D. Pedersen, I. Wilkie, & P. Mellett (Eds.), *Hypnosis: The Fourth European Congress at Oxford* (pp. 18–28). London: Whurr.

Evans, F. J. (1990). Behavioral responses during sleep, In R. R. Bootzin, J. F. Kihlstrom, & D. L. Schacter (Eds.), *Sleep and cognition* (pp. 77–87). Washington, DC: American Psychological Association.

Evans, F. J., & Graham, C. (1980). Subjective random number generation and attention deployment during acquisition and overlearning of a motor skill. *Bulletin of the Psychonomic Society, 15,* 391–394.

Evans, F. J., Gustafson, L. A., O'Connell, D. N., Orne, M. T., & Shor, R. E. (1966). Response during sleep with intervening waking amnesia. *Science, 152,* 666–667.

Evans, F. J., Gustafson, L. A., O'Connell, D. N., Orne, M. T., & Shor, R. E. (1969). Sleep-induced behavioral response: Relationship to susceptibility to hypnosis and laboratory sleep patterns. *Journal of Nervous and Mental Disease, 148,* 467–476.

Eysenck, H. J. (1955). *Dimensions of personality.* London: Routledge & Kegan Paul.

Eysenck, H. J. (1981). *The causes and effects of smoking.* London: Maurice Temple Smith.

Frankel, F. H., & Orne, M. T. (1976). Hypnotizability and phobic behavior. *Archives of General Psychiatry, 33,* 1259–1261.

Frischholz, E. J., Spiegel, D., Spiegel, H., Balma, D. L., & Markell, C. S. (1982). Differential hypnotic responsivity of smokers, phobics, and chronic-pain control patients: A failure to confirm. *Journal of Abnormal Psychology, 91,* 269–272.

Gerschman, J., Burrows, G. D., Reade, P., & Foenander, G. (1979). Hypnotizability and the treatment of dental phobic behavior. In G. D. Burrows, D. R. Collison, & L. Dennerstein (Eds.), *Hypnosis, 1979.* Amsterdam: Elsevier/ North-Holland.

Graham, X. R., Wright, G. W., Toman, W. J., & Mark, C. B. (1975). Relaxation and hypnosis in the treatment of insomnia. *American Journal of Clinical Hypnosis, 18,* 39–51.

Hammer, A. G., Evans, F. J., & Bartlett, M. (1963). Factors in hypnosis and suggestion. *Journal of Abnormal and Social Psychology, 67,* 15–23.

Hilgard, E. R. (1965). *Hypnotic susceptibility.* New York: Harcourt, Brace & World.

Hilgard, E. R. (1973). The domain of hypnosis, with some comments on alternative paradigms. *American Psychologist, 28,* 972–982.

Hilgard, E. R. (1977). *Divided consciousness: Multiple controls in human thought and action.* New York: Wiley.

Hilgard, J. R. (1970). *Personality and hypnosis: A study of imaginative involvement.* Chicago: University of Chicago Press.

Holroyd, J. (1980). Hypnosis treatment for smoking: An evaluative review. *International Journal of Clinical and Experimental Hypnosis, 28,* 341–357.

Horne, R. L., Evans, F. J., & Orne, M. T. (1982). Random number generation, psychopathology and therapeutic change. *Archives of General Psychiatry, 39,* 680–683.

Horne, R. L., Evans, F. J., & Orne, M. T. (1983, October). *Hypnotizability and treatment outcome in hospitalized psychiatric patients.* Paper presented at the annual meeting of the Society for Clinical and Experimental Hypnosis, Boston.

Hull, C. L. (1933). *Hypnosis and suggestibility: An experimental approach.* New York: Appleton-Century-Crofts.

John, R., Hollander, B., & Perry, C. (1983). Hypnotizability and phobic behavior: Further supporting data. *Journal of Abnormal Psychology, 92,* 390–392.

Kihlstrom, J. F., & Evans, F. J. (1979). Memory retrieval processes during posthypnotic amnesia. In J. F. Kihlstrom & F. J. Evans (Eds.), *Functional disorders of memory* (pp. 179–218). Hillsdale, NJ: Erlbaum.

Laurence, J.-R., & Perry, C. (1981). The "hidden observer" phenomenon in hypnosis: Some additional findings. *Journal of Abnormal Psychology, 90,* 334–344.

Lavoie, G., & Sabourin, M. (1980). Hypnosis and schizophrenia: A review of experimental and clinical studies. In G. D. Burrows & L. Dennerstein (Eds.), *Handbook of hypnosis and psychosomatic medicine.* Amsterdam: Elsevier/North-Holland.

Margolis, C. G. (1983, May). *Hypnosis for nausea and cachexia in adults with cancer.* Paper presented at the annual meeting of the American Psychiatric Association, New York.

Markowsky, P. A., & Evans, F. J. (1978, October). *Occasional lateness for appointments in hypnotizable subjects.* Paper presented at the 30th Annual Meeting of the Society for Clinical and Experimental Hypnosis, Asheville, NC.

Murray-Jobsis, J. (1983). *Hypnotic responsiveness in severely disturbed patients.* Paper presented at the 35th Annual Meeting of the Society for Clinical and Experimental Hypnosis, Boston.

Nace, E. P., Warwick, A. M., Kelley, R. L., & Evans, F. J. (1982). Hypnotizability and outcome in brief psychotherapy. *Journal of Clinical Psychiatry, 43,* 129–133.

Orne, M. T., & Evans, F. J. (1966). Inadvertent termination of hypnosis with hypnotized and simulating subjects. *International Journal of Clinical and Experimental Hypnosis, 14,* 61–78.

Perry, C. W., Evans, F. J., O'Connell, D. N., Orne, E. C., & Orne, M. T. (1978). Behavioral response to verbal stimuli administered and tested during REM sleep: A further investigation. *Waking and Sleeping, 2,* 35–47.

Perry, C., Gelfand, R., & Marcovitch, P. (1979). The relevance of hypnotic susceptibility in the clinical context. *Journal of Abnormal Psychology, 88,* 592–603.

Perry, C., & Mullen, G. (1975). The effects of hypnotic susceptibility on reducing smoking behavior treated by an hypnotic technique. *Journal of Clinical Psychology, 31*, 498–505.

Pettinati, H. M. (1982). Measuring hypnotizability in psychotic patients. *International Journal of Clinical and Experimental Hypnosis, 30*, 404–416.

Pettinati, H. M., Horne, R. L., & Staats, J. S. (1986). Hypnotizability in patients with anorexia nervosa and bulimia. *Archives of General Psychiatry, 42*, 1014–1016.

Pettinati, H. M., Wade, J. H., Horne, L. R., & Staats, J. M. (1990). Hypnotizability of psychiatric inpatients according to two different scales. *American Journal of Psychiatry, 147*, 69–75.

Prince, M. (1929). *Clinical and experimental studies in personality*. Cambridge, MA: Sci-Art.

Salierno, C. A., Evans, F. J., & Evans, B. J. M. (1984, April). *Random number generation as an objective measure of clinical progress in emotionally disturbed adolescents*. Paper presented at the 55th Annual Meeting of the Eastern Psychological Association, Baltimore.

Shor, R. E. (1960). The frequency of naturally occurring "hypnotic-like" experiences in the normal college population. *International Journal of Clinical and Experimental Hypnosis, 8*, 151–163.

Shor, R. E., & Orne, E. C. (1962). *Harvard Group Scale of Hypnotic Susceptibility, Form A*. Palo Alto, CA: Consulting Psychologists Press.

Spiegel, H. (1970). A single-treatment method to stop smoking using ancillary self-hypnosis. *International Journal of Clinical and Experimental Hypnosis, 18*, 235–250.

Spiegel, H. (1974). The grade 5 syndrome: The highly hypnotizable person. *International Journal of Clinical and Experimental Hypnosis, 22*, 303–319.

Spiegel, H., & Spiegel, D. (1978). *Trance and treatment: Clinical uses of hypnosis*. New York: Basic Books.

Suita, J. (1982, August). *Randomness and hypnotic susceptibility*. Paper presented at the Ninth International Congress of Hypnosis and Psychosomatic Medicine, Glasgow, Scotland.

Tellegen, A., & Atkinson, G. (1974). Openness to absorbing and self-altering experiences ("absorption"), a trait related to hypnotic susceptibility. *Journal of Abnormal Psychology, 83*, 268–277.

Weitzenhoffer, A. M., & Hilgard, E. R. (1959). *Stanford Hypnotic Susceptibility Scale, Forms A and B*. Palo Alto, CA: Consulting Psychologists Press.

Weitzenhoffer, A. M., & Hilgard, E. R. (1962). *Stanford Hypnotic Susceptibility Scale, Form C*. Palo Alto, CA: Consulting Psychologists Press.

Zeltzer, L., & LeBaron, S. (1983, May). *The effectiveness of behavioral intervention for reducing nausea and vomiting in children and adolescents receiving chemotherapy*. Paper presented at the annual meeting of the American Psychiatric Association, New York.

HYPNOSIS AS PSYCHOLOGICAL REGRESSION

CHAPTER 6

Hypnosis as a Special Case of Psychological Regression

MICHAEL R. NASH
University of Tennessee

INTRODUCTION

This chapter presents a psychoanalytic theory of hypnosis. This perspective is developed from current psychoanalytic thinking on the nature of shifts in psychological functioning during intensive uncovering therapies, dreaming, reverie, fantasy, and pathological conditions. Hypnosis is viewed as involving a special case of psychological regression, marked by characteristic changes in the experience of self, relationship, and information processing.

Freud, like many of his contemporaries in the turn-of-the-century psychiatric community, recognized that the shifts in behavior and experience of normal subjects during hypnosis resemble those observed in pathological conditions associated with neurosis. Early on, Freud hinted that these shifts during hypnosis might be characterized as changes in *how* the psyche functions (Freud, 1900/1953, pp. 101–102). But he chose to focus his attention on the hypersuggestibility of the hypnotic subject, and to explain this "credulous submissiveness" in terms of libidinal fixation or regression in the transference: an unconscious fixation of the subject's libido to the figure of the hypnotist, through the medium of the masochistic component of the sexual instinct (Freud, 1905/1960). Furthermore, Freud posited not only that suggestibility is a reanimation of the

This is a revised and expanded version of a paper entitled: "Hypnosis as a Window on Regression," (1988) *Bulletin of the Menninger Clinic, 52,* 383–403.

adult's relationship with a parent, but that it recapitulates "the relation of the individual member of the primal horde to the primal father" (Freud, 1921/1955, p. 127). Thus Freud defined hypnosis as a double regression: a reinstatement of childlike gullibility and the re-emergence of a vaguely remembered cultural primitiveness—a kind of ontogenetic *and* cultural regression. Though Freud's earlier clinical descriptions of shifts in psychic content and process during hypnosis were the ones destined to be confirmed by later researchers, his emphasis on libidinal explanations held sway over psychiatry and psychology for many years.

Following Freud's lead, analysts continued to emphasize libidinal fixation or regression as the core feature of hypnosis. Ferenczi (1909/1980) actually used the words "maternal hypnosis" and "paternal hypnosis" to describe the particular types of early libidinal ties to which the subject may be regressed. Schilder's (Schilder, 1956) view of hypnosis was even more clearly wedded to drive theory, as he identified two sources of hypnotic responsiveness: "goal-inhibited eroticism" and submission to authority. Importantly, however, Schilder did introduce the idea that not all of the subject's ego is immersed in the libidinal regression, and that a central part of the ego remains unaffected. Kubie and Margolin (1944) began to introduce into theories of hypnosis ideas borrowed from ego psychology: "boundaries", "perception," "adaptation," and "organization of conscious-ness." But hypersuggestibility and the dramatic shifts in experience and relationship undergone during hypnosis were still attributed to a reinstate-ment of infantile personality organization within the arena of the transference. The common thread in these libidinal theories is that the hypnotic subject undergoes an authentic ontogenetic transformation or regression to an infantile mode of drive gratification vis-à-vis the hypnotist. Shifts in the way the subject experiences self and others are thus construed as a re-emergence of normal infantile psychological structures.

In 1959, Merton Gill and Margaret Brenman published one of the most seminal and sophisticated treatments of hypnosis theory. They maintained that "a regressed state can not be considered equivalent to an earlier state of developmental organization" (Gill & Brenman, 1959, p. 212). While carefully noting the almost childlike compliance of hypnotic subjects, Gill and Brenman maintained that what is central to hypnosis is not a libidinal regression, but a shift in ego functioning. Reasoning from their own clinical research findings, Gill and Brenman concluded that dramatic and measurable changes in experience accompany hypnosis: changes in self-awareness, voluntariness, bodily experience, absorption, and availability of affect, as well as a movement from secondary- to primary-process thinking. All of these functions are ego-based, and changes in their operation during hypnosis may reflect shifts in various parts of the ego and diminution in its differentiation.

Importantly, Gill and Brenman viewed this shift or regression in ego functioning as occurring only in a subsystem of the ego. Like Schilder, they posited that a portion of the ego remains largely unaffected by hypnosis. Furthermore, Gill and Brenman concluded that hypnosis might be viewed as "regression in service of the ego" (Kris, 1952). That is, during hypnosis, the modulated regressive shifts in a subsystem of the ego enables the individual to make use of primary process in the service of creative problem solving and adaptation. Gill and Brenman's theory was still burdened, however, by the failure of psychoanalysis to define more precisely what is meant by "psychological regression." In addition, their attempt to integrate "hypnosis as transference" with "hypnosis as ego regression" was not wholly satisfactory.

The final two major contributors to our psychoanalytic understanding of hypnosis are Erika Fromm and Elgin Baker. Baker has focused much of his research and theory on how hypnosis affects the personality organization of severely disturbed patients (Baker, 1981). In so doing, he has illuminated the central role the ego plays in hypnosis.

Erika Fromm and her laboratory colleagues have made great strides in clarifying the fate of the ego during hypnosis (Fromm, Lombard, Skinner, & Kahn, 1987–1988; Fromm, 1979). Though her work is far too extensive to review here, her concept of "ego receptivity" is particularly central to a psychoanalytic understanding of hypnosis. Basing this construct on rigorously derived empirical data from her research work with self-hypnosis and heterohypnosis, Fromm posits that ego functioning during hypnosis is neither passive (as the libidinal theorists would have it) nor active (vigilant and task-oriented). Rather, it is "receptive": Voluntarism, critical judgment, and deliberate control of internal emotional experiences are temporarily relinquished, and the subject allows unconscious and preconscious material to emerge freely. This ego receptively embraces Pat Bowers's notion of "effortless experiencing" during hypnosis (Bowers, 1978), and it certainly resembles some of Freud's thinking about free association (Freud, 1900/1953, pp. 101-102). The beauty of the concept of ego receptivity is that it explains two broad characteristics of hypnotic response: hypersuggestibility (receptivity to outside stimuli) and shifts in experience (receptivity to "inner" stimuli).

THEORETICAL CONCEPTS AND PRINCIPLES

In this section, I first discuss the nature of psychological regression and identify the specific type of regression relevant to hypnosis. Second, I present a definition of hypnosis based on psychological regression. Finally,

I outline the changes in behavior and experience we may expect to find if indeed regression is operative during hypnosis.

The Nature of Psychological Regression

Freud distinguished two types of psychological regression—"temporal" and "topographic"—each based on a different biologically based metaphor (Freud, 1909/1957, 1917/1957). Much of the confusion in psychoanalytic theorizing about hypnosis stems from the proclivity of later theorists to use the term "regression" globally, obscuring the important distinctions Freud recognized long ago.

Temporal Regression

Freud rooted his concept of temporal regression in a theory of human development: that with maturation there is an orderly and lawful progression from less organized structures to more complex, advanced structures. Importantly, Freud also maintained that these early abandoned stages in human development do not perish. Freud believed that under some circumstances (e.g., during hypnosis), these early modes of relating may be reanimated. In fact, he viewed this type of regression as the essence of mental disease (Freud, 1915/1957). Temporal regression, then, is a lawful undoing of development, a reverse movement in time that faithfully retraces the path of maturation. It is likely that Freud's profound interest in archeology also influenced his thinking here. After all, in archeology it is easy to show that remnants of old architectural structures *do* persist beneath the new ones. Though obscured, they can be uncovered, sometimes in pristine form.

No one seriously argues Freud's point that psychological development moves from simpler to more complexly organized states. But there is disagreement about whether old stages persist in the psychic structure. Some contemporary psychoanalysts and cognitive-developmental psychologists maintain that early stages in human development do persist and that returning to an earlier psychophysiological matrix is possible, even necessary, when treating seriously impaired patients (Balint, 1968; Bion, 1977, Langer, 1970; Werner, 1948). Others argue that the psychic structure of the disturbed adult differs from that of a child, and that developmentally previous stages are not retrievable in their "pure" form because they have been unalterably changed (Gill & Brenman, 1959; Peterfreund, 1978; Piaget, 1973; Spitz, 1965).

Topographic Regression

As Freud saw it, topographic regression has nothing to do with time or development. Like temporal regression, topographic regression is a reversal— but one in space, not in time. Freud derived the metaphor of topographic regression from the system of the reflex arc in neurology and physiology. He postulated that under normal circumstances neural excitation flows from sensory and perceptual neural structures to higher-level thought and response structures. Topographic regression is a reversal in this process. It is a reverse movement along a path "from the region of thought-structures to that of sensory perceptions" (Freud, 1905/1960, p. 162); "in this process thoughts are transformed into images" (Freud, 1917/1957, p. 227); it is a backward course that results in a transformation of thoughts into visual imagery (Freud, 1933/1964). Working largely from his observations about free association, dreaming, and hypnosis, Freud observed that the regressive shift from thought to imagery is also accompanied by a change in *how* experience is organized and processed (primary instead of secondary processing). Thus during a topographic regression, a new balance is struck between conscious and unconscious, self and other, emotional expression and restraint.

A Definition of Hypnosis as Psychological Regression

Hypnosis is a condition during which a subsystem of the ego undergoes a topographic regression, resulting in characteristic changes in the experience of self and other. These changes may include a shift from secondary to primary processing; greater ego receptivity; increased availability of affect; displacement and condensation in the relationship with the hypnotist; an enhanced capacity for regression in service of the ego; distortions in the experience of the body; and a change in the experience of volition. This definition relies heavily upon the work of earlier ego-psychological theorists, especially Gill and Brenman (1959) and Fromm (1979). Topographic regression is posited to be the primary and distinguishing characteristic of hypnosis, with transference phenomena being one of several aspects of this shift in ego functioning.

What are the implications of the above-stated definition of hypnosis as a topographic regression in a subsystem of the ego? Based on research evidence to be described in the next section, my premise is that the regression in hypnosis is topographic, not temporal, and that the changes in behavior, experience, and relationship we observe with hypnosis are manifestations of a shift in how the subject processes information. If hypnosis is indeed a form of topographic regression, then we may expect to observe measurable changes in seven areas of experience when comparing hypnotic to normal nonhypnotic response: (1) changes in thought processes in the direction of prelogical, symbolic, and primary-process mentation (Gill, 1972; Gill & Brenman, 1959); (2) enhanced capacity to enlist primary-process material in the service of creativity and adaptation (i.e., regression in service of the ego—Hartmann, 1939/1958; Kris, 1952; Schafer, 1958); (3) increased availability of affect, marked by more vivid and intense emotion (Gill & Brenman, 1959); (4) fluctuations in how the body is experienced; (5) responses more frequently experienced as occurring involuntarily, in a manner similar to the experience of neurotic symptoms; (6) displacement and condensation in the relationship with the hypnotist; and (7) evidence of increased ego receptivity (Fromm, 1979). Finally, if the topographic regression obtains in only a subsystem of the ego, then under some circumstances hypnotic behaviors should reveal the operation of some nonparticipatory monitoring function of the individual.

RESEARCH AND APPRAISAL

Why Not Temporal Regression?

In sharpening our definition of hypnosis as a form of psychological regression, it is helpful to identify ways in which hypnosis is *not* regression. Indeed, if we carefully examine the research evidence for a temporal regression during hypnosis, we find no compelling reason to believe that hypnotic subjects return to a developmentally previous mode of psychophysiological, cognitive, or interpersonal functioning. It is true that with suggestions to regress to childhood, highly hypnotizable adults will exhibit dramatic changes in behavior and demeanor. Early theorists, influenced by Freud's work, embraced these performances as compelling evidence of an actual or at least partial regression to a past psychophysiological state (Erickson & Kubie, 1941; Ferenczi, 1909/1980; Kubie & Margolin, 1944; Weitzenhoffer, 1957). But as Spanos and his colleagues have pointed out, the pattern of research findings is disturbingly familiar: An early study reports a genuine reinstatement of childlike psychological processes, but later, more carefully controlled studies either fail to replicate these findings or demonstrate that they are due to demand characteristics (Spanos, Ansari, & Stamm, 1979). There are four processes that could conceivably be temporally regressed during hypnosis: physiology, cognition, perception, and personality. What follows is a brief overview of the research in each of thse areas (a more thorough treatment of this topic can be found in Nash, 1987).

The Return of Childhood Physiological Patterns

Some case studies in the 1930s, 1940s, and 1950s seemed to suggest that following hypnotic age regression suggestions, adults experienced a return of childlike neurophysiological patterning and reflexive responding (Erickson, 1937; Gidro-Frank & Bowersbuch, 1948; McCranie,

Crasilneck, & Teter, 1955). But despite newly developed neurological and neurophysiological assessment techniques, no adequately designed study has been carried out to test this hypothesis further. At this point there is no convincing evidence to support a return of early physiological functioning during hypnosis.

The Return of Childhood Cognitive Processes

Beginning in the 1920s (Young, 1926), researchers have examined whether childhood cognitive functioning may return during hypnotic age regression. There are three categories of evidence that might support a temporal regression in the arena of cognition: (1) especially clear recall of remote events during hypnosis; (2) a return to childhood levels of cognitive ability and achievement; and (3) a return of developmentally earlier Piagetian stages of cognitive complexity. Investigators using appropriate experimenter-blind conditions and motivational control groups have found no evidence that increased accuracy of recall is uniquely attributable to hypnotic age regression procedures, even when the subjects themselves are certain that what they have reported is true (Barber, 1961; O'Connell, Shor, & Orne, 1970). When researchers test for a return of childhood levels of cognitive ability on standardized intelligence measures, they find that the intellectual functioning of hypnotically regressed subjects is essentially adult; it is no more childlike than that of nonhypnotized role-playing controls (Barber, 1962; Roberts, 1984; Sarbin & Farberow, 1952). Finally, all five adequately designed studies that have compared the performance of hypnotically age-regressed adults to that of role-playing adults and actual children on Piagetian tasks have found that the cognitive functioning of hypnotized adults does not resemble that of children (Bynum, 1977; O'Brien et al., 1977; O'Connell Et Al, 1970; Roberts, 1984; P. S. Silverman & Retzlaff, 1986).

Return of Childhood Perceptual Processes

An interesting study (Parrish, Lundy, & Leibowitz, 1969) suggests that hypnotically age-regressed adults may be particularly susceptible to making childlike misattributions to visual illusions. Four subsequent attempts at replication have failed (Ascher, Barber, & Spanos, 1972; Perry & Chisholm, 1973; Porter, Woodward, Bisbee, & Fenker, 1972). Researchers have failed to find a childlike quality to hypnotic perceptual processes, even when regression is directly suggested.

Return of Childhood Personality Processes

Some early work suggested that hypnotically age-regressed subjects will give childlike responses on personality measures, such as the Rorschach, the Thematic Apperception Test (TAT), and word association tasks (Spiegel, Shor, & Fishman, 1945; Mercer & Gibson, 1950; Kline & Guze, 1951; Kline & Haggerty, 1953; Reiff & Scheerer, 1959). However, later, better-controlled studies found the psychological protocols of hypnotically age-regressed and control subjects to be easily distinguishable from those of actual children (Crasilneck & Michael, 1957; Gordon & Freston, 1964; Schofield & Reyher, 1974; Staples & Wilensky, 1968). When hypnotically age-regressed performances were somewhat childlike, nonhypnotized, role-playing subjects could do just as well.

In sum, even when hypnotized subjects are explicitly told to return to a previous age, their responses do not resemble those of actual children. Though hypnotic subjects report subjectively compelling and sometimes profoundly moving childhood experiences, their mental and physiological activity remains essentially adult. The case for a genuine temporal regression taking place during hypnosis appears untenable. Whatever is regressed about hypnosis, it does not seem to involve a return of old psychic structures; it does not seem to involve an undoing of development.

Research Evidence Relevant to Hypnosis as a Topographic Regression in a Subsystem of the Ego

As noted earlier, seven implications follow on an assumption that hypnosis involves a topographic regression. In this section I review the hypnosis research literature bearing on the seven areas of functioning that should undergo specific and measurable changes during hypnosis if the present theoretical premise is correct: a relative shift from secondary- to primary-process thinking; evidence of regression in service of the ego; increased availability of affect; fluctuations in how the body is experienced; changes in the experience of volition; displacement and condensation in the relationship with the hypnotist; and increased ego receptivity.

Primary and Secondary Process during Hypnosis

Some interesting and rigorously standardized scales that operationalize manifestations of primary- and secondary-process thinking have been derived from the projective assessment literature. Not surprisingly, several hypnosis studies have involved administration of projective tests along with hypnotic procedures to determine whether hypnotic protocols show more evidence of imagistic and primary-process mentation than nonhypnotic baseline protocols of the same subjects, or nonhypnotic protocols of other subjects. West, Baugh, and Baugh (1963) used the Rorschach and Draw-A-Person tests in a within-subject design (with and without hypnosis). Even though the 10 subjects were not prescreened for hypnotizability, the experimenters found more primary-process mentation when subjects were tested during hypnosis. In a much more tightly controlled study, using nonhypnotized as well as simulating controls, Wiseman and Reyher (1973) found that using a Rorschach card to induce a dream during hypnosis led to hypnotic subjects' eliciting more primary-process mentation than either nonhypnotized or simulating subjects. In a related study, Levin and Harrison (1976) administered a Rorschach card-induced dream and a TAT story to 28 highly hypnotizable females under counterbalanced conditions (with and without hypnosis). There was indeed a shift to more primary-process material in the hypnosis condition as compared to the nonhypnosis condition.

Two other studies examined the production of primary-process material during hypnosis. Hammer, Walker, and Diment (1978) posited that subjective responses to a poem spoken aloud to 10 hypnotized subjects would contain increased primary-process thinking when compared to responses of nonhypnotized controls. Systematic content analysis of introspective reports revealed more primary-process thinking during hypnosis. The response of two nonhypnotized control groups consisting of highly hypnotizable subjects indicated that primary-process thinking during hypnosis was not an effect of demand characteristics. In a similar content analysis of the hypnotic, day, and nocturnal dreams of 16 subjects (medium to high in hypnotizability) during a 6-week period, Barrett (1979) found that hypnotic dreams differed from daydreams and were more similar to nocturnal dreams in terms of emotional themes and cognitive distortions. This finding provides some additional evidence of a link between hypnosis and the emergence of primary-process thinking.

The programmatic research of Erika Fromm and her colleagues at the University of Chicago has focused primarily on ego functioning during hypnosis (Fromm, Oberlander, & Gruenewald, 1970; Gruenewald, Fromm, & Oberlander, 1972; Oberlander, Gruenewald, & Fromm, 1970). Thirty-two highly hypnotizable subjects were administered the entire Rorschach test with, and without, hypnosis (order was counterbalanced). The Holt and Klopfer methods of scoring were used. Once again, more primary-process material was produced in the hypnosis condition across a series of indices of primitive mentation, across all experimenters, and across order of conditions.

In a study originating in the perceptual literature, Walker, Garrett, and Wallace (1976) conducted tests to determine whether eidetic-like imagery could be experienced by hypnotized subjects. When a standard hypnotic procedure was administered to 20 highly hypnotizable adults who had shown no eidetic imagery in pretesting, 2 (10%) of the subjects displayed eidetic-like imagery during hypnosis. Four subsequent experiments replicated the results of this study, finding eidetic-like imagery during hypnosis in high- but not in low-hypnotizability subjects (Crawford, Wallace, Katsuhiko, & Slater, 1985; Wallace, 1978). These authors concluded that hypnosis may facilitate imaginal processing of information, with a shift from a sequential, verbal, and logical mode during the nonhypnotized state to a more visual, holistic style during hypnosis.

Thus, there is substantial reason to believe that changes in thought processes do occur during hypnosis, and that these changes are consistent with a topographic regression; that is, hypnosis involves a shift to more nonlogical, symbolic, imagistic, and primary-process mentation. But this research literature is not without some difficulties. First, the methodological complexity of working with dependent measures derived from projective procedures has limited the quantity and scope of published studies. Second, although some researchers examining primary-process were careful to include control procedures to assess the effects of demand characteristics (e.g., Wiseman & Reyher, 1973; Hammer et al., 1978), more such experiments are needed if we are to definitively rule out the possibility that increases in primary-process mentation are merely attempts on the part of hypnotic subjects to please the experimenter.

Regression in Service of the Ego

"Regression in service of the ego" has been defined as "a partial temporary lowering of the level of psychic functioning [in which the ego permits] relatively free play to the primary-process thinking in order to accomplish its adaptive tasks" (L. H. Silverman, 1965, p. 232). Thus regression in service of the ego involves two features: First, there is a relaxation of defenses, with a consequent increase in primary-process mentation; second, the process itself leads to creative problem solving and adaptive responding. We have already established that there is good reason to believe that hypnosis involves an increase in primary-process mentation. The question then becomes this: Does this shift in thought processes enable hypnotic subjects to be more creative or adaptive in their responding?

Three well-designed studies using the Holt et al, (1970) Rorschach-based measure of adaptive regression have examined this question, and the answer seems to be no. Wiseman and Reyher (1973) found persuasive evidence for an increase in primary-process mentation during the hypnotic condition, but no elevations on adaptiveness of response. Levin and Harrison (1976) found that adaptive regression scores did appear to have two factors: (1) a primary-process factor and (2) a control and defense factor. There was indeed an increased incidence of primary-process material during hypnosis, but there was no shift in the control and defense factor. That is, the increase in adaptive functions characteristic of regression in service of the ego was again not evident during hypnosis, despite a significant increase in primary-process. Fromm and her colleagues (Fromm et al., 1970; Gruenewald et al., 1972; Oberlander et al., 1970) found no effect for hypnosis on Holt et al.'s (1970) adaptive regression scale. Adaptive regression was just as likely to appear in the nonhypnotized as in the hypnotized condition. The subjects' adaptive regression scores were associated more with general psychological adjustment than with whether they were hypnotized or not. Some well-adjusted subjects did reveal enhanced adaptive functioning in the hypnotic condition, but poorly adjusted subjects seemed to rely even more heavily on maladaptive styles of coping during hypnosis.

Although regression in service of the ego is not necessarily a core feature of all topographic regressions (after all, regressions in neurotic and psychotic patients are decidedly not adaptive), this concept *is* key to a psychoanalytic understanding of how hypnosis works clinically. The three studies reviewed were unanimous in their failure to detect increments in adaptation during or after hypnosis. Because of its central role in psychoanalytic explanations of how hypnosis is mutative, and because these three studies all used only Holt et al.'s Rorschach-based adaptive regression scale, I believe that the concept of regression in service of the ego deserves another look. Any researcher wishing to do so would be well advised to explore ways of more directly operationalizing regression in service of the ego in terms of tangible increments in coping, mastery, and creativity.

Increased Availability of Affect

If hypnosis does involve a topographic regression, then defenses against emotion should be relaxed with a parallel increase in availability of personally relevant affect. It is indeed true that even in laboratory studies, hypnotic subjects respond dramatically to suggestions of sadness or happiness (Bull & Gidro-Frank, 1950). But a major problem with these observations is that the emotion of hypnotic subjects may not really be so remarkable: The dramatic performances may be a function of experimental demand characteristics rather than of hypnosis per se (Orne, 1962).

Four very rigorously designed studies used the "real–simulator" design to determine whether demand characteristics could be ruled out as an explanation of emotional response during hypnosis (Bryant & McConkey, 1989; Damaser, Shor, & Orne, 1963; Hepps & Brady, 1967; Sheehan, 1969). When hypnotic emotions were compared with simulated emotions, they looked essentially similar in terms of heart rate, skin conductance, muscle activity, and certain projective measures of anxiety. As Bryant and McConkey (1989) point out, "this similarity does not indicate that the [response of hypnotized subjects is] due to demand characteristics, but it does not allow us to rule out that possibility" (p. 315). In other words, if we are to more confidently identify and understand changes in the experience of emotions during hypnosis, we must examine aspects of emotion that are not so easily feigned by nonhypnotized subjects who are faking hypnosis.

There is some evidence that if very subtle aspects of emotional response are examined, or if personally relevant and meaningful material is recalled, hypnotic emotional response does differ from simulated emotional response. Weiss, Blum, and Gleberman (1987) focused on the onset latency and the fluctuation of muscular contraction associated with facial expression. They did observe measurable differences between hypnotic and simulated emotions of anxiety and pleasure.

In recent programmatic research, my colleagues and I found that although hypnotically age-regressed adults are no more childlike than controls, they may have freer access to more intense emotions. In these studies (Nash, Johnson, & Tipton, 1979; Nash, Lynn, Stanley, Frauman, & Rhue, 1985), hypnotized and nonhypnotized control subjects were given suggestions to regress to age 3 and were asked to imagine themselves in various home situations. To index the regressive component of responses, we used dependent measures (derived from object relations theory) that were germane to the interpersonal, affect-laden experience of the subject. Specifically, the experimental procedures assessed how subjects related to their transitional objects (e.g., teddy bears, blankets). Children's interactions with their transitional objects are fairly well defined in terms of three qualities: (1) spontaneity—the transitional object is necessary during loneliness or depression; (2) specificity—the object is singular in nature (i.e., other objects are not accepted or required); and (3) intensity—the transitional object is excitedly cuddled, loved, and sometimes mutilated (Gaddini & Gaddini, 1970; Rudhe & Ekecrantz, 1974; Winnicott, 1953). Our hypnotically age-regressed subjects were significantly more spontaneous, specific, and emotionally intense in relation to their transitional objects than were the nonhypnotized controls.

Initially, we suggested that under some circumstances there might be a partial reinstatement of archaic, interpersonally relevant affective processes during hypnotic age regression. But our follow-up study (Nash, Drake, Wiley, Khalsa, & Lynn, 1986) defined some limitations on the nature of the presumed regression. To determine whether the transitional object reported by a hypnotically age-regressed subject was the same as the subject had had as a child, we independently interviewed the mothers of both the hypnotized and control subjects used in the earlier study. Despite the similarity to children in their emotional response to transitional objects, hypnotized subjects were significantly less able than nonhypnotized controls to identify their specific childhood transitional objects correctly (23% accuracy for hypnotized subjects, compared to 70% accuracy for controls). Furthermore, all recollections obtained during hypnosis were incorporated into posthypnotic recollections, regardless of accuracy. We concluded that hypnotic age regression may enhance access to important emotional material (a topographic regression), but that it does not imply an accurate reliving of a specific event.

Fluctuations in Body Experience

The ego is considered first and foremost a body ego (Freud, 1923/1961). If hypnosis involves a topographic regression, one would expect hypnotized subjects to report fluctuations in their experiences of their bodies. Although reports of altered body experiences are not universal among hypnotized subjects, some subjects spontaneously report feelings of shrinking, swelling, or loss of equilibrium. Gill and Brenman (1959) cited these occurrences and claimed that they become more dynamically important with time. Freundlich and Fisher (1974) found that depersonalization and body distortions were more pronounced during hypnosis, and that the extent of distortion was positively correlated with hypnotic susceptibility. In studies of common unsuggested sequelae to hypnosis, distortions in body awareness were found even during routine experimental administration of standard hypnotic scales (Crawford, Hilgard, & MacDonald, 1982). More distortions were reported by highly hypnotizable subjects, and more negative transient experiences of a general nature were reported following individual (as opposed to group) administration. Four cases of apparently spontaneous depersonalization following termination of hypnosis have been reported (Haber, Nitkin, & Shenker, 1979; J. R. Hilgard, Hilgard, & Newman, 1961; Starker, 1974; Wineberg & Straker, 1973). Although no definitive study of regressive body experience has been undertaken, future researchers may wish to assess body experience as an index of topographic regression.

Changes in the Experience of Volition

A topographic regression involves a relaxation of executive ego functions involving planning, organization, intention, and personal responsibility. This is seen most clearly with neurotic patients who describe symptoms as "happening to me" with little or no recognition of their own participation. If hypnosis is indeed a topographic regression, we would expect an attenuation of the hypnotic subject's sense of "I-ness" or volition.

What is meant by a shift in the experience of volition is not that the hypnotic subject is an automaton, as very early theorists would have had it. Indeed, as the Lynn, Rhue, and Weekes (1990) literature review demonstrates, hypnotized subjects' response is not involuntary in the sense that the subjects are unable to resist suggestions. Will and volition do play a role in hypnotic response, and subjects are able to refuse to comply, with or without explicit permission. Nor does a shift in the experience of volition mean that the suggested response occurs automatically, without any effort on the part of the subject to make it happen. There is reason to believe that many hypnotic subjects bring about their response via purposeful, goal-directed strategies and actions (Lynn et al., 1990). From a psychoanalytic perspective, what is meant by a shift in experience of volition is what Shor termed "nonconscious involvement." Obviously behaviors (e.g., responding to an arm-lowering suggestion) are carried out only because the hypnotic subject wills the behavior to happen. The hypnotic subject wants to, and is, moving his or her arm down, but at the same time is fashioning the conscious experience of simply holding the arm steady. The wish to comply is somehow not fully represented in awareness. The experience of "it happened by itself" is the hallmark of a regressive shift in the experience of volition, whether we are speaking of a hypnotic procedure or a neurotic symptom.

Just as is the case with neurotic patients, hypnotic subjects may be unaware of the personal and situational factors that influence their behavior. Reports of nonvolition during hypnosis do not appear to reflect diminished control over behaviors, but instead reveal an experienced separation between intent (to comply) and awareness of that intent. That hypnotic subjects can and do refuse to comply with some suggestions is consistent with the idea that the topographic regression only involves a subsystem of the ego. Reports of this type of shift in the experience of volition correlate with behavioral and subjective aspects of hypnotic responsiveness (E. R. Hilgard, 1977, 1979; Kihlstrom, Evans, Orne, & Orne, 1980). It appears that the experience of nonvolition can be manipulated by the phrasing of suggestions, and that rapport factors may play an important role in the nature and extent of a shift in the experience of volition (Lynn, Nash, Rhue, Frauman, & Sweeney, 1984).

Displacement and Condensation in the Relationship with the Hypnotist

Freud viewed hypnotic phenomena as manifestations of a libidinal regression in the relationship with the hypnotist, such that the hypnotic subject returns to an infantile mode of relating (a temporal regression). Thus for Freud all hypnotic phenomena flow from this basic property of hypnosis as transference. Gill and Brenman (1959) amended this view by identifying hypnotic phenomena as arising from both transference regressions *and* shifts in ego functioning. A view of hypnosis as topographic regression is somewhat more revisionist. I posit that what we recognize as transference-based phenomena during hypnosis are products of a topographic regression. That is, during hypnosis the shift from secondary- to more primary-process thinking leads the subject to make the kinds of interpersonal connections that are so common in dreaming: displacement and condensation. The hypnotist becomes the repository of the subject's important and sometimes archaic interpersonal schema, not because hypnosis renders the subject a psychic infant, but because hypnosis involves a shift in the balance between defense and expression, control and gratification, secondary process and primary process. Such a shift increases the probability that nonlogical and highly personalized attributions will be made about the hypnotist via displacement and condensation. The relevant metaphor, then, is not adult hypnotic subject as infant, but rather adult hypnotic subject as dreamer.

Only within the past few years have empirical investigations directly addressed the special relationship between hypnotist and subject. Two investigators have offered particularly thoughtful and measurable working definitions of this relationship. Shor (1979) defined "archaic involvement" with the hypnotist as "the extent to which there occurred a temporary displacement or 'transference' onto the . . . hypnotist of core personality emotive attitudes . . . most typically in regard to parents" (p. 133). Sheehan and Dolby (1979) suggested that "when transference is operable, the subject can be assumed to respond beyond the role demands of the hypnotic test situation as they are normally defined and to interact with the hypnotist in an especially motivated and personally meaningful way" (p. 573). Although these definitions place a different emphasis on past versus contemporary components of a relationship, they have generated some interesting empirical work on the nature of relationship during hypnosis.

Citing Shor's hypothesis, Bitter (1975) defined transference as the semantic similarity between the hypnotist and the more similar parent (as measured by semantic differentials). Bitter administered a semantic differential measure concerning the experimenter to 86 females both before and after hypnosis. When the results were compared with pre- and postmeasures of 34 nonhypnotized control subjects, they indicated that perceived similarity between the hypnotist and either parent did not facilitate hypnotic response. In addition, the hypnotic procedure itself did not enhance perceived similarity between the hypnotist and either parent. Transference, at least as measured by semantic differentials, did not appear to be an important feature of hypnosis in this study.

In a carefully designed double-blind study, Frauman, Lynn, Hardaway, and Molteni (1984) examined subliminal activation of symbiotic fantasies as a way to help subjects more fully experience the archaic positive aspects of the hypnotic relationship. Before hypnosis, the experimental group received subliminally presented symbiotic stimulation ("Mommy and I are one"); a control group received a neutral message ("People are walking"). Comparisons of subsequent hypnotic performance revealed that the experimental treatment did indeed result in increased ratings of rapport with the hypnotist. Subjects in the "Mommy" group were also marginally more responsive to hypnosis than were controls, indicating the importance of relationship factors in hypnosis.

In related work, 20 items presumed to index archaic involvement with the hypnotist were adopted directly from Shor's descriptions of how transferential experiences of archaic involvement are reported posthypnotically by subjects (Nash & Spinler, 1989). Each of these items was transformed into a self-rated Likert-type scale, yielding a 20-item scale to be administered following hypnosis. Findings indicated significant positive correlation between hypnotizability and posttreatment scores on this measure (R = .52). Factor analysis suggested three clusters of variables relevant to archaic involvement and hypnotic response: (1) perceived power of the hypnotist, (2) positive emotional bond to the hypnotist, and (3) fear of negative appraisal. All three factors correlated significantly with hypnotic susceptibility.

Sheehan (1971, 1980; Sheehan & Dolby, 1979) examined the extent to which good hypnotic subjects evidence an especially motivated interaction with the hypnotist, along with increased involvement in the experience of suggested events. Using appropriate imagination, task motivation, and simulating control groups, Sheehan found that hypnotic subjects characteristically participated more personally in hypnotic dream experiences than did control subjects. Hypnotized subjects more often reported dreams in which they perceived the hypnotist in a positive light and spontaneously expressed feeling protected, cared for, and supported. This special commitment superseded demand characteristics and was sensitive to manipulations for reducing rapport. Sheehan interpreted these findings less in terms of analytic theory and more in terms of a special "motivated cognitive commitment" to the hypnotist and the hypnotic task. Either way, Sheehan's research suggests the importance of relationship factors in hypnosis and offers new ways to investigate an often elusive phenomenon. Work by Levitt and Baker (1983) underscores a similar association between relationship factors and hypnotic performance in a clinical population.

Ego Receptivity and Hypnosis

Erika Fromm identifies three modes of ego functioning:

1. *Ego passivity*. An experience of choicelessness. The person helplessly submits to the demands coming from the instincts and the external environment. Examples of ego passivity are certain neurotic and psychotic symptomatology, catastrophic reactions, and certain drug states.

2. *Ego activity*. A problem-solving mode. The person is ready and able to manipulate the environment via a high level of attention, activity, reality orientation, and logic.

3. *Ego receptivity*. A relaxed and uncritical mode. The person diverts attention from critical judgment and strict adherence to reality testing, so as to allow unconscious and preconscious material to emerge. Examples of ego receptivity include daydreaming, reverie, and free association.

Fromm posits that the regressive shifts in ego functioning during hypnosis are such that the subject moves from an ego-active to a more ego-receptive mode. This would explain the hypnotic subject's freer access to inner experience, as well as his or her extraordinary receptivity to external stimuli (hypersuggestibility). It is not so much that ego activity stops or is even attenuated during hypnosis; rather, the focus of awareness shifts to a realm of effortless ongoing experience that is dominated by sensory, imagistic, and nonlogical inputs. Monitoring, reality testing, and task-oriented vigilance continue, but outside of awareness.

In a longitudinal study of 33 highly hypnotizable subjects, Fromm and her colleagues carefully examined close to 900 separate journal entries, one for each daily self-hypnosis session for each subject (Fromm et al., 1987–1988). Results suggested a strong link between ego receptivity and hypnosis. Reports of absorption, subjective depth, vividness of imagery and hypnotic susceptibility were correlated with predominance of ego receptivity experiences in the journals and openness to internal self-initiated experiences in general. Clearly, Fromm's groundbreaking work on self-hypnosis offers a new methodology for exploring the parameters of the regressive shifts taking place during hypnosis. This is a new and promising area for future research.

Why Regression Is a Subsystem of the Ego and Not the Entire Ego

If the concept of topographic regression does capture the nature of hypnotic experience, it is perfectly clear that this regression does not encompass the entire "I-ness" of the subject. On this point, the social-psychological explanation of hypnosis as role enactment (Sarbin, 1950) and the present psychoanalytic explanation of hypnosis as topographic regression in a subsystem of the ego are in accord. Whether on the stage or in day-to-day living, we are induced by social cues and contexts to enact certain roles. We may purposefully or inadvertently become inattentive to incompatible roles or cues as we enact a certain way of relating or appearing, but these cues are nonetheless processed (after all, an actor will leave the stage if the fire alarm is sounded). From a social-psychological perspective, as the cues change, our performance changes. From a psychoanalytic perspective, it appears that even during the most compelling hypnotic performances, there is a portion of the ego that does not engage, that remains apart, that does not participate in the regression. If hypnosis were a topographic regression across the entire ego, it would be like dreaming or a psychotic state, with little or no chance for the subject to initiate, focus, change, or terminate the experience because the *entire* ego is a participant. From a social-psychological, analytic, or neodissociation perspective, it is clear that hypnotic subjects do respond to cues that are incompatible with their hypnotic role—whether we examine hidden-observer phenomena, duality in hypnotic age regression, or differential effects of prehypnosis instructions.

CONCLUSIONS

Too often in science, we fail to explicitly identify a conceptual "dead end." I believe the weight of the evidence is such that we can now say with some certainty that hypnosis does not involve a temporal regression. Whatever change in usual functioning may be involved in hypnosis, it is not the lawful backward retracing of development that is required by the concept of temporal regression. There may be some superficial resemblances between an infant state and the adult hypnotized state, but, as this chapter suggests, these resemblances are in fact superficial. Peterfreund (1978) illustrates how equating infant and adult states based on superficial resemblances can be grossly misleading:

> A man who has suffered a cerebrovasular accident and is therefore unable to speak may be said to be suffering from aphasia. But he is not in the same state as an infant of two months who cannot speak. . . . [It would be] fallacious to describe [him] as having "regressed" to an earlier state of "normal aphasia." (p. 439)

Similarly, during hypnosis adult subjects are exceedingly responsive to suggestion. Though this hypersuggestibility may crudely resemble the compliant gullibility of very small children, adult hypnotic behavior and experience remain quite distinct from those of children. It would be a mistake to attribute the hypnotic subject's hypersuggestibility to a reinstatement of an infantile psychological mode of functioning.

But if I am "throwing the baby" out of hypnosis, I want to keep the "bath water." That is, just because the concept of temporal regression fails to capture what hypnosis is, it does not invalidate the explanatory value of another type of psychological regression rooted in a more rigorous empirical tradition: topographic regression. Hypnotized subjects are not adults responding like children, but adults responding like topographically regressed adults by exhibiting more imagistic, primary-process material, perhaps making more adaptive use of this material, displaying more spontaneous and intense emotion, experiencing unusual body sensations, undergoing changes in the experience of volition, displacing core attributes about important others onto the hypnotist, and maintaining a posture of receptivity to inner and outer experience. In this sense hypnosis is like dreaming. After all, both hypnosis and dreaming can involve a dramatic change in subjective experience, but with the difference that in hypnosis a portion of the ego remains apart from the experience. Monitoring and executive functions are not so fundamentally ablated, but suspended—held outside of awareness.

REFERENCES

Ascher, L. M., Barber, T. X., & Spanos, N. P. (1972). Two attempts to replicate the Parrish–Lundy–Leibowitz experiment on hypnoticage regression. *American Journal of Clinical Hypnosis, 14*, 178–185.

Baker, E. L. (1981). An hypnotherapeutic approach to enhance object relatedness in psychotic patients. *International Journal of Clinical and Experimental Hypnosis, 124*, 136–147.

Balint, M. (1968). *The basic fault: Therapeutic aspects of regression.* London: Tavistock.

Barber, T. X. (1961). Experimental evidence for a theory of hypnotic behavior: II. Experimental controls in hypnotic age-regression. *International Journal of Clinical and Experimental Hypnosis, 181–193.*

Barber, T. X. (1962). Hypnotic age regression: A critical review. *Psychosomatic Medicine, 24*, 286–299.

Barrett, D. (1979). The hypnotic dream: Its relation to nocturnal dreams and waking fantasies. *Journal of Abnormal Psychology, 88*, 584–591.

Bion, W. R. (1977). *Seven servants.* New York: Jason Aronson.

Bitter, E. J. (1975). An empirical investigation of the relationship between hypnosis and transference (Doctoral dissertation, University of Montana, 1974). *Dissertation Abstracts International, 35*(10), 5099B.

Bowers, P. G. (1978). Hypnotizability: Creativity, and the role of effortless experiencing. *International Journal of Clinical and Experimental Hypnosis, 26*, 184–202.

Bryant, R. A., & McConkey, K. M. (1989). Hypnotic emotions and physical sensations: A real–simulating analysis. *International Journal of Clinical and Experimental Hypnosis, 37*, 305–319.

Bull, N., & Gidro-Frank, L. (1950). Emotions induced and studied in hypnotic subjects: Part II. The findings. *Journal of Nervous and Mental Diseases, 112*, 97–120.

Bynum, E. (1977). Hypnotic age regression: An experimental investigation (Doctoral dissertation, Pennsylvania State University, 1977). *Dissertation Abstracts International, 38*(5), 2394B–2395B.

Crasilneck, H. B., & Michael, C. M. (1957). Performance on the Bender under hypnotic age regression. *Journal of Abnormal Psychology, 54*, 319–322.

Crawford, H. J., Hilgard, J. R., & MacDonald, H. (1982). Transient experiences following hypnotic testing and special termination procedures. *International Journal of Clinical and Experimental Hypnosis, 30*, 117–126.

Crawford, Wallace, Katsuhiko, & Slater (1985). *Eidetic-like imager in hypnosis: Rare but there.* Unpublished manuscript.

Damaser, E. C., Shor, R. E., & Orne, M. T. (1963). Physiological effects during hypnotically requested emotions. *Psychosomatic Medicine, 25,* 334–343.

Erickson, M. H. (1937). Development of apparent unconsciousness during hypnotic reliving of a traumatic experience. *Archives of Neurological Psychiatry, 38,* 1282–1288.

Erickson, M. H., & Kubie, L. S. (1941). The successful treatment of a case of acute hysterical depression by a return under hypnosis depression by a return under hypnosis to a critical phase of childhood. *Psychoanalytic Quarterly, 10,* 583–609.

Ferenczi, S. (1980). Introjection and transference. In E. Jones (Trans.), *First contributions to psychoanalysis* (pp. 35–93). New York: Brunner/Mazel. (Original work published 1909)

Frauman, D. C., Lynn, S. J., Hardaway, R., & Molteni, A. (1984). Effect of subliminal symbiotic activation on hypnotic rapport and susceptibility. *Journal of Abnormal Psychology, 93,* 481–483.

Freud, S. (1953). The interpretation of dreams. In J. Strachey (Ed. and Trans.), *The standard edition of the complete psychological works of Sigmund Freud* (Vols. 4–5, pp. 1–627). London: Hogarth Press. (Original work published 1900)

Freud, S. (1955). Group psychology and the analysis of the ego. In J. Strachey (Ed. and Trans.), *The standard edition of the complete psychological works of Sigmund Freud* (Vol. 18, pp. 69–143). London: Hogarth Press. (Original work published 1921)

Freud, S. (1957). Five lectures on psycho-analysis. In J. Strachey (Ed. and Trans.), *The standard edition of the complete psychological works of Sigmund Freud* (Vol. 12, pp. 9–56). London: Hogarth Press. (Original work published 1909)

Freud, S. (1957). Thoughts for the times on war and death. In J. Strachey (Ed. and Trans.), *The standard edition of the complete psychological works of Sigmund Freud* (Vol. 14, pp. 275–300). London: Hogarth Press. (Original work published 1915)

Freud, S. (1957). A metapsychological supplement to the theory of dreams. In J. Strachey (Ed. and Trans.), *The standard edition of the complete psychological works of Sigmund Freud* (Vol. 14, pp. 222–235). London: Hogarth Press. (Original work published 1917)

Freud, S. (1960). Jokes and their relation to the unconscious. In J. Strachey (Ed. and Trans.), *The standard edition of the complete psychological works of Sigmund Freud* (Vol. 8, pp. 9–236). London: Hogarth Press. (Original work published 1905)

Freud, S. (1961). The ego and the id. In J. Strachey (Ed. and Trans.), *The standard edition of the complete psychological works of Sigmund Freud* (Vol. 19, pp. 12–59). London: Hogarth Press. (Original work published 1923)

Freud, S. (1964). New introductory lectures on psycho-analysis. In J. Strachey (Ed. and Trans.), *The standard edition of the complete psychological works of Sigmund Freud* (Vol. 22, pp. 7–182). London: Hogarth Press. (Original work published 1933)

Freundlich, B., & Fisher, S. (1974). The role of body experience in hypnotic behavior. *International Journal of Clinical and Experimental Hypnosis, 22,* 68–83.

Fromm, E. (1979). The nature of hypnosis and other altered states of consciousness: An ego-psychological theory. In E. Fromm & R. E. Shor (Eds.), *Hypnosis:*

Developments in research and new perspectives (2nd ed., pp. 81–103). Chicago: Aldine.

Fromm, E., Lombard, L., Skinner, S. H., & Kahn, S. (1987–1988). The modes of the ego in self-hypnosis. *Imagination, Cognition and Personality, 7*, 335–349.

Fromm, E., Oberlander, M. I., & Gruenewald, D. (1970). Perceptual and cognitive processes in different states of consciousness: The waking state and hypnosis. *Journal of Projective Techniques and Personality Assessment, 34*, 374–387.

Gaddini, R., & Gaddini, E. (1970). Transitional objects and the process of individuation: A study in three different social groups. *Journal of the American Academy of Child Psychiatry, 9*, 347–365.

Gidro-Frank, L., & Bowersbuch, M. K. (1948). A study of the plantar response in hypnotic age regression. *Journal of Nervous and Mental Disease, 107*, 443–458.

Gill, M. M. (1972). Hypnosis as an altered and regressed state. *International Journal of Clinical and Experimental Hypnosis, 20*, 224–237.

Gill, M. M., & Brenman, M. (1959). *Hypnosis and related states: Psychoanalytic studies in regression.* New York: International Universities Press.

Gordon, J. E., & Freston, M. (1964). Role-playing and age regression in hypnotized and nonhypnotized subjects. *Journal of Personality, 32*, 411–419.

Gruenewald, D., Fromm, E., & Oberlander, M. I. (1972). Hypnosis and adaptive regression: An ego-psychological inquiry. In E. Fromm & R. E. Shor (Eds.), *Hypnosis: Research developments and perspectives* (pp. 495–509). Chicago: Aldine-Atherton.

Haber, C. H., Nitkin, R., & Shenker, I. R. (1979). Adverse reactions to hypnotherapy in obese adolescents: A developmental viewpoint. *Psychiatric Quarterly, 51*, 55–63.

Hammer, A. G., Walker, W., & Diment, A. D. (1978). A nonsuggested effect of trance induction. In F. H. Frankel & H. S. Zamansky (Eds.), *Hypnosis at its bicentennial: Selected papers* (pp. 91–100). New York: Plenum.

Hartmann, H. (1958). *Ego psychology and the problem of adaptation* (D. Rapaport, Trans.). New York: International Universities Press. (Original work published 1939)

Hepps, R. B., & Brady, J. P. (1967). Hypnotically induced tachycardia: An experiment with simulating controls. *Journal of Nervous and Mental Diseases, 145*, 131–137.

Hilgard, E. R. (1977). *Divided consciousness: Multiple controls in human thought and action.* New York: Wiley.

Hilgard, E. R. (1979). Divided consciousness in hypnosis: The implications of the hidden observer. In E. Fromm & R. E. Shor (Eds.), *Hypnosis: Developments in research and new perspectives* (2nd ed., pp. 45–79). New York: Aldine.

Hilgard, J. R., Hilgard, E. R., & Newman, M. (1961). Sequelae to hypnotic induction with special reference to earlier chemical anesthesia. *Journal of Nervous and Mental Disease, 133*, 461–478.

Holt, R. R., Eagle, C., Havel, J., Goldberger, L., Phillip, A., Rabkin, J., & Safrin, R. (1970). *Manual for scoring of primary-process manifestations in Rorschach responses* (rev. 10th ed.). New York: Research Center for Mental Health, New York University.

Kihlstrom, J. F., Evans, F. J., Orne, E. C., & Orne, M. T. (1980). Attempting to breach posthypnotic amnesia. *Journal of Abnormal Psychology: 89*, 603–616.

Kline, M. V., & Guze, H. (1951). The use of a projective drawing technique in the investigation of hypnotic age regression and progression. *British Journal of Medical Hypnosis, 3*(2), 10–21.

Kline, M. V., & Haggerty, A. D. (1953). A hypnotic experimental approach to the genesis of occupational interests and choice: III. Hypnotic age regression and the TAT: A clinical case study in occupational identification. *International Journal of Clinical and Experimental Hypnosis, 1,* 18–31.

Kris, E. (1952). *Psychoanalytic explorations in art.* New York: International Universities Press.

Kubie, L. S., & Margolin, S. (1944). The process of hypnotism and the nature of the hypnotic state. *American Journal of Psychiatry, 100,* 611–622.

Langer, J. (1970). Werner's comparative organismic theory. In P. H. Mussen (Ed.), *Carmichael's manual of child psychology* (3rd ed., Vol. 1, pp. 733–771). New York: Wiley.

Levin, L. A., & Harrison, R. H. (1976). Hypnosis and regression in the service of the ego. *International Journal of Clinical and Experimental Hypnosis, 24,* 400–418.

Levitt, E. E., & Baker, E. L. (1983). The hypnotic relationship—another look at coercion, compliance, and resistance: A brief communication. *International Journal of Clinical and Experimental Hypnosis, 31,* 125–131.

Lynn, S. J., Nash, M. R., Rhue, J. W., Frauman, D. C., & Sweeney, C. (1984). Nonvolition, expectancies, and hypnotic rapport. *Journal of Abnormal Psychology, 93,* 295–303.

Lynn, S. J., Rhue, J. W., & Weekes, J. R. (1990). Hypnotic responsiveness: A social cognitive analysis. *Psychological Review, 97,* 169–184.

McCranie, E. J., Crasilneck, H. B., & Teter, H. R. (1955). The EEG in hypnotic age regression. *Psychiatric Quarterly, 29,* 85–88.

Mercer, M., & Gibson, R. W. (1950). Rorschach content in hypnosis: Chronological age level regression. *Journal of Clinical Psychology, 6,* 352–358.

Nash, M. R. (1987). What, if anything, is regressed about hypnotic age regression? A review of the empirical literature. *Psychological Bulletin, 102,* 42–52.

Nash, M. R., Drake, S. D., Wiley, S., Khalsa, S., & Lynn, S. J.(1986). Accuracy of recall by hypnotically age-regressed subjects. *Journal of Abnormal Psychology, 95,* 298–300.

Nash, M. R., Johnson, L. S., & Tipton, R. D. (1979). Hypnotic age regression and the occurrence of transitional object relationships. *Journal of Abnormal Psychology, 88,* 547–555.

Nash, M. R., Lynn, S. J., Stanley, S., Frauman, D., & Rhue, J. (1985). Hypnotic age regression and the importance of assessing interpersonally relevant affect. *International Journal of Clinical and Experimental Hypnosis, 33,* 224–235.

Nash, M. R., & Spinler, D. (1989). Hypnosis and transference: A measure of archaic involvement with the hypnotist. *International Journal of Clinical and Experimental Hypnosis, 37,* 129–144.

Oberlander, M. I., Gruenewald, D., & Fromm, E. (1970, September). *Content and structural characteristics of thought processes in hypnosis.* Paper presented at the meeting of the American Psychological Association, Miami Beach, FL.

O'Brien, R. M., Kramer, C. E., Chiglinsky, M. A., Stevens, G., Nunan, L., & Fritzo, J. (1977). Moral development examined through hypnotic and task motivated age regression. *American Journal of Clinical Hypnosis, 19,* 209–213.

O'Connell, D. N., Shor, R. E., & Orne, M. T. (1970). Hypnotic ate regression: An empirical and methodological analysis. *Journal of Abnormal Psychology Monographs, 76*(3, Pt. 2).

Orne, M. T. (1962). On the social psychology of the psychological experiment: With particular reference to demand characteristics and their implications. *American Psychologist, 17*, 776–783.

Parrish, M., Lundy, R. M., & Leibowitz, H. W. (1969). Effect of of hypnotic age regression on the magnitude of the Ponzo and Poggendorff illusions. *Journal of Abnormal Psychology, 74*, 693–698.

Perry, C., & Chisholm, W. (1973). Hypnotic age regression and the Ponzo and Poggendorff illusions. *International Journal of Clinical and Experimental Hypnosis, 21*, 192–204.

Peterfreund, E. (1978). Some critical comments on psychoanalytic conceptualizations of infancy. *International Journal of Psycho-Analysis, 59*, 427–441.

Piaget, J. (1973). *The child and reality: Problems of genetic psychology* (A. Rosin, Trans). New York: Grossman.

Porter, J. W., Woodward, J. A., Bisbee, C. T., & Fenker, R. M. (1972). Effect of hypnotic age regression on the magnitude of the Ponzo illusion: A replication. *Journal of Abnormal Psychology, 79*, 189–194.

Reiff, R., & Scheerer, M. (1959). *Memory and hypnotic age regression: Developmental aspects of cognitive function explored through hypnosis.* New York: International Universities Press.

Roberts, D. (1984). Hypnotically induced ate regression versus age regression in response to task motivation instructions on five developmental tasks (Doctoral dissertation, Hofstra University). *Dissertation Abstracts International, 45*(5), 1594B.

Rudhe, L., & Ekecrantz, L. (1974). Transitional phenomena: The typical phenomenon and its development. *Acta Psychiatrica Scandinavica, 50*, 381–400.

Sarbin, T. R. (1950). Contributions to role-taking theory: I. Hypnotic behavior. *Psychological Review, 57*, 255–270.

Sarbin, T. R., & Farberow, N. L. (1952). Contributions to role-taking theory: A clinical study of self and role. *Journal of Abnormal Psychology, 47*, 117–125.

Schafer, R. (1958). Regression in the service of the ego: The relevance of psychoanalytic concept for personality assessment. In G. Lindzey (Ed.), *Assessment of human motives* (pp. 119–148). New York: Holt, Rinehart & Winston.

Schilder, P. F. (1956). The nature of hypnosis. Translation by Gerda Corvin. New York: International Union Press.

Schofield, L. J., & Reyher, J. (1974). Thematic productions under hypnotically aroused conflict in age regressed and waking states using the real–simulator design. *Journal of Abnormal Psychology, 83*, 130–139.

Sheehan, P. W. (1969). Artifical induction of posthypnotic conflict. *Journal of Abnormal Psychology, 74*, 16–25.

Sheehan, P. W. (1971). Countering preconceptions about hypnosis: An objective index of involvement with the hypnotist [Monograph]. *Journal of Abnormal Psychology, 78*, 299–322.

Sheehan, P. W., & Dolby, R. M. (1979). Motivated involvement in hypnosis: The illusion of clinical rapport through hypnotic dreams. *Journal of Abnormal Psychology, 88*, 573–583.

Shor, R. E. (1979). A phenomenological method for the measurement of variables important to an understanding of thenature of hypnosis. In E. Fromm & R. E. Shor (Eds.), *Hypnosis: Developments in research and new perspectives* (2nd ed., pp. 105–135). New York: Aldine.

Silverman, L. H. (1965). Regression in the service of the ego: A case study. *Journal of Projective Techniques and Personality Assessment, 29,* 232–244.

Silverman, P. S., & Retzlaff, P. O. (1986). Cognitive stage regression through hypnosis: Are earlier cognitive stages retrievable? *International Journal of Clinical and Experimental Hypnosis, 34,* 192–204.

Spanos, N. P., Ansari, F., & Stamm, H. J. (1979). Hypnotic age regression and eidetic imagery: A failure to replicate. *Journal of Abnormal Psychology, 88,* 88–91.

Spiegel, H., Shor, J., & Fishman, S. (1945). An hypnotic ablation technique for the study of personality. *Psychosomatic Medicine, 7,* 273–278.

Spitz, R. A. (1965). *The first year of life: A psychoanalytic study of normal and deviant development of object relations.* New York: International Universities Press.

Staples, E. A., & Wilensky, H. (1968). A controlled Rorschach investigation of hypnotic age regression. *Journal of Protective Techniques, 32,* 246–252.

Starker, S. (1974). Persistence of a hypnotic dissociative reaction. *International Journal of Clinical and Experimental Hypnosis, 22,* 131–137.

Walker, N. S., Garrett, J. B., & Wallace, B. (1976). Restoration of eidetic imagery via hypnotic age regression: A preliminary report. *Journal of Abnormal Psychology, 85,* 335–337.

Wallace, B. (1978). Restoration of eidetic imagery via hypnotic age regression: More evidence. *Journal of Abnormal Psychology, 87,* 673–675.

Weiss, F., Blum, G. S., & Gleberman, L. (1987). Anatomically based measurement of facial expressions in simulated versus hypnotically induced affect. *Motivation and Emotion, 11,* 67–81.

Weitzenhoffer, A. M. (1957). *General techniques of hypnotism.* New York: Grune & Stratton.

Werner, H. (1948). *Comparative psychology of mental development.* Chicago: Follett.

West, J. V., Baugh, V. S., & Baugh, A. P. (1963). Rorschach and Draw-A-Person responses of hypnotized and nonhypnotizedsubjects. *Psychiatric Quarterly, 37,* 123–127.

Wineburg, E. N., & Straker, N. (1973). An episode of acute, self-limiting depersonalization following a first session of hypnosis. *American Journal of Psychiatry, 130,* 98–100.

Winnicott, D. W. (1953). Transitional objects and transitional phenomena: A study of the first not-me possession. *International Journal of Psycho-Analysis, 34,* 89–97.

Wiseman, R. J., & Reyher, J. (1973). Hypnotically induced dreams using the Rorschach inkblots as stimuli: A test of Freud's theory of dreams. *Journal of Personality and Social Psychology, 27,* 329–336.

Young, P. C. (1926). An experimental study of mental and physical functions in the normal and hypnotic states: Additional results. *American Journal of Psychology, 37,* 345–356.

HYPNOSIS AS
RELAXATION

CHAPTER 7

Anesis

WILLIAM E. EDMONSTON, JR.
Colgate University

INTRODUCTION

Historically, clinically, experimentally, and physiologically, relaxation precedes and forms the fundamental basis of subsequent phenomena associated with the term hypnosis. Individuals relax through a number of diverse manipulations and rituals. Some relax by lying down and progressively and sequentially reducing tension in the musculature. Others prefer to listen to soft music or the soft, repetitive words of another suggesting the gentle beginnings of an altered state. Still others relax through jogging or strenuous exercise. Regardless of the method employed, the goal is the same—relaxation. And the consequences of the relaxation so achieved are feelings of pleasantness and unreality; heightened responsivity to exogenous and endogenous suggestion; the assumption of brief life roles not otherwise assumed in the helter-skelter of everyday living; the dissociation of parts of our cognitive, sensory, and motor activities; the diminution of ego controls; and an occasional amnesic period.

From the ancient Hindu practices through modern Transcendental Meditation (TM), humans have considered relaxation/sleep-like conditions to have curative features and to equate with a condition of altered consciousness popularly labeled hypnosis. Elsewhere, I have traced the historic practices that preceded and formed a conceptual basis of modern-day hypnotic inductions and practices (Edmonston, 1986). A number of these historical precedents—for example, the uses of water (magnetized or otherwise) and metal objects—have little place in hypnosis as practiced today. Others (e.g., laying on of hands) are used to a limited extent, while still others (eye fixation, soothing verbalizations) form rituals around which most modern induction techniques are constructed. One, and only one, of the historical procedures associated with the development

197

of hypnosis and the hypnotic condition has maintained its presence in both our clinical and experimental work: the association of physical and cognitive relaxation with what we call hypnosis and should call *anesis*.

Why have relaxation and the procedures for bringing about relaxation been the sustaining element in the history of hypnotic induction? Why should almost 6,000 years of recorded history continually reaffirm the powerful association between relaxation techniques and what we eventually came to label hypnosis? Could it be that the symbiosis of these two concepts in history portends an unspoken equivalence that both ancients and moderns recognized, but could not articulate? Are they two concepts or one concept with different labels, depending upon the viewer?

Anesis as Theory

At the outset of writing *Hypnosis and Relaxation* (Edmonston, 1981), I had no intention of developing a theory of hypnosis. *Hypnosis and Relaxation* evolved from experimental data demonstrating that the responses of subjects during hypnosis did not differ from those elicited during a condition of simple relaxation. As it turned out, this observation was clear whether one looked at the clinical or the experimental literature. The equation of neutral hypnosis—the phase of the hypnotic process that follows induction and precedes the issuing of and response to suggestions—with the condition of relaxation became even more obvious from the few studies using nonhypnotic relaxation comparison groups. Even then, I did not consider this equation a theory in the sense of a set of formal hypotheses, axioms, and the like. At the time of its publication, I considered *Hypnosis and Relaxation* to be a simple, straightforward statement of clinical and experimental observation. I chose, therefore, to base the conclusion of *anesis* on observation and experimentation, rather than on speculation, intuition, or rationalistic explanation.

From the data, I concluded:

> The relaxation of hypnosis is *prerequisite* to all of the theories in the field. The relaxation precedes, must come first, *before* the various theoretical explanations can begin to weave their hypothetical webs. . . . It [relaxation] is the mechanism for the disinhibition; the hypersuggestibility; the circumventing of the ego mechanisms; the regressions in the ego's service; the effectiveness of the attitudes, motivations, and the role-playing of the subjects and the 'demand characteristics' of the situations; the dissociations and the dividing of the consciousness; and, yes, the production of the so-called hypnotic phenomena themselves. (Edmonston, 1981, p. 210)

Yet, as reviews started to appear, I found that I had created a ripple in the relatively calm sea of sociocognitive writings that presently claim the domain of hypnosis. Reviewers (e.g., Moon, 1982) seemed greatly concerned that the so-called characteristics of hypnosis other than relaxation were not equally addressed. The most often mentioned of these were role playing, attention focusing, imagery, and dissociation. Added to this list might also have been the motivational interpretation of the 1960s, the emergent primary processes of the indestructible psychoanalytically based viewpoints, and the subjective experiences of perceptual and memory distortion occasioned by the social demand characteristics of the hypnotic situation.

How, then, are we to compare the relaxation hypothesis with other theories of hypnosis? And where does suggestibility fit into the equation? We must proceed first with a consideration of the other theories.

Comparisons with Other Theories

Hypnosis as Partial Sleep

The theoretical position to which *anesis* has the greatest affinity is Pavlov's, contained in his observation that "Inhibition, ordinary sleep and hypnosis are one and the same process" (1923, p. 604). Pavlov conceived of human hypnosis (he called it "suggested sleep") as residing on a continuum from full wakefulness to total sleep, the progression being marked by the inverse relationship between cortical excitation and cortical inhibition (see Edmonston, 1967, 1981, for detailed accounts of Pavlov's writings). According to Pavlov, the irradiation of cortical inhibition is progressive, affecting first motor responses and only later more vegetative responses, whose control resides more in subcortical areas. As inhibition spreads subcortically, the individual eventually drifts into total sleep. Thus, hypnosis, being on this continuum of inhibition, should affect certain types of responses (particularly voluntary motor responses) to a greater extent than others. This has been shown to be the case in a series of studies on conditioned responses of finger withdrawal (Plapp & Edmonston, 1965), eyeblinks (Plapp, 1967), electrodermal changes (Edmonston, 1968, 1979; Edmonston & Pessin, 1966), and heart rate (Edmonston, 1981), which follow a voluntary–involuntary control path through human responsiveness. This progressive loss of responsivity with hypnotic induction is manifested in an early loss of what Pavlov called the "speech motor analyzer," which is the first to be inhibited with induction and the last to be disinhibited with the termination of hypnosis (see Platonov, 1955/ 1959). One of the earliest clinical signs of hypnosis *is* the disinclination of the subject to speak, along with the loss of muscle tone apparent in the drooping of the head, the slouching of the shoulders, and the general lethargy of the body.

Pavlov also perceived changes in speech function not only as an indication of the beginning stages of hypnosis, but as an integral part of the induction. He accounted for the ability of the human subject to respond to later suggestions while in the repose of hypnosis through rapport zones of cortical excitation, symbiotic with the larger areas of inhibition. Thus, the cortical condition during hypnosis is a mosaic of inhibited and excited foci, the latter forming the link between the hypnotist and the subject.

Very clearly, Pavlov's writings did not equate hypnosis with deep sleep, as Hull (1933), Bass (1931), and others misinterpreted them. Even as early as 1851 Wood made it clear that there was a difference between natural sleep, in which "*all* nervous centres . . . repose," and magnetism (hypnosis), in which "sensations and volition are chiefly affected" (p. 433), the rest retaining their excitation phase. Over a century later, Das (1958) made the same observation: "It has never been claimed by Pavlov or Pavlovians that hypnosis is sleep" (p. 85). Why, then, have investigators from Bass and Hull onward been so ready to disregard Pavlov's theory? Early on, it was probably due to misinterpretation and the fact that a major investigator (Clark Hull) had declared hypnosis not to be sleep. However, now that Pavlov's ideas have been better understood (see Platonov, 1955/1959; Edmonston, 1981), the resistance to the idea of inhibitory organismic changes being the basis of and initial phase in the total process of hypnosis is more of a puzzle. For Pavlov, as for myself, the induction of hypnosis is a process of *inhibition*, the end point of which—relaxation—forms the fundamental basis of all other understandings. The elicitation of the phenomena of hypnosis becomes possible and is enhanced through the inhibitory mechanisms of relaxation. If anything, it is a process of momentary, relative *disinhibition* that occurs when the hypnotic subject carries out the suggestions of the hypnotist. Thus, a two-step process is hypothesized. The first and fundamental step is the relaxation, followed by fluctuating levels of alertness dictated by the activity requirements of subsequent suggestions. Puységur observed the same two-step process in Victor Race over 200 years ago (Puységur, 1837).

Cognitive Theory

As indicated below, the 1960s saw a deluge of articles based on the notion that response to suggestion could be elicited by instructions exhorting subjects to perform as instructed. Barber (Barber & Calverley, 1962, 1963b) claimed that his results displaced trance state theories of hypnosis by showing that the traditional trance induction procedures were unnecessary to produce responsiveness to suggestion. However, studies from different laboratories (E. R. Hilgard, 1965; E. R. Hilgard & Tart, 1966; Edmonston & Robertson, 1967) showed that the equation of motivational instructions and a traditional relaxation induction was premature.

In the 1970s, Barber produced a series of items outlining an alternative paradigm to the "trance paradigm," labeled "cognitive–behavioral theory" (Barber, 1979; Barber & Ham, 1974; Barber, Spanos, & Chaves, 1974; Barber & Wilson, 1977). Again, his focus has been on the nature of the instructions given to subjects prior to their being tested on various scales of suggestibility, including another measuring instrument, the Creative Imagination Scale (CIS; Wilson, 1976; Barber & Wilson, 1977; Wilson & Barber, 1978). Like the Barber Suggestibility Scale (BSS; Barber & Calverley, 1963a), the CIS does not require an induction procedure before the 10 challenge items of the scale are administered to individuals. Thus, like the BSS, the CIS predicts from nonhypnotic behavior to hypnotic behavior, or the degree to which an individual will respond to suggestions while hypnotized.

In order to test his theory, Barber developed a set of instructions called "think-with" instructions. In many respects, these instructions (see Barber & Wilson, 1977) are much like the instructions previously labeled "task-motivating," in that they exhort the individual to put aside negative thoughts ("This will never work," "This is ridiculous") and "to focus . . . thinking and to use . . . imagination creatively to produce certain effects and to experience certain events" (Barber & Wilson, 1977, p. 46). The instructions are quite explicit, giving the subjects specific examples of not only the types of test items likely to be administered, but also the nature of the responses the subject might give. In addition, it is made quite clear that a passive condition will *not* be effective: "[N]othing will happen [as a result of closing the eyes and passively awaiting the suggested phenomena], because only my mind, my own thoughts, can make a T.V. screen appear before my eyes" (Barber & Wilson, 1977, p. 46). The use of the words "mind," "thoughts," and "thinking" apparently qualify such instructions as a cognitive approach to the mystery of hypnosis.

According to Barber's data (Barber & Wilson, 1977), group-administered think-with instructions produced significantly higher CIS scores than did a "traditional" induction or a briefly instructed control group, although DeStefano (1976) was unable to match these results with the BSS. Furthermore, Barber, Wilson, and Scott (1980) did demonstrate that a traditional induction significantly enhanced performance on the BSS (a "hypnotist-centered" scale), whereas performance on the CIS (a "subject-centered" scale) was no better than that of a perfunctorily instructed control group. In addition, McConkey, Sheehan, and White (1979) had previously shown that although the CIS is positively related (r = .28) to the Harvard Group Scale of Hypnotic Susceptibility (HGSHS), "imagination alone is insufficient to account for [subjects'] capacity to respond well to hypnotic test suggestions" (p. 273). Mitchell and Lundy (1986) also showed that induction instructions composed of imagery suggestions alone were no more "effective in producing measured behavioral responses" (p. 98) than relaxation instructions, and that the latter were *more* effective in facilitating the subjective report of hypnotic involvement. If the cognitive, "think-with" component of hypnotic behavior were regnant, it should equally affect the entire spectrum of measurement scales, and not just those specifically designed for highlighting thought provoked activity. It is not that the individual's cognitions are unimportant in the total process, but the contention that subject cognitions are the essence of hypnosis does not tell the whole story.

That individuals think and talk to themselves, and that these intraindividual conversations have behavioral consequences, are truisms born of personal experience. No doubt, following the years of sterile behaviorism, a return to cognitive, mind-oriented explanations of behavior was warranted. The question we must ask ourselves now is: Should our headlong rush to cognitive and sociological interpretations blind us to fundamental and extensive consistencies in the historical, experimental, and clinical literature?

It seems to me that once again we have a horse-and-cart problem, if we adopt the "Hamlet hypothesis" ("There is nothing good or bad, but thinking makes it so"). By trying to explain hypnosis solely on the basis of subjective cognitions, without *first* positing a condition or state that precedes and provides the agar in which the subjective ideas can develop and thus influence the hypnotic phenomena (suggested challenges), we invert the temporal sequence of events. It is when the hurried, tension-laden cognitions of everyday living are set aside in calm relaxation that the focused attention of other task-oriented cognitions can become regnant and weave their influence over suggested responses and otherwise unusual phenomena.

This is not a new idea, for it dates at least as far back as Mesmer's early years. Mesmer was astonished to hear the effects of his procedures "attributed in a vague manner to imagination" (Mesmer, 1781) and later pronounced by the 1784 commission to be due "to the excitement of the imagination" (see Hull, 1933, p. 8). Why was he astonished? It was obvious that his patients' imaginations were affected by his techniques. But for Mesmer the effects of animal magnetism were not dependent upon imagination, but vice versa. Imaginative forces germinated in the fertile soil of magnetism, much as the cognitions of present-day subjects develop in the loam of *anesis*. The condition of *anesis* (relaxation, hypnosis) does not detract from our understandings of the responses to hypnotic suggestions being heavily influenced by subject cognitions. There is little conflict here, merely a temporal sequence that needs explicit recognition (a second cognition).

One final note regarding cognitive theory in general and Barber's studies in particular is in order. Once *anesis* has been achieved, three defining characteristic changes occur: (1) the subjective impression of nonvoluntariness, (2) *spontaneous* amnesia, and (3) *hyper*suggestibility. Regarding the last of these, few investigations have taken the time and effort to test, not simple suggestibility, but *hyper*suggestibility. That individuals will respond to suggestion without being hypnotized has never been in question, although some, like Barber, have made great moment of the fact that subjects will respond to the suggestions contained in hypnotic susceptibility scales without the prior presentation of an induction procedure. The results of such tests of suggestibility (*sans* an induction procedure) have been held to fault other theoretical understandings of hypnosis, particularly trance state theories. However, suggestibility is *not* hypnosis and hypnosis is *not* suggestibility, as I have explicated elsewhere (Edmonston, 1989). The two should not be confused. Changes in one form a marker for the other. As Reyher (1977) put it, "suggestibility is increased simply upon the subject's adoption of a passive–receptive, open-minded attitude" (p. 69). What is pertinent to this discussion and to the interpretation of relaxation as the fundamental basis of hypnosis is that responsivity to suggestion is enhanced through relaxation; the fact that we can demonstrate suggestibility through other instructional sets does not abrogate the relaxation hypothesis. (See also my discussion of neodissociation theory below.)

Psychoanalytic Theory

Psychoanalytic theory is the indestructible theory, for there will always be an unconscious—a part of us that influences our behaviors in ways that surprise and at times distress us. However, the question is not whether the unconscious and its attendant components influence hypnotic behavior, but what is it about hypnosis that makes a psychoanalytic understanding of its vicissitudes appealing to some investigators? For some, the concept of the unconscious is important and necessary, but what mechanism allows for the unconscious to assume the upper hand in hypnosis—for the emergence of primary-process thinking, of a regression and enhanced ego receptivity to the suggestions of the situation? The answer is: the relaxation that is fundamental to hypnosis.

Ego strength is conceived of as a linear function reciprocally related to primary-process, id functions. As ego strength weakens, primary-process thinking directs increasing amounts of behavior, so that there is hypothesized a relationship between depth of hypnosis and emergence of primary process: The deeper the hypnosis, the more primary-process thinking (Fromm, 1979). But the emergence of the unconscious, primitive state is not a sudden bursting forth of repressed images, as it might be in an obsessed patient; it does not break out of control and overwhelm the individual into a state of panic or worse. In the hypnotic situation, the ebb of ego control is a gradual process occurring in a somewhat stepwise fashion, the tempo of which is dictated by the soothing words of the hypnotist. The unconscious is *allowed* to come forward; it is not suddenly released by a magical signal, causing the patient to experience a rush of id impulses. Fromm's formulation of "deeper hypnosis, more primary-process thinking" clearly implies a gradual involvement in hypnosis. This gradual involvement comes about through the ritual of induction and its consequences, *anesis*. Relaxation, the fundamental of hypnosis, is the basic mechanism that allows and enhances all that follows and is understood in psychoanalytic terms.

Coming from a therapeutic tradition, psychoanalytic theory shares much with other therapy-derived techniques. Autogenic training (H. A. Schultz & Luthe, 1959), progressive relaxation (Jacobson, 1929), and behavior therapy (Wolpe, 1958, 1969) all begin with exercises or instructions that enhance the relaxed condition of the patient. It is *following* the achievement of relaxation that the therapeutic effectiveness of autogenic training is developed. It is *following* relaxation that psychoanalytic hypnotherapy is able to work with the patient's unconscious processes. The imagery of free association emerges in classical psychoanalysis *following* the development of a low state of arousal. Why the couch? Relaxation is the basic principle underlying present-day behavior therapies also. Even Wolpe (1958), whose original behavior therapy relied on hypnotic techniques, was cognizant of the pretherapeutic role played by relaxation— "those . . . who can relax will make progress" (p. 41). Behavior therapies and the psychoanalytic theory of hypnosis rest on the same foundation: relaxation.

Neodissociation Theory

E. R. Hilgard (1977a), discussing hypnotic talent, perceived two components to hypnosis, both lying on a continuum of personal involvement. This continuum of involvement in responsiveness to suggestions somewhat parallels the earlier work of Sidis (1898) on suggestibility, in which he drew a distinction between "normal" suggestion and "abnormal" suggestion. The latter takes place in the condition of hypnosis; the former does not. Hilgard's first component of responses to suggestions "require[s] little in the way of hypnotic procedures and talent to produce" (E. R. Hilgard, 1977a, p. 57). The second component, on the other hand, is exemplified by the hypnotically talented subjects who actually experience hallucinations, age regressions, and the like.

The distinction between suggestibility and hypnosis has not always been kept in clear perspective. As I stated above and discussed in detail elsewhere (Edmonston, 1989), suggestibility is *not* hypnosis, and hypnosis is *not* suggestibility. Hypnosis *enhances* suggestibility; it is not defined by it. Consequently, Hilgard is quite right to point out that the state–nonstate issue is a nonissue when discussing suggestibility (his first component). No state change need be hypothesized to account for responsiveness to suggestion. Nonstate theories win the day, hands down.

However, if one is to consider Hilgard's second component, a hypothesized change in state becomes appropriate, even mandatory. The question is not whether or not a change in the condition of the individual being hypnotized has occurred, but what the fundamental nature of the change is. Is it a dissociation, "a shift in cognitive [executive] controls," "a shift in perceptual or observational functions" (E. R. Hilgard, 1977a, p. 58), all expressed in such events as the voluntary becoming involuntary and the involuntary being made partially voluntary; or is it something yet more fundamental that allows the dissociations described by neodissociation theory?

The dissociation process does not initiate hypnosis, much as it is not the rise of the primary process in psychoanalytic thinking that gives rise to hypnosis. The dissociations occur in the context of *anesis*. Hypnotic induction procedures disrupt ongoing memory patterns, cognitively disorient the subject, reduce muscular feedback, and create a shift in executive function, so that the dissociations needed for participation in more advanced hypnotic phenomena are achieved. "The altered background for receiving suggestions, the state of hypnosis, is one of felt changes from normal in that the usual orientation to reality has been disturbed and familiar reality testing does not go on" (E. R. Hilgard, 1977b, p. 227). The initial altered background allowing the dissociated responses to suggestion—much as it allows the emergence of the unconscious for the psychoanalysts—is the relaxation fundamental to hypnosis.

Role Theory

"The play's the thing," or so the contextualist position of role theory maintains: "[B]oth the hypnotist and the subject are actors, both enmeshed in a dramatic plot, both striving to enhance their credibility" (Coe & Sarbin, 1977, p. 12). Using the metaphors of drama, role theory understands hypnosis as a social dialogue between two individuals of differing role-taking abilities, with different understandings of the context, who lose themselves in the distinctions between reality and pretense. Like Orne's simulator control subjects, role takers are so involved in the role of the hypnotized subject as defined and constantly redefined by the hypnotist that an observer, casual or otherwise, would be hard pressed to detect the drama underlying the performance. But the inability to make such distinctions (simulated from real, role-enacted from pretense) does not relieve the role theorist from the obligation to consider that it is a change in condition (relaxation) that makes such pretense appear genuine. This is not simply because traditional hypnosis has historically been related to relaxation, but also because role playing and simulation have their limitations within the context of hypnosis. Properly evaluated, pretense and reality can be distinguished. As Reyher (1973) pointed out, if one wants to understand the effect of alcohol on functioning, one does not have a sober individual pretend to be, role play, or simulate intoxication. The visual and auditory aspects of such role playing are easily enacted. However, the real test is to have an inebriated person attempt to simulate sobriety. Touching one's finger to one's nose, picking up a dime from the pavement, and walking a straight line are not so easily accomplished once the change in condition—the sedation of alcohol—has taken place (ask anyone who has been stopped for driving while intoxicated). Reyher (1973), by the same token, found that hypnotized subjects simulating wakefulness were easily selected from a group of nonhypnotized ("awake") subjects. "Simulation of an altered state while [a subject] is in the waking state is not as sensitive to differences between the two states as is the simulation of the waking state while [the subject] is in an altered state" (Reyher, 1973, p. 35).

Just as wakefulness cannot be feigned while one is asleep, it cannot be adequately role-played while one is hypnotized. (See also my discussion in Edmonston, 1981.) It would seem that pretense in this context is unidirectional, and that the condition of wakefulness is the basic condition from which all role playing proceeds. Role theory must presume some base condition from which roles are enacted and can be enacted. Wakefulness is that condition, for we cannot credibly enact wakefulness from other, less alert conditions. Or are our concepts of reality so fluid that we can make no comparisons among behaviors? Are we to assume that when we engage in wakeful behaviors, we are but enacting the role of an awake individual? Is the same true for sleeping, eating, dreaming, dying? If so, where is the stability of reality? What is real and what is pretense? For there can be no pretense without reality. Pretense *assumes* a reality to play on, a condition from which to role-play another scenario. We know by comparison, not by merely describing a superfluidity of existence in which there are no anchors for our understanding.

For the individual, the paramount anchor is the self. Think about it. The one stable thing in life is your individual concept of self. No matter how happy or how sad, how well or how ill, you feel it is still the same "you" who has, considers, and perceives these conditions. Though your experiences have grown and your body has aged through the years, you are still the same person who peers into the mirror each morning, *despite* the obvious changes in appearance and abilities. Though you are now 6 feet tall, it is still the same you as when you were 3 feet tall. And this wakeful, stable self can and does note condition changes while enacting the various roles Sarbin and Coe have made central to their formulation of hypnosis. But role enactments are behavioral changes in the context of perceived changes in condition. The so-called role playing of the hypnotic subject is in response to a basic change in condition which cannot itself be reversed by pretense. That change is relaxation—the fundamental of hypnosis. Like the cognitions, the dissociations, and the emerging primary processes, role enactments are given license through *anesis*—the relaxation of neutral hypnosis.

THEORETICAL CONCEPTS AND PRINCIPLES

The arguments that precede and follow this brief section are prerequisite to understanding the principles and concepts listed here. Too often, a simple listing of theoretical principles is at best misinterpreted and at worst trivialized and quickly dismissed by the reader who has not come fully to grips with its development and the data base in which the principles took root.

Anesis is a two-step process: (1) relaxation, followed by (2) the fluctuating levels of alertness dictated by the activity requirements of subsequent suggestions. The three basic characteristics of *anesis*—(1) *hyper*suggestibility, (2) *spontaneous* amnesia, and (3) the subjective impression of nonvoluntariness—are facilitated by the relaxation that precedes all hypnotic phenomena. Thus, the relaxation of *anesis* precedes, facilitates, and is prerequisite to all other aspects of hypnosis set forth by other theories. It enhances disinhibition, appropriate attitudes and motivations, reduced ego functioning, dissociations, role playing, and hypersuggestibility.

RESEARCH AND APPRAISAL

The Role of Control Groups in Defining Hypnosis

We define our concepts by comparison. For some, hypnosis is defined as not being sleep, or not being a waking state. For others, the definition of hypnosis precludes both a waking and a sleep state, relegating the concept to a location somewhere on a continuum between what are popularly considered to be end points on a sleep–wakefulness linear dimension (Pavlov, 1928; Platonov, 1955/1959; see Edmonston, 1981, for a summary). During the 19th century and the early part of the 20th century, hypnosis was considered some form of sleep because, by comparison, individuals mesmerized by Puységur and hypnotized by Braid appeared to be asleep. Thus, hypnosis was defined by comparison—the comparison of the appearance of the hypnotized individual with individuals in a condition of sleep.

Probably the first comparison made toward the definition of hypnosis was with wakefulness—another fluid condition (like sleep) treated as if it were a simple category. Both the ancients and moderns noticed that upon induction, the induced appeared different from the inducer, and since the inducer considered himself or herself to be awake, in full control of faculties, and voluntarily behaving, a definition by comparison was drawn: Hypnosis is not wakefulness. More modern research methodologies have drawn upon this first, rather crude comparison by using as control groups "awake" individuals (the condition is often never defined beyond that simple word). Soon variations on this theme appeared: Investigators began using time-control awake groups who sat (or lay) quietly for the same amount of time it took to render a hypnotic induction to the experimental (hypnotized) group. A later refinement was to read to the control subjects a dull passage of "nonemotional" material intended to control for the verbal auditory stimulation provided by the hypnotist in presenting the formal induction.

By the 1960s another comparison was being made with hypnosis. "Task-motivated" groups, in which the individuals were exhorted to perform the suggested tasks of the experiment to the best of their abilities, were used either as intra- or as interindividual control groups. Weitzenhoffer and Sjoberg (1961) used such a comparison group, and concluded that the hypnotic induction was critical, for it brought "about a change in the individual which is subsequently reflected in . . . behavior with respect to suggestions" (p. 215). Rosenhan and London (1963), Slotnick and London (1965), and Smith (1969) also showed that the effectiveness of motivational instructions depended upon being paired with a hypnotic induction.

Barber and his associates, however, argued that task-motivational instructions and hypnotic induction (the traditional, relaxation-based format) were equally effective in increasing responses to certain kinds of suggestions (Barber & Glass, 1962; Barber & Calverley, 1962, 1963a, 1963b, 1965a, 1965b), although Barber and Calverley (1965a, 1965b) themselves also demonstrated that the simple addition of relaxation suggestions (nonhypnotic) to defining the situation as hypnosis produced increased levels of performance.

If a deep-sleep control condition was considered the appropriate control condition for Pavlov's theory, and task-motivational instructions were felt to be the most suitable control for a motivational theory of hypnosis, then the newly developed "think-with" instructions have become the comparison model for the cognitive theories. However, as I have discussed above, the effectiveness of this set of instructions appears dependent upon the type of scale used as a measurement. With the CIS, enhanced performance over a traditional, relaxation-centered induction is claimed (Barber & Wilson, 1977); however, with the BSS that conclusion is less tenable (DeStefano, 1976).

Orne (1971, 1979) developed yet another comparison strategy in response to the oft-expressed concern that subjects and patients "slip in and out" of hypnosis, depending upon whether the performance called for is "hypnotic" or not. Orne's simulator model avoids such an interpretation of the data by having individuals who are unhypnotizable simulate, or pretend that they are hypnotized and act accordingly. Such a comparison maneuver could also serve for the role theorists, for Orne's data have supported—again by comparison—the contention that hypnosis is neither hoax nor pretense on the part of traditionally hypnotized individuals. Through his studies Orne has focused on the subjective quality of hypnotic performance—a definition that is "descriptive rather than explanatory" (Orne, 1977, p. 19), as with role-playing interpretations of hypnosis.

However, the logic of the "slip-in, slip-out" hypothesis is seldom carried to its conclusion: namely, that the categories of human behavior are already explicated, and that when hypnotized individuals act in a manner similar to that seen when they are awake, they must indeed be awake, and vice versa. Such thinking would make any comparison group almost superfluous, by defining different behaviors in terms of preconceived categories. Orne's simulator model put to rest this pseudoproblem of slipping in and slipping out, but it was Reyher's (1973) work that demonstrated, within the context of simulator comparisons, that there may be something more overtly apparent happening when an individual is hypnotized. Hypnotized subjects in his experiments could not deceive observers when the subjects attempted to simulate wakefulness while hypnotized. On the other hand, individuals experienced in hypnosis could not distinguish Orne's simulators from truly hypnotized subjects. Hypnosis can be adequately simulated by nonhypnotized subjects, but wakefulness cannot be adequately simulated by hypnotized subjects.

Neither the psychoanalytic nor the neodissociation accounts of hypnosis has produced a comparison maneuver specific to its interpretations, although one could imagine such a maneuver. For example, one might utilize severely neurotic or psychotic individuals as control subjects for a psychoanalytic theory control group. Both of these groups, according to that theory, have reduced ego functioning and more apparent primary-process operating in both overt behavior and ideation. Neither possible comparison, I fear, has been given adequate consideration, although psychotic individuals are believed to be notoriously poor candidates for hypnosis and could be conceptualized as having a minimum of ego control, or a maximum of intrapsychic dissociation. Similarly, patient populations might serve to control for the effects of naturally occurring dissociations on hypnotic functioning. Drug-induced state changes could also be used to assess the degree of dissociation created in the hypnotic situation. Using either group as a control maneuver for either theory, one might predict that such control groups (psychologically disturbed individuals or drug-influenced individuals) would prove quite different from an experimental group composed of individuals instructed with a traditional, relaxation-centered induction procedure.

Nonhypnotic Relaxation Comparisons

Comparison groups, then, are our key to understanding and defining hypnosis, but none of the comparisons noted above (deep sleep, wakefulness, task motivation, and simulator controls) was adequate to test the role of relaxation in hypnosis. While the controversies of these comparison models kept us busy, the direction suggested by the historical relationship between hypnosis and relaxation lay dormant. Once a nonhypnotic relaxation comparison began to be used and properly understood, a clearer understanding of traditional, neutral hypnosis became possible. As I pointed out in *Hypnosis and Relaxation* (Edmonston, 1981), once I stopped focusing on the nonuniqueness of hypnosis in comparison with a nonhypnotic relaxation control, and realized that *not* being different from a control maneuver was as important as (if not more so) than being different, the fundamental underpinning of hypnosis (i.e., relaxation) became apparent. It all began with a series of studies of Pavlov's theory, which predicted that responses on a voluntary–involuntary continuum would be progressively less and less influenced by hypnotic induction (see Edmonston, 1979). This proposition was demonstrated with behavioral responses such as finger withdrawal (Plapp & Edmonston, 1965) and eyelid conditioning (Plapp, 1967).

 As I moved into the area of electrodermal response (EDR) conditioning, heart rate, and oral temperature, I introduced a nonhypnotic relaxation control group for comparison with traditional, neutral hypnosis (Edmonston, 1979, 1981; Cogger & Edmonston, 1971). Although the main data continued to support the hypotheses derived from Pavlov's writings, the comparisons between the hypnosis and the relaxation groups were what drew my attention. It seemed that much of the basic physiology of the individual reacted in the same way to both traditional hypnotic induction instructions and nonhypnotic instructions to become deeply relaxed but not "hypnotized."

 Plapp (1967) pointed out that the relaxation suggestions which characterized most hypnotic inductions could be the probable cause for the

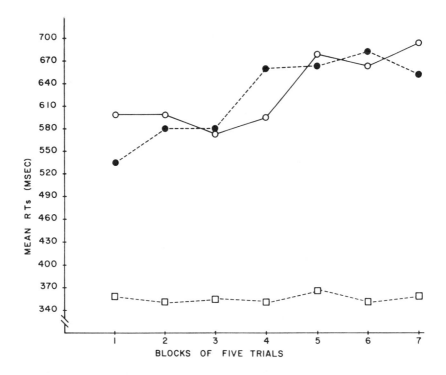

FIGURE 7.1. Mean reaction times (RTs) of relaxation control (solid circles, dashed line), relaxation induction (open circles, solid line) and alert induction (squares, dashed line) groups. From "The Effects of Neutral Hypnosis on Conditioned Responses: Implications for Hypnosis as Relaxation" by W. E. Edmonston, Jr., in E. Fromm and R. E. Shor (Eds.), *Hypnosis: Developments in Research and New Perspectives* (2nd ed., pp. 415–455). New York: Aldine. Copyright 1979 by E. Fromm and R. E. Shor. Reprinted by permission.

finding that reaction time (RT) was significantly slower in hypnotized subjects and did not demonstrate the progressive increase in speed of reaction seen in waking subjects. A colleague and I (Ham & Edmonston, 1971) followed that observation with a study of RT using an alert induction *à la* Liebert, Rubin, and Hilgard (1965); a Stanford Hypnotic Susceptibility Scale, Form A (SHSS: A) induction (Weitzenhoffer & Hilgard, 1959); and relaxation instructions that precluded either being hypnotized or falling asleep. Figure 7.1 (Edmonston, 1979) presents our results. No significant difference in RT was found between the two latter groups; both differed from the alert group. These findings are important for two reasons: (1) Once more, in yet another response realm, relaxation and traditional hypnosis were not different as measured; and (2) an alert "induction" created a condition *different* from that seen in traditional, neutral hypnosis. Rader (1972) obtained similar results when testing the motivational aspects of hypnosis: The RTs of his hypnosis group were significantly slower than those of a hypnosis-plus-motivation group, which was "probably as alert as the alert hypnosis induction group in the Ham and Edmonston study" (p. 101).

It is surprising, given the emphasis on eye fixation as an attention-holding maneuver in many induction procedures (see Edmonston, 1986), that more attention has not been paid to these portions of the central nervous system. Strosberg and Vics (1962) found systematic physiologic changes in eyes during hypnosis, which they attributed to the relaxation that was occurring. Friedman, Taub, Sturr, Church, and Monty (1986) also attributed part of their findings to some component of the hypnotic induction process. While assessing the relationship between luminance threshold and speed of sensory information processing, they opined that the relaxation component of hypnotic induction may have accounted for their negative results.

Although a few other investigators studied eye movements during the 1960s (Lorens & Darrow, 1962; Amadeo & Shagass, 1963; Antrobus, Antrobus, & Singer, 1964), it was not until the 1970s that Weitzenhoffer, who proposed slow eye movements (SEMs) as an involuntary indicator of hypnosis (Weitzenhoffer, 1969, 1971; Weitzenhoffer & Brockmeier, 1970), reported SEM patterns similar to those in Stage 1 sleep in hypnosis. A colleague and I (Dunwoody & Edmonston, 1974) confirmed his data and extended them, again with the use of a nonhypnotic relaxation control group. Our findings showed that SEMs as a parameter are not unique to traditionally induced hypnosis, but are related to the fundamental of hypnosis—relaxation.

The similarity of traditional, neutral hypnosis to relaxation has also been reported from other laboratories. In fact, data from a classic early study, long overlooked, supported the conclusion of *anesis*. Dorcus, Brintnall, and Case (1941) found that hypnotized subjects left to their own devices after the experimenter had been called from the room stayed, on the average, 28 minutes, while a group told simply to lie down, close their eyes, and relax left the room in an average of 23 minutes (see Barber, 1979). Here, then, was an early behavioral indication that people act similarly in both situations, implying that underlying attitudinal distinctions are not made between hypnosis and relaxation. That clinical patients also perceive hypnosis as predominantly relaxation was shown in a clinical survey study (see Edmonston, 1977a), as well as in Crawford, Hilgard, and Macdonald's (1982) study of transient experiences following administration of the HGSHS and the SHSS:C (Shor & Orne, 1962; Weitzenhoffer & Hilgard, 1962). These authors found that in 72% of their subjects, feelings of relaxation and being rested followed the individual scale—a figure consistent with the 60% found by J. R. Hilgard (1974) and 81% found by Coe and Ryken (1979) earlier. Whether clinical patients or college student experimental subjects are employed, hypnosis and relaxation are perceived as highly similar.

Some of the data comparing hypnosis and nonhypnotic relaxation have come from the realm of behavior therapy. Paul (1969a, 1969b), for example, showed that either nonhypnotic relaxation or hypnosis was effective in reducing tension, stress, and anxiety, measured both subjectively and physiologically. Others in the 1970s also started using a relaxation control group in their studies (McAmmond, Davidson, & Kovitz, 1971; Bullard & DeCoster, 1972; Reyher & Wilson, 1973; Peters & Stern, 1973; Mather & Degun, 1975; Tebecis, Provins, Farnbach, & Pentony, 1975; Coleman, 1976; Morse, Martin, Furst, & Dubin, 1977; Benson et al., 1978). McAmmond et al. (1971) found that both hypnosis and relaxation reduced a skin conductance response to pain in the dental situation. Although Bullard and DeCoster (1972) reported that the vividness of subjects' reported experiences on the BSS was not different between the two conditions of hypnosis and relaxation, objective scores did favor hypnosis. A possible reason for this finding was the anxiety engendered by the term, hypnosis, in the case of the hypnotized group. Reyher and Wilson (1973) provided support for such an interpretation when they found that subjects manifested a significantly higher anxiety level when experimental procedures were presented as "hypnosis" (compared to a "relaxation" presentation).

Gruzelier and Brow (1985), noting that the number of nonspecific EDRs is positively related to both arousal and anxiety, found no difference between a hypnosis and a relaxation group on electro-dermal and spontaneous fluctuations (EDSFs) and level of skin conductance, although responses to an orienting stimulus were more affected by the hypnosis condition than by the relaxation condition. Since the relaxation group consisted of listening to a story, rather than a series of instructions to become deeply relaxed but not hypnotized, the meaning of the latter finding is not fully clear. The authors themselves point out that relaxation does have effects on habituation, as seen in Walrath and Hamilton (1975) and Morse et al. (1977), mentioned below.

Peters and Stern (1973) found the same significant increase in skin temperature and peripheral vasodilatation as did Reid and Curtsinger (1968) and Timney and Barber (1969), but with one crucial difference. These increases could not be distinguished from the same increases found in a control group instructed simply to "sit and relax." Cardiovascular functioning was also one measure used by Mather and Degun (1975) in an intrasubject design comparing hypnotized to relaxed conditions. Again, neither a significant decrease in heart rate nor response to a suggestion to awaken on time differentiated between the two groups. (See also Wagstaff, 1976, for a critique of this article.) Groups engaged in TM, hetero-hypnosis, or sitting quietly could not be distinguished on heart rate or self-reported phenomenological data, but could be differentiated on respiration rate (TM and hypnosis significantly slower) and skin temp-erature (control group higher) (Barmark & Gaunitz, 1979). *None* of the measures distinguished between the relaxation of TM and that of hypnosis.

Other physiological measures have been the focus of studies comparing hypnosis directly with relaxation. Tebecis et al. (1975) reported significantly greater electroencephalographic (EEG) theta activity in hypnotized and nonhypnotic relaxation groups (they mislabeled their relaxation group "awake") than in an awake control group (correctly labeled), but no significant difference between the two experimental groups. Walrath and Hamilton (1975) also could not distinguish among meditation, autohypnosis, and relaxation groups in autonomic arousal. It decreased significantly in all three from a baseline period to a treatment period. Benson et al.(1978) had similar findings in the clinical context of anxiety neuroses, and Morse et al. (1977), taking a physiological shotgun approach, could discern no differences among meditative relaxation, autohypnosis, and heterohypnosis on respiration rate, pulse rate, blood pressure, skin resistance, EEG, and electromyogram (EMG). Equally important was the finding that all of these measures were higher in an alert group than in any of the relaxation conditions. "Relaxation–hypnosis and meditation [nonhypnotic relaxation] can be considered similar on both physiological and subjective levels" (Morse et al., 1977, p. 321). Similar findings were reported by Mount, Walters, Rowland, Barnes, and Payton (1978). In Norway the same inability to distinguish between two groups, one receiving the SHSS:A induction items and the other receiving time-matched instructions to relax, on blood pressure was noted (Sletvold, Jensen, & Gotestam, 1986). Regarding EMG measurements, Charles-worth and Doughtie (1982) could find no difference between learned and hypnotic relaxation on a postinstructional EMG measure.

Morse et al.'s comment (1977) above is much like Coleman's (1976) starting hypothesis, which turned out to be his final conclusion: "[T]he only difference between relaxation procedures and hypnotic induction procedures is the name given them" (p. 13). Using EEG and EMG measures and three self-report scales, Coleman found that nonhypnotic relaxation did not differ from hypnosis, although both differed signifi-cantly from a control set. In addition to his physiological and subject report findings, Coleman also discovered that both relaxation groups scored significantly higher on hypnotic responsivity than the control group, but did not differ from each other.

Clinical Considerations

Before I comment on the similarities in therapeutic effectiveness of hypnosis and relaxation, a brief look at one study that tried to separate the relaxation from the cognitive components of the hypnotic situation is in order, because it calls to our attention one fundamental aspect of clinical practice: Despite the particular mix of imagery and relaxation used, it is the latter that the clinician attempts to achieve in his or her patient to enhance therapeutic effectiveness. Mitchell and Lundy (1986) employed three induction methods: (1) a relaxation technique derived from the SHSS:C; (2) an imagery induction derived from Gibbons's (1979) hyperempiric and Liebert et al.'s (1965) alert inductions; and (3) a combined induction, which contained elements of both relaxation and alert imagery. The authors found no difference among the inductions on objectively measured behavioral responses, but did find that the relaxation and the combined groups produced significantly greater subjective reports of hypnosis.

Although the combined group scored higher than the relaxation group on three subjective measures, Mitchell and Lundy (1986) concluded that relaxation enhances the subjective experience of hypnosis, and that "the fact that relaxation instructions were present in both conditions that were superior to the imagery condition would appear to support Edmonston's position" (1986, p. 105). The authors pointed out that such a conclusion is not one of absolute clarity. Separating imagery from relaxation is no mean task, especially since we may be dealing with a cross-augmentation effect. However, let us keep in mind that in the induction process itself many clinicians use suggested imagery to enhance relaxation. This act alone signals that what clinicians perceive as regnant is not the imagery, but the relaxation, which once achieved can be turned back on the imaginative mechanisms to produce cognitions that are therapeutic. Hypnotherapeutics and the manner in which they are practiced give us some clues as to what the effective component in the process may be.

In *Hypnosis and Relaxation* (Edmonston, 1981), I reviewed the striking similarities in therapeutic effectiveness between nonhypnotic relaxation techniques (e.g., TM, behavior therapies) and hypnosis. In the treatment of hypertension, migraine headache, addictions (to drugs, alcohol, and tobacco), insomnia, and anxiety, the general therapeutic finding was the same: Nonhypnotic relaxation yields results similar to those of hypnosis. I will not attempt to review all of the literature covered in *Hypnosis and Relaxation* here, but briefly note studies that have appeared since its publication. For example, in the treatment of hypertension, Friedman and Taub (1982) were able to replicate their previous findings (1977, 1978) of decreased blood pressure through relaxation, as were Southam, Agras, Taylor, and Kraemer (1982), who showed that relaxation treatment had a measurable positive effect in the natural environment as well as in the clinic setting.

In the realm of pain and headache treatment, Mills and Farrow (1981) reported the relaxation inherent in TM to be more efficient than non-TM relaxation in reducing verbal reports of distress, although both groups of subjects had similar pain sensation scores and heart rate and EDR measures. Cogan and Kluthe (1981) found 20 minutes of Lazarus's relaxation training to be superior to finger-tapping distraction, patterned breathing, or a no-treatment control condition in reducing ratings of intensity to ischemic pain.

Stern, Brown, Ulett, and Sletten (1977) found that hypnotic analgesia, acupuncture and morphine produced significantly decreased pain ratings for both cold-pressor and ischemic pain. Van Gorp, Meyer, and Dunbar (1985) reported similar results on cold-pressor-induced pain, and Tripp and Marks (1986), who directly compared hypnosis and relaxation, found the two procedures to be comparable in the cold-pressor test.

One area of pain control wherein various relaxation therapies have been applied is that of headache. Since my review (Edmonston, 1981), Friedman and Taub (1984) used a relaxation control group, along with four hypnosis groups, a biofeedback group, and a wait-list control group to assess changes in the frequency and intensity of migraine symptoms and amount of medication used. All of the treatments produced a reduction of symptoms and medication, without any distinction appearing across treatment groups. Since the authors deliberately added the relaxation group to test the propositions of the hypnosis–relaxation equation, these findings clearly indicate, at least in the clinical area of migraine headache control, an equivalency of effectiveness between hypnosis and relaxation. Similarly, Spinhoven (1988) found an equivalency of effectiveness in his review of the literature on various maneuvers for headache control, as did Bassman (1983) for primary symptoms.

Smoking is probably one of the most explored areas of the application of clinical hypnosis to addictions (see Table 5.8 in Edmonston, 1981). More recently, Schubert (1983) used two treatment techniques differing only in whether or not hypnosis or relaxation preceded the therapeutic suggestions. At the completion of treatment, 55% of the hypnosis and 74% of the relaxation group had ceased smoking. At 4-month follow-up, the figures were 55% and 58%, respectively. Two conclusions can be drawn: First, and more important, hypnosis and relaxation produce almost identical results in the treatment of cigarette addiction (and these results are significantly better than untreated individuals); second, relaxation may be more generally applicable with respect to the population in which success may be expected.

Again, again, and again, clinical applications of relaxation and hypnosis yield no appreciable differences in their effectiveness. Why?

Because, at base, they are one and the same process, and are so perceived by the clinical patient (see Edmonston, 1977a).

Physiological Considerations

Quite often in our search for understanding human behaviors, we are confounded by voluntary acts, and so we are unable to differentiate between what the individual chooses to do and what is involuntarily thrust upon the individual. Although we recognize the boundaries of this involuntary–voluntary dichotomy to be in large part ethereal, it does allow us the means (albeit somewhat difficult to define with certainty) to distinguish between willful, enacted behaviors and those that are not the consequence of some intention to act. We have seen the importance of such a dichotomizing of behavior in the research testing Pavlov's theory (see above). Orne's simulator model is of the same ilk, and I will discuss the notion of nonvoluntariness, to which Weitzenhoffer (1980, 1989) has recently called attention (see below).

One escape from the intrusion of voluntary acts into our attempts to understand hypnosis (and other behaviors as well) has been a flight to the measurement of those physiological processes not usually considered under the voluntary control of the individual (e.g., heart rate, EEG, EDR, etc.). Although we now have methods by which many of these physiological processes can be made accessible to manipulation by the individual being measured, such processes remain unmanipulable by most of us without special training and special equipment. With that caveat—that most people do not have the training or the special electronics to make the involuntary voluntary—let us turn our attention to physiological measures of the conditions of hypnosis and relaxation as yielding a clue to the nature of the relationship we have seen developing in the preceding pages of this chapter. The data already covered in the section on relaxation control groups are not reiterated here, nor is much of the literature reviewed in *Hypnosis and Relaxation* (Edmonston, 1981), except by brief notation.

Hypnosis

The studies noted below involve measurements taken during neutral hypnosis, or instances in which the neutral hypnosis portion of the study could be teased out of the general domain of the study. This is important, because we are interested in the condition of hypnosis *not* confounded by additional suggestions and instructions, often therapeutic in nature. In this restricted context, then, a number of studies have suggested a relationship among EEG patterns often seen in Stage 1 sleep and hypnosis (Barker & Burgwin, 1948, 1949; Darrow, Henry, Gill, Brenman, & Converse, 1950; Platonov, 1955/1959; Marenina, 1959). But by and large, a relationship between the deeper stages of sleep and hypnosis has not been forthcoming (Evans, 1979) until recently, when Saletu (1987) reported significant increases in delta and theta activity during hypnosis, with a concomitant decrease in alpha and beta productivity.

One pattern that occurs on the continuum from wakefulness to deep sleep appears regularly in the context of hypnosis—the Stage 1 sleep production of alpha rhythms (8–13 Hz), particularly the slower alpha frequencies. Most studies have not concentrated on alpha production during neutral hypnosis, but rather on alpha production as it relates to hypnotic responsivity. The results are a confounding potpourri, as Evans (1979) has pointed out. The few studies measuring alpha density (a relaxed pattern) in hypnosis (rather than hypnotic susceptibility) have produced a picture of increased alpha density with hypnosis (e.g., Brady & Rosner, 1966; Edmonston & Grotevant, 1975; Melzack & Perry, 1975). In addition, Tebecis et al. (1975) showed increased theta activity in hypnosis and relaxation conditions, both of which differed from an awake condition but not from each other.

Some of the hypnosis data on EDR and EDSF have already been presented above. Several studies (Barber & Coules, 1959; Stern, Edmonston, Ulett, & Levitsky, 1963; Tart, 1963) have shown that basal skin resistance (BSR) drops dramatically upon the termination of hypnosis (skin resistance is inversely related to arousal), although it did not appear to change in the process of hypnotic induction. This finding suggests that the physiology recognizes the condition produced as different from ordinary wakefulness. Tart (1963), a colleague and I (Edmonston & Pessin, 1966), and Tebecis and Provins (1976) all reported a general rise in BSR with hypnosis. The findings on EDSF are much more uniform, indicating a significant decrease during hypnosis that is different from that seen in the usual control groups (Stern et al., 1963; O'Connell & Orne, 1968; Pessin, Plapp, & Stern, 1968; and Edmonston, 1968, 1979).

The data on respiration, its close associate metabolism, cardiovascular functioning, and body temperature show reasonably consistent decreases in the first three measures and increases in the fourth during hypnosis (see Edmonston, 1981, for a more detailed explication).

Relaxation

How, then, do the data above (increased alpha production, BSR, peripheral blood flow, and body temperature; decreased EDSF, respiration rate, basal metabolic rate, heart rate, and systolic blood pressure) compare with those found in nonhypnotic relaxation? Quite well, when we look at similar data associated with TM. Wallace (1970), Wallace, Benson, and Wilson (1971), Beary and Benson with Klemchuk (1974), and Benson et al. (1978) found increased alpha production and BSR, together with decreased respiration rate, O_2 consumption, and heart rate. These authors measured neither EDSF nor peripheral blood flow, but did, in contrast to the data in hypnosis, find no changes in body temperature (measured rectally) and systolic blood pressure. West (1979) did measure EDSF and found a significant decrease in both EDSF and skin conductance with 6 months of regular meditation. Christoph, Luborsky, Kron, and Fishman (1978) also found lowered heart and respiratory rates, but no blood pressure changes. On the other hand, Agras, Southam, and Taylor (1983) demonstrated the relaxation literature to be as variable as that in hypnosis. They found that 15 months of relaxation practice significantly lowered diastolic blood pressure, and at least one other study (Pollack & Zeiner, 1979) found no change in heart rate, respiration rate, or skin conductance when comparing relaxation to sitting quietly. Puente (1981), however, showed reduced respiration and heart rates during both TM and Benson's relaxation response technique (Benson, Beary, & Carol, 1974). Similarly, Pollack and Zeiner (1979) found progressively decreased heart rate, skin conductance, and respiration rate elicited by three types of relaxation conditions.

The few inconsistent findings in the relaxation literature, like those in the hypnosis literature, can often be attributed to methodological differences between studies, rather than any fundamental deviation from the common trend of the physiology of the trophotropic response (increased alpha production and BSR, and a decrease in respiratory and heart rate). Taneli and Krahne (1987), in a detailed study of EEG in TM, reported increased alpha production (particularly toward the anterior), with trains of theta appearing as the TM progressed.

Two areas of measurement applied to relaxation have not received much attention in the hypnosis literature: blood chemistry and biochemical changes. Wallace et al. (1971) found decreased blood pH with concomitant increases in base excess and decreases in blood lactate during TM. With respect to hypnosis, Lovett-Doust (1953) found reduced O_2 saturation on hypnotic induction, whereas no changes were found in nonprotein nitrogen, urea, uric acid, sugar, creatinine, hemoglobin percent, red blood cells, polymorphonuclear percent, lymphocytes, eosinophils, transitionals, basophils (Goldwyn, 1930), and leukocytes (Goldwyn, 1930; Wittkower, 1929). Nor have investigators shown much interest in the biochemistry of hypnosis, except Kiecolt-Glaser et al. (1986; see below).

However, biochemical changes accompanying relaxation have been the focus of several recent studies. Since a biochemical response can be either compensatory for previous homeostatic imbalances or, as well, a reflection of one's present state, response to some sort of stress probe is often a preferred way of ascertaining biochemical changes. Hoffman et al. (1982) used orthostatic and isometric muscular stress as such a probe, and found an increase of norepinephrine plasma levels with the practice of TM for 30 days. This significant increase in plasma norepinephrine was hypothesized to be due to the greater sympathetic system effort needed to overcome the relaxation response, to counteract orthostatic stress, and to perform the isometric work.

The parasympathetic mode of autonomic nervous system functioning during relaxation is also reflected biochemically by an increase in saliva translucency and a decrease in saliva protein (Morse et al., 1982). Platelet monoamine oxidase is affected as well by relaxation (Kralik, Ho, Mathew, & Claghorn, 1983).

The blood chemistry of meditating subjects was further probed by Jevning, Pirkle, and Wilson (1977) when they assayed 13 plasma neutral and acidic amino acids in 28 individuals. All of the plasma amino acids were stable, except one—phenylalanine, which was elevated in well-practiced individuals and significantly increased during the 20-minute period of actual TM. Even the practice of TM for as little as 3 to 4 months increased phenylalanine levels. Why plasma phenylalanine? Jevning et al. offered one explanation. Phenylalanine is not only required for protein synthesis; it is also the precursor of tyrosine, which in turn is hydroxylated to form norepinephrine, a cortical neurotransmitter. Relaxation reduces the turnover of this transmitter, which in turn would leave higher levels of phenylalanine circulating in the peripheral blood system. Thus, a reduction of cortical activity is signaled by the increase of phenylalanine in the blood.

These and a number of other articles on biochemical indices of meditation have been reviewed by Delmonte (1985). This review focused on the question of the efficacy of meditation in bringing about biochemical changes, in comparison with, for example, eyes-closed rest. Although meditation itself does not seem to be much more effective than eyes-closed rest, there are "reported decreases in growth hormone, lactate, cortisol, dopamine-beta-hydroxylase, aldosterone, triiodothyronine, cholesterol erythrocyte metabolism, hepatic blood flow, forearm respiration, salivary pH, and salivary proteins, and reported increases in salivary translucency, salivary minerals, phenylalanine, 5-hydroxyindole-3-acetic acid, prolactin, cardiac output, forearm blood flow, non hepatic, and nonrenal blood flow" (Delmonte, 1985, p. 561). The basic argument in the field of TM study is not whether these changes are due to relaxation or not (this is reasonably well established), but which form of relaxation is more efficient in bringing them about. Comparative studies with the biochemistry of hypnosis need to be done in order to determine whether hypnosis and relaxation are as similar at this level as at the behavioral, physiological, and clinical levels.

Kiecolt-Glaser et al. (1986) did include hypnosis as one form of relaxation training used with medical students to evaluate "the psychosocial modulation of cellular immunity" prior to the stress of examinations. Since

TABLE 7.1. Comparisons of Physiological Effects in Neutral Hypnosis, Nonhypnotic Control, and Nonhypnotic Relaxation (A Summary of Edmonston's 1981 Review)

Physiological parameter	(1) Neutral hypnosis: Effect	(2) Nonhypnotic control: Effect compared to (1)	(3) Nonhypnotic relaxation: Effect compared to (1)
Heart rate	Decrease	1 > 2	1 > 3
Respiration	Decrease	1 > 2	1 = 3
EEG			
Alpha	Increase	1 > 2	1 = 3
Theta	Increase	1 > 2	1 = 3
Metabolism	Decrease	1 > 2	1 = 3
Blood chemistry: Arterial oxygen saturation	Decrease	1 > 2	Not known
Body temperature	Unpredictable	As for 1	As for 1
Blood pressure			
Systolic	Decrease	1 > 2	1 = 3
Diastolic	Unpredictable	As for 1	As for 1
Peripheral blood flow	Increase	1 > 2	1 = 3
Electrodermal			
Basal skin resistance	Increase	1 > 2	1 = 3
Spontaneous fluctuations	Decrease	1 > 2	1 = 3
Reaction time	Decrease	1 > 2	1 = 3
Eye movements: SEM	Present	Not present	Present

Note. From "Neutral Hypnosis, Progressive Muscular Relaxation, and the Relaxation Response: A Review" by A. Humphreys, 1984, *British Journal of Experimental and Clinical Hypnosis, 2,* 19–27. Copyright 1984 by *British Journal of Experimental and Clinical Hypnosis.* Reprinted by permission.

the experimental (relaxation) group was composed of a variety of relaxation techniques, it was not possible to tease out the relative effectiveness of the techniques, but the authors did report that frequency of relaxation practice in any form may enhance the immunological response of the organism.

Summary

Humphreys (1984) summarized my 1981 review of physiologic comparisons among neutral hypnosis, nonhypnotic relaxation, and a nonhypnotic control condition (see Table 7.1). The conclusion to be drawn is obvious in the far right-hand column, where virtually all of the comparisons show an equivalency. Now to these studies still more have been added that yield essentially the same finding. In addition, the developing dimension of biochemical measurement has been added to our arsenal of compelling evidence for a basic physiological similarity between hypnosis and relaxation. Put more directly: "the physiology of hypnosis appears to be similar to that of any other relaxed state" (Evans, 1981, p. 454). Our next problem is to explore briefly the conceptual problems associated with the term relaxation itself.

Relaxation and Alertness

Given the findings above, and particularly those of Jevning et al. (1977) of a biochemical indication of reduced cortical activity, Pavlov's views of cortical inhibition may not be so out of tune with the present *Zeitgeist*. We now have numerous indications—clinical, experimental, physiological, biochemical—that hypnosis and relaxation share the same set of perceptual and bodily changes. However, in light of the earlier exploration of the varied understandings of hypnosis, a brief look at how we conceptualize relaxation is in order.

The question of what constitutes relaxation for the human organism is not new, although interest seems to have peaked during this century, beginning with the works of Jacobson (1929) and J. H. Schultz (1932). As Davidson and Schwartz (1976) pointed out, two of the most famous psychologists of the last century, William James and Sigmund Freud, never really focused on the condition of relaxation, although for the latter such a condition preceded and facilitated the major psychoanalytic technique of free association.

Certainly, we can partially define relaxation through measurement of the consequences of various techniques purportedly producing the condition. Much of this literature has already been discussed above, in *Hypnosis and Relaxation* (Edmonston, 1981), and in Davidson and Schwartz's (1976) article. What we seem to be dealing with is a state of low arousal, depicted physiologically by Stage 1 sleep EEG patterns and by reduced metabolic activity, heart rate, respiration rate, muscle tension (EMG), skin conductance, and spontaneous fluctuations in the EDR. The last two measures are often taken as measures of "cognitive" relaxation (in contrast to muscular or somatic relaxation), in that they are used as indicators of anxiety and emotional activity. The whole basis of many behavior therapies is the incompatibility of relaxation with conditions of anxiety (e.g., Wolpe, 1958), so that the reduction of bodily activity aids in the reduction of cognitive activity. Yet it has been argued that individuals who are physically fatigued may still report that their "mind is racing," preventing the onset of sleep, for example. Might it be that physical fatigue, muscular tiredness, is not the same as bodily relaxation? That the condition of extreme fatigue is as wakefulness in that the body is temporarily unable to achieve the relaxation that precedes recuperating sleep? A hard day at the office often elicits the need to "unwind" before the more vegetative, parasympathetic functions of eating and sleeping can be achieved. We unwind by relaxing.

Although we conceptualize two types of relaxation—cognitive and motor—and develop our theorizing and our experiments accordingly, we may only be viewing two faces of the same basic process, where either or both will suffice to define the concept. Think about your own experience after a period of strenuous physical work involving the striate musculature. To achieve relaxation, you engage in a nonphysical ("mental," if you will) activity. You may sit and read or watch TV or have a pleasant conversation with another, or just mentally review or think about things. You unwind and relax through cognitive action. Now, think about your own experience after a long day of "mental," nonphysical activity—reading or writing in a sedentary position. What do you do to relieve the mental fatigue, the "mushy mind" feeling? You *exercise*! That's right. You engage in strenuous physical work or exercise, and *relax*.

The relationship between what Davidson and Schwartz (1976) have called somatic and cognitive relaxation may be more apparent than real, in that our physical being does not operate dichotomously. Of course we utilize both outgoing and incoming stimuli in our moment-to-moment adjustments to the environments, both internal and external, but it is the totality of our condition to which we are ultimately responsive. As human beings, we tend to break things down into apparent component parts in order to understand their functioning better (including ourselves), and as an aid to conceptualizing experimental approaches to understanding. However, whether we are studying the central nervous system or the apparent paradox of relaxation, we must keep before us the artificiality of our conceptualizations and not lose sight of the totality of functioning we are attempting to assess. No doubt "the experience of relaxation will probably be more profound" (Davidson & Schwartz, 1976, p. 412) when both muscular and cognitive relaxations are present, but either or both are the roads to the experience of relaxation.

Perhaps this is why a real distinction between hypnosis and relaxation cannot be made. In the usual hypnotic induction techniques, both cognitive and muscular approaches are utilized, so that the cognitive images enhance the muscular relaxation and the somatic relaxation enhances the furtherance of imagery and other therapeutic maneuvers. That the two conceptualized types of relaxation are inseparable within ourselves was hinted at by Paul's work (1969a, 1969b), in which he found progressive relaxation *and* hypnotic techniques to affect both somatic and cognitive processes. Recall also the patients' predominant perception of hypnosis in my clinical survey study; it was of relaxation (Edmonston, 1977a). Relaxation, as *anesis*, involves both cognitive and somatic components, either of which will suffice for the report of relaxation having taken place.

But if hypnosis is relaxation, how do we understand the so-called "alert trance" phenomena? As I pointed out in *Hypnosis and Relaxation* (Edmonston, 1981), the conceptionalizations of active and passive hypnosis are not new, beginning probably with Puységur and continuing with the recent work of Bányai and her collaborators (Bányai & Hilgard, 1976; Bányai, Mészáros, & Greguss, 1981) and that of Malott (1984). Most of the early distinctions between active and passive hypnosis dealt with the observations that initially the subject or patient was passive as hypnosis was achieved, and later, within the hypnotic condition, became active in order to carry out the demands of suggestion. We know now that this arousal in the context of hypnosis is a relative matter. Reyher (1973) showed that hypnotized subjects cannot adequately project the image of wakefulness.

Other studies purporting to deal with active and passive hypnosis were in fact dealing with individual differences in the subjects, rather than two distinct types of trance (White, 1937; Kratochvíl & Shubat, 1971); while other research either lacked sound methodology (e.g., Oetting, 1964; Vingoe, 1968) or actually produced findings that showed that traditional hypnosis and alert hypnosis were *different*, not similar (Liebert et al., 1965). (See Edmonston, 1981, for a detailed discussion.)

Bányai and Hilgard (1976) produced data from a comparison between the performances on the SHSS:A and SHSS:B of subjects who had been exposed to two quite different "induction" procedures—alerting instructions while pedaling an exercise bike, and traditional hypnotic induction instructions while seated comfortably. Although the mean responsiveness scores yielded no difference between the two induction techniques, "secondary consequences of induction" (e.g., general appearance and movement characteristics) indicated more of a difference than the mean response scores implied. Regarding the latter, the authors reported that "those who preferred the traditional induction were, in general, higher scorers than those who preferred the alert induction" (Bányai & Hilgard, 1976, p. 222). These considerations and the methological dilemma posed by the physical activity/alert procedure cast doubt, I felt, on consideration of "alert trance" as being the equivalent of traditional hypnosis, and, in particular, of this one data set "disproving" a relaxation–hypnosis equation. If we were to take the latter approach to data in our field, for example, we could affirm nothing about anything, for we can always find (as exemplified in the literature covered above) at least one data set that runs counter to the general trends. What we must do when confronted with contrary evidence is to look at methodological differences and the fine details of the study or studies in question, to ascertain whether the data that on the surface appear so contrary are really so. This is what I did in *Hypnosis and Relaxation* with the data on alert trance up until 1980.

Bányai has replicated her 1976 results with 94 subjects (Bányai et al., 1981), using the active/alert/pedaling "induction." On Stanford-like challenges, the two groups gave "essentially the same" average behavioral responses; however, with respect to cognitive test items (hypnotic dream, hallucinations, *amnesia*) a significant difference was found, favoring the traditional induction.

The subjects also reported experiencing an altered state of consciousness. I have no quarrel with that. My contention is that the altered state of consciousness engendered through an active/alert set of activities and instructions is not hypnosis as traditionally understood. That there are different kinds of altered states of consciousness is not at issue; what is at issue is what altered state we should call hypnosis and what we should not.

However, differences between the two procedures in Bányai et al.'s data (1981) were even more marked in the electrophysiological measurements. General EEG records did not change in comparison with an awake control period, but visual evoked potentials (VEPs, particularly a P70 component) did, displaying a significant decrease in the traditional group and no change in the active/alert group. Mészáros, Bányai, and Greguss (1981) studied these types of measurements further and concluded that the basic characteristic of hypnosis is the modification of selective attention—a point Stern et al. (1963) discussed earlier. Suppressed VEPs, by and large, indicate reduced cortical anticipatory activity (as we might expect from the relaxation of hypnosis), and attentional factors certainly undergo modification during hypnosis.

Read in detail, these studies (Bányai & Hilgard, 1976; Bányai et al., 1981) are not as convincing as the conclusion drawn from them may sound: "[R]elaxation and decreased activity do not constitute the essence of hypnosis" (Bányai et al., 1981, p. 464). Because this conclusion is based on behavioral Stanford challenges, it gives us pause to reflect on how we have begun to define hypnosis since the general acceptance of the various forms of the SHSS (and the HGSHS) as measures of *hypnotic susceptibility*. Despite the fact that the forms of the SHSS do not take into sufficient account two historical bases of traditional hypnosis—nonvoluntariness and amnesia (see Weitzenhoffer, 1980)—we persist in trying to define a hypothetical construct (hypnosis) with consequential conditions only, ignoring the logical need to make explicit the antecedent conditions as well. Hilgard himself has pointed out that hypnosis "cannot be defined simply as a response to suggestion" (E. R. Hilgard, 1973, p. 973). Different antecedent conditions with the same consequences do not a definition make. This is the logical fallacy of identical predicates: "I am a man; Christ was a man; therefore, I am Christ." For our field, it might read: "Active/alert instructions yield high Stanford scores; relaxation instructions yield high Stanford scores; therefore, active/alert instructions are equivalent to relaxation instructions; in addition, relaxation is not hypnosis." However, as we will see presently, there is a way of resolving the logical confusion created by the adherents of active/alert instructions.

Meanwhile, Bányai and her colleagues were not the only ones utilizing a set of alerting instructions in the context of hypnosis. Kratochvíl and Zezulka (1980) compared an activating induction involving the subject walking in a figure-8 design while hearing suggestions for heightening activity and wakefulness, with a traditional set of suggestions issued to the subject in a comfortable armchair. Their data showed, regardless of the preconception of the process the subjects were exposed to (active vs. sleep), that those receiving alerting instructions scored higher (probability "very close to statistical significance at the 5% level"— Kratochvíl & Zezulka, 1980, p. 56) on the eight criteria measures assessed. Thus, their study provides more data suggesting that traditional inductions and alerting inductions produce different effects.

Just as Bányai and Hilgard's (1976) procedure made it impossible for observer/scorers to be "blind" to the experimental procedure assigned a particular subject, the same was true of Kratochvíl and Zezulka's (1980) study and part of Malott's (1984) work. The latter study, however, did pit a verbal induction for alertness against a traditional induction, both with the subjects in a comfortable chair (in addition to a group pedaling and a group pedaling and hearing alerting instructions). Malott's findings are very instructive, particularly if we keep in mind the notion that relaxation may be achieved either cognitively or somatically. A verbal alerting induction alone was significantly less effective than a traditional hypnotic induction, as measured by the SHSS:A or SHSS:B. Put another way, verbal alerting instructions alone produce a *different* result from traditional hypnotic instructions. Malott, therefore, has shown that alerting instructions do not produce the same behavioral result as traditional, relaxation-centered inductions.

However, other of Malott's findings still bear further consideration, for they may lead us to understand why an active/alert condition may produce behavioral results similar to those obtained through a traditional induction. Although the pedaling-alone condition resulted in marginally higher scores than verbal alerting alone, pedaling in combination with alerting instructions produced scores as high as did the traditional induction, much the same as was found in Bányai's work (Bányai & Hilgard, 1976; Bányai et al., 1981). This is critical. Contrast verbal instructions for alertness with verbal instructions for hypnosis and you find a *difference* in outcome measures. Contrast physical activity (whether with or without verbal alerting instructions) with verbal instructions for hypnosis and you get *similar* outcomes. Relaxation can be entered by either route.

In 1981 and again in 1984, I argued that "alert trance" and *anesis* differ in kind rather than in degree, as Humphreys (1984) had countered. Perhaps they differ in kind with respect to *verbal* antecedents, but differ in degree when physical activity is added to the formula. Perhaps the so-called "alert trance" is in reality a cognitively relaxed state achieved through muscular activity, for as Moon pointed out, "the appearance of a subject undergoing Bányai's bicycle technique . . . looked far from unrelaxed, despite vigorous (but rhythmical) pedaling "(1982, p. 59). Bányai herself (Bányai et al., 1981) remarked on the vacant facial expressions and seemingly unfocused gaze of her pedalers, although, in contrast to the relaxation induction subjects, the pedalers' posture was tense and their movements were accelerated. And we know that joggers jog to *relax*. Perhaps the rapprochement between these two apparently disparate understandings of hypnosis lies in their basic similarity—relaxation, through passive or active manipulations. To paraphrase J. R. Hilgard (1974), there are multiple pathways to hypnosis, including physical activities and verbal relaxation instructions, and they all lead to one condition: the basic fundamental condition of *anesis*.

CONCLUSION

As I have tried to point out throughout this chapter, relaxation is the basis for all that follows in hypnosis: for the cognitions, for the emerging primary process, for the dissociations, and for the roles others have proposed as defining the hypnotic situation. Even when we assess some of the unique characteristics of hypnosis—as distinct from the theoretical explanations—the relaxation that is hypnosis plays a prodromal and facilitory role. For example, Braid (1855/1970) wrote of two types of *spontaneous* amnesia accompanying hypnosis, one accessible through rehypnotization, the other irreversible (see also Sidis, 1898). Aside from the fact that spontaneous amnesias have practically disappeared from the vocabulary of hypnosis (see Edmonston, 1989), amnesia is facilitated by the basic condition of hypnosis (relaxation). Recall is an active process. The passivity of relaxation, be it cognitive or somatic, is not compatible with the active process of recall without further, disinhibitory instructions. Amnesias that may occur spontaneously may be only a natural outcome of the relaxation and thus a disinclination toward the active recall that relaxation engenders.

The relaxation that is hypnosis has the same relationship to the experience of the nonvoluntariness that some have noted accompanies hypnosis (e.g., Weitzenhoffer, 1980). Again, it is an active–passive polarity. The experience of voluntariness is incompatible with the experience of relaxation; thus the latter enhances the former's opposite. Relaxation is perceived as passive, voluntariness as active. But the experience of nonvoluntariness *is* compatible with the relaxation of hypnosis.

Finally, at least since the time of Liébeault and Bernheim, suggestibility has played a major role in our conceptualizations about hypnosis. It was Hull (1933), however, who proposed that it was not suggestibility per se with which we should be concerned, but hypersuggestibility, which itself is enhanced by the relaxation of hypnosis. As I have pointed out elsewhere (Edmonston, 1989), suggestion misleads the senses by disrupting the central nervous system's interpreting mechanisms. Cortical alertness, the antithesis of the relaxation inherent in hypnosis, sharpens the senses, focuses the individual on anticipated action, arouses the sympathetic nervous system, brings forth the ergotropic response, and by and large reduces suggestion's effectiveness. However, the disinhibition of lower nervous system centers through the cortical inhibition posed by Pavlov (and noted in the Stage 1 sleep-like EEGs during hypnosis) heightens the potential for sensory misinterpretation and thereby makes suggestions more potent, as measured in the hypersuggestibility of hypnosis. It is the trophotropic response of relaxation that forms the groundwork for hypersuggestibility.

Thus, much of what we observe in modern-day hypnosis is attributable to the relaxation inherent in the condition. This is why I have argued for a more accurate label of what hypnosis is. I have proposed (Edmonston, 1981) to replace the outmoded term hypnosis with *anesis*, the noun form of the Greek verb *aniesis* ("to relax, to let go"), because it accurately describes and summarizes the literature just reviewed. These data do not support the continued use of the term hypnosis, or even neutral hypnosis. They direct us to a new beginning of understanding; they direct us to anesis.

REFERENCES

Agras, W. S., Southam, M. A., & Taylor, C. B. (1983). Long-term persistence of relaxation-induced blood pressure lowering during the working day. *Journal of Consulting and Clinical Psychology*, 51, 792–794.

Amadeo, M. & Shagass, C. (1963). Eye movements, attention, and hypnosis. *Journal of Nervous and Mental Disease*, 136, 139–145.

Antrobus, J. S., Antrobus, J. S., & Singer, J. L. (1964). Eye movements accompanying day dreaming, visual imagery, and thought suppression. *Journal of Abnormal and Social Psychology*, 69, 244–253.

Bányai, E. I., & Hilgard, E. R. (1976). A comparison of active-alert hypnotic induction with traditional relaxation induction. *Journal of Abnormal Psychology*, *85*, 218–224.

Bányai, E. I., Mészáros, I., & Greguss, A. C. (1981). Alteration of activity level: The essence of hypnosis or a byproduct of the type of induction? In G. Adám, I. Mészáros, & E. I. Bányai (Eds.), *Advances in physiological sciences: Vol. 17. Brain and behavior* (pp. 457–465). Elmsford, NY: Pergamon Press.

Barber, T. X. (1979). Suggested ("hypnotic") behavior: The trance paradigm versus an alternative paradigm. In E. Fromm & R. E. Shor (Eds.), *Hypnosis: Developments in research and new perspectives* (2nd ed., pp. 217–271). New York: Aldine.

Barber, T. X., & Calverley, D. S. (1962). "Hypnotic behavior" as a function of task motivation. *Journal of Psychology*, *54*, 363–389.

Barber, T. X., & Calverley, D. S. (1963a). "Hypnotic-like" suggestibility in children and adults. *Journal of Abnormal and Social Psychology*, *66*, 589–597.

Barber, T. X., & Calverley, D. S. (1963b). The relative effectiveness of task-motivating instructions and trance-induction procedures in the production of "hypnotic-like" behavior. *Journal of Nervous & Mental Disease*, *137*, 107–116.

Barber, T. X., & Calverley, D. S. (1965a). Empirical evidence for a theory of "hypnotic" behavior: Effects on suggestibility of five variables typically induced in hypnotic induction procedures. *Journal of Consulting Psychology*, *29*, 98–107.

Barber, T. X., & Calverley, D. S. (1965b). Empirical evidence for a theory of "hypnotic" behavior: The suggestibility-enhancing effects of motivational suggestions, relaxation–sleep suggestions, and suggestions that the subject will be effectively "hypnotized." *Journal of Personality*, *33*, 256–270.

Barber, T. X., & Coules, J. (1959). Electrical skin conductance and galvanic skin response during "hypnosis." *International Journal of Clinical and Experimental Hypnosis*, *7*, 79–92.

Barber, T. X., & Glass, L. B. (1962). Significant factors in hypnotic behavior. *Journal of Abnormal and Social Psychology*, *64*, 222–228.

Barber, T. X., & Ham, M. W. (1974). *Hypnotic phenomena*. Morristown, NJ: General Learning Press.

Barber, T. X., Spanos, N. P., & Chaves, J. F. (1974). *Hypnosis, imagination, and human potentialities*. Elmsford, NY: Pergamon Press.

Barber, T. X., & Wilson, S. C. (1977). Hypnosis, suggestions and altered states of consciousness: Experimental evaluations of the new cognitive–behavioral theory and the traditional trance-state theory of "hypnosis." *Annals of the New York Academy of Sciences*, *296*, 34–47.

Barber, T. X., Wilson, S. C., & Scott, D. S. (1980). Effects of a traditional trance induction on response to "hypnotist-centered" versus "subject-centered" test suggestions. *International Journal of Clinical and Experimental Hypnosis*, *28*, 114–126.

Barker, W., & Burgwin, S. (1948). Brain wave patterns accompanying changes in sleep and wakefulness during hypnosis. *Psychosomatic Medicine*, *10*, 317–326.

Barker, W., & Burgwin, S. (1949). Brain wave patterns during hypnosis, hypnotic sleep, and normal sleep. *Archives of Neurology and Psychiatry*, *62*, 412–420.

Barmark, S. M., & Gaunitz, S. C. B. (1979). Transcendental Meditation and heterohypnosis as altered states of consciousness. *International Journal of Clinical and Experimental Hypnosis*, *27*, 227–239.

Bass, M. J. (1931). Differentiation of the hypnotic trance from normal sleep. *Journal of Experimental Psychology, 14*, 382–399.

Bassman, S. W. (1983). *The effects of indirect hypnosis, relaxation, and homework on the primary and secondary psychological symptoms of women with muscle-contraction headache.* Unpublished doctoral dissertation, University of Cincinnati.

Beary, J. F., & Benson, H., with Klemchuk, H. P. (1974). A simple psychophysiologic technique which elicits the hypometabolic changes of the relaxation response. *Psychosomatic Medicine, 36*, 115–120.

Benson, H., Beary, J. F., & Carol, M. P. (1974). The relaxation response. *Psychiatry, 37*, 37–46.

Benson, H., Frankel, F. H., Apfel, R., Daniels, M. D., Schniewind, H. E., Nemiah, J. C., Sifneos, P. E., Crassweller, K. D., Greenwood, M. M., Kotch, J. B., Arns, P. A., & Rosner, B. (1978). Treatment of anxiety: A comparison of the usefulness of self-hypnosis and a meditational relaxation technique. *Psychotherapy and Psychosomatics, 30*, 229–242.

Brady, J. P., & Rosner, B. S. (1966). Rapid eye movements in hypnotically induced dreams. *Journal of Nervous & Mental Disease, 143*, 28–35.

Braid, J. (1970). The physiology of fascination and the critics criticised. In M. M. Tinterow (Ed.), *Foundations of hypnosis from Mesmer to Freud* (pp. 365–389). Springfield, IL: Charles C Thomas. (Original work published 1855)

Bullard, P. D., & DeCoster, D. T. (1972). The effects of hypnosis, relaxation, and reinforcement on hypnotic behaviors and experiences. *American Journal of Clinical Hypnosis, 15*, 93–97.

Charlesworth, E. A., & Doughtie, E. B. (1982). Modification of baseline by differential task presentation as either hypnosis or "learned" relaxation. *Perceptual and Motor Skills, 55*, 1131–1137.

Christoph, P., Luborsky, L., Kron, R., & Fishman, H. (1978). Blood pressure, heart rate, and respiratory responses to a single session of relaxation: A partial replication. *Journal of Psychosomatic Research, 22*, 493–501.

Coe, W. C., & Ryken, K. (1979). Hypnosis and risks to human subjects. *American Psychologist, 34*, 673–681.

Coe, W. C., & Sarbin, T. R. (1977). Hypnosis from the standpoint of a contextualist. *Annals of the New York Academy of Sciences, 296*, 2–13.

Cogan, R., & Kluthe, K. B. (1981). The role of learning in pain reduction associated with relaxation and patterned breathing. *Journal of Psychosomatic Research, 25*, 535–539.

Cogger, W. G., Jr., & Edmonston, W. E., Jr. (1971). Hypnosis and oral temperature: A re-evaluation of experimental techniques. *British Journal of Clinical Hypnosis, 2*, 76–80.

Coleman, T. R. (1976). A comparative study of certain behavioral, physiological, and phenomenological effects of hypnotic induction and two progressive relaxation procedures (Doctoral dissertation, Brigham Young University). *Dissertation Abstracts International*, (University Microfilms No. 76-2561).

Crawford, H. J., Hilgard, J. R., & Macdonald, H. (1982). Transient experiences following hypnotic testing and special termination procedures. *International Journal of Clinical and Experimental Hypnosis, 30*, 117–126.

Darrow, C. W., Henry, E. C., Gill, M., Brenman, M., & Converse, M. (1950).

Frontal–motor parallelism and motor–occipital in-phase activity in hypnosis, drowsiness, and sleep. *Electroencephalography and Clinical Neurophysiology, 2,* 355.

Das, J. P. (1958). The Pavlovian theory of hypnosis: An evaluation. *Journal of Mental Science, 104,* 82–90.

Davidson, R. J., & Schwartz, G. E. (1976). The psychobiology of relaxation and related states: A multi-process theory. In D. I. Mostofsky (Ed.), *Behavior control and modification of physiological activity* (pp. 399–442). Englewood Cliffs, NJ: Prentice-Hall.

Delmonte, M. M. (1985). Biochemical indices associated with meditation practice: A literature review. *Neuroscience and Biobehavioral Reviews, 9,* 557–561.

DeStefano, R. F. (1976). *The "inoculation" effect in think-with instructions for "hypnotic-like" experiences.* Unpublished doctoral dissertation, Temple University.

Dorcus, R. M., Brintnall, A. K., & Case, H. W. (1941). Control experiments and their relation to theories of hypnotism. *Journal of General Psychology, 24,* 217–221.

Dunwoody, R. C., & Edmonston, W. E., Jr. (1974). Hypnosis and slow eye movements. *American Journal of Clinical Hypnosis, 16,* 270–274.

Edmonston, W. E., Jr. (1967). Stimulus–response theory of hypnosis. In J. E. Gordon (Ed.), *Handbook of clinical and experimental hypnosis* (pp. 345–387). New York: Macmillan.

Edmonston, W. E., Jr. (1968). Hypnosis and electrodermal responses. *American Journal of Clinical Hypnosis, 11,* 16–25.

Edmonston, W. E., Jr. (1977a). Neutral hypnosis as relaxation. *American Journal of Clinical Hypnosis, 20,* 69–75.

Edmonston, W. E., Jr. (Ed.). (1977b). *Conceptual and investigative approaches to hypnosis and hypnotic phenomena.* New York Academy of Sciences, Annals, Vol. 296.

Edmonston, W. E., Jr. (1979). The effects of neutral hypnosis on conditioned responses: Implications for hypnosis as relaxation. In E. Fromm & R. E. Shor (Eds.), *Hypnosis: Developments in research and new perspectives* (2nd ed., pp. 415–455). New York: Aldine.

Edmonston, W. E., Jr. (1981). *Hypnosis and relaxation: Modern verification of an old equation.* New York: Wiley.

Edmonston, W. E., Jr. (1986). *The induction of hypnosis.* New York: Wiley.

Edmonston, W. E., Jr. (1989). Conceptual clarification of hypnosis and its relationship to suggestibility. In A. V. Gheorghiu, P. Netter, H. J. Eysenck, & R. Rosenthal (Eds.), *Suggestibility: Theory and research* (pp. 69–78). Berlin: Springer-Verlag.

Edmonston, W. E., Jr., & Grotevant, W. R. (1975). Hypnosis and alpha density. *American Journal of Clinical Hypnosis, 17,* 221–232.

Edmonston, W. E., Jr., & Pessin, M. (1966). Hypnosis as related to learning and electrodermal measures. *American Journal of Clinical Hypnosis, 9,* 31–51.

Edmonston, W. E., Jr., & Robertson, T. G., Jr. (1967). A comparison of the effects of task motivational and hypnotic induction instructions on responsiveness to hypnotic suggestibility scales. *American Journal of Clinical Hypnosis, 9,* 184–187.

Evans, F. J. (1979). Hypnosis and sleep: Techniques for exploring cognitive activity during sleep. In E. Fromm & R. E. Shor (Eds.), *Hypnosis: Developments in research and new perspectives* (2nd ed., pp. 139–183). New York: Aldine.

Evans, F. J. (1981). Sleep and hypnosis: Accessibility of altered states of consciousness. In G. Adam, I. Mészáros, & E. I. Bányai (Eds.), *Advances in physiological sciences: Vol. 17. Brain and behavior* (pp. 453–456). Elmsford, NY: Pergamon Press.

Friedman, H., & Taub, H. A. (1977). The use of hypnosis and biofeedback procedures for essential hypertension. *International Journal of Clinical and Experimental Hypnosis, 25,* 335–347.

Friedman, H., & Taub, H. A. (1978). A six-month follow-up of the use of hypnosis and biofeedback procedures in essential hypertension. *American Journal of Clinical Hypnosis, 20,* 184–188.

Friedman, H., & Taub, H. A. (1982). Accessibility—A necessary control for studies of essential hypertension: A brief communication. *International Journal of Clinical and Experimental Hypnosis, 30,* 4–8.

Friedman, H., & Taub, H. A. (1984). Brief psychological training procedures in migraine treatment. *American Journal of Clinical Hypnosis, 26,* 187–200.

Friedman, H., Taub, H. A., Sturr, J. F., Church, K. L., & Monty, R. A. (1986). Hypnotizability and speed of visual information processing. *International Journal of Clinical and Experimental Hypnosis, 34,* 234–241.

Fromm, E. (1979). The nature of hypnosis and other altered states of consciousness: An ego-psychological theory. In E. Fromm & R. E. Shor (Eds.) *Hypnosis: Developments in research and new perspectives* (2nd ed., pp. 81–103). New York: Aldine.

Gibbons, D. E. (1979). *Applied hypnosis and hyperempiria.* New York: Plenum.

Goldwyn, J. (1930). The effect of hypnosis on basal metabolism. *Archives of Internal Medicine, 45,* 109–114.

Gruzelier, J. H., & Brow, T. D. (1985). Psychophysiological evidence for a state theory of hypnosis and susceptibility. *Journal of Psychosomatic Research, 29,* 287–302.

Ham, M. W., & Edmonston, W. E., Jr. (1971). Hypnosis, relaxation, and motor retardation. *Journal of Abnormal Psychology, 77,* 329–331.

Hilgard, E. R. (1965). *Hypnotic susceptibility.* New York: Harcourt, Brace & World.

Hilgard, E. R. (1973). The domain of hypnosis, with some comments on alternative paradigms. *American Psychologist, 28,* 972–980.

Hilgard, E. R. (1977a). The problem of divided consciousness. *Annals of the New York Academy of Sciences, 296,* 48–59.

Hilgard, E. R. (1977b). *Divided consciousness: Multiple controls in human thought and action.* New York: Wiley.

Hilgard, E. R., & Tart, C. T. (1966). Responsiveness to suggestions following waking and imagination instructions and following induction of hypnosis. *Journal of Abnormal and Social Psychology, 71,* 196–208.

Hilgard, J. R. (1974). Sequelae to hypnosis. *International Journal of Clinical and Experimental Hypnosis, 22,* 281–298.

Hoffman, J. W., Benson, H., Arns, P. A., Stainbrook, G. L., Landsberg, L., Young, J. B., & Gill, A. (1982). Reduced sympathetic nervous system responsivity associated with the relaxation response. *Science, 215,* 190–192.

Hull, C. L. (1933). *Hypnosis and suggestibility: An experimental approach.* New York: Appleton-Century-Crofts.

Humphreys, A. (1984). Neutral hypnosis, progressive muscular relaxation, and the relaxation response: A review. *British Journal of Experimental and Clinical Hypnosis, 2,* 19–27.

Jacobson, E. (1929). *Progressive relaxation.* Chicago: University of Chicago Press.

Jevning, R., Pirkle, H. C., & Wilson, A. F. (1977). Behavioral alteration of plasma phenylalanine concentration. *Physiology and Behavior, 19,* 611–614.

Kiecolt-Glaser, J. K., Glaser, R., Strain, E. C., Stout, J. C., Tarr, K. L., Holliday, J. E., & Speicher, C. E. (1986). Modulation of cellular immunity in medical students. *Journal of Behavioral Medicine, 9,* 5–21.

Kralik, P. M., Ho, B. T., Mathew, R. J., & Claghorn, J. L. (1983). Kinetic evaluation of platelet monoamine oxidase following relaxation in chronic anxiety. *Acta Psychiatrica Scandinavica, 67,* 315–318.

Kratochvíl, S., & Shubat, N. (1971). Activity–passivity in hypnosis and in the normal state. *International Journal of Clinical and Experimental Hypnosis, 19,* 140–145.

Kratochvíl, S., & Zezulka, K. (1980). The influences of preconception and induction technique on active hypnotic behavior. In M. Pajntar, E. Roskar, & M. Lavric (Eds.), *Hypnosis in psychotherapy and psychosomatic medicine* (pp. 53–57). Kranj, Czechoslovakia: Slovakian Society for Clinical and Experimental Hypnosis.

Liebert, R. M., Rubin, N., & Hilgard, E. R. (1965). The effects of suggestions of alertness in hypnosis on paired-associate learning. *Journal of Personality, 33,* 605–612.

Lorens, S. A., & Darrow, C. W. (1962). Eye movements, EEG, and EKG during mental manipulation. *Electroencephalography and Clinical Neurophysiology, 14,* 739–746.

Lovett-Doust, J. W. (1953). Studies on the physiology of awareness: Oximetric analysis of emotion and the differential planes of consciousness seen in hypnosis. *Journal of Clinical and Experimental Psychopathology, 14,* 113–126.

Malott, J. M. (1984). Active–alert hypnosis: Replication and extension of previous research. *Journal of Abnormal Psychology, 93,* 246–249.

Marenina, A. I. (1959). Further investigations on the dynamics of cerebral potentials in the various phases of hypnosis in man. In *The central nervous system and human behavior: Translations from the Russian medical literature* (pp. 645–649). Bethesda, MD: U.S. Department of Health, Education and Welfare.

Mather, M. D., & Degun, G. S. (1975). A comparison study of hypnosis and relaxation. *British Journal of Medical Psychology, 48,* 55–61.

McAmmond, D. M., Davidson, P. O., & Kovitz, D. M. (1971). A comparison of the effects of hypnosis and relaxation training on stress reactions in a dental situation. *American Journal of Clinical Hypnosis, 13,* 233–242.

McConkey, K. M., Sheehan, P. W., & White, K. D. (1979). Comparison of the Creative Imagination Scale and the Harvard Group Scale of Hypnotic Susceptibility, Form A. *International Journal of Clinical and Experimental Hypnosis, 27,* 265–277.

Melzack, R., & Perry, C. (1975). Self-regulation of pain: The use of alpha-feedback and hypnotic training for the control of chronic pain. *Experimental Neurology, 46,* 452–469.

Mesmer, F. A. (1781). *Précis historique des faits relatifs au magnétisme animal jusqu'en avril 1781*. London: Author.

Mészáros, I., Bányai, E. I., & Greguss, A. C. (1981). Evoked potential, reflecting hypnotically altered state of consciousness. In G. Adám, I. Mészáros, & E. I. Bányai (Eds.), *Advances in physiological sciences: Vol. 17. Brain and behavior* (pp. 467–475). Elmsford, NY: Pergamon Press.

Mills, W. W., & Farrow, J. T. (1981). The Transcendental Meditation technique and acute experimental pain. *Psychosomatic Medicine, 43*, 157–164.

Mitchell, G. P., Jr., & Lundy, R. M. (1986). The effects of relaxation and imagery inductions on responses to suggestions. *International Journal of Clinical and Experimental Hypnosis, 34*, 98–109.

Moon, T. (1982, November 5). [Review of *Hypnosis and relaxation: Modern verification of an old equation*]. *Bulletin of the British Society of Experimental and Clinical Hypnosis*, pp. 51–60.

Morse, D. R., Martin, J. S., Furst, M. L., & Dubin, L. L. (1977). A physiological and subjective evaluation of meditation, hypnosis, and relaxation. *Psychosomatic Medicine, 39*, 304–324.

Morse, D. R., Schacterle, G. R., Furst, M. L., Goldberg, J., Greenspan, B., Swiecinski, D., & Susek, J. (1982). The effect of stress and meditation on salivary protein and bacteria: A review and pilot study. *Journal of Human Stress, 8*, 31–39.

Mount, G. R., Walters, S. R., Rowland, R. W., Barnes, P. R., & Payton, T. I. (1978). The effects of relaxation techniques on normal blood pressure. *Behavioral Engineering, 5*, 1–4.

O'Connell, D. N., & Orne, M. T. (1968). Endosomatic electrodermal correlates of hypnotic depth and susceptibility. *Journal of Psychiatric Research, 6*, 1–12.

Oetting, E. R. (1964). Hypnosis and concentration in study. *American Journal of Clinical Hypnosis, 7*, 148–151.

Orne, M. T. (1971). The simulation of hypnosis: Why, how, and what it means. *International Journal of Clinical and Experimental Hypnosis, 19*, 183–210.

Orne, M. T. (1977). The construct of hypnosis: Implications of the definition for research and practice. *Annals of the New York Academy of Sciences, 296*, 14–33.

Orne, M. T. (1979). On the simulating subject as a quasi-control group in hypnosis research: What, why, and how. In E. Fromm & R. E. Shor (Eds.), *Hypnosis: Developments in research and new perspectives* (2nd ed., pp. 519–565). New York: Aldine.

Paul, G. L. (1969a). Physiological effects of relaxation training and hypnotic suggestion. *Journal of Abnormal Psychology, 74*, 425–437.

Paul, G. L. (1969b). Inhibition of physiological responses to stressful imagery by relaxation training and hypnotically suggested relaxation. *Behaviour Research and Therapy, 7*, 249–256.

Pavlov, I. P. (1923). The identity of inhibition with sleep and hypnosis. *Scientific Monthly, 17*, 603–608.

Pavlov, I. P. (1928). *Lectures on conditioned reflexes: Twenty-five years of objective study of the higher nervous system activity (behavior) of animals*. (W. H. Gantt, Ed. and Trans.). New York: Liveright.

Pessin, M., Plapp, J. M., & Stern, J. A. (1968). Effects of hypnosis induction and attention direction on electrodermal responses. *American Journal of Clinical Hypnosis, 10*, 198–206.

Peters, J. E., & Stern, R. M. (1973). Peripheral skin temperature and vasomotor responses during hypnotic induction. *International Journal of Clinical and Experimental Hypnosis, 21,* 102–108.

Plapp, J. M. (1967). Hypnosis, conditioning, and physiological responses (Doctoral dissertation, Washington University). *Dissertation Abstracts International,* (University Microfilms No. 67-9406).

Plapp, J. M., & Edmonston, W. E., Jr. (1965). Extinction of a conditioned motor response following hypnosis. *Journal of Abnormal and Social Psychology, 70,* 378–382.

Platonov, K. I. (Ed.). (1959). *The word as a physiological and therapeutic factor: Problems of theory and practice of psychotherapy on the basis of the theory of I. P. Pavlov* (2nd ed., D. A. Myshne, Trans.). Moscow: Foreign Languages Publishing House. (Original work published 1955)

Pollack, M. H., & Zeiner, A. R. (1979). Physiological correlates of an experimental relaxation procedure with comparisons to uninstructed relaxation and sitting. *Biological Psychology Bulletin, 5,* 161–170.

Puente, A. E. (1981). Psychophysiological investigations on Transcendental Meditation. *Biofeedback and Self-Regulation, 6,* 327–342.

Puységur, A. M. J., Chastenet, Marquis de. (1837). *An essay of instruction on animal magnetism* (J. King, Trans.). New York: J. C. Kelley.

Rader, C. M. (1972). Influence of motivational instructions on hypnotic and nonhypnotic reaction time performance. *American Journal of Clinical Hypnosis, 15,* 98–101.

Reid, A. F., & Curtsinger, G. (1968). Physiological changes associated with hypnosis: The effect of hypnosis on temperature. *International Journal of Clinical and Experimental Hypnosis, 16,* 111–119.

Reyher, J. (1973). Can hypnotized subjects simulate waking behavior? *American Journal of Clinical Hypnosis, 16,* 31–36.

Reyher, J. (1977). Clinical and experimental hypnosis: Implications for theory and methodology. *Annals of the New York Academy of Sciences, 296,* 69–85.

Reyher, J., & Wilson, J. G. (1973). The induction of hypnosis: Indirect vs. direct methods and the role of anxiety. *American Journal of Clinical Hypnosis, 15,* 229–233.

Rosenhan, D., & London, P. (1963). Hypnosis in the unhypnotizable: A study in rote learning. *Journal of Experimental Psychology, 65,* 30–34.

Saletu, B. (1987). Brain function during hypnosis, acupuncture, and Transcendental Meditation. In B. Taneli, C. Perris, & D. Kemali (Eds.), *Advances in biological psychiatry: Vol. 16. Neurophysiological correlates of relaxation and psychopathology* (pp. 18–40). Basel: S. Karger.

Schubert, D. K. (1983). Comparison of hypnotherapy with systematic relaxation in the treatment of cigarette habituation. *Journal of Clinical Psychology, 39,* 198–202.

Schultz, H. A., & Luthe, W. (1959). *Autogenic therapy: A psychophysiological approach to psychotherapy.* New York: Grune & Stratton.

Schultz, J. H. (1932). *Das Autogene Training.* Stuttgart: Thieme Verlag.

Shor, R. E., & Orne, E. C. (1962). *Harvard Group Scale of Hypnotic Susceptibility.* Palo Alto, CA: Consulting Psychologists Press.

Sidis, B. (1898). *The psychology of suggestion.* New York: D. Appleton.

Sletvold, H., Jensen, G. M., & Gotestam, G. (1986). Blood pressure responses to hypnotic and nonhypnotic suggestions in normotensive subjects. *Pavlovian Journal of Biological Science, 21*, 32–35.

Slotnick, R. S., & London, P. (1965). Influence of instructions on hypnotic and non-hypnotic performance. *Journal of Abnormal Psychology, 70*, 38–46.

Smith, W. H. (1969). The effects of hypnosis and suggestion on auditory threshold. *Journal of Speech and Hearing Research, 12*, 161–168.

Southam, M. A., Agras, W. S., Taylor, C. B., & Kraemer, H. C. (1982). Relaxation training: Blood pressure lowering during the working day. *Archives of General Psychiatry, 39*, 715–717.

Spinhoven, P. (1988). Similarities and dissimilarities in hypnotic and nonhypnotic procedures for headache control: A review. *American Journal of Clinical Hypnosis, 30*, 183–194.

Stern, J. A., Brown, M., Ulett, G. A., & Sletten, I. (1977). A comparison of hypnosis, acupuncture, morphine, Valium, aspirin, and placebo in the management of experimentally induced pain. *Annals of the New York Academy of Sciences, 296*, 175–193.

Stern, J. A., Edmonston, W. E., Jr., Ulett, G. A., & Levitsky, A. (1963). Electrodermal measures in experimental amnesia. *Journal of Abnormal and Social Psychology, 67*, 397–401.

Strosberg, I. M., & Vics, I. I. (1962). Physiologic changes in the eye during hypnosis. *American Journal of Clinical Hypnosis, 4*, 264–267.

Taneli, B., & Krahne, W. (1987). EEG changes of Transcendental Meditation practitioners. In B. Taneli, C. Perris, & D. Kemali (Eds.) *Advances in biological psychiatry: Vol. 16. Neurophysiological correlates of relaxation and psychopathology* (pp. 41–71). Basel: S. Karger.

Tart, C. T. (1963). Hypnotic depth and basal skin resistance. *International Journal of Clinical and Experimental Hypnosis, 11*, 81–92.

Tebecis, A. K., & Provins, K. A. (1976). Further studies of physiological concomitants of hypnosis: Skin temperature, heart rate, and skin resistance. *Biological Psychology, 4*, 249–258.

Tebecis, A. K., Provins, M. A., Farnbach, R. W., & Pentony, P. (1975). Hypnosis and EEG. *Journal of Nervous and Mental Disease, 161*, 1–17.

Timney, B. N., & Barber, T. X. (1969). Hypnotic induction and oral temperature. *International Journal of Clinical and Experimental Hypnosis, 17*, 121–132.

Tripp, E. G., & Marks, D. (1986). Hypnosis, relaxation, and analgesia suggestions for the reduction of reported pain in high- and low-suggestible subjects. *Australian Journal of Clinical and Experimental Hypnosis, 14*, 99–113.

Van Gorp, W. G., Meyer, R. G., & Dunbar, K. D. (1985). The efficacy of direct versus indirect hypnotic induction techniques on reduction of experimental pain. *International Journal of Clinical and Experimental Hypnosis, 33*, 319–328.

Vingoe, F. J. (1968). The development of a group alert–trance scale. *International Journal of Clinical and Experimental Hypnosis, 16*, 120–132.

Wagstaff, G. F. (1976). A note on Mather and Degun's "A comparative study of hypnosis and relaxation." *British Journal of Medical Psychology, 49*, 299–300.

Wallace, R. K. (1970). Physiological effects of Transcendental Meditation. *Science, 167*, 1751–1754.

Wallace, R. K., Benson, H., & Wilson, A. F. (1971). A wakeful hypometabolic physiologic state. *American Journal of Physiology, 221*, 797–799.

Walrath, L. C., & Hamilton, D. W. (1975). Autonomic correlates of meditation and hypnosis. *American Journal of Clinical Hypnosis, 17*, 190–197.

Weitzenhoffer, A. M. (1969). Hypnosis and eye movements: A possible SEM correlate of hypnosis. *American Journal of Clinical Hypnosis, 11*, 221–227.

Weitzenhoffer, A. M. (1971). Ocular changes in passive hypnosis. *American Journal of Clinical Hypnosis, 14*, 102–121.

Weitzenhoffer, A. M. (1980). Hypnotic susceptibility revisited. *American Journal of Clinical Hypnosis, 22*, 130–146.

Weitzenhoffer, A. M. (1989). *The practice of hypnotism*. New York: Wiley.

Weitzenhoffer, A. M., & Brockmeier, J. D. (1970). Attention and eye movements. *Journal of Nervous and Mental Disease, 151*, 130–142.

Weitzenhoffer, A. M., & Hilgard, E. R. (1959). *Stanford Hypnotic Susceptibility Scale: Forms A and B*. Palo Alto, CA: Consulting Psychologists Press.

Weitzenhoffer, A. M., & Hilgard, E. R. (1962). *Stanford Hypnotic Susceptibility Scale: Form C*. Palo Alto, CA: Consulting Psychologists Press.

Weitzenhoffer, A. M., & Sjoberg, B. M. (1961). Suggestibility with and without "induction of hypnosis." *Journal of Nervous and Mental Disease, 132*, 204–220.

West, M. A. (1979). Physiological effects of meditation: A longitudinal study. *British Journal of Social and Clinical Psychology, 18*, 219–226.

White, R. W. (1937). Two types of hypnotic trance and their personality correlates. *Journal of Psychology, 3*, 279–289.

Wilson, S. C. (1976). *An experimental investigation evaluating the Creative Imagination Scale and its relationship to "hypnotic-like" experiences*. Unpublished doctoral dissertation, Heed University, Hollywood, FL.

Wilson, S. C., & Barber, T. X. (1978). The Creative Imagination Scale as a measure of hypnotic responsiveness: Applications to experimental and clinical hypnosis. *American Journal of Clinical Hypnosis, 20*, 235–249.

Wittkower, E. (1929). Uber Affektiv-Somatische Veranderungen. II. Mitteilung: Die Affektleukozytose. *Klinische Wochenschrift, 8*, 1082.

Wolpe, J. (1958). *Psychotherapy by reciprocal inhibition*. Stanford, CA: Stanford University Press.

Wolpe, J. (1969). *The practice of behavior therapy*. Elmsford, NY: Pergamon Press.

Wood, A. (1851). Contributions towards the study of certain phenomena, which have recently dominated experiments in electro-biology. *Monthly Journal of Mental Science, 12*, 407–435.

PART THREE

CLINICAL PERSPECTIVES

The Locksmith Model: Accessing Hypnotic Responsiveness

JOSEPH BARBER

UCLA Neuropsychiatric Institute

INTRODUCTION

Of the many qualities that fascinate and beguile the observer of hypnosis, one that particularly mesmerizes me is the sometimes inexplicable and therefore seemingly magical nature of "hypnotic cures." Although most people have unreasonably high expectations about the therapeutic possibilities of hypnosis, one reason why these high expectations are maintained is that hypnosis does seem capable of relieving people's suffering in sometimes inexplicable ways.

No one can be indifferent, for instance, to the experience of observing a hysterically mute man suddenly speaking after hearing hypnotic suggestions that inspire him to do so. No one can maintain an air of detachment when in the presence of a woman comfortably undergoing surgery, without chemical anesthesia, with only the quiet assurance of words to defend her against the dreadful pain of the surgeon's knife. How can we understand such apparently "magical" phenomena?

The first clinical case in which I used hypnosis was that of a 31-year-old man who was experiencing the distress of sexual dysfunction; his symptoms included fragile erection and premature ejaculation. To my complete surprise, after one treatment involving hypnotic suggestion, he reported complete relief of symptoms. Follow-up at 1 year confirmed the lasting character of this relief. Some years later I treated a 63-year-old woman whose presenting complaint was that she had smoked at least two packs per day since age 13; she now felt the need to stop, but felt completely unable to do so. After one treatment involving hypnotic suggestion, she was completely free of her addiction/compulsion. Follow-up at 1 and 5 years confirmed that the change was stable.

Neither of these cases represents a problem that one expects can be successfully managed in one treatment. And, indeed, though this can happen, it is not ordinarily the case. Not every hysterical patient's symptoms change with hypnotic intervention. Not every mute person speaks when hypnotized and told to do so. Not everyone can undergo surgery with hypnoanesthesia. No reasonable person expects magical cures, but they do occur sufficiently often to both warrant our attention, and to illustrate what is important and perhaps unique about hypnosis. Hypnosis is well known for being used successfully in the psychotherapeutic treatment of troubling behavior (such as habits and compulsions), affective disorders (including phobias and certain anxiety disorders, such as post-traumatic stress disorder), psychophysiological syndromes (including hypertension, urticaria, asthma, and other disorders whose etiology involves autonomic hyperreactivity), pain (both acute and chronic), and dissociative disorders (including psychogenic amnesia and multiple personality disorder). In addition, it is used adjunctively in psychotherapeutic treatment of more complex disorders where symptom alteration is not the primary goal (T. X. Barber, 1978; Bowers & Kelly, 1979; Di Piano & Salzberg, 1979; E. R. Hilgard & Hilgard, 1983; Mott, 1982; Perry, Gelfand, & Marcovitch, 1979; Watkins, 1971). We must be intrigued by a psychological treatment that can quickly—and (here is the point) *so inexplicably*—relieve the suffering patient of the burden of his or her symptoms. How does this happen? In this discussion of the role of hypnosis in facilitating such change, I focus on the interaction between the intrapsychic and the interpersonal elements of the hypnotic experience: the altered state of consciousness and the psychotherapeutic relationship.

Whenever we address the question of therapeutic change, we need to consider the myriad of possibilities—including coincidence. Was the change likely to occur at that time in the patient's life for reasons apart from treatment, and the clinician was coincidentally fortunate to be a part of it? Was the change a function of the patient's expectation about psychotherapy? Was it a response to the clinician's attention and concern? Was the change in the patient a function of the significant modification of the clinician's own behavior because he or she was using hypnotic techniques? Or was the change in fact a function of the use of hypnosis? If so, was the change a function of the subjective experience of being hypnotized? Of receiving particular therapeutic suggestions while experiencing hypnosis? Did the patient's experience of the therapeutic relationship contribute, slightly or significantly, to the change? All of these factors certainly have their effects. But there are certain clinical phenomena, most dramatically demonstrated by medical applications of hypnosis, that are unique to hypnosis; it is these phenomena that most alert us to the need to attend to the mechanisms of its efficacy.

Esdaile's (1846/1957) report of thousands of minor surgeries and 345 major surgeries, employing hypnotic suggestion as the sole anesthetic, and A. A. Levitan's (personal communication, 1989) report of hypnoanesthesia being used in a series of 23 major surgical procedures, illustrate that there is something remarkable about hypnosis. The literature on clinical hypnosis is replete with reports of the medical application of this psychological treatment. These reports describe the treatment of traumatic burns (Ewin, 1978, 1980); management of pain, both in adults (J. Barber, 1986; Crasilneck & Hall, 1985; E. R. Hilgard & Hilgard, 1983) and in children (J. R. Hilgard & LeBaron, 1984; Zeltzer & LeBaron, 1982); reduction of postoperative bleeding (Benson, 1971); management of nausea and appetite loss secondary to chemotherapy (J. Barber & Gitelson, 1980); and management of asthma, Raynaud's disease, hypertension, and other psychophysiological syndromes (Crasilneck & Hall, 1985; Goldsmith, 1986).

What is it about the experience of hypnosis that is curative? It is widely believed that the suggestions themselves are the effective elements. But to account for the effect of suggestions, we need to attend to two other features of the hypnotic experience: (1) the salutary effect of the subjective experience of the hypnotic state or condition, and (2) the healing power of the hypnotherapeutic relationship. It is in understanding the interaction between these factors that we may come to an understanding of the phenomenon of hypnosis, and in particular to understand something of its nature as a healing influence. In this chapter, I suggest that the natural variations in the ways people experience hypnosis require that the therapist undertake a "locksmith approach" to engaging both hypnotic and curative capacities. I explain this approach in more detail later in the chapter.

This model expresses the following assumptions:

1. Psychotherapeutic cures involve alterations in both cognitive and affective processes. Such alterations require shifts in one's ability to attend to experience that is not within a person's ordinary awareness, and to capacities for change that are not within volitional control.

2. Hypnosis allows access to not-conscious (not necessarily only unconscious) experience.

3. In an altered state in which one can both be conscious and simultaneously have access to not-conscious processes, one can alter assumptions, meanings, perceptions, memories, and learned associations. Therefore, one can bring about change in behavior and experience.

4. As a process, hypnosis circumvents ordinary defensive processes, as well as normal nondefensive cognitive structures that serve the healthy

function of keeping out-of-conscious material or automated cognitive connections out of awareness, thereby facilitating a patient's attention to material that is meaningful in the context of treatment.

5. The therapeutic relationship that develops as a part of the experience of hypnosis is an essential element in this process of circumvention, by altering the relation of the patient to self or others in a way that creates a safe context for internal change.

6. Having such an altered experience itself changes one's assumptions and expectations of the possibilities for new affect and behavior. The therapeutic relationship facilitates the development of the altered consciousness, which in a positive feedback loop facilitates the further development of the relationship, and so on.

7. People vary in their abilities and in their readiness to develop the altered state. The hypnotic process and the relationship must be varied idiosyncratically to unlock the naturally occurring capacities for dissociative and other curative unconscious processes.

THEORETICAL CONCEPTS AND PRINCIPLES

Description of Hypnosis

Hypnosis is an altered state of consciousness in which the individual's imagination creates vivid reality from suggestions offered either by someone else, by suggestions inferred from environmental cues, or by suggestions initiated by the individual himself or herself. This condition allows the individual to be inordinately responsive to such suggestions, so that he or she is able to alter perception, memory, and physiological processes that under ordinary conditions are not readily susceptible to conscious control.

The efficacy of hypnosis is sometimes argued in the context of the "state–nonstate" question, in which its effects are assumed to be either a function of an alteration in consciousness or a function of interpersonal factors (E. R. Hilgard & Hilgard, 1983). The locksmith model assumes that the efficacy of hypnosis is a function of both the alteration in state *and* interpersonal factors (e.g., the psychotherapeutic relationship). The proportion of effect of these two variables is itself variable, depending on the individual and the circumstance. Sometimes a psychotherapist will determine that fuller attention should be given to elaborating the change in state of consciousness, whereas in another case the determination will be to focus more fully on interpersonal issues.

Hypnosis is often discussed as if it were "Hypnosis with a capital H," as if it exists somehow outside the natural spectrum of psychology. Recent research demonstrates, however, that hypnosis is more a *process* than a *thing*. For instance, the experiential analysis technique (EAT) of Sheehan and McConkey (1982) demonstrates the varying and intricate nature of the hypnotic experience, beneath what may be a deceptively simple surface of behavior. For example, a subject participating in a hypnotic experiment may be hypnotized and given emotionally neutral suggestions. The subject may behave in routine fashion, responding in an emotionally neutral fashion. Exploration of the subject's internal experience with the EAT, however, reveals that the subject may have idiosyncratically interpreted some of the "neutral" suggestions in response to his or her own inclinations, and consequently may be experiencing significant inner turmoil and distress. Even if a hypnotized subject appears to the observer to behave in a quiescent or passive manner, the EAT provides a demonstration of the considerably active cognitive nature of the hypnotic experience for that subject. A hypnotized subject tends to seek actively to understand and make personally relevant and meaningful interpretations of the suggestions, so that he or she may have a significantly different experience from another subject in the experiment who is given precisely the same suggestions. Hypnosis is a complex constituent of the still more complex process of human perception and cognition. Occasionally, our attention to the unusual and unique features of the hypnotic experience can make us forget that it is a normal human psychological experience. Principles of psychology that help us to understand other aspects of human consciousness must be consonant with principles that seek to illuminate hypnosis, and vice versa.

Sheehan and McConkey's (1982) investigations, as well as those of Pekala and his colleagues (Pekala & Kumar, 1984, 1987; Pekala & Nagler, 1989), demonstrate that the development of hypnotic experience involves development of an altered state of consciousness. The alteration seems to include an alteration in one's ordinary sense of reality and a shift to an alternate perspective. This new perspective embodies both cognitive and affective features, as permitted by one's deepest needs for safety and contact, and guided by one's imagination. The reduction of one's usual defenses may occur, permitting greater than usual levels of emotional contact. Moreover, alterations in other, nondefensive co-conscious[1] structures that regulate the inclusion of cognition and affect ordinarily existing outside consciousness all contribute to the experience that hypnosis is an exceptional state of mind. Furthermore, these characteristics of hypnosis contribute in a major way to therapeutic change—aside from the effects of therapeutic suggestion itself—by providing the patient with an alternate and unusual sense of self and relation to the world. Because hypnosis can create a reduction in one's attention to external reality (Pekala & Kumar, 1984; Pekala & Nagler, 1989)[2], whatever happens seems to take place in an abstracted way, or can be experienced as if "this is all that matters," and is not automatically integrated into one's ordinary life. Events, as well as one's emotional response to those events, take on a perspective that can seem "larger than life." In an unusual state, unusual things can happen: A patient, for instance, may experience renewed hopefulness about the possibilities for change.

Another critical aspect of hypnotic experience is dissociation. Every example of prototypical hypnotic behavior includes either the sense of nonvolitionality (a lack of awareness of one's self as the agent of the experience) or a lack of awareness of a stimulus. Both experiences involve dissociation. An example of the first is arm levitation, whereby an individual experiences an automatic lifting of his or her arm. an example of the second, hypnotic deafness, involves the lack of awareness of audition. Almost from the beginning of the investigation of hypnotic phenomena in the 19th century, dissociation has been recognized as a salient feature of hypnosis (and even its *sine qua non*). Janet (1907) recognized that hypnotic phenomena were dissociative in character, and understood them to involve a process of compartmentalization of consciousness. More recently, Kihlstrom (1984) has suggested that such phenomena involve processing of material to co-consciousness—not only repression of material to the unconscious, as Freud characterized the phenomenon. Recognition of the similarities between dissociative phenomena found in certain pathological conditions (primarily hysterical syndromes), and those dissociative phenomena demonstrable in the context of hypnosis, requires us to place hypnosis within the spectrum of natural human experience (although hypnosis does not itself represent a pathological phenomenon). Dissociation is a common phenomenon outside the context of hypnosis, which suggests that most humans have the capacity for dissociation. The question for the hypnotherapist is how to access this capacity.

E. R. Hilgard's theory of hypnosis also asserts dissociation to be a central component. His neodissociation theory provides a cognitive explanation for dissociative hypnotic phenomena (E. R. Hilgard, 1986). This theory suggests that information flowing in and out of consciousness can become compartmentalized, or dissociated, away from ordinarily used cognitive pathways; consequently, the individual becomes consciously unaware of that information. (Thus, a patient is able to not-consciously feel the pain of surgery when responding to hypnotic suggestions for analgesia; or an individual is unable to recall an item from memory until a hypnotic cue is given, eliminating the amnesia.) The "hidden observer" is a metaphor created by E. R. Hilgard to refer to the phenomenon whereby a hypnotized subject, experiencing hypnotic deafness or hypnotic analgesia (or other dissociative phenomena) and asked to access information from a "hidden" part of consciousness, can accurately report what he or she otherwise cannot hear or feel. This feature of the hypnotic experience is confirmatory evidence that parallel cognitive processing (e.g., co-consciousness) is occurring in such circumstances. The phenomenon of the "hidden observer" (E. R. Hilgard, 1986) both raises the issue of dissociation to dramatically interesting levels, and requires us to take into account the remarkable capacity of some people to know and not to know at the same time. Although I refer to Hilgard's neodissociation theory as a means of explaining significant aspects of the hypnotic process (notably dissociation), there still exist questions about the nature of the process that permits an individual somehow to compartmentalize a portion of experience outside ordinary consciousness. It is this capacity that may play a significant role in symptom alteration. When it is suggested to a patient that the symptom will disappear (or will not be bothersome any more), the patient experiences—sometimes immediately—a diminution in the symptom. Presumably, this is accomplished largely through dissociating awareness of the symptom, whether the symptom is the cue that activates habitual nail biting or the pain of surgery or the affective stimulus that evokes a phobic response.

This condition of altered consciousness is further distinguished by what Shor (1959) called a "reduction in the generalized reality orientation": a lessening of awareness of the elements within one's environment that are ordinarily perceived as constituting reality (thus enabling a markedly altered perspective). And, finally, the hypnotic condition is characterized by a tendency toward "archaic involvement"; that is, the subject is inclined to relate to the hypnotist/therapist in ways that "echo back to the love relationships of early life" (Shor, 1979, p. 110). This quality contributes significantly to the unusually rapid and sometimes intense development of the therapeutic relationship in the hypnotic context. The relational elements of the hypnotic experience are certainly not well understood. Yet, as Diamond (1987) suggests, it is the understanding of these particular elements that will bring the important and essential subtleties of the hypnotic experience within our conceptual grasp.

In summary, this discussion of hypnotic process focuses on two principles: altered consciousness (including dissociation and a reduction in reality orientation) and altered interpersonal process (including archaic involvement).

Kihlstrom has contributed a further refinement to our understanding of the cognitive processes underlying the various phenomena of hypnosis, such as posthypnotic behavior, amnesia, perceptual alterations, the "hidden observer," and other phenomena that are essentially dissociative in character. He suggests that co-conscious processes, which can also become accessible to consciousness, are to be distinguished from unconscious processes. It is likely that hypnosis accesses these *out-of*-consciousness processes, rather than only *un*conscious repressive processes, as was suggested by Freud in his disagreement with Janet. Contemporary discussion of hypnosis and consciousness continues to focus almost solely on unconscious processes (E. R. Hilgard, 1986; Kihlstrom, 1984).

Demonstration of out-of-consciousness or other intrapsychic features of the hypnotic experience does not, of course, obviate other, interpersonal determiners of hypnotic behavior (Orne, 1959, 1962; Sarbin & Coe, 1972; Spanos & Hewitt, 1980); such components have to be encompassed in any description or model or theory of hypnosis. A social or role-playing theory of hypnosis might account for the same therapeutic changes by reference to (1) expectancy for change on the part of patients; (2) motivated voluntary compliance to responding; and (3) in the furtherance of the roles played by patients, rationalizing or confabulating of their accounts of the hypnotic experience so that the reports, as well as the behavior, comply with the hypnotherapist's suggestions. (There is significant evidence of the action of expectancy and compliance, but little to support the hypothesis that subjects tend to confabulate experiential reports in a clinical context.) Since the experience of hypnosis occurs in an interpersonal environment, these nonhypnotic factors operate simultaneously with hypnotic ones. Such factors enrich the experience and add power to the effectiveness of hypnosis as well. A patient's expectation, for example, that a psychotherapist has the skill to enable the patient to experience hypnosis can facilitate the process. The patient's relief and gratitude that the psychotherapist is taking time with the patient, and evincing genuine interest in the patient's experience and emotions, can enable the patient to be more trusting and less vigilant; this also can facilitate the process of hypnosis.

Orne's (1959, 1962) inquiry into the essential, as distinguished from the social-contextual, nature of hypnosis revealed that contextual factors create artifactual features of the hypnotic experience. For instance, recognizing that one is participating in an experiment labeled as "hypnotic" calls up all the beliefs, expectations, and feelings one carries about hypnosis, and these factors may themselves create alterations in one's experience and behavior, independent of the effects of the hypnotic experience itself. Thus, such interpersonal processes—as distinguished from alteration of consciousness or other intrapsychic processes—play a significant role in the essential experience of hypnosis.

The development of the simulator model as a quasi-control for experimental investigation of hypnosis has revealed yet more fully the complex interpersonal nature of the hypnotic experience (Orne, 1979). Evidence that hypnotic responsiveness can be modified—even among very low responders—partly by instructing subjects how to respond hypnotically does make one cautious about interpreting the simulator evidence. Nonetheless, experiments using this model have demonstrated, as have

Sheehan and McConkey's (1982) experiments with the EAT, the complex interaction of contextual and essential features of the hypnotic experience. Both Orne's and Sheehan and McConkey's work further demonstrates how critical phenomenological analysis is to an understanding of hypnosis, and how miniscule are the data available to us about a hypnotic subject's experience if we attend only to an observation of the subject's behavior. The experience of hypnosis is not as simple as once was thought.

The hypnotic experience is often thought of primarily as a cognitive one; as a consequence, attention to the affective dimension is neglected (Diamond, 1987). If we are to understand the ways in which hypnosis can best be used in psychotherapy, we need to attend more fully to the affective dimension of the hypnotic experience. The patient is powerfully affected, largely unconsciously, by the healing experience of contact with a benevolent parental figure. Although this is a significant factor in all psychotherapeutic interaction, it may develop more quickly and its intensity may be greater when the experience of hypnosis is involved. This alteration itself can lead to disorienting or otherwise disturbing perceptual distortions, as well as to powerful affective responses. This alteration demands the psychotherapist's careful management of the changing boundaries between patient and psychotherapist, as required by the nature of the psychotherapy.

Hypnosis in Psychotherapy

Theories focusing on the altered state of consciousness and the altered interpersonal involvement in hypnosis both attempt to account for the way hypnosis allows access to unconscious processes. Cognitive theories focus on the engagement of co-consciousness or compartmentalization; psychodynamic theories focus on access to "primary-process" material, particularly as it is manifested in altered experience of self and one's relation to the world, and use the therapeutic relationship as the vehicle by which such alteration is experienced.

In describing the use of hypnosis in the context of psychotherapy, reference is often made to "hypnotherapy." Such a term can be easily misconstrued. Because hypnosis is a psychological technique or clinical application, rather than a therapy in and of itself, its appropriate and intelligent use requires that hypnosis be integrated into a larger psychotherapeutic context. Hypnotic technique may be integrated with behavior therapy (Clarke & Jackson, 1983), psychodynamic or psychoanalytic therapy (Baker, 1986; Copeland, 1986; Diamond, 1986), group therapy (Greenberg, 1977), family therapy (Araoz & Negly-Parker, 1988; Ritterman, 1983; Sargent, 1986), and gestalt therapy (J. Barber, 1985, 1986). Hypnosis is used in three principal ways: to alter symptoms, to explore or uncover repressed memories, and to affect the therapeutic relationship.

Symptom Alteration

Most patients think of hypnosis primarily as an agent of symptom alteration. This is not unreasonable, although most patients' expectations in this regard may be unrealistically high. Perception and memory can be altered by hypnotic suggestion; so, too, can affect. All are involved, for instance, in reducing the anxiety of a phobic context. Learned associations, like habits, can be disrupted and replaced. It is important to note, however, that symptoms that are chronic and/or characterological in nature have not been shown to be particularly amenable to treatment by hypnosis (e.g., overeating, alcoholism, and other substance abuse; Wadden & Anderton, 1982). Presumably, this is because, although these symptoms may have once involved learned associations, their chronicity has imbedded them into the patient's sense of self, and their primary feature is no longer associational.

Exploration or Uncovering

Another common use for hypnosis is in uncovering repressed memories (Wilson, Greene, & Loftus, 1986). There is much evidence to indicate that repressed memory is amenable to de-repression by hypnotic suggestion. It is also well demonstrated, however, that there is a significant likelihood of memory distortion (Sheehan & Tilden, 1986). Although the veracity of "facts" uncovered by hypnosis is not clear in any particular case, in the context of psychotherapy the personal meaning of such unconscious "memories" is very important, and such uncovering can provide "grist for the mill." Consequently, hypnosis is also valuable for exploring less conscious aspects of experience. In the context of hypnosis, a patient with little insight into an issue may be guided through a series of emotionally meaningful experiences from which insight and understanding may be gained (J. Barber, 1986; Diamond, 1986; Edelstien, 1981). A further use of hypnosis is in discovering innovative or creative solutions to life problems. Sometimes patients are "stuck," and are unable to "think outside the circle" to come to a desirable solution to a problem. By altering ordinary assumptions and expectations, the hypnotic experience can allow a freshened and imaginative sense of problem-solving possibilities.

Affecting the Therapeutic Relationship

Altering the therapeutic relationship is an inevitable result of the hypnotic experience, whether the psychotherapist intends this or not (Baker, 1986; Copeland, 1986; Diamond, 1986; Sheehan & McConkey, 1982). The therapist's awareness of this phenomenon may render such an experience useful rather than problematic, however. Such awareness is essential in obviating potential problems arising from sudden development in the patient of feelings toward the psychotherapist that may range from love to hate. The suddenness and intensity with which these feelings can arise can be disorienting and frightening to the patient. A psychotherapist who is aware of these possibilities and who understands the basis for these feelings can avoid a crisis in the therapeutic relationship, and can help the patient make significant growth in the domain of human relationships. This particular use of hypnosis can be of great value in the treatment of patients with personality disorders—individuals who have significant difficulty in forming relationships with others (Baker, 1986; Copeland, 1986).

Even if the psychotherapist does not intend to use hypnosis in this way, it is imperative that he or she be mindful of the fact that the patient will develop feelings that, without the psychotherapist's help, may be painful and difficult for the patient to understand. The psychotherapist can be helpful in such instances by taking such a phenomenon into account; by accommodating to it, he or she can integrate it into the therapeutic work.

Deciding When and Why to Use Hypnosis

When thinking whether or not (or why) to use hypnotic techniques in the context of psychotherapy, a consideration one might make is whether or not the circumventing of defenses that often accompanies the hypnotic experience is desirable. A traveler coming upon a "Road Closed" sign may feel tempted to take a detour around the sign and continue along the closed road; if the traveler is familiar with the terrain, he or she may thus get home more quickly than by turning around and taking another, longer (perhaps better-marked) route. But in doing so, the traveler also risks ending up in a ditch. Warning signs and psychological defenses are in place for a reason. However, if a therapist is respectful of them, circumventing defenses can sometimes be an efficient way to accelerate the progress of therapy. For example, if a patient evidences repressed memory, hypnotic suggestion may be used to release that memory quickly. The time-saving value of this may be obvious. But, clearly, circumventing defenses can also be a hazardous undertaking. It depends, of course, on the level of personality organization of the patient, as well as on the consequences to the patient of reducing the efficacy of certain defenses. One must have a guideline, in a given case, to determine whether the benefit of releasing repressed memory will outweigh the possible harm. The psychotherapist must know the "terrain" of the patient.

A patient is made vulnerable by the context of psychotherapy. The psychotherapist seeking to wend his or her way through the patient's defensive structure in order to unlock the patient's hypnotic capacities needs to be cautious. Because the patient's ego defenses are reduced in the hypnotic condition, the patient is rendered more vulnerable to ego wound. Consequently, using hypnosis requires even more conscientious vigilance and responsible care on the part of the psychotherapist than is required in the context of nonhypnotic therapy. Hypnotherapy requires significantly heightened interest, empathy, and respect for the patient's experience.

Hypnotic Responsiveness

Assuming one has determined that hypnotic treatment may be beneficial to a patient, one then encounters the question of whether a particular patient will be responsive to hypnotic treatment. This is an issue that is part of an essential and difficult theoretical controversy about hypnosis: the controversy over the relationship between the efficacy of hypnotic treatment and hypnotic responsiveness (also referred to as "hypnotic susceptibility" and "hypnotizability"). One's interpretation of the phenomenon of varying responsiveness to hypnotic treatment is essentially linked, as we shall see, to one's interpretation of the basis for hypnotic mechanisms. If a patient is (or is not) responsive, is this a function of that individual's basic capacity to respond, of the efficacy of particular hypnotic procedures, or of features of the hypnotic relationship? Historically, focus has usually been placed on the concept of an individual's trait of "susceptibility" to hypnotic suggestion. In this discussion, I would like to focus attention on the interplay among the hypnotic relationship, hypnotic procedures, and individual capacities, all of which contribute to an individual's responsiveness to hypnotic treatment.

Clearly, there are demonstrable individual differences in response to hypnotic suggestion, just as there are in any other psychological or physiological response system. What is not clear is the following: How do we predict a particular individual's capacity to respond to hypnotic suggestions? Furthermore, how much hypnotic capacity is necessary for clinical treatment? (How do we account for the widespread achievement of hypnotic analgesia among Esdaile's or Levitan's patients, described above?)

Few clinicians use tests of hypnotic responsiveness (Cohen, 1989), and there are compelling reasons for this (J. Barber, 1989; Diamond, 1989). However, some argue convincingly that clinicians should use tests, such as the Stanford Hypnotic Clinical Scale (SHCS; E. R. Hilgard & Hilgard, 1983) or the Hypnotic Induction Profile (Spiegel, 1974), to screen patients when considering the use of hypnotic treatment (Frankel, 1976, 1989; Spiegel, 1989). But there is significant evidence that patients of even measurably low hypnotic responsiveness can experience change following hypnotic treatment (J. Barber, 1980). This change may be a result of getting through defenses against hypnotic responsiveness (Erickson, 1967). Alternatively, it may reflect nonhypnotic factors, such as the power of the therapeutic relationship (Baker, 1986; Diamond, 1984,

1987; Edelstien, 1981). However, intrapsychic and relational factors are not mutually exclusive. Management of the therapeutic relationship is one means the therapist can employ to move beyond intrapsychic barriers. This perspective holds that most people are capable of experiencing hypnosis, and that "low responders" are, for a variety of psychological reasons, inhibited from accessing and expressing this capacity. Most people are capable of experiencing a satisfactory clinical response to hypnotic treatment, whether they are responding primarily to hypnotic suggestion per se, to other intrapsychic factors (such as imaginative ability), to therapeutic effects of the relationship, or to some combination of all of these. From this perspective, triaging patients on the basis of hypnotic responsiveness scores would deny some the opportunity, however unexpected, for treatment success.

Tests of hypnotic responsiveness tell us how *readily* a patient is able to achieve the hypnotic state, and how readily he or she *may* respond to particular hypnotic suggestions (e.g., the suggestions on the test). But, clinically, what we need to know is whether a patient may have access to unused capacities that may ultimately allow the development of this state. The primary capacity is imaginative involvement (J. R. Hilgard, 1970).

The scale of Imaginative Absorption from Tellegen's Multidimensional Personal Questionnaire (Tellegen & Atkinson, 1974) informs us, among other things, about a patient's familiarity and comfort with imaginal experience. The correlation between scores on the Tellegen scale and Weitzenhoffer and Hilgard's (1959) Stanford Hypnotic Susceptibility scale, Form A (SHSS:A) is modest but reliable. Although a patient's response to the Tellegen scale does not provide the same information we obtain from the SHSS:A, it does offer an impression about his or her hypnotic responsiveness. If an individual responds "true" to certain items on the Tellegen scale that reflect dissociative experience, one can have some confidence that he or she has a significant capacity for dissociation—and thus for hypnotic responsiveness (A. Tellegen, personal communication, 1989).

To the extent that an individual's cognitive world is characterized by the endorsed items on the scale, his or her capacity for absorption to a dissociative degree is high, and predicts the likelihood of his or her responding to hypnotic suggestions. Aside from the value of this prediction, however, the psychotherapist is informed impressionistically about ways the patient experiences his or her imaginal world, and is therefore better informed about how to use suggestion with the patient. Moreover, another advantage of this scale is that its use in psychotherapy does not create a "testing" context in which the patient may fail, and thereby become dispirited or pessimistic about the prospect of responding to hypnotic suggestions (and of obtaining help).

Even if we do not have confidence in a predictable relationship between hypnotic responsiveness and response to clinical hypnotic treatment, it can be clinically useful to have some estimate of a patient's responsiveness—if not to determine our choice of using hypnosis, perhaps to inform us about how best to use hypnosis with a particular individual. For example, an individual of low hypnotic responsiveness will probably have greater difficulty in responding, and may be more limited in what he or she can experience hypnotically. Informed of this, the psychotherapist can be alert to identify possible sources of inhibition of hypnotic responsiveness, and can expect to move at a slower pace and with lower expectations for achieving certain hypnotic phenomena. Tests of hypnotic responsiveness are one means of estimating such responsiveness, of course; however, they carry the disadvantage of offering the clear message to the patient that he or she is either succeeding or failing at being responsive to hypnotic suggestion (which may be demoralizing and countertherapeutic, particularly in the case of a patient who is not responsive). They also may not actually inform us about capacities that have been inhibited from expression, as we shall see.

Experimental Origins of This Perspective

I initially became interested in clinical applications of hypnosis in the context of the treatment of chronic pain. A brief description of my experience may help to clarify the perspective I am going to offer concerning hypnosis.

I was participating in the experimental investigation of neurophysiological mechanisms of analgesia, and it was becoming clear that the response to analgesic agents as disparate as opioid medication and acupuncture was subserved by a common neurophysiological system— what was then called the "central pain inhibitory system" (now understood to be subserved by a class of neurotransmitters called the endorphins). I wondered, though, whether hypnotic analgesia might be mediated by a different neurophysiological mechanism. I reasoned, for instance, that hypnotic analgesia is different from both opioid and acupuncture analgesia in the respect that it can be rapidly initiated and rapidly terminated, and can last for undetermined (even quite lengthy) periods of time.

We experimentally tested the hypothesis that hypnotic analgesia was mediated by the same mechanism as had been identified for both opioid and acupuncture analgesia. This experiment required that I learn how to activate hypnotic analgesia (of which I had had no prior experience). Reviewing the literature, I learned how analgesia is typically suggested. I was made aware of the established belief that hypnotic analgesia is not commonly attainable, and is likely in only a fraction of the population. This was somewhat vexing to me, because, of course, it meant that I would need to test many subjects in order to obtain data from a sufficient number of successfully analgesic subjects.

I wondered, though, whether attention to the refinement of hypnotic technique might make some difference in the rate of success of obtaining analgesia. I thought, for instance, that by applying the approach of empathically entering the subject's phenomenal world, and using techniques such as indirect suggestion, permissiveness, and utilization (derived from Erickson's work), one might increase the probability of successful induction of analgesia. These techniques generally avoid direct hypnotic statements; they seek to accommodate the subject's present experience (whatever it may be), and to lead the subject in a more natural, less intrusive fashion toward the desired hypnotic experience.

This hypothesis was actually a consequence, I now realize, of my own skepticism: I did not believe that one could elicit hypnotic analgesia by simply saying to the subject, in effect, "You will not feel pain." Consequently, over time I developed a very careful and deliberate induction, and included suggestions for analgesia that would be appropriate to the experimental design. I created these suggestions by imagining that I was working with a difficult hypnotic subject—that is, an individual who found development of a hypnotic experience to be an unfamiliar and troublesome encounter. My mindset, as I developed the induction, involved something of the following: "These suggestions are to be given so that a relatively vigilant, distrustful person, uncomfortable with attention to his or her imaginal world, might be more inclined to respond. Moreover, multiple alternative approaches will be used with each subject, in case one approach is not sufficient. Finally, my demeanor will communicate that success in achieving hypnotic responsiveness is to be expected."

Although I had not yet thought of the metaphor of the locksmith, I did feel an optimism that I could somehow intuit the subject's defenses against hypnotic experience, and find a way around or through those defenses. Because the resulting induction (which was called "rapid induction analgesia," or RIA) contained very vague and permissive suggestions, it was possible to use it in a relatively unvarying way; consequently, this induction became the hypnotic treatment that was subsequently used throughout the experiment. Although RIA was relatively unvarying (and therefore "standard" across subjects), it was given in a manner that was intended to sound highly idiosyncratic, spoken meaningfully to each subject as if each word was intended solely to be heard by that subject. Each suggestion was given several times, each time using a different hypnotic approach.

Our results indicated that hypnotic analgesia was not reversed by an opioid antagonist, which suggested that hypnotic analgesia did not depend upon the endogenous opioid system for effect. Equally interesting, however, was the finding that each subject, not just an otherwise predictable fraction of our sample, was able to demonstrate quite dramatic increases in pain threshold following hypnotic suggestion for analgesia (J. Barber & Mayer, 1977).

It is very regrettable that I did not measure hypnotic responsiveness, in order to assess the relationship between responsiveness and analgesia; I had not expected that it would be a relevant issue in this experiment. One can only presume that this sample of medical, dental, and graduate students reflected a range of hypnotic responsiveness, and included individuals of low responsiveness. During the experiment, I was quite surprised with each succeeding subject that we continued to obtain such dramatic changes in sensory pain threshold. I did not know how to understand it, given the expectation that such analgesia would be obtained in only a few subjects. These findings led me to believe that the unexpected results might be attributable to the efficacy of the particular hypnotic technique used in the experiment, since it was different from techniques described in the experimental literature on hypnotic analgesia.

The oral surgeons who offered technical assistance in the experiment were interested in the clinical dental application of this technique. Clinical trials of RIA were made in a dental setting, where, again, hypnotic analgesia was obtained far more frequently than one would have expected (J. Barber, 1977). This finding seemed to provide further support for the hypothesis that hypnotic analgesia could be obtained, independent of hypnotic responsiveness.

Subsequent laboratory findings supported the hypothesis that hypnotic technique, not hypnotic responsiveness, determined the likelihood of hypnotic effect. In these studies, Fricton and Roth (1985) and I (J. Barber, 1976) both examined the relation between hypnotic responsiveness and hypnotic analgesia, using RIA. Alman and Carney (1980) examined the relation between hypnotic responsiveness and posthypnotic behavior, using RIA modified to a nonpain context. Each found no significant relationship when a hypnotic style was used that stressed empathic entry into the subject's phenomenal world via indirect and permissive suggestions. However, a significant body of evidence developed from the laboratories of a number of hypnotic investigators—including the work of E. R. Hilgard and Morgan (1975), E. R. Hilgard and Hilgard (1983), and J. R. Hilgard and LeBaron (1982)—that suggests a reliable relationship between hypnotic responsiveness and the evocation of hypnotic phenomena, including, but not restricted to, analgesia. I was intrigued by, but could not be satisfied by, this apparent new evidence to the contrary.

I was deeply puzzled. I was operating from the premise that the analgesia I observed—analgesia to very high levels of noxious electrical stimulation in the laboratory, and analgesia to ordinarily quite painful procedures in the dental clinic—was attributable to hypnotic suggestion. But let us consider that such is not the case—that analgesia in these circumstances can result from nonhypnotic factors (Frischholz, Spiegel, & Spiegel, 1981; J. R. Hilgard & LeBaron, 1984).

In an effort to investigate this possibility, a colleague and I undertook another experiment, in which a careful distinction was made in the measurement of the pain experience between sensory pain and affective pain,[3]; we found what may be an explanation for the disparity in results of earlier investigations (Price & Barber, 1988). We found, as one would expect, that highly responsive subjects were able to significantly reduce their perception of sensory pain, and that less responsive subjects were not. In relation to the hypothesized relationship between responsiveness and analgesia, however, we unexpectedly found that relatively unresponsive subjects were as able as highly responsive subjects to reduce their experience of affective pain. One might hypothesize that highly responsive subjects engaged hypnotic capacities in order to reduce the sensory pain, and that unresponsive subjects, responding to similar suggestions in the hypnotic situation, were unable to engage hypnotic capacities but were able to reduce their suffering by engaging nonhypnotic capacities (e.g., distraction).[4] This explanation accommodates the data of this investigation and may also help to account for the disparate results of studies referred to above, some of which indicated a relationship between hypnotic analgesia and hypnotic responsiveness, and some of which did not. However, in the case of hypnotic analgesia for acute surgical pain, this explanation is unsatisfying, since no known nonhypnotic capacities (e.g., distraction) are effective in significantly reducing such profound levels of pain.

Any theory of hypnosis that seeks to explain psychological (if not hypnotic) analgesia produced by relatively unresponsive individuals must also accommodate the experience of Esdaile (1846/1957), and Levitan (personal communication, 1989), described earlier, whose successful use of hypnoanesthesia was more widespread than would be predicted, given the assumptions of the normal distribution of hypnotic capacity. We cannot presume that each of their patients was highly responsive. Can we then postulate that there are nonhypnotic processes that could have created such profound analgesia? Perhaps. But Esdaile did not suggest that his patients were merely distracted by the pain, or that they were suffering in compliant silence; rather, he was impressed that they were *not* suffering from the pain of surgery. Videotape recordings of Levitan's patients reveal his patients to be relaxed and comfortable during surgery. Levitan's patients were selected not for experimental reasons, but out of medical considerations: Chemoanesthesia would have constituted a serious risk to their health. Again, we can assume that all of his patients were not highly responsive to hypnosis; therefore, again, we are confronted with the need to include such dramatic analgesic effects among nonresponding individuals in any theory of hypnosis. We do not yet have a satisfying explanation for apparently hypnotic experience and behavior with individuals who are not highly responsive, except, as I have discussed, to suggest that responsiveness can be accessed under certain conditions. The question of the relationship between hypnotic analgesia and hypnotic responsiveness still remains to be fully answered.

Hypnotic responsiveness is only one domain we can attend to when considering the nature of the hypnotic effect. As with any other clinical treatment, we cannot know why someone changes following hypnotic treatment. Change following treatment does not, of course, mean that the treatment caused the change. If we are incautious about interpreting our "successes," we are likely to develop superstitious behavior.

Most psychotherapeutic success does not come about in one treatment or in dramatic fashion, although some psychotherapists seek to understand how it might (Gustafson, 1986). Most psychotherapeutic success evolves from a number of small, incremental (though significant) changes. However, one characteristic of hypnotic treatment, and one advantage of it, is that it often does result in dramatically sudden rather than incremental change. When successful change comes as a surprise, as it does in the case of unresponsive individuals, we are challenged to understand what the causal agent might have been, if not hypnosis.

The Locksmith Model

As investigators attending to hypnotic phenomena, we are faced with this question: Is hypnotic responsiveness a stable trait of the individual, or is it a cluster of capacities that can be accessed, sometimes with great difficulty? If hypnotic capacities can be variably accessed, what are the relevant issues? What features of the hypnotic experience do we need to attend to? The perspective proposed here is that the capacity for imaginative involvement is crucial for development of the hypnotic experience, and that the hypnotic relationship is the means by which we can engage that capacity in patients.

Focusing on subject characteristics, such as hypnotic responsiveness or defensiveness, is essential to our inquiry about hypnosis; still, a narrow focus only on the subject can prevent us from attending to the essentially interactive nature of the phenomenon of hypnosis. Hypnosis is not simply the transmission of suggestions by one person and the reception of these by another. Both Diamond (1984) and Bányai (1985) have demonstrated that the personal qualities of the hypnotist, and the real and transferential relationship that develops between the hypnotist and subject, are critical components of the hypnotic process. Bányai's experimental work demonstrates the two-way interaction quite elegantly: it illustrates that the experience and behavior of the hypnotized subject affect the experience and behavior of the hypnotist/researcher, creating a feedback of interaction.

As clinicians, we certainly are familiar with the experience of rapidly developed affect on the part of the patients with whom we have done hypnotic treatment. However, we might be less clearly conscious about the effect of such treatment on the experience of our own affect—particularly our feelings toward the patients. The same forces that determine how psychotherapist and patient relate in a nonhypnotic context continue to exert themselves, although in a more rapid and intense manner, when hypnosis is involved. The sometimes sudden, "magical" change that can occur in the context of hypnotic treatment may be due at least partly to the experience of this very powerful alliance between psychotherapist and patient.

Although hypnotic responsiveness plays a significant role in determining the likelihood and degree of clinical hypnotic effect, and in the ease with which it may be obtained, it may also be that such responsiveness can be idiosyncratically activated by certain factors in the clinical context. A measurably low hypnotic responsiveness may predict, in a given case, the low probability of obtaining a hypnotic effect. However, if it is important to the patient that he or she experience a significant hypnotic effect, perhaps there are ways (however unlikely) in which this can be accomplished. Such a circumstance more clearly and more often obtains in the emergency or hospital setting, where suffering is acute and profound, and where a patient's deepest adaptive resources can be called upon for action. A seriously burned individual who arrives in the hospital emergency room, suffering the agony of pain and fear, may be more likely to respond to a physician's reassuring suggestions for comfort and well-being than the person would be in other, less dire circumstances. If it is true that there are no atheists in foxholes, where one's ordinary intellectual defenses are irrelevant, perhaps it is also true that there are no unhypnotizable patients in emergency rooms, where acute suffering renders one's ordinary intellectual defenses similarly irrelevant.

This phenomenon is not usually a simple one, however. If a patient's suffering renders him or her panicked and out of control, or if the patient is highly disorganized and defensive, then the physician must be particularly adept to make suggestions effective. In such a circumstance, however, the physician can establish a relationship by communicating an effective concern (i.e., "You are in the hospital; lie still while I take care of you"). Sometimes pharmacological sedation provides the fastest and most effective means of providing comfort to the patient until reorganization of cognitions develops, thus allowing for the creation of a therapeutic relationship.

It the patient is suffering, but total panic has not occurred, then there is an excellent opportunity (if the practitioner knows how to use it) for rapidly developing a relationship, supported by the patient's regressive needs and the clinician's authoritatively helpful (and perhaps life-saving) actions.

Motivation for change and the effect of the psychotherapeutic relationship are two obvious elements that can create change. Perhaps these and other elements present in the hypnotherapeutic setting can liberate or "unlock" a capacity for hypnotic responsiveness that remains otherwise inaccessible and dormant, just as nonhypnotic capacities for response to psychotherapeutic treatment can be unlocked. This is one explanation for the findings of lack of relationship between measured responsiveness and apparent hypnotic effect, described above.

A locksmith is skilled at opening locks. Some locks have very simple, very straightforward mechanisms requiring very simple, very straightforward keys. After assessing what kind of key is needed, the locksmith can fashion such a simple key with ease. Some locks, however, involve more subtle and intricate mechanisms requiring very subtle, very intricate keys. The locksmith can also fashion such a complex key, but with more care and perhaps with more difficulty, and perhaps with failed attempts along the way. By comparison with a mechanical lock, a human's consciousness-altering "mechanisms" are ludicrously complex, involving not only intrapsychic locking mechanisms, but mechanisms of interactive feedback with the locksmith as well. But this comparison does illuminate the similar process of assessing characteristics to determine what kind of key will be successful. If we do not take it too literally, the metaphor of the locksmith can guide our thinking about the assessment of an individual patient's consciousness-altering "mechanisms," and what needs must be met in order to unlock them. It can also inspire us to continue working with the lock even when our first attempts fail.

When relating to a patient whose hypnotic responsiveness is not high, or when confronted with a patient whose hypnotic responsiveness is high but whose hypnotic experience is unsatisfying or inconsequential, we might hypothesize that the patient is defending against the experience of hypnosis for any of a variety of possible reasons. For instance, felt loss of control is a very common motivator for a patient to defend against the hypnotic experience. If a patient experiences only a fragile sense of autonomy, then fear of increased dependence may be another. If a patient realizes, however vaguely, that he or she is holding significant repressed emotion, then fear of liberating (and experiencing) that emotion may be yet another. These hypotheses represent potential approaches—keys, in terms of the metaphor— to meeting the patient's needs, so that he or she may be more readily receptive to the hypnotic experience.

The psychotherapist encountering these situations is confronted with the necessity of judging whether it is beneficial or harmful for the patient to risk the loss of control or autonomy, or risk facing emotional pain. One might argue that in certain cases, employing hypnosis—at least at that point in the therapeutic process—may be inappropriate. Sometimes, in fact, the introduction of the issue of hypnotic treatment can raise such issues more quickly and more clearly, and for that reason alone can accelerate the pace of psychotherapy.

If, for instance, I judge that hypnotic treatment is appropriate, and, furthermore, if I determine that it is both safe and beneficial either to confront or to circumvent the patient's defenses toward the experience of hypnotic treatment, then I imagine myself as a "psychological locksmith," whose goal it is to avoid the patient's defensive maneuvers (and nondefensive inhibitions as well) and to unlock the hypnotic capacities that can activate a change in the patient's experience, which then may lead to therapeutic change.

Although the early experimental literature on modifiability of hypnotic responsiveness reported that the changes in responsiveness were relatively modest (Diamond, 1974, 1977; Sachs, 1971), there is more recent evidence to support a more optimistic attitude toward such modification (Gfeller, Lynn, & Pribble, 1987; Spanos, Brett, Menary, & Cross, 1987; Spanos, Robertson, Menary, & Brett, 1986). These investigations demonstrate that hypnotic responding is closely related to (if not determined by) imaginal abilities, the capacity to relinquish reality-bound thinking, and the capacity for relating to the hypnotist (the same characteristics referred to earlier as essential to the development of a hypnotic experience). Furthermore, these investigations illuminate the complexity of the hypnotic response: They lend experimental support to the view that hypnotic responsiveness is mutable, and, more particularly, that such mutability is dependent upon alterations in an individual's attitudes toward hypnosis and in his or her characteristic ways of relating to the hypnotist.

Adding to the complexity of understanding the relationship between hypnotic responsiveness and clinical outcome, however, is the fact that in a clinical context it is difficult to determine with certainty whether a patient is in fact hypnotized. And perhaps it is the case that when a clinician believes that he or she, through thoughtful circumvention of defenses and other inhibitions, has accessed a "low responder's" hypnotic capacities and has evoked responses from the patient that appear to be hypnotic in character and quality—perhaps these responses are not actually hypnotic in nature, after all, but merely mimic hypnosis. Perhaps the psychotherapist has inadvertently taught the patient, in effect, how to simulate hypnosis. And perhaps the therapeutic change that occurs is not a function of the patient's having been hypnotized at all. Perhaps there is a nonhypnotic effect that can best be produced in "unhypnotizable" patients in the context of trying to produce hypnotic effects. It would be ironic if the best (or the only) way to produce such effects in patients who are unable to experience hypnosis is to behave as if they are able. However, this is the strategy actually employed by many clinicians who use hypnosis.

Imagine for a moment that the seriously burned individual referred to earlier was the subject of a hypnosis experiment the day before the accident, and that the person was found to be generally unresponsive to hypnotic suggestion. What possible circumstances could an experiment create that could generate the degree and kind of comforting and life-sustaining motivation that would be generated by the trauma of the following day? On the one hand, we have to adjust our theories to accommodate experimental findings; on the other, we must recognize that such experimental findings cannot represent the full picture of the subject. Experimental findings can be excellent and necessary guides, but they do not necessarily represent therapeutic limits, because experiments are themselves limited in the degree to which they can replicate meaningful human experience in the laboratory.

The extreme circumstances of the emergency medical setting may represent the most likely ones in which to observe rare and unlikely responsiveness to hypnotic suggestion. Consequently, clinicians who work in other, less dramatic settings are less likely to obtain hypnotic response from hypnotically unresponsive patients. However, if the assumptions above bear any resemblance to reality, then we can expect that clinicians may be more effective in obtaining such responses when they are better able to engage the processes that underlie response in emergency settings. What might those processes be? How can we better engage them in such prosaic settings as the psychotherapist's office?

One feature that can characterize the hypnotic experience is that of a sense of profundity, solemnity, and depth: Nothing in the world matters at that moment except the experience of the patient. This is one of the characteristics of an emergency situation as well. Consequently, when endeavoring to engage a patient in a hypnotic experience, I often try to convey the deeply important, even crucial nature of that moment with the patient, and to join with the patient in the experience. While I am trying to understand the patient's internal world at that moment, to empathize with the patient's experience at that moment, I can simultaneously communicate my attention to the importance of that moment to the patient.

Although one's experiences as a clinician need to be very carefully evaluated to identify possibly confounding elements, such experiences are nonetheless valid bases for reasoning. Diamond (1987) relates clinical anecdotes, familiar to many psychotherapists using hypnosis, about "low responders" who ultimately achieve hypnotic effects following certain meaningful experiences in relation to the psychotherapist. Such clinical experience inspires the optimism of the would-be locksmith. One cannot logically argue that such an effect is not actually "hypnotic" simply because the patient was previously unresponsive to hypnotic suggestion, especially if such clinical experiences bear the characteristics of hypnosis. It may be difficult, in any single case, to determine whether an effect is hypnotic in nature or is a function of contextual factors. Such difficulty does not, however, mean that the effect is not hypnotic. We may not be able to determine in any given case whether the effect is hypnotic.

I do not want to overemphasize the importance or relevance of any particular attitude toward or communication to a patient in this context. The profundity of the experience need not necessarily be conveyed by an air of solemnity. With children, for instance (and even occasionally with adults), humor may be a salient feature of the interaction, with the profundity of the circumstance conveyed by the *intensity* of the therapist's involvement. There may be a variety of attitudes that will help a patient to be responsive. The operating principles, I believe, for engaging the patient and accessing the potential for therapeutic response are an empathic communication of hopefulness and a nearly limitless quantity of patience.

The following clinical vignette may illustrate this discussion: An 81-year-old man, a very active and extremely successful businessman with more liveliness and energy than many men half his age, sought psychotherapy to help him become, in his own words, less "psychologically blocked." He had undergone 6 years of psychoanalysis on two different occasions, many years earlier, and reported that he had not learned anything about himself. "I totally failed in my analysis," he said, and added, in his typically wry way, "but I think my analyst learned a lot." What he wanted from psychotherapy, he said, was to be able to recall the events and emotions of his childhood, because at the death of his wife 3 years previously, he had become aware of the degree to which he was emotionally repressed, and of the degree to which he was unable to recall his childhood with any clarity or emotional vividness. He felt he was missing a lot from his life. He believed that hypnotic treatment would be helpful in accomplishing this task.

Why would an 81-year-old man seek psychotherapy for the purpose of recalling his childhood? I believed that he had more compelling reasons for doing so than he was expressing, probably more than he consciously knew. Because of his frequent references to his wife's death; because he often made reference to how youthful he felt and how difficult it was to believe he was 81; and because he expressed interest in various projects that, realistically, were to be several years in the making, I inferred that one of his motivations for seeking therapy was a fear of his own death. I assumed his wife's death had brought home to him that he, too, was mortal, and vividly confronted him with his loneliness. (Throughout his life, he had never had close friends. His wife had been his best, perhaps his only friend.) I believed he wanted to recall his childhood partly in order to reconstitute for himself the experience of being a child again, thereby obtaining the distance from death that this would bring, as well as the possibility of being nurtured and taken care of in the way a child can be. Consequently, I believed that a benign emotional connection with me would be salutary to him, and would make the prospect of an effective hypnotic experience more probable. Although I thought that hypnosis might in fact serve to facilitate recall of his childhood, I believed that this actually was of secondary importance. However, I also thought that a hypnotic experience might facilitate the development of a good emotional connection with me. My goal, therefore, was to use the experience of hypnosis to that end, and to integrate hypnotic techniques with nonhypnotic psychotherapeutic techniques of high contact, mirroring, and alliance—all to the purpose of facilitating the development of our relationship.

Although I do not ordinarily administer a test of hypnotic responsiveness, I thought that the "scientific" connotation of the test would be helpful in establishing a sound basis in the client's mind for our work, and that his responses to the test would provide a relatively neutral arena for the beginning of our interaction. He obtained a score of 1 on the SHCS, responding positively only to the first item, which involved the suggestion that his outstretched hands would automatically move together. His very competitive and achievement-oriented (and highly self-critical) nature was demonstrated by his great disappointment in his performance. He responded more fully to dissociative items on the Tellegen scale of Imaginative Absorption, which led me to believe that he had a good capacity for imaginative absorption, but was defending himself against the access to that capacity in the context of hypnosis. (A retest on the SCHS 1 week later yielded the same response, to the first item only.)

As a tentative first step toward acknowledging characteristics about him that he had not described to me (particularly his defensiveness), I conjectured aloud to him that he had ample capacity to experience hypnosis, but that he was cautiously protecting himself from harmful or painful emotional experiences, and that such protection precluded full response to hypnotic suggestion. He did not experience any guarding, he said, but he would trust my judgment on that. "After all," he said, "you must know your business!" (I took this to be an admonition that I *must know* my business. I also took this to be confirmation of my hypothesis that he wanted to be taken care of to a greater extent than he was able to consciously acknowledge.)

This man was unusually bright, articulate, witty, uncommonly charming, vigilant, and guarded. He did not acknowledge feeling sad or troubled in any way, other than by expressing his wish to have better recall of his childhood. He alternated between attempts at emotional contact and efforts to maintain emotional distance with me. I enjoyed being with him, and at the same time found myself slightly guarded against his sometimes barbed witticisms. At the end of the first meeting, I asked him what the experience of talking with me about very personal issues was like. "Are you fishing for compliments?" he said, smiling, yet communicating, I thought, a critical or contemptuous response to my question. In addition to his vigilance, he was suspicious. Consequently, my intention with him at the outset of treatment (and continuing on) was to be as personally present as I could be, in order to obviate any phoniness he would be likely to sense if I were not genuine in my contact with him. I felt affection for him and compassion for his fear of emotional vulnerability, and so my demeanor with him reflected these feelings. I gently communicated to him my admiration for his courage at facing his problems and for his willingness to experience hypnosis, thereby risking a loss of control of his usual way of being. He sometimes was able to tolerate and even enjoy my contact with him, but he sometimes suddenly reverted to critical comments, such as "Well, what are we doing here, anyway? I still don't have any childhood memories!"

At the second, third, and fourth treatment appointments, we alternated between hypnotic induction attempts and more dynamically oriented nonhypnotic therapy for the purpose of enhancing our contact and increasing his awareness of affect. He met the hypnotic induction attempts with interest; however, either he fell asleep in response to the suggestions for comfort and relaxation, or he interrupted my suggestions with declarations that nothing was happening. I responded to each of his declarations with interest and regard for his experience, and curiosity about the "nothingness." Each time he was able (though minimally) to become interested in his own experience, and to evince some optimism about continuing. One might argue that four occasions of minimal hypnotic responsiveness should have been ample evidence (particularly in light of the low responsiveness score) that this patient was not a good candidate for hypnotic treatment. However, because of his responses to the Tellegen scale, and because he impressed me as a highly imaginative man, able to become engaged in his fantasies (he was a marvelously compelling story teller), I was confident that he was capable of experiencing hypnosis, but that he was strongly defended against the experience. I thought that this lack of hypnotic responsiveness was just one diagnostic indicator of this patient's fearful, untrusting, vigilant, and repressed attitudes toward his own emotional experience, as well as toward his emotional contact with others. I was optimistic that he would begin responding hypnotically when he felt safe enough to do so. I felt confident that I could "pick the lock" under which both his hypnotic responsiveness and his emotional responsiveness were kept.

Because I judged that the experience of hypnosis would enable him to be less defensive and more able to engage his imaginal world, thereby facilitating access to memories and fantasies, and because I believed that he now had enough experience with me to tentatively trust my benevolence, I determined to continue my efforts. However, I decided to try a different approach to hypnotic induction.

Toward the end of the fourth treatment appointment, following yet another disappointing induction attempt, I suggested to him that he was now ready to experience hypnosis, but of a different kind than he had previously prepared himself for. (This suggested, I hoped, that he was unprepared to defend against this kind.) I then told him very earnestly that arm levitation was an experience he was now ready for, and that when this occurred he was to try his very best to ignore it, and to attend instead to the uncommonly heavy and steadfast feelings of his left hand. (This was intended to convey a sense of the inevitability and the automaticity of the levitation experience, as well as a sense that his own "steadfastness" was continuing. It was also intended to provide him with a kind of internal conflict of attention that would not be counterproductive.) I then gave suggestions for right-arm levitation, and he quickly responded. I maintaining all the while an attitude of controlled fascination and of benevolent, hopeful curiosity about his experience. I suggested that he not close his eyes (as he had become accustomed to doing during induction), but continue staring at his heavy left hand, in order to detect whether anything at all was happening to that arm. I continued, interspersing confusing suggestions that generally and vaguely led to the idea that he was able to experience a very light (and therefore safe) state of hypnosis—one that would not permit a very great emotional response, "just a mild one." I also suggested that when he felt the emotions rising to the surface, he could feel free either to block them or to allow them to flow, so long as he felt safe; I further suggested that his natural curiosity would lead him to wish he could continue the experience.

He was very pleased and excited when discussing this experience later. He asked me how he could practice this on his own at home, and I gave him suggestions for developing arm levitation on his own. As might be expected of him, when he returned for the next appointment he expressed disappointment that, when attempting arm levitation on his own, he was only able to achieve levitation of about 2 inches in elevation— thereby indicating, in his mind, complete lack of success. I told him that this response seemed cruelly characteristic of his customary self-defeating style, and, also told him how genuinely remarkable his "mere 2 inches" of levitation was (by comparison with his ordinary experience of not levitating at all).

In subsequent treatment appointments, I continued to offer and to maintain as much emotional contact as he could tolerate, and sometimes used hypnotic suggestions to reduce his discomfort with this contact. He eventually became more and more at ease with me (although greater ease one day might be met with less ease the next). He began to recall his nightly dreams, which he had not done for many years; he also began to respond more and more fully to hypnotic inductions, and was able to experience vivid fantasies of early childhood experiences that contained significant affective charge. He began to have fantasies of, or to remember, significant experiences of sadness, loneliness and deprivation in his childhood. During hypnotic treatments, he became able to experience arm levitation, arm catalepsy, and response to posthypnotic suggestions, including suggestions for specific amnesias. In general, he became more emotionally open and made greater contact with me, and reported that he was able to be intermittently more emotionally available to his family. He reported much satisfaction with this "unexpected" result.

After 32 treatment appointments, he was able to weep openly in my presence, and also experienced uncontrollable weeping with his son as he disclosed meaningful material about his life. He was also able to express deeply felt guilt over the death of his wife. He felt that his emotional inaccessibility to his wife had contributed to a lack of emotional connection throughout their long marriage, and had ultimately led to her death. It was partly this guilt that had provoked the fear of his own death (as if death might be a punishment to him for his lapses toward his wife). And he was able to discuss his fear of dying. He did so, initially with great hesitancy and trepidation, then with more openness. He was very pleased and satisfied by his "new" self, and was able to experience, in his words, "more joy in life."

The experience of this patient illustrates some of the complexity of the psychotherapeutic experience and, even more so, of the hypnotherapeutic experience. Initial objective assessment suggested that this patient would not be a likely candidate for hypnotic treatment. Indeed, this patient's responses to hypnotic suggestion were not adequate for hypnotic treatment. However, with other psychotherapeutic experience that led the patient to a more secure foundation for relating to me, and perhaps in response to my own stubborn hopefulness, he was eventually able to access his hypnotic capacities and respond in a fully adequate fashion.

Close examination of this case reveals no magical cure. What is noteworthy, however, is the patient's unexpected (on the basis of responsiveness assessment) successful development of a clinically useful hypnotic experience. "Magic" is invoked when a clinician "happens" to find the right key (especially if this occurs on a first treatment attempt). From the perspective of the locksmith, lack of treatment success means that one has not yet found (or fashioned) the right key—not that there is no lock and no key. Some patient's locks are so incredibly intricate, so rusty and stiff from disuse, and sometimes so ingeniously booby-trapped that it may not be prudent to attempt to find the right key. Unlike a competent locksmith, a competent psychotherapist cannot expect to open every lock. On the other hand, it may be tempting to relent too soon in one's efforts. A clinician may perform a procedure (e.g., a hypnotic induction), find a lack of response from the patient, and feel frustrated. Defending against the frustration, he or she may then conclude that the patient does not have the capacity to respond, and may move on to other treatments (or other patients). Making peace with one's lack of effect, and trying again (and perhaps again and again), may be vitally important—not only because a renewed attempt may be more appropriate for that patient, but because such persistence communicates to the patient that the clinician is optimistic, confident, committed to helping, and not yet discouraged. (Perhaps one reason for the unexpected effectiveness of RIA was that, in each subject or patient, several different forms of each suggestion were given. Furthermore, several attempts were made in the event that the first did not succeed, with the implication that yielding to failure was not expected.)

RESEARCH AND APPRAISAL

As noted earlier, both Diamond (1984) and Bányai (1985) have demonstrated that the personal qualities of the hypnotist, and the real and transferential relationship that develops between the hypnotist and subject, are critical components of the hypnotic process. Banyai's experimental work demonstrates the two-way interaction quite specifically, illustrating that the experience and behavior of the hypnotized subject affect the experience and behavior of the hypnotist/researcher, thus creating a feedback of interaction.

Other recent experimental investigations of the phenomenology of hypnosis (Pekala & Kumar, 1984, 1987; Pekala & Nagler, 1989) allow us to objectively describe features of the hypnotic experience. These observations lend support to a theory advanced by Shor (1962), which posits that the hypnotic experience is characterized by an altered state of consciousness; a reduction of the generalized reality orientation; and an alteration in the transferential relationship, called "archaic involvement."

The earlier discussion concerning the relationship between hypnotic responsiveness and response to clinical hypnotic treatment has cited research that lends support, either directly or indirectly, to the locksmith model (Alman & Carney, 1980; J. Barber, 1976, 1977, 1980; J. Barber & Mayer, 1977; Diamond, 1974, 1977; Esdaile, 1846/1957; Fricton & Roth, 1985; A. A. Levitan, personal communication, 1989; Price & Barber, 1988). Likewise, I have discussed some of the evidence supporting the alternative thesis—namely, that hypnotic responsiveness is a relatively stable, unvarying trait, and is the best predictor of the efficacy of hypnotic treatment (Frankel, 1976; Frischholz et al., 1981; Gottfredson, 1973; E.

R. Hilgard & Hilgard, 1983; E. R. Hilgard & Morgan, 1975; J. R. Hilgard & LeBaron, 1982).

The evidence that is of most crucial importance, and that to date is lacking, is evidence that speaks specifically to the issue of hypnotic responsiveness and the efficacy of hypnotic treatment in psychotherapy. The trend toward phenomenological analysis of hypnotic processes makes more likely the possibility of scientific inquiry into the two-way interaction of the hypnotherapist and patient. Bányai's work, and the investigations of Sheehan and McConkey, have generated the most significant experimental evidence of the importance of that interaction. The work of Baker and Diamond has yielded the most significant clinical evidence. The research to date clearly supports the hypothesis that natural variations in the ways people experience hypnosis require a locksmith approach to engaging hypnotic capacities. When we understand more about how to engage those capacities predictably and systematically, we will be able to grasp more fully the nature of the magic of therapeutic change.

CONCLUSION

There is reason to believe that hypnotic responsiveness is not a fixed and stable trait. But how best to use hypnosis with an individual has to be discovered: It is necessary to understand the complex and idiosyncratic determinants of hypnotic responsiveness for that individual. This chapter has described a model for thinking about how hypnotic responsiveness can be "unlocked," how the "right" circumstances for accessing a person's potential can be created. Creating safe and supportive circumstances allows an individual to overcome habitual cognitive styles and/or defenses, and thus promotes the development of the special condition of hypnosis.

Acknowledgments. I am grateful to Cheri Adrian, PhD, once again, for the special intelligence and generosity she brought to our discussion of the ideas contained in this chapter. I am also grateful to Sam LeBaron, MD, PhD, for his very helpful comments on the chapter.

NOTES

1. "Co-consciousness" refers to a process of "lateral" dissociation or segmentation of memory or affect into "secondary," parallel consciousness (as opposed to a "verticle" segmentation into the unconscious)—for instance, the processes underlying the "hidden-observer" phenomenon, described below.

2. We (J. Barber & Price, 1991) found a relationship between decreasing awareness of external reality and increasing absorption in the hypnotic experience (and increase in perceived hypnotic depth).

3. "Sensory pain" is the component of the pain experience that provides the individual with information such as the body location of the pain; the intensity of the pain; whether the pain is constant or intermittent, lacinating or dull, hot or cold; and so on. "Affective pain" (also called "suffering") is the component of the pain experience that provides the individual with information concerning the degree of unpleasantness of the pain. All pain experience is constituted of both elements.

4. V. Gheorghiu (personal communication, 1986) suggests that response to waking suggestion, rather than hypnotic suggestion, is an important factor to remember when trying to understand such phenomena.

REFERENCES

Alman, B. M., & Carney, R. (1980). Consequences of direct and indirect suggestions on success of posthypnotic behavior. *American Journal of Clinical Hypnosis, 23*, 112–118.

Araoz, D. L., & Negly-Parker, E. (1988). *The new hypnosis in family therapy*. New York: Brunner/Mazel.

Baker, E. L. (1986). Applications of clinical hypnosis with psychotic patients. In E. Dowd & J. Healy (Eds.), *Case studies in hypnotherapy* (pp. 222–234). New York: Guilford Press.

Bányai, E. I. (1985). *On the interactive nature of hypnosis: A social psychophysiological approach*. Paper presented at the 10th International Congress of Hypnosis and Psychosomatic Medicine, Toronto.

Barber, J. (1976). *The efficacy of hypnotic analgesia for dental pain in Individuals of both high and low hypnotic susceptibility*. Unpublished doctoral dissertation, University of Southern California.

Barber, J. (1977). Rapid induction analgesia: A clinical report. *American Journal of Clinical Hypnosis, 19*, 138–147.

Barber, J. (1980). Hypnosis and the unhypnotizable. *American Journal of Clinical Hypnosis, 23*, 4–9.

Barber, J. (1985). Hypnosis and awareness: Integrating hypnosis and Gestalt therapy. In Zeig, (Ed.), *Ericksonian Psychotherapy, Vol. 1*. New York: Brunner/ Mazel.

Barber, J. (1986). The case of Superman: Integrating hypnosis and gestalt therapy in the treatment of dyssomnia. In E. Dowd & J. Healy (Eds.), *Case studies in hypnotherapy* (pp. 46–60). New York: Guilford Press.

Barber, J. (1989). Predicting the efficacy of hypnotic treatment. *American Journal of Clinical Hypnosis, 32*, 10–11.

Barber, J., & Gitelson, J. (1980). Cancer pain: Psychological management using hypnosis. *Cancer, 30*, 130–136.

Barber, J., & Mayer, D. (1977). Evaluation of the efficacy and neural mechanism of a hypnotic analgesia procedure in experimental and clinical dental pain. *Pain, 4*, 41– 48.

Barber, T. X. (1978). "Hypnosis," suggestions, and psychosomatic phenomena: A new look from the standpoint of recent experimental studies. *American Journal of Clinical Hypnosis, 21*, 13–27.

Benson, V. B. (1971). One hundred cases of post-anesthetic suggestion in the recovery room. *American Journal of Clinical Hypnosis, 14*, 9–15.

Bowers, K. S., & Kelly, P. (1979). Stress, disease, psychotherapy, and hypnosis. *Journal of Abnormal Psychology, 88*, 490–505.

Clarke, J. C., & Jackson, J. A. (1983). *Hypnosis and behavior therapy: The treatment of anxiety and phobias.* New York: Springer.

Cohen, S. B. (1989). Clinical uses of measures of hypnotizability. *American Journal of Clinical Hypnosis, 32*, 4–9.

Copeland, D. R. (1986). The application of object relations theory to the hypnotherapy of developmental arrests: The borderline patient. *International Journal of Clinical and Experimental Hypnosis, 34*, 157–168.

Crasilneck, H. B. & Hall, J. A. (1985). *Clinical hypnosis: Principles and applications* (2nd ed.). New York: Grune & Stratton.

Diamond, M. J. (1974). Modification of hypnotizability: A review. *Psychological Bulletin, 81*, 180–198.

Diamond, M. J. (1977). Hypnotizability is modifiable: An alternative approach. *International Journal of Clinical and Experimental Hypnosis, 25*, 147–166.

Diamond, M. J. (1984). It takes two to tango: The neglected importance of the hypnotic relationship. *American Journal of Clinical Hypnosis, 26*, 1–13.

Diamond, M. J. (1986). When the knight regains his armor: An indirect, psychodynamically based brief hypnotherapy of an ego-dystonic sexual impulse disorder. In E. Dowd & J. Healy (Eds.), *Case studies in hypnotherapy* (pp. 71–82). New York: Guilford Press.

Diamond, M. J. (1987). The interactional basis of hypnotic experience: On the relational dimensions of hypnosis. *International Journal of Clinical and Experimental Hypnosis, 35*, 95–115.

Diamond, M. J. (1989). Is hypnotherapy art or science? *American Journal of Clinical Hypnosis, 32*, 11–12.

Di Piano, F. A., & Salzberg, H. C. (1979). Clinical applications of hypnosis to three psychosomatic disorders. *Psychological Bulletin, 86*, 1223–1235.

Edelstien, M. G. (1981). *Trauma, trance, and transformation.* New York: Brunner/Mazel.

Erickson, M. H. (1964). Initial experiments investigating the nature of hypnosis. *American Journal of Clinical Hypnosis, 7*, 152–162.

Erickson, M. H. (1967). Deep hypnosis and its induction. In J. Haley (Ed.), *Advanced techniques of hypnosis and psychotherapy: Selected papers of Milton H. Erickson, M.D.* (pp. 7–31). New York: Grune & Stratton.

Esdaile, J. (1957). *Hypnosis in medicine and surgery* (Introduction and supplementary reports by W. S. Kroger). New York: Julian Press. (Original work published 1846)

Ewin, D. M. (1978). Clinical use of hypnosis for attenuation of burn depth. In F. H.

Frankel & H. S. Zamansky (Eds.), *Hypnosis at its bicentennial* (pp. 155–162). New York: Plenum Press.

Ewin, D. M. (1980). Hypnosis in burn therapy. In G. D. Burrows & L. Dennerstein (Eds.), *Handbook of hypnosis and psychosomatic medicine* (pp. 269–276). Amsterdam: Elsevier/North-Holland.

Frankel, F. H. (1976). *Hypnosis: Trance as a coping mechanism.* New York: Plenum Press.

Frankel, F. H. (1989). Hypnosis is a multi-dimensional event. *American Journal of Clinical Hypnosis, 32,* 13–14.

Fricton, J. R., & Roth, P. (1985). The effects of direct and indirect hypnotic suggestions for analgesia in high and low susceptible subjects. *American Journal of Clinical Hypnosis, 27,* 226–231.

Frischholz, E. J., Spiegel, H., & Spiegel, D. (1981). Hypnosis and the unhypnotizable: A reply to Barber. *American Journal of Clinical Hypnosis, 24,* 55–58.

Gfeller, J. D., Lynn S. J., & Pribble, W. E. (1987). Enhancing hypnotic susceptibility: Interpersonal and rapport factors. *Journal of Personality and Social Psychology, 52,* 586–595.

Goldsmith, S. (1986). *Psychotherapy of physical symptoms.* New York: University Press of America.

Gottfredson, D. (1973). Hypnosis as an anesthetic in dentistry (Doctoral dissertation, Brigham Young University). *Dissertation Abstracts International, 33,*(7), 3303B.

Greenberg, I. A. (Ed.). (1977). *Group hypnotherapy and hypnodrama.* Chicago: Nelson-Hall.

Gustafson, J. P. (1986). *The complex secret of brief psychotherapy.* New York: Norton.

Hilgard, E. R. (1986). *Divided consciousness: Multiple controls in human thought and action* (expanded ed.). New York: Wiley.

Hilgard, E. R., & Hilgard, J. R. (1983). *Hypnosis in the relief of pain* (rev. ed.). Los Altos, CA: William Kaufmann.

Hilgard, E. R., & Morgan, A. H. (1975). Heart rate and blood pressure in the study of laboratory pain in man under normal conditions and as influenced by hypnosis. *Acta Neurologiae Experimentalis, 35,* 741–759.

Hilgard, J. R. (1970). *Personality and hypnosis: A study of imaginative involvement.* Chicago: University of Chicago Press.

Hilgard, J. R., & LeBaron, S. (1982). Relief of anxiety and pain in children and adolescents with cancer: Quantitative measures and clinical observations. *International Journal of Clinical & Experimental Hypnosis, 30,* 417–442.

Hilgard, J. R., & LeBaron, S. (1984). *Hypnotherapy of pain in children with cancer.* Los Altos, CA: William Kaufmann.

Janet, P. (1907). *The major symptoms of hysteria.* New York: Macmillan.

Kihlstrom, J. F. (1984). Conscious, subconscious, unconscious: A cognitive perspective. In K. S. Bowers, and D. Meichenbaum (Eds.), *The unconscious reconsidered* (pp. 149–211). New York: Wiley.

Mott, T. (1982). The role of hypnosis in psychotherapy. *American Journal of Clinical Hypnosis, 11,* 263–269.

Orne, M. T. (1959). The nature of hypnosis: Artifact and essence. *Journal of Abnormal and Social Psychology, 58,* 277–299.

Orne, M. T. (1962). On the social psychology of the psychological experiment: With particular reference to demand characteristics and their implications. *American Psychologist, 17*, 776–783.

Orne, M. T. (1979). On the simulating subject as a quasicontrol group in hypnosis research: What, why, and how. In E. Fromm & R. E. Shor (Eds.), *Hypnosis: Developments in research and new perspectives* (2nd ed., pp. 519–565). Chicago: Aldine.

Pekala, R. J., & Kumar, V. K. (1984). Predicting hypnotic susceptibility by a self-report phenomenological state instrument. *American Journal of Clinical Hypnosis, 27*, 114–121.

Pekala, R. J., & Kumar, V. K. (1987). Predicting hypnotic susceptibility via a self-report instrument: A replication. *American Journal of Clinical Hypnosis, 30*, 57–65.

Pekala, R. J., & Nagler, R. (1989). The assessment of hypnoidal states: Rationale and clinical application. *American Journal of Clinical Hypnosis, 31*, 231–236.

Perry, C., Gelfand, R., & Marcovitch, P. (1979). The relevance of hypnotic susceptibility in the clinical context. *Journal of Abnormal Psychology, 88*, 592–603.

Price, D. D., & Barber, J. (1988). A quantitative analysis of the efficacy of hypnotic analgesia. *Journal of Abnormal Psychology, 96*, 46–51.

Ritterman, M. (1983). *Using hypnosis in family therapy.* San Francisco: Jossey-Bass.

Sachs, L. B. (1971). Construing hypnosis as modifiable behavior. In A. B. Jacobs & L. B. Sachs (Eds.), *Psychology of private events* (pp. 65–71). New York: Academic Press.

Sarbin, T. R., & Coe, W. C. (1972). *Hypnosis: A social psychological analysis of influence communication.* New York: Holt, Rinehart & Winston.

Sargent, G. A. (1986). Family systems and family hypnotherapy. In E. Dowd & J. Healy (Eds.), *Case studies in hypnotherapy* (pp. 83–98). New York: Guilford Press.

Sheehan, P. W., & McConkey, K. M. (1982). *Hypnosis and experience: The exploration of phenomena and process.* Hillsdale, NJ: Erlbaum.

Sheehan, P. W., & Tilden, J. (1986). The consistency of occurrences of memory distortion following hypnotic induction. *International Journal of Clinical and Experimental Hypnosis, 34*, 122–137.

Shor, R. E. (1959). Hypnosis and the concept of the generalized reality-orientation. *American Journal of Psychotherapy, 13*, 582–602.

Shor, R. E. (1962). Three dimensions of hypnotic depth. *International Journal of Clinical and Experimental Hypnosis, 10*, 23–28.

Shor, R. E. (1979). A phenomenological method for the measurement of variables important to an understanding of the nature of hypnosis. In E. Fromm & R. E. Shor (Eds.), *Hypnosis: Developments in research and new perspectives* (2nd ed., pp. 105–135). Chicago: Aldine.

Spanos, N. P., Brett, P. J., Menary, E. P., & Cross, W. P. (1987). A measure of attitudes toward hypnosis: Relationships with absorption and hypnotic susceptibility. *American Journal of Clinical Hypnosis, 30*, 139–150.

Spanos, N. P., & Hewitt, E. C. (1980). The hidden observer in hypnotic analgesia: Discovery or experimental creation? *Journal of Personality and Social Psychology, 3*, 1201–1214.

Spanos, N. P., Robertson, L., Menary, E. P., & Brett, P. J. (1986). Component analysis of a cognitive skill training package for the enhancement of hypnotic suggestibility. *Journal of Abnormal Psychology, 95*, 350–357.

Spiegel, H. (1974). *Manual for Hypnotic Induction Profile.* New York: Soni Medica.

Spiegel, H. (1989). Should therapists test for hypnotizability? *American Journal of Clinical Hypnosis, 32*, 15–16.

Tellegen, A., & Atkinson, G. (1974). Openness to absorbing and self-altering experiences ("absorption"), a trait related to hypnotic susceptibility. *Journal of Abnormal Psychology, 83*, 268–277.

Wadden, T. A., & Anderton, C. H. (1982). The clinical use of hypnosis. *Psychological Bulletin, 91*, 215–243.

Watkins, J. G. (1971). The affect bridge: A hypnoanalytic technique. *International Journal of Clinical and Experimental Hypnosis, 19*, 21–27.

Weitzenhoffer, A. M., & Hilgard, E. R. (1959). *Stanford Hypnotic Susceptibility Scale, Forms A and B.* Palo Alto, CA: Consulting Psychologists Press.

Wilson, L., Greene, E., & Loftus, E. F. (1986). Beliefs about forensic hypnosis. *International Journal of Clinical and Experimental Hypnosis, 34*, 110–121.

Zeltzer, L., & LeBaron, S. (1982). Hypnosis and nonhypnotic techniques for reduction of pain and anxiety during painful procedures in children and adolescents with cancer. *Journal of Pediatrics, 101*, 1032–1035.

CHAPTER 9

Ericksonian Hypnotherapy: A Communications Approach to Hypnosis

JEFFREY K. ZEIG and PETER J. RENNICK
Milton H. Erickson Foundation

INTRODUCTION

Jay Haley (1963) maintained that any theory of human behavior must take hypnosis into account. Hypnosis *is* a fascinating phenomenon that underscores the profound effects possible in interpersonal communication. It is astonishing that one person can elicit in another such effects as hallucination, automatic movements, and disorientation in time. Many traditional theories have tried to explain these effects in terms of the internal state of the hypnotic subject, and, in doing so, to distinguish hypnosis from other "states."

In contradistinction to such traditional approaches, it is the thesis of this chapter that Milton Erickson was the father of an interpersonal communications approach to hypnosis and psychotherapy. He was a pioneer who explored the parameters of how communication, especially indirect communication, could elicit and maximize previously dormant potentials (Zeig, 1987) and foster therapeutic results. Toward that end he originated and developed a hypnotherapy whose essential feature is not formal trance, which may or may not be employed, but rather an interpersonally focused communication system unique to the individuals involved, and aimed primarily (this is the "hypnotic" element) at tapping unconscious capabilities and responsiveness.

An initial brief examination of the historical context and theoretical environment—against which Milton Erickson's hypnosis and hypnotherapy can be seen—provides a useful introduction to the principles elaborated in greater detail in the central part of this chapter. Consequently, we first examine some differences in the way psychotherapy and hypnosis have evolved; consider the major efforts to define hypnosis; and then offer an alternate view of hypnosis based on an interactional perspective.

Evolution of Psychotherapy and Hypnosis

Psychotherapy evolved as a discipline concerned with the inner workings of individuals. Understanding the "whys and wherefores" of the individual psyche was the preoccupation of psychotherapy for its first 70 years. Subsequently, in the 1960s, a revolution occurred in which there was a shift from a focus on what happened inside the individual to a focus on the system in which the individual operated and played a part. Relationships—what happened *between* people rather than inside them— increasingly took a primary position in the minds of clinicians (Zeig, 1987).

Hypnosis had a similar beginning. Practice, theory, and research have historically centered on elucidating the nature of hypnosis as it existed within individuals. Most investigations in the 20th century have tried to determine the nature of hypnosis as a phenomenon (a "thing") within the hypnotized subject. Unfortunately, hypnosis has not evolved in parallel with the field of psychotherapy; for the most part, a systemic orientation to hypnosis has been lacking. (For an exception, see Haley, 1963.) Research and theorizing about hypnosis are still largely "stuck" in the view of hypnosis as a phenomenon within an individual, rather than a process between people.

It is interesting to note historically that hypnosis often has occupied an important position at the beginning of a theorist's career. For example, Freud initially made much use of hypnosis, but rejected it as unreliable in order to pursue his burgeoning psychoanalytic methods. Other experts such as Joseph Wolpe, Fritz Perls, and Eric Berne were familiar with hypnosis, but diverged from its use in order to develop their theories of human behavior and intervention (Zeig, 1985). Hypnosis served as an important building block in all of these major psychological theories. But now, by limiting investigation into the systemic dynamics of hypnosis, the field of hypnosis may be limiting itself.

Before moving on to further examination of hypnosis as an interactional process, we first explore the question of how hypnosis has been defined.

What Is Hypnosis?

Zeig (1988, pp. 354–357) has explored the problem of defining hypnosis and summarized definitions proposed by major theorists. We borrow liberally here from that passage.

When defining a process such as hypnosis, one can be either objective or subjective. Moreover, a process such as hypnosis can be defined according to its appearance, its function, its etiology, its history, or its process; in terms of its relationship to other phenomena; or as something that happens among individuals. Psychological phenomena, such as hypnosis, are usually defined from the perspective of a pre-existent theory. Traditionally, this has been a theory of individual psychology, such as behaviorism or psychoanalysis. Circularly, the established definition of the phenomenon is then perpetuated by the theory.

Definitions are neither benign nor "neutral"; on the contrary, they influence, and usually focus and limit, subsequent thinking. For example, a therapist's definition of hypnosis will influence treatment planning. A therapist who takes an objective approach to hypnosis is most likely to utilize a preset script for induction and programming as a method of therapy. Most experts have attempted to define hypnosis objectively from the perspective of their pre-existing underlying theory of personality and its language. In current literature, there are eight traditional definitions of hypnosis:

1. Janet, near the turn of the century, and more recently Ernest Hilgard (Hilgard, 1977), have defined hypnosis in terms of dissociation.
2. Social psychologists Sarbin and Coe (1972) have described hypnosis in terms of role theory. Hypnosis is a role that people play; they act "as if" they were hypnotized.
3. T. X. Barber (1969) defined hypnosis in terms of nonhypnotic behavioral parameters, such as task motivation and the act of labeling the situation as hypnosis.
4. In his early writings, Weitzenhoffer (1953) conceptualized hypnosis as a state of enhanced suggestibility. Most recently (Weitzenhoffer, 1989, Vol. 1, p. 13), he has defined hypnotism as "a form of influence by one person exerted on another through the medium or agency of suggestion."
5. Psychoanalysts Gill and Brenman (1959) described hypnosis by using the psychoanalytic concept of "regression in the service of the ego."
6. Edmonston (1981) has assessed hypnosis as being merely a state of relaxation.
7. Spiegel and Spiegel (1978) have implied that hypnosis is a biological capacity.

8. Erickson (Erickson, Rossi, & Rossi, 1976) is considered the leading exponent of the position that hypnosis is a special, inner-directed, altered state of functioning.

An Alternative View of Hypnosis

The definitions above are attempts to objectify hypnosis. Zeig (1988, p. 356) has proposed that hypnosis can be defined subjectively and phenomenologically from the perspective of the patient, and interactionally as a process between individuals. The attempt to establish an objective and quantifiable definition is bypassed, which may be just as well, since previous attempts to objectify hypnosis have been unsuccessful. This is not to say we should not attempt to define hypnosis. Rather, the definition can be flexible.

This fluid approach may be the bane of objectivists who want to know "the real thing" in operational terms. However, for clinicians, flexibility is a necessity, and the "blinders" that are an inevitable concomitant of an established theoretical position often work against the goals of the therapy.

Zeig (1988) has pointed out that hypnosis as a process is more qualitatively similar to other subjective emotional experiences. The experience of love, for example, differs from person to person; what is love to one is not to the next. Most people would avoid attempts to empirically objectify "love" and to distinguish it from other emotional states. Hypnosis can be similarly treated. Consequently, it may be more beneficial to define hypnosis in multiple ways that reflect complex and changing psychodynamic, interpersonal, and situational variables. Zeig (1988) suggests that hypnosis can be defined from the perspectives of the observer, the patient, and the therapist as follows:

1. From the observer's position, hypnosis can be defined as a context for effective influence communication.

2. From the patient's point of view, hypnosis can be experienced as a state of focused awareness on whatever is immediately relevant, in which previously unrecognized psychological and physiological potentials are accessed to some avolitional extent.

3. From the therapist's position, hypnosis can be conceived of as a dissociative responsiveness to injunction in a context defined as hypnosis.

It may be unnecessary to have a single definition of hypnosis. Hypnosis is a multifaceted phenomenon that entails a system of interaction between people. Perhaps by widening definitions to take into account a variety of perspectives, we can demystify hypnosis and place it into the realm of interesting interpersonal processes of influence.

Note that in all three of the perspectives above, the concept of trance is irrelevant. Zeig (1988) has noted that this position is based on an indirect approach whereby the hypnotherapist mainly presents "covert injunctions" to the patient, which also can be called "indirect suggestions," "minimal cues," "multilevel communications," "demand characteristics" (Orne, 1959), or "one-step-removed communication."

And though it may initially seem to be an extreme position, it may be best at this juncture in the evolution of hypnosis to discard the idea of trance and to make trance irrelevant to hypnosis. By doing so, we can more easily view hypnosis as an interpersonal process. This may seem to run counter to Erickson's belief that hypnosis is a separate, unique state; as we will see, however, closer examination of his work reveals his frequent use of naturalistic methods or "hypnotherapy without formal trance." And though trance per se may be irrelevant, indirection is a process relevant to social influence and lies at the core of Ericksonian hypnotherapy—an idea that is developed further below.

Erickson, in fact, demonstrated a flexible approach to defining hypnosis, and sometimes he did not define hypnosis by using the concept of trance. For example, Theodore Sarbin (personal communication, November 30, 1989) has described meeting Erickson in the late 1930s, when he (Sarbin) was a graduate student. As a student querying a master, he asked Erickson, "What is hypnosis?" Expecting a reply couched in terms of neurological constructs, dissociation, or the like, Sarbin was surprised when Erickson offered, without elaboration, the following reply: "Hypnosis is a tool."

THEORETICAL CONCEPTS AND PRINCIPLES

Erickson's Clinical Epistemology

Books are to be call'd for, and supplied, on the assumption that the process of reading is not a half sleep, but, in the highest sense, an exercise, a gymnast's struggle; that the reader is to do something for himself, must be on the alert, must himself or herself construct indeed the poem, argument, history, metaphysical essay—the text furnishing the hints, the clue, the start or framework.

—Walt Whitman,
Democratic Vistas (1871/1982, pp. 992–993)

Whitman refers here to a relationship between "the reader" and "the text," characterized on the reader's part by active construction of the content of "the book." This is a relationship quite analogous to that which Milton Erickson elicited from his patients. Erickson frequently alluded to the fact that the therapist is responsible for creating the climate and conditions conducive to change, but the patient must supply the important thinking and doing that achieve it (Zeig, 1980b).

And, although it may initially seem quixotic to say so, this may not be the only similarity between Whitman and Erickson. In a real sense, Milton Erickson initiated an entirely new direction in American psychotherapy and hypnosis, much as Walt Whitman 100 years earlier had recast and revitalized American poetry. Theirs was a passion for the unique within the ordinary, for the idiosyncratic, for the specialness of the individual. Erickson operationalized this respect for individual differences by carefully tailoring the hypnotherapy to fit the beliefs and values of the patient. Indeed, acceptance of the patient's behavior, symptoms, and resistances was extended to utilization of these as the foundation for the construction of effective interventions.

The importance of the individual in Erickson's approach needs to be fully understood. This is not simply an aspect of a humanistic attitude. The temptation to intellectual analysis, to explanatory theorizing, to fitting the client to the therapist's framework continues apace in contemporary psychotherapy. Unexamined assumptions and foregone conclusions, in the mind of either the therapist or the client, about the meaning and solution of problems remain among the more serious obstacles to the successful resolution of problems.

Erickson refused to be seduced by the siren song of preconceived, established, or conventional notions about hypnosis and psychotherapy. From the outset he seems to have adopted a radical clinical epistemology in which the individual person was to be the beginning and the end of the therapy. This required him to invent a new theory for each patient and to evolve tools (hypnosis was one) adaptable to a range of individual differences.

Haley (1982) has pointed out: "One way to describe his [Erickson's] contribution to the present revolution in the field of therapy is to point out that his position about what to do in therapy was exactly the opposite of what was done by traditional theorists" (p. 19). Similarly, Erickson's contribution to hypnosis is the opposite of what was done by hypnosis theorists. Whereas traditional theorists started with a theory and then developed a definition, principles of practice, and research, Erickson started with a conception of how to promote interpersonal influence. He evolved his principles from practice, rather than allowing theory to guide practice.

In the following paragraphs, we briefly summarize the most fundamental of Erickson's ideas and procedures that flowed from this epistemology. Erickson used hypnosis as a communicational strategy for the achievement of therapeutic goals. The elements described in the following sections pervaded his work in trance induction and utilization, in hypnosis without formal trance, and in research. A true appreciation of the depth and range of his accomplishments in these areas can only be obtained by a thorough reading of his collected papers (Erickson, 1980).

The Goal of Ericksonian Hypnotherapy

> The induction and maintenance of a trance serve to provide a special psychological state in which patients can reassociate and reorganize their inner psychological complexities and utilize their own capacities in a manner in accord with their own experiential life.
> —Milton Erickson,
> *The Collected Papers* (1980, Vol. 4, p. 38)

This sentence clearly and succinctly expresses the essential activity of hypnosis as Erickson conceived it: The therapist's task is to elicit in the patient a process of *inner resynthesis*, from which effective results can proceed (Erickson, 1980, Vol. 4, p. 38). Fundamentally, what develops in hypnosis does not derive from the presented suggestions per se, but from how the patient internally processes and idiosyncratically utilizes these suggestions. The passive patient assumed by traditional methods is here replaced by an internally involved and active individual.

Zeig (1985) has described traditional hypnosis as "outside-in" and Ericksonian methods as "inside-out." In traditional methods, the hypnotist puts suggestions *into* a passive subject. In Ericksonian approaches, ideas often are presented indirectly so that the therapy evolves from within the patient. The numerous associations stimulated by the indirect technique "drive" more effective behavior. As a result, changes happen primarily to the credit of the patient, not the therapist.

The philosophies of utilization and tailoring, and the various methods of indirection (all of which are summarized below), were Erickson's solutions to the question of how to stimulate constructive inner processes. But the central aspect of his hypnosis was the development of inherent interpersonal responsiveness. Through hypnosis a therapist can ascertain the extent and style of the patient's responsiveness, and can then help the patient develop even greater responsiveness and cooperation. Zeig (1988, p. 358) has asserted that the success of the therapy is proportional to the degree of developed responsiveness to minimal cues (indirect techniques).

The Means: Promoting Interpersonal Influence

Indirection: Utilizing Injunctions

With the concept of "indirection," we come to the heart of Erickson's understanding of how to influence patients effectively. Though he cannot be credited with either creating or being the first to recognize and utilize indirect suggestion (Erickson, 1980, Vol. 1, pp. 452 ff.), he can be acknowledged to have employed it more extensively, inventively, and methodically than anyone before him, so that indirection has become synonymous with things Ericksonian.

Essentially, the Ericksonian approach to hypnotherapy is "R and R": accessing *responsiveness*, especially to minimal cues, in order to get the patient in touch with *resources* that can be harnessed to promote change. In a communications analysis, being indirect entails building responsiveness. Indirection is a natural outgrowth of effective hypnotizing.

Building Interpersonal Responsiveness

In building interpersonal responsiveness, it is not enough merely to elicit responsive behavior. With hypnotherapy, the therapist induces responsiveness to "minimal cues." The use of indirect (multiple-level) technique is integral to achieving hypnosis.

Let us clarify this idea of minimal cues. If within the framework of hypnosis a patient is commanded to lift his or her right arm and merely lifts it, that response is not necessarily hypnosis. However, if the therapist says to the patient, "I would like you to directly realize in a way that is *uplifting* that hypnosis is really an experience that is *right* for you in a way that you can find *handy*," and then the patient somewhat avolitionally lifts his or her right arm, that is considered an essentially hypnotic response (Zeig, 1985, p. 394). Alternatively, if the therapist says, "In hypnosis I would like you to really understand that you can find yourself *headed down* into a comfortable state," and the patient moves his or her head down in dissociative (automatic) response to the implied injunction, that is judged as hypnosis. In this sense, an Ericksonian therapist obscures cues and makes them indirect, so that the patient's responses become more and more autonomously generated. This is especially true in trance induction.

In fact, before proceeding with complex therapeutic suggestions, Erickson usually worked with a patient to establish to the best of their mutual ability—to the best of the patient's intrinsic limits—a responsiveness to minimal cues. Such responsiveness is not only integral to hypnosis;

it is the key that unlocks the door to the constructive capacities of the unconscious, as we clarify below. In Erickson's psychotherapy, responsiveness to minimal cues was the ground in which future suggestions were planted. They were placed in a fertilized bed of responsive behavior (Zeig, 1985, p. 394).

Finally, we would point out that elicitation of responsiveness in the patient implies an interaction of minimal cues between patient and therapist; that is, the therapist is likewise learning to be responsive (albeit with deliberation) to the patient's ongoing unconscious expression of minimal cues, and continuously adjusting accordingly. What ensues is a dance-like sequence in which the therapist follows in order to lead, utilizing the patient's previous steps, and offering a slight modification of an established movement, from which a new step can evolve, sometimes "spontaneously," but always to the credit of the patient.

After Erickson elicited cooperative responsiveness to minimal cues through his formal and informal induction procedures, he then proceeded to address therapeutic goals. Often therapy was achieved by using strategies that entailed the principles of utilization and accessing resources.

Utilization

As we have indicated, making use of the patient's responsiveness and learnings requires respecting the fact that patients differ as personalities and realizing that techniques must be customized to fit individual needs and situations (Erickson, 1980, Vol. 1, p. 15). Differences between patients, as well as changes within each patient's own trance experience, made Erickson sensitive to the need for "fluidity of changes in technique . . . from one type of approach to another as indicated" (Erickson, 1980, Vol. 1, p. 16). Consequently, he developed and recommended the use of a "naturalistic approach," by which he meant "the acceptance and utilization of the situation encountered without endeavoring to psychologically restructure it. In doing so, the presenting behavior of the patient becomes a definite aid and actual part in inducing trance, rather than a possible hindrance" (Erickson, 1980, Vol. 1, p. 168). Utilization of the patient's language, behavior, and particular view of reality conveyed acceptance and respect, promoted rapport and a working alliance, and provided the foundation and raw material from which effective interventions could be built.

For example, comfortable and ready acceptance by Erickson of one patient's compulsive need to pace back and forth in his office allowed the patient to accept slight but incrementally increased modifications of his pacing, until he was finally able to sit down and enter a deep trance (Erickson, 1980, Vol. 1, p. 181). Drawing upon another patient's successful experience as a florist as the basis for a lengthy description of the growth and development of a tomato plant, interspersed with suggestions for pain-free comfort, enabled Erickson to induce a deep trance in that patient, who was suffering greatly from terminal cancer (Haley, 1973, pp. 300 ff.). Brutally honest agreement with another patient's conviction of her own ugliness had the paradoxical effect of assuring the patient of a genuine and effective treatment to come (Haley, 1973, pp. 115 ff.).

Accepting and utilizing a patient's psychological states, understandings, as well as his or her symptoms and resistances, promoted more rapid trance induction, the development of more salutary trance states, and an easier acceptance of therapy (Erickson, 1980, Vol. 1, p. 176). The techniques of behavioral matching, naturalistic induction, symptom prescription, and strategic use of trance phenomena, as we will discuss below, all flowed organically from this fundamental idea of utilizing "what the patient brings."

Accessing Latent Resources

Because the degree of responsiveness to minimal cues varies among individuals, it makes sense that with Ericksonian hypnosis individual differences are stressed. The rote application of techniques characteristic of traditional approaches is avoided.

Individual differences also exist in regard to inherent resources and ways in which these can be accessed. Once a patient's responsiveness to minimal cues has been established, the induction is over and the therapist's efforts are directed toward eliciting resources. This is basically a matter of looking into the reality situation for aspects that can be used in the process of achieving goals.

Often trance phenomena are resources that are ascertained hypnotically. Zeig (1988) has stated that "Whatever hypnotic phenomena the patient does best [are] resource[s] that can be used to accomplish the therapy." For example, if the patient can do time distortion, painful periods of time can be shortened, and/or times in which comfort is experienced can be expanded. If the patient can do age regression, reorientation can be achieved to a pain-free time of life.

Resources can be found in the patient's presenting problem, in his or her past experiences, and in the social environment; here again we see the principle of utilization at work. For Erickson, the word "resources" was in large measure a function of the unconscious mind and each individual's lifelong learnings accumulated therein. It is as if the patient is viewed as supersaturated. As a catalyst, the therapist provides indirect suggestions so that effective behavior crystallizes around stimulated ideas within the patient. The therapist guides associations to elicit previously dormant resources. Every depressed patient has a history of changing mood. Every anxious patient has a history of being calm. The therapist elicits and contextualizes the constructive history of unrecognized learnings within the patient and helps the patient bring these learning into the foreground.

Activating resources can also be accomplished, as Erickson recognized, through the use of therapeutic tasks by which therapy can be taken outside the consulting room and put back into the patient's life situation (Erickson, 1980, Vol. 4, p. 148). A number of therapists have emphasized his pioneering use of such tasks (cf. C. H. Lankton, 1988).

Direction and Indirection

To stimulate internal processing by an individual of what had personal meaning, Erickson developed many types of indirect suggestion. Rossi (see Erickson, 1980, Vol. 1, p. 452) presented 12, and S. R. Lankton and Lankton (1983) described 11, including the interspersal approach, truisms, compound and contingent suggestions, shock and surprise, implication, binds, and multiple-level communications. Erickson also experimented extensively with direct and traditional, ritualistic techniques. He concluded, after many thousands of subjects, that "the simpler and more permissive and unobtrusive is the technique, the more effective it has proved to be, both experimentally and therapeutically in the achievement of significant results" (Erickson, 1980, Vol. 1, p. 15).

But we hasten to add, because there has been confusion on this point, that Erickson's precise use of indirect methods did not preclude the use of direct approaches. As Zeig (1985) has pointed out, for Erickson, indirection was only of value in the relationship to the patient. Zeig (1980a, p. 26) has described what he believes to be one of the principles that Erickson used: "The degree of indirection used is directly proportional to the amount of anticipated resistance." In other words, it does not pay to be indirect if direct techniques will accomplish the goal.

Erickson did not often talk about how to construct therapeutic implications. Rather, he seemed to think, "Where is the patient in relation to therapeutic goals? How can I create a context that can help the patient achieve these goals?" Usually the prepared ground was comprised of fertile indirect suggestions. Erickson's anecdotes, symbols, binds, tasks, and so forth were simply ways of indirectly presenting common-sense ideas to make them come alive (Zeig, 1985). The paradox of indirect forms of communication (injunctions) lies in their ability to compel and to influence, while being at the same time "just ordinary conversation."

Conscious and Unconscious Levels of Awareness

Far from Breuer and Freud's (1893–1895/1955) intimidating concept of the unconscious as an abscess in need of draining, Erickson reframed the unconscious mind as wiser and more perceptive than the conscious mind (Erickson & Rossi, 1979, p. 302). He saw it as a vast repository of unrecognized potentials, some of which are autonomously utilized each day, while others remain dormant. Activation of untapped or underutilized capabilities could be accomplished, Erickson recognized, by speaking directly to the unconscious mind through the medium of metaphors, stories, puns, jokes, even "word salad." To depotentiate and disrupt the limiting mental sets of the conscious mind and to access unconscious potentials, he specifically developed his interspersal and confusion techniques, and made subtle use of vocal dynamics and nonverbal ways of communicating.

"One of the greatest advantages of hypnotherapy lies in the opportunity to work independently with the unconscious without being hampered by the reluctance, or sometimes actual inability, of the conscious mind to accept therapeutic gains" (Erickson, 1980, Vol. 4, p. 40). Also, working separately with the unconscious mind provides an opportunity to "temper and control the patient's rate of progress and thus to effect a reintegration . . . acceptable to the conscious mind" (Erickson, 1980, Vol. 4, p. 41). Though this separation has obvious advantages when therapy is dealing with repressed, traumatic material, one of Erickson's contributions was his technique of inducing hypnosis by eliciting a dissociation between the activities of the patient's conscious and unconscious minds. Erickson found hypnosis useful to the extent that it allowed the operations of the patient's conscious mind to recede and the functions of the unconscious mind to surface.

In this regard, though Erickson acknowledged that conscious insight might be helpful in some cases, in the early years he stood virtually alone in his assertion that solutions could be developed by the unconscious mind without full conscious comprehension of the problem by either the therapist or the patient. Often he thought it advisable to keep the conscious mind distracted from the unconscious mind's activity, as in his frequent use of amnesia suggestions just prior to reorienting the patient from trance. Confusion to disrupt conscious sets became a customary way of inducing, and amnesia a customary way of concluding, therapeutic trance.

Teleological Orientation

Erickson admonished his patients and students that life is lived in the present and directed toward the future, and that therapy is likewise lived in the present and directed toward the future (Zeig, 1985). Ericksonian therapy is geared toward the future. Goals are established and treatment is directed toward achieving them strategically. "The *sine qua non* of psychotherapy should be the present and the future adjustment of the patient, with only that amount of attention to the past necessary to prevent a continuance or a recurrence of past maladjustment" (Erickson, 1980, Vol. 4, p. 171). Erickson saw the past as finished, unalterable. And though understanding connections between prior events and present problems might be "somewhat educational" (Zeig, 1980b, p. 268), it was not at all essential for positive therapeutic change to occur. Of far greater practical value, for him, was getting the patient to do things now and in the future.

A microcosm of Erickson's whole approach to therapy, and one of his more important contributions to hypnosis, can be found in his technique of "pseudo-orientation in time." This involved the hypnotic projection of an individual into an imagined future, followed by a review of how that future would be accomplished, and by posthypnotic suggestions to do what was thus indicated. With this technique, Erickson was utilizing hypnosis to create a self-fulfilling prophecy within the patient; this enabled the patient to use the future to determine the present, instead of allowing the past to determine the future.

An orientation to the future can also be seen in the techniques of "seeding" of future suggestions and building constructive responses in small steps, which Erickson developed. This was a process of "divide and conquer": If a patient presented the problem of losing 40 pounds, Erickson would quickly reorient the patient to losing 1 pound. Breaking goals down into minimal sequential steps can be an effective strategy for change. If a therapist can predict subsequent steps, he or she can seed them prior to presenting them. This is essentially a matter of priming responsive behavior. Erickson regularly seeded concepts prior to presenting them. This technique is akin to the literary technique of foreshadowing. The possibilities of seeding are numerous, and Erickson was ingenious in using this method (Zeig, 1990).

Hypnosis with and without Formal Trance

Beahrs (1971) has pointed out that although Erickson "is the acknowledged leader of medical hypnosis, he used formal trance induction in less than ten percent of his work" (p. 73). Despite this fact, and though Erickson blurred "the boundary between waking and hypnotic techniques," Beahrs makes clear that "subtle hypnotic techniques are carefully integrated into Erickson's therapy." As we have attempted to demonstrate in the foregoing sections, Erickson's naturalistic use of indirection in psychotherapy—that is, hypnotherapy without formal trance—was a natural outgrowth of exploring ways of influencing patients through the careful use of communicational patterns flexible enough to avoid conscious interference and compelling enough to elicit unconscious responsiveness.

Consider Erickson's comments on his intervention with a 14-year-old girl with serious academic and behavioral problems:

It was to get [her] from within herself to make response behavior that would be corrective of her situation and her condition that I proceeded as I did. *Hypnosis is essentially that sort of concept, i.e., a way to offer stimuli of various kinds that will enable patients in response to those stimuli to utilize their own experiential learning.* (Erickson, 1980, Vol. 2, p. 316; italics added)

Importantly, though he spoke here of hypnosis, no trance was induced. In commenting on his work with a young, recently married couple who shared the lifelong problem of enuresis, he outlined a therapy that was hypnotic while jettisoning "trance"; at the same time, a context for change was designed through explicit, compelling directions in which indirection played a pivotal part. It was, he recognized, a therapy woven of paradoxes, but here is Erickson's description in his own words:

Concerning the evasive reply given to the patients about the use of hypnosis, by which they were compelled to assume fully their own responsibilities, the fact remains that the entire procedure was based upon an indirect use of hypnosis. The instructions were so worded as to *compel without demanding the intent attention of the unconscious*. The calculated vagueness of some of the instructions forced their unconscious minds to assume responsibility for their behavior. (Erickson, 1980, Vol. 4, p. 102; italics added)

In another case, Erickson warned against "often too ready a dependence upon hypnosis itself and the immediate use of some well-known structured form of hypnotic approach" (Erickson, 1980, Vol. 4, p. 192), rather than meeting patients and problems on their own terms.

These case examples serve to illustrate that whatever else it may be, Ericksonian hypnosis can be described as responsive behavior elicited from one person by another, thus shifting the focus from an intrapsychic to an interpersonal context. Furthermore, Erickson's interventions utilizing hypnosis without formal trance can be seen to have been carefully engineered "mazes"—prearranged communicational environments into which unaware patients willingly walked, and within which their attention was captured and focused as the meaning of and the rules regarding their particular reality shifted and were reconstituted.

Peering behind the apparently magical results he achieved, we can observe Erickson the dramatist at work, weaving from the patient's own responses a personalized series of customarily indirect messages bound to culminate in a particular denouement or turning point, inevitably involving an internally achieved transformation for the main character. And, though *what* hypnosis is and is not within an individual has been a problem for theorists and researchers, the real problem for Ericksonian psychotherapy has always been *how* to elicit responsive behavior in the direction of positive change. Dispensing with formal trance may seem to water down the concept of hypnosis, but for clinicians hypnosis is primarily an interpersonal influence process and a tool for change, not a reified concept.

To summarize Ericksonian psychotherapy and hypnosis, we could say that it is an interpersonal context energized by a careful utilization of the patient's realities and motivations and the therapist's active efforts to elicit and develop the patient's inherent resources. Within this communication system, injunctions are strategically employed by the therapist to build responsiveness (especially to minimal cues) from the patient in the direction of therapeutic goals. Consequently, we would suggest that formal trance induction and utilization are optional, not integral, aspects of hypnotherapy—branches of the tree, not the tree itself. Getting to the forest behind the trees seems to require a focused flexibility: a keeping of one eye on the target goal, and the other on individualizing a variety of means of getting there. This binocularity typified Erickson throughout his innovative career.

Different Perspectives on Ericksonian Practice

The overview presented above is by no means the only effort to articulate an Ericksonian perspective. Erickson's methods have motivated a variety of theorists and practitioners to elaborate their own models of his approaches. Each has tended to emphasize one or another feature of his multilayered and generative work. Below, we briefly present and describe the following five streams of Ericksonian practice: (1) Haley's strategic model; (2) the Mental Research Institute's (MRI's) interactional model; (3) the Erickson–Rossi development of hypnosis; (4) neuro-linguistic programming (NLP); and (5) post-Ericksonian hypnotherapists.

Haley's Strategic Model

Jay Haley (1967, 1973) was the first to offer an organized presentation of some of Erickson's essential ideas and to recognize him as the father of brief strategic approaches to psychotherapy. Originally he emphasized Erickson's active position as a therapist, de-emphasizing hypnosis in favor of the use of directives to get patients to *do* something. By accepting what the patient had to offer (including his or her symptoms and resistances), and utilizing these, Erickson created a brief treatment based on cooperation, positive redefinition, and indirectly elicited behavior.

Continuing to introduce and elaborate Erickson's work, Haley (1976) characterized it as focused on the present, on interactions, and on symptoms as communications that serve an interpersonal function. Change occurs primarily as a result of intense relationships of the kind Erickson created with patients to secure their cooperation (or rebellion) in the direction of symptom removal or amelioration. Further examination of Erickson's work through the family life cycle revealed its strongly strategic nature: His interventions were carefully aimed to elicit behavioral change, not to stimulate insight or uncover hidden causes.

Expanding ideas derived from interactions with Erickson and Gregory Bateson, to name a few, Haley (1976) created a strategic approach to family therapy characterized by its brief and pragmatic approach to developmental issues and by the active role of the therapist in providing directives for change. More recently, and in collaboration with Cloe Madanes, Haley (1984) has developed other Ericksonian and strategic methods, including devising directives to stimulate change via "benevolent ordeals," and the use of directive tasks to rearrange problematic relationship hierarchies in families (Madanes, 1981, 1984).

The Interactional Model of the Mental Research Institute

Like Haley, the MRI practitioners have de-emphasized the direct use of hypnosis. Their interactional model is derived from the seminal theoretical work of Gregory Bateson as well as the innovative techniques of Milton Erickson. They have generated a number of highly practical and influential concepts, most significantly the idea of "hooks," later elaborated as "the position the patient takes" (Fisch, Weakland, & Segal, 1982); the concepts of first and second-order change (Watzlawick, Weakland, & Fisch, 1974); the concepts of symmetric and complementary relationships (Watzlawick, Beavin, & Jackson, 1967); and the notions of indicative and injunctive communication (Watzlawick, 1985). In addition, they expanded on the techniques of reframing and symptom prescription (Watzlawick et al., 1974).

This work has greatly extended our understanding of interactional patterns, especially within families. In their systemic and solution-oriented approach to psychological problems, expediting change through the "illogical" and the "unexpected," the MRI group has extracted essential aspects of Erickson's indirect use of hypnosis.

Clearly aligned with this pragmatic approach is the work of deShazer (1985), whose brief therapy model, applying invariant prescriptions, emphasizes utilization of the patient's strengths, a future focus, and an "as simple as effectively possible" orientation to interventions.

The Erickson–Rossi Development of Hypnosis

Ernest Rossi has been Erickson's Boswell. There are four books in which Rossi explains Erickson's therapeutic work (Erickson et al., 1976; Erickson

& Rossi, 1979, 1981, 1989), as well as three volumes of Erickson's seminars, workshops, and lectures (Rossi, Ryan, & Sharp, 1983; Rossi & Ryan, 1985, 1986). Whereas Haley and the MRI group have focused on the interpersonal aspects of Erickson's approach, Rossi has developed more of the intrapsychic dimension of Erickson's hypnosis and psychotherapy.

In the works cited above, Rossi examined in considerable detail two essential components of Erickson's work: the forms of indirect suggestion and the utilization approach to hypnotherapy. The nature of the therapeutic trance is elaborated as a highly motivated, inner-directed, altered state of functioning in which active unconscious learning is acquired. As Weitzenhoffer pointed out in his introduction to *Hypnotic Realities* (Erickson et al., 1976), "How to facilitate, activate, cultivate, and . . . utilize unconscious levels of functioning" (p. xix) forms the central focus of Erickson's approach and consequently, of Rossi's explications. Subsequently, Rossi has developed important contributions linking hypnosis to neurophysiological possibilities (Rossi, 1986; Rossi & Cheek, 1988).

Neurolinguistic Programming

Richard Bandler and John Grinder have elucidated Erickson by drawing concepts from transformational grammar as the backbone of their approach. They have delineated the concepts of pacing and leading, particularly detailing the microdynamic structure of the indirect methods Erickson used (Bandler & Grinder, 1975; Grinder, DeLozier, & Bandler, 1977). In other writings they have developed their own model, NLP, emphasizing the sensory-based elements of perceptions and representations (Dilts, Grinder, Bandler, DeLozier, & Cameron-Bandler, 1979; Dilts, 1983). Recognition and utilization of an individual's sensory processes for accessing experience or memories provide a means for achieving hypnotic and therapeutic results. In their concepts of anchoring, reframing, and changing personal history, they have attempted to structure and extend Erickson's hypnotic work (Grinder & Bandler, 1981, 1982).

Post-Ericksonian Hypnotherapists

In the years since Erickson's death, a number of his students and others stimulated by his work have offered new frameworks for understanding his approaches and extending his methods. Space limitations allow only brief reference to the significant contributions of these practitioners.

Stephen R. Lankton and Carol H. Lankton (1983) have focused on Erickson's use of trance, its induction, and its utilization; they see indirection, conscious–unconscious dissociation, and utilization of the client's behavior as typifying Erickson's hypnosis. They have constructed a valuable model of metaphor ("multiple embedded metaphor"), which structures stories to elicit trance phenomena and retrieve resources. In addition, working from a systemic framework, they have applied Ericksonian hypnotherapy to work with families (S. R. Lankton & Lankton, 1986).

Stephen Gilligan (1987) emphasized Erickson the hypnotherapist, detailing cooperation strategies that underlay Erickson's use of therapeutic trance; in particular, he has illuminated the confusion techniques Erickson originated. William O'Hanlon (1987) has offered a well-organized primer of Ericksonian hypnotherapy and strategic psychotherapy, one of the first attempts to highlight their many interconnections. He has also provided a helpful digest of the major frameworks of Ericksonian approaches. In addition, collaborating with James Wilk (O'Hanlon & Wilk, 1987) and with Michelle Weiner-Davis (O'Hanlon & Weiner-Davis, 1989), he has combined Ericksonian approaches with those of Haley, the MRI, and the Brief Family Therapy Center in Milwaukee to consolidate the central ideas and methods of a brief, solution-oriented therapy.

We should mention the following important work: Araoz (1982) has applied hypnosis to sexual issues; Ritterman (1983) developed the use of hypnosis with families; Dolan (1985) indicated Ericksonian techniques for working with resistant, chronic patients; Yapko (1988) elaborated a variety of directives for treating depression; and Mills and Crowley (1988) have explored the use of metaphor, especially with children.

Finally, a growing number of studies focused on clinical applications of Ericksonian techniques to a variety of problems and populations, including the following: chemical dependency treatment (Lovern & Zohn, 1982; McGarty, 1985); social practices (Baker, 1982); Asian-Americans (Kim, 1983); pain (Williams, 1983); preschool children (Honig & Wittmer, 1985); agoraphobics (Edgette, 1985); family therapy and mediation (Sargent & Moss, 1987); erectile dysfunction (Schweitzer, 1986); sexual orientation confusion (Wolf & Klein, 1987); and art therapy (Gantt, 1985). Blending Ericksonian approaches has been the focus of other work: with psychoanalytic psychotherapy (Cohen, 1982; Pollens, 1986); with Milan therapy (Matthews, 1984); with general medical problems (Corley, 1982; Mun, 1982); and with cancer treatment (Rosen, 1985). Rosen (1982) has developed Erickson's use of therapeutic anecdotes. Perhaps these citations, drawn at random from several quarters, will give some indication of the range of interest in Ericksonian ideas in the last several years.

RESEARCH AND APPRAISAL

It may be worthwhile to preface our comments on research in Ericksonian approaches by summarizing Erickson's remarks at the end of a 1944 (Erickson, 1980, Vol. 2) experimental study, because of the light they throw on the relationship between *how* one hypnotizes and *what* one believes hypnosis to be, on the one hand, and the kinds of results one can expect to obtain from their application in a research context, on the other.

First, Erickson pointed out that "rigidly controlled experimental procedures . . . cannot provide for unexpected spontaneous developments extending beyond the desired experimental situation. Often such unanticipated developments constitute the more significant findings" (1980, Vol. 2, p. 49). Second, he objected to the expectation in so many studies of the subject's becoming simply an instrument of the hypnotist (1980, Vol. 2, p. 50). And finally, he emphasizes that "time and effort are required to permit a development of any profound alteration in behavior" (1980, Vol. 2, p. 50). Such changes cannot be produced on command.

We can note here not only the way in which clinical and experimental dimensions are recursively entwined, but also some of the reasons why Erickson, an indefatigable researcher, turned to the "naturalistic" or "field observations" method. He adopted this approach as a way of avoiding the contaminating influence of the subject's wish to please the researcher by helping him to obtain certain results. Erickson's field studies over a 50-year period record a variety of startling results, demonstrating what can be done when extensive efforts are applied to understand and perspicaciously utilize an individual's frame of reference and personal motivation.

Such efforts remain unprecedented and unreplicated in the entire history of hypnosis, and expose the limitations of much standardized, direct, suggestion-based research. Erickson was no opponent of carefully controlled and statistically oriented research; he made use of such approaches himself. But he continually recognized and drew attention to their limitations in evoking frequently fragile and subtle hypnotic phenomena. His own methods endure as a significant record of achievement and a model of what is possible.

In 1962, he summarized his interest in and indicated a future direction for research:

> In brief, we need to look upon research in hypnosis not in terms of what we can think and devise and hypothesize, but in terms of what we can, by actual observation and notation, discover about the unique, varying, and fascinating kind of behavior that we can recognize as a state of awareness that can be directed and utilized in accord with inherent but unknown laws. (Erickson, 1980, Vol. 2, p. 350)

Although this statement articulates a still worthy (if yet to be realized) goal, it also clarifies the fact that Erickson's interest, even as a researcher, was as usual focused on the individual manifestation of unique capabilities, rather than the things in common an experimental group could demonstrate.

Turning our attention to recent controlled experimental studies, most of which have dealt with the question of the value of indirect over direct suggestions, we find a contradictory situation. J. Barber (1980) demonstrated that so-called unsusceptible, unhypnotizable subjects were indeed responsive to hypnotic treatment when a naturalistic, indirect approach was utilized. These results, combined with his earlier 100% effectiveness in reducing dental pain (J. Barber, 1977; J. Barber & Mayer, 1977) by means of indirect hypnosis, would lend support to the greater efficacy of an Ericksonian approach. However, Gillett and Coe (1984) obtained dissimilar results, and Van Gorp, Meyer, and Dunbar (1985) not only failed to replicate Barber's outcomes, but found the analgesic effect limited to traditional procedures.

Similarly conflicting results emerge when we compare Alman and Carney's (1980) and Stone and Lundy's (1985) findings that behavioral responses to suggestions were enhanced by indirect wording, with the opposite results demonstrated by Lynn, Neufeld, and Matyi (1987) and Matthews, Bennett, Bean, and Gallagher (1985), who found no evidence for the superiority of indirect suggestions. Woolson (1986), however, comparing direct and Ericksonian induction procedures, found that although susceptibility scores between the two were close, a greater number of the Ericksonian group subjects were rated as medium or highly susceptible. He comments that his study's results confirm Erickson's original purpose in developing indirect methods as a way of bypassing patients' resistances, in that the indirectly induced subjects were not as aware of their hypnotized state as were the direct subjects.

More recently, Matthews and Mosher (1988) reported that subjects who received the indirect approach felt more deeply hypnotized than when they received the direct approach, while at the same time replicating the earlier Matthews et al. (1985) findings of no difference between indirect and direct hypnotic procedures. Hollander, Holland, and Atthowe (1988), on the other hand, addressing the issue of hypnotizability, produced results showing that subjects did show increased hypnotic ability when an indirect, Ericksonian format was employed.

Murphy (1988) also offered results appearing to rule out any significant difference between indirect and direct suggestions for two simple forms of indirect suggestions studied, but he cautioned that his investigatin was too limited to be an adequate test. More importantly, his structural–linguistic model of the complex forms of indirect suggestion ("both direct suggestion and presupposition elements occur in all complex indirect suggestion structures" [p. 26]) perhaps points a useful route out of the "either–or" bind into which research on this issue has gotten itself during the past two decades. Otani's (1989) study also highlighted the complexity and subtlety of Erickson's hypnotic techniques and use of indirection by submitting two of his trance induction transcripts to Markov chain analysis. Although Otani obtained new information regarding the macrodynamics of suggestion, which is worthy of attention in future investigations of hypnotic processes, it would certainly appear that no final conclusions can be drawn at this time regarding the advantage of indirect over direct forms of suggestion.

In another area of research relevant to Erickson's ideas, we cite a recent article by Kihlstrom (1987). Surveying the latest findings of a large number and variety of consciousness studies, he concludes:

> One thing is now clear: Consciousness is not to be identified with any particular perceptual–cognitive functions such as discriminative response to stimulation, perception, memory, or the higher mental processes involved in judgement and problem-solving. All of these processes can take place outside of phenomenal awareness. (p. 237)

Kihlstrom goes on to clarify that complex psychological functioning does not depend on, and largely goes on outside of, conscious awareness. These conclusions corroborate Erickson's long-standing concept of a powerful and generative unconscious, the repository of a vast range of unrecognized capabilities.

Finally, we would suggest that because a number of models of Ericksonian hypnosis have only recently been developed, it may be some time before they are adapted to experimental purposes. While recognizing the vital importance of research, we also need to remember that Ericksonian psychotherapy is only a little over a decade old. It was only in 1980 that the word "Ericksonian" came into vogue when it was used in the title of that year's International Congress on Ericksonian Approaches to Hypnosis and Psychotherapy, organized by the Milton H. Erickson Foundation. Also, its clinically based and highly individualized procedures do not lend themselves readily to the standardized approach required by most controlled studies.

Nonetheless, the research efforts cited above offer directions for future development.

CONCLUSION

One of the important developments in psychotherapy has been the development of the systemic approach, which initially entailed working with families. The systemic approach has taken a discretely different orientation from the original individual-based methods of psychotherapy. Traditional hypnosis has been stuck in looking at the individual in an attempt to objectify hypnosis.

This chapter has attempted to present fundamental tenets of an interactional and phenomenological approach to hypnosis by exploring aspects of Milton Erickson's use of hypnosis. Within this communications approach, "trance" is irrelevant. Rather, hypnosis can be understood as an interpersonal process designed to generate specialized responsiveness and to elicit resources in the direction of therapeutic goals.

Acknowledgments. We wish to express appreciation to Brent Geary and Stephen Gilligan for reading drafts of this chapter and supplying corrections that were included in the final revision.

REFERENCES

Alman, B. M., & Carney, R. E. (1980). Consequences of direct and indirect suggestions on success of posthypnotic behavior. *American Journal of Clinical Hypnosis, 22*(2), 112–118.

Araoz, D. L. (1982). *Hypnosis and sex therapy.* New York: Bruner/Mazel.

Baker, E. (1982). Therapeutic social practices. *Advances in Descriptive Psychology, 2,* 209–232.

Bandler, R., & Grinder, J. (1975). *Patterns of the hypnotic techniques of Milton H. Erickson, M.D.* (Vol. 1). Cupertino, CA: Meta.

Barber, J. (1977). Rapid induction analgesia: A clinical report. *American Journal of Clinical Hypnosis, 19*(3), 138–147.

Barber, J. (1980). Hypnosis and the unhypnotizable. *American Journal of Clinical Hypnosis, 23*(1), 4–9.

Barber, J., & Mayer, D. (1977). Evaluation of the efficacy and neural mechanism of a hypnotic analgesia procedure in experimental and clinical dental pain. *Pain, 4,* 41–48.

Barber, T. X. (1969). *Hypnosis: A scientific approach.* New York: Brunner/Mazel.

Beahrs, J. O. (1971). The hypnotic psychotherapy of Milton H. Erickson. *American Journal of Clinical Hypnosis, 14*(2), 73– 90.

Breuer, J., & Freud, S. (1955). Studies on hysteria. In J. Strachey (Ed. and Trans.), *The standard edition of the complete psychological works of Sigmund Freud* (Vol. 2, pp. 1–305). London: Hogarth Press. (Original work published 1893–1895)

Cohen, S. B. (1982). Ericksonian techniques and psychoanalysis. In J. K. Zeig (Ed.), *Ericksonian approaches to hypnosis and psychotherapy* (pp. 173–180). New York: Brunner/Mazel.

Corley, J. B. (1982). Ericksonian techniques with general medicine problems. In J. K. Zeig (Ed.), *Ericksonian approaches to hypnosis and psychotherapy* (pp. 287–291). New York: Brunner/Mazel.

Dilts, R. B. (1983). *Application of neuro-linguistic programming.* Cupertino, CA: Meta.

Dilts, R. B., Grinder, J., Bandler, R., DeLozier, J., & CameronBandler, L. (1979). *Neuro-linguistic programming I.* Cupertino, CA: Meta.

Dolan, Y. (1985). *A path with a heart: Ericksonian utilization with resistant and chronic clients.* New York: Brunner/Mazel.

Edgette, J. H. (1985). The utilization of Ericksonian principles of hypnotherapy with agoraphobics. In J. K. Zeig (Ed.), *Ericksonian psychotherapy: Vol. 2. Clinical applications* (pp. 286–291). New York: Brunner/Mazel.

Edmonston, W. E., Jr. (1981). *Hypnosis and relaxation: Modern verification of an old equation.* New York: Wiley.

Erickson, M. H. (1980). *The collected papers of Milton H. Erickson on hypnosis* (4 vols., Rossi, Ed.). New York: Irvington.

Erickson, M. H., & Rossi, E. (1979). *Hypnotherapy: An exploratory casebook.* New York: Irvington.

Erickson, M. H., & Rossi, E. (1981). *Experiencing hypnosis.* New York: Irvington.

Erickson, M. H., & Rossi, E. (1989). *The February man.* New York: Irvington.

Erickson, M. H., Rossi, E., & Rossi, S. (1976). *Hypnotic realities.* New York: Irvington.

Fisch, R., Weakland, J., & Segal, L. (1982). *Tactics of change.* San Francisco: Jossey-Bass.

Gantt, L. (1985). Ericksonian hypnosis and art therapy. *American Journal of Art Therapy, 23*(4), 125.

Gill, M. M., & Brenman, M. (1959). *Hypnosis and related states: Psychoanalytic studies in regression.* New York: International Universities Press.

Gillett, P. L., & Coe, W. C. (1984). The effects of rapid induction analgesia (RIA), hypnotic susceptibility, and severity of discomfort on reducing dental pain. *American Journal of Clinical Hypnosis, 27*, 81–90.

Gilligan, S. (1987). *Therapeutic trances: The cooperation principle in Ericksonian hypnotherapy.* New York: Brunner/Mazel.

Grinder, J., & Bandler, R. (1981). *Trance-formations: Neuro-linguistic programming and the structure of hypnosis.* Moab, UT: Real People Press.

Grinder, J., & Bandler, R. (1982). *Reframing: Neuro-linguistic programming and the transformation of meaning.* Moab, UT: Real People Press.

Grinder, J., DeLozier, J., & Bandler, R. (1977). *Patterns of the hypnotic techniques of Milton H. Erickson, M.D.* (Vol. 2). Cupertino, CA: Meta.

Haley, J. (1963). *Strategies of psychotherapy.* New York: Grune & Stratton.

Haley, J. (1967). *Advanced techniques of hypnosis and therapy.* New York: Grune & Stratton.

Haley, J. (1973). *Uncommon therapy: The psychiatric techniques of Milton H. Erickson, M.D.* New York: Norton.

Haley, J. (1976). *Problem-solving therapy.* San Francisco: Jossey-Bass.

Haley, J. (1982). The contribution to therapy of Milton H. Erickson, M. D. In J. K. Zeig (Ed.), *Ericksonian approaches to hypnosis and psychotherapy* (pp. 5–25). New York: Brunner/Mazel.

Haley, J. (1984). *Ordeal therapy.* San Francisco: Jossey-Bass.

Hilgard, E. R. (1977). *Divided consciousness: Multiple controls in human thought and action.* New York: Wiley.

Hollander, H. E., Holland, L., & Atthowe, J. M. (1988). Hypnosis: Innate ability or learned skills? In S. R. Lankton & J. K. Zeig (Eds.), *Research, comparisons and medical applications of Ericksonian techniques* (Ericksonian Monograph, No. 4, pp. 37–53). New York: Brunner/Mazel.

Honig, A., & Wittmer, D. (1985). Toddler bids and teacher responses. *Child Care Quarterly, 14*(1), 14–29.

Kihlstrom, J. F. (1987). The cognitive unconscious. *Science, 237,* 1445–1452.

Kim, S. (1983). Ericksonian hypnotic framework for Asian-Americans. *American Journal of Clinical Hypnosis, 25*(4), 235–241.

Lankton, C. H. (1988). Task assignments: Logical and otherwise. In J. K. Zeig & S. R. Lankton (Eds.), *Developing Ericksonian therapy: State of the art* (pp. 257–279). New York: Brunner/Mazel.

Lankton, S. R., & Lankton, C. H. (1983). *The answer within: A clinical framework of Ericksonian hypnotherapy.* New York: Brunner/Mazel.

Lankton, S. R., & Lankton, C. H. (1986). *Enchantment and intervention in family therapy.* New York: Brunner/Mazel.

Lovern, J., & Zohn, J. (1982). Utilization and indirect suggestion in multiple-family group therapy with alcoholics. *Journal of Marital and Family Therapy, 8*(3), 325–333.

Lynn, S. J., Neufeld, V., & Matyi, C. (1987). Inductions versus suggestions: Effects of direct and indirect wording on hypnotic responding and experience. *Journal of Abnormal Psychology, 96,* 76–79.

Madanes, C. (1981) *Strategic family therapy.* San Francisco: Jossey-Bass.

Madanes, C. (1984). *Behind the one-way mirror.* San Francisco: Jossey-Bass.

Matthews, W. (1984). Ericksonian and Milan therapy: An intersection between circular questioning and therapeutic metaphor. *Journal of Strategic and Systemic Therapies, 3*(4), 16–25.

Matthews, W. J., Bennett, H., Bean, W., & Gallagher, M. (1985). Indirect vs. direct hypnotic suggestions—an initial investigation: A brief communication. *International Journal of Clinical and Experimental Hypnosis, 33*(3), 219–223.

Matthews, W. J., & Mosher, D. L. (1988). Direct and indirect hypnotic suggestion in a laboratory setting. *British Journal of Experimental and Clinical Hypnosis, 5*(2), 63–71.

McGarty, R. (1985). Relevance of Ericksonian psychotherapy to the treatment of chemical dependency. *Journal of Substance Abuse Treatment, 2*(3), 147–151.

Mills, J., & Crowley, R. (1988). *Therapeutic metaphors for children and the child within.* New York: Brunner/Mazel.

Mun, C. T. (1982). Ericksonian approaches in general practice. In J. K. Zeig (Ed.), *Ericksonian approaches to hypnosis and psychotherapy* (pp. 292–298). New York: Brunner/Mazel.

Murphy, M. B. (1988). A linguistic–structural model for the investigation of indirect suggestion. In S. R. Lankton & J. K. Zeig (Eds.), *Research, comparisons and medical applications of Ericksonian techniques.* New York: Brunner/Mazel.

O'Hanlon, W. H. (1987). *Taproots: Underlying principles of Milton Erickson's therapy and hypnosis.* New York: Norton.

O'Hanlon, W., & Wilk, J. (1987). *Shifting contexts: The generation of effective psychotherapy.* New York: Guilford Press.

O'Hanlon, W. H. & Weiner-Davis, M. (1989). *In search of solutions: A new direction in psychotherapy*. New York: Norton.

Orne, M. T. (1959). The nature of hypnosis: Artifact and essence. *Journal of Abnormal and Social Psychology, 58*, 277–299.

Otani, A. (1989). An empirical investigation of Milton H. Erickson's approach to trance induction: A Markov chain analysis of two published cases. In S. R. Lankton (Ed.), *Ericksonian hypnosis: Application, preparation and research* (pp. 55–68). New York: Brunner/Mazel.

Pollens, M. (1986). Ericksonian hypnosis and psychoanalytic psychotherapy: The anatomy of an effective partnership. *Journal of Contemporary Psychotherapy, 16*(1), 39–51.

Ritterman, M. (1983). *Using hypnosis in family therapy*. San Francisco: Jossey-Bass.

Rosen, S. (1982). *My voice will go with you*. New York: Norton.

Rosen, S. (1985). Hypnosis as an adjunct to chemotherapy in cancer. In J. K. Zeig (Ed.), *Ericksonian psychotherapy: Vol. 2. Clinical applications* (pp. 387–397). New York: Brunner/Mazel.

Rossi, E. L. (1986). *The psychobiology of mind–body healing: New concepts of therapeutic hypnosis*. New York: Norton.

Rossi, E. L., & Cheek, D. (1988). *Mind–body therapy: Ideodynamic healing in hypnosis*. New York: Norton.

Rossi, E. L., & Ryan, M. (1985). *The seminars, workshops and lectures of Milton H. Erickson: Vol. 2. Life reframing in hypnosis*. New York: Irvington.

Rossi, E. L., & Ryan, M. (1986). *The seminars, workshops and lectures of Milton H. Erickson: Vol. 3. Mind–body communication in hypnosis*. New York: Irvington.

Rossi, E. L., Ryan, M., & Sharp, F. (1983). *The seminars, workshops, and lectures of Milton H. Erickson: Vol. 1. Healing in hypnosis*. New York: Irvington.

Sarbin, T. R., & Coe, W. C. (1972). *Hypnosis: A social psychological analysis of influence communication*. New York: Holt, Rinehart & Winston.

Sargent, G., & Moss, B. (1987). Ericksonain approaches in family therapy and mediation. *Mediation Quarterly, 14–15*, 87–100.

Schweitzer, H. (1986). Ericksonian sports metaphors in the treatment of secondary erectile dysfunction. *Journal of Sex Education and Therapy, 12*(1), 65–68.

Spiegel, H., & Spiegel, D. (1978). *Trance and treatment: Clinical uses of hypnosis*. New York: Basic Books.

Stone, J. A., & Lundy, R. M. (1985). Behavior compliance with direct and indirect body movement suggestions. *Journal of Abnormal Psychology, 94*, 256–263.

Van Gorp, W. G., Meyer, R. G., & Dunbar, K. E. (1985). The efficacy of direct and indirect hypnotic induction techniques on reduction of experimental pain. *International Journal of Clinical and Experimental Hypnosis, 33*, 319–328.

Watzlawick, P. (1985). Hypnotherapy without trance. In J. K. Zeig (Ed.), *Ericksonian psychotherapy: Vol. 1. Structure* (pp. 5–14). New York: Brunner/Mazel.

Watzlawick, P., Beavin, J. H., & Jackson, D. D. (1967). *Pragmatics of human communication: A study of international patterns, pathologies, and paradoxes*. New York: Norton.

Watzlawick, P., Weakland, J., & Fisch, R. (1974). *Change: The principles of problem formation and problem resolution*. New York: Norton.

Weitzenhoffer, A. M. (1953). *Hypnotism: An objective study of suggestibility*. New York: Wiley.

Weitzenhoffer, A. M. (1989). *The practice of hypnotism* (2 vols.). New York: Wiley.

Whitman, W. (1982). Democratic vistas. In *Complete poetry and collected prose* (pp. 992–993). New York: The Viking Press. (Original work published 1871)

Williams, J. A. (1983). Ericksonian hypnotherapy of intractable shoulder pain. *American Journal of Clinical Hypnosis, 26*(1), 26–29.

Wolf, T., & Klein, F. (1987). Ericksonian hypnosis and strategic interventions for sexual orientation confusion. *Journal of Homosexuality, 14*(1–2), 67–76.

Woolson, D. A. (1986). An experimental comparison of direct and indirect Ericksonian hypnotic induction procedures and the relationship to secondary suggestibility. *American Journal of Clinical Hypnosis, 29*(1), 23–28.

Yapko, M. D. (1988). *When living hurts: Directives for treating depression.* New York: Brunner/Mazel.

Zeig, J. K. (1980a). Symptom prescription techniques: Clinical applications using elements of communication. *American Journal of Clinical Hypnosis, 23*(1), 23–33.

Zeig, J. K. (Ed.). (1980b). *A teaching seminar with Milton H. Erickson.* New York: Brunner/Mazel.

Zeig, J. K. (1985). *Experiencing Erickson.* New York: Brunner/Mazel.

Zeig, J. K. (Ed.). (1987). *The evolution of psychotherapy.* New York: Brunner/ Mazel.

Zeig, J. K. (1988). An Ericksonian phenomenological approach to therapeutic hypnotic induction and symptom utilization. In J. K. Zeig & S. R. Lankton (Eds.), *Developing Ericksonian therapy: State of the art* (pp. 353–375). New York: Brunner/Mazel.

Zeig, J. K. (1990). Seeding. In J. K. Zeig & S. G. Gilligan (Eds.), *Brief therapy: Myths, methods, and metaphors* (pp. 221–246). New York: Brunner/ Mazel.

THE SOCIOCOGNITIVE
PERSPECTIVE

Role Theory: Hypnosis from a Dramaturgical and Narrational Perspective

WILLIAM C. COE
California State University Fresno
THEODORE R. SARBIN
University of California Santa Cruz

INTRODUCTION

Our construction of hypnosis was developed out of a growing dissatisfaction with popular theories, which interpreted hypnotic phenomena within metapsychological frameworks supporting such concepts as trance, mental states, animal magnetism, and so on. When role theory was first advanced as a social-psychological theory to account for hypnosis, the prevailing view was that the perplexing performances of the subject or client were attributable to a special state of affairs within the brain or mental apparatus. The purported mental state could not be observed directly, but was inferred from the subject's performance and the subject's *account* of the performance. In a leap of logic, mentalistic explanations of hypnosis took the subject's performance and account as evidence for the purported mental state—a condition that, among other things, had motivational properties. The overt motoric and verbal actions of the laboratory subjects and clinical patients were made to do double duty in mentalistic explanations. Not only was the mental state the *cause* of the performance; the performance was *evidence* that a mental state existed. The logical fallacy was overlooked, not only by practitioners whose primary interests were in healing the sick, but also by theorists and researchers working within the mentalistic framework.

In addition to the logical fallacy, the conventional theories (circa 1930s) contained the premise that the mental state was supposedly brought about through the medium of an "induction." Typically, the induction was composed of sentences formulated and uttered by the hypnotist, some of which were patently counterfactual, such as "You are drifting away," "You are now 5 years old," and "Your body is floating through space." Mentalistic explanations, under the influence of the mechanistic doctrine that all behavior could be accounted for in terms of the transmittal of forces, assumed that the induction released a force that operated on the mental or brain machinery. This view, not unique to theorists of hypnosis, cast the subject or client in the role of a passive organism, a person devoid of agency. The "good" subject was described as "susceptible" to the force somehow released by the hypnotist's verbal and gestural behaviors. Investigators who constructed scales to assess individual differences made the claim that they were measuring "susceptibility" to hypnosis, thus reflecting the underlying premise that the hypnotic subject was a passive object acted upon by unidentified forces.

Our early efforts to construct a more satisfactory theory flowed from the postulate that the transaction between the hypnotic subject and the hypnotist could be seen as a social encounter. "Role," the metaphor that best captured the observations, was borrowed from the theater. It is close to the truth to say that we saw the hypnotic interaction as a theatrical performance in which both the hypnotist and the subject enacted reciprocal roles. The role metaphor served as a potent reminder that subjects in experiments and clients in therapy are not automata, not exclusively organisms, but also agents. Even when they are participants in the hypnotic encounter, they continue to engage in actions to meet the requirements of their personal agendas, including goals, purposes, and values.

In our early attempts at constructing a more useful theory, we focused on dramaturgical metaphors. We were careful to make clear to potential critics that the role of hypnotized subject was not a stereotyped, mechanical set of actions. Rather, we saw the role as an opportunity for subjects to demonstrate individual differences in their performances. The prevailing image for us was that of an actor on the stage interacting with a director, other actors, and an audience. Although this imagery may have influenced some critics to interpret our conception as role playing, sham, faking, or dissimulation, we argued forcefully that the actions of hypnotic subjects were serious efforts at adopting and enacting a social role. We underscored the seriousness of the actions by emphasizing "role enactment," a term that calls up images of men and women going about the business of meeting the requirements of social life—for example, a parent's enacting his or her role vis-à-vis a child. Our view is captured by Shakespeare's often-quoted line "'All the world's a stage," and by the framework advanced by the social philosopher George Herbert Mead, whose seminal writings on role taking have influenced several generations of social scientists.

Implied, but not always expressed in our earlier writings, was the recognition that enactments of the hypnotic role were not context-free. Although our entry into the subdiscipline of hypnosis occurred at a time when positivism was at its zenith, we were aware of restrictions imposed by the use of laboratory methods and mechanistic models. The recognition that *contexts* influenced hypnotic performance directed us to identify features of the context that would help in understanding the phenomena and in constructing a general theory. As described below, our approach centered on the actions of the hypnotist and the subject as a more or less self-contained dramatic encounter. In the 1950 formulation (Sarbin, 1950), the quality of hypnotic role enactment was attributed to three contextual variables: favorable motivation (congruence of self and role), accuracy of role perception, and performance skills. After the publication of a general theory of role taking that was applicable to all forms of social conduct (Sarbin, 1956), six variables were identified that influenced the quality of hypnotic role enactment: (1) role expectations of the subject, (2) the accuracy of the subject's locating of self in the miniature social structure, (3) motoric and imaginal skills, (4) role demands generated by specific features of the experimental or clinical situation, (5) the congruence of the hypnotic role with the subject's self-conceptions, and (6) the guiding and reinforcing properties of the subject's audience.

In more recent times, we have expanded the search for contextual elements that would help illuminate the universally observed individual differences in hypnotic responsiveness (Sarbin, 1977, 1986). In a later section of this chapter, we point to more recent refinements of our explanatory framework. The variable that we identified earlier as "self–role congruence" has been recast as the congruence of the hypnotic role performance with the subject's ongoing self-narrative. In this augmentation of our theory, we have found it useful to entertain the hypothesis that the subject's account of his or her conduct may reflect the withholding of secrets, the artful practice of deception, and/or the intricate strategy of self-deception.

CONCEPTS AND PRINCIPLES

Hypnosis as Dramaturgy

The development of our theory, as noted before, flowed from a deliberate construction of hypnosis as dramaturgy. That is to say, the two chief

participants in the hypnotic encounter—the hypnotist and the subject—
are actors who make use of their skills, purposes, and beliefs to fashion
their role performances. With this dramaturgical metaphor as a framework, we set out to construct a set of variables that would help to explain
the counterexpectational behavior identified as hypnosis. It is important to
accent the observation that the subject engages in actions that are contrary
to expectations. Theorists of hypnosis are not interested in accounting for
conduct that meets ordinary expectations, such as a person's compliance
with a request to be seated. They are primarily interested in counterexpectational conduct, such as subjects' claims that they cannot remember a
recent event, or they see a nonexistent person, or they report no pain under
conditions that ordinarily call for pain responses.

In this respect, hypnotic performances and the performances of stage
actors are parallel. Both actors engage in counterexpectational conduct. In
the film *Rain Man*, Dustin Hoffman is an actor trying to convince the
audience that he is an autistic patient; in the typical experiment,
well-disposed subjects engage in actions to convince their audiences that
they are under the influence of hypnosis. The counterexpectational
conduct is legitimated by the theatrical frame in one instance, and by the
laboratory or clinical frame in the other.

In our earlier work (Sarbin & Coe, 1972), we attempted to clarify how
the six role theory variables could apply to hypnotic performers, whether
in the clinic, the professional stage, or the laboratory.

Role Concepts and Hypnosis

One's performance of a given role is considered under the concept of "role
enactment." It is at this point that other people will judge the convincing-
ness or appropriateness of our actions in a given situation. The accuracy of
hypnotic enactment is characteristically judged from objective and/or subjective scores on standardized hypnotic responsiveness scales (e.g., Barber,
1965; Barber & Wilson, 1977; Hilgard & Crawford, 1979; Morgan &
Hilgard, 1979a, 1979b; Shor & Orne, 1962; Spanos, Radtke, Hodgins,
Stam, & Bertrand, 1983; Weitzenhoffer & Hilgard, 1959, 1962, 1967).
Sometimes it is judged on the basis of depth reports (Tart, 1979), and
sometimes on the hypnotist's impression of the subject's degree of response
(London, 1962; Orne & O'Connell, 1967). The classical behaviors of the
hypnotic role include catalepsies, compulsive posthypnotic behaviors, sensory and motoric changes, and so on. We have accounted for these changes
in terms of role variables and the side effects of organismic involvement.
More recently, reports of highly responsive subjects that are counterfactual
and uttered with high degrees of conviction have become the primary
evidence in support of special-state conceptualizations of hypnosis (Coe,
1978, 1980a; Coe & Sarbin, 1977; Sarbin & Coe, 1972, 1979).

Role Location

The process of role location is that of seeking answers to such questions as "Who is he or she?" or "Who are you?" and the reciprocal questions "Who am I?" and "What is expected of me?" In the usual hypnosis laboratory or clinical situation, the hypnotist bombards subjects with cues that lead them to locate their roles as that of hypnotic subjects. Since the task of correctly locating the role of hypnotist is a simple one, locating the hypnotic subject role is usually held constant in hypnosis studies. Nevertheless, there is evidence that perceived characteristics of the hypnotist can affect hypnotic responsiveness. Coe et al. (1970) and Balaschak, Blocker, Rossiter, and Perin (1970) both manipulated the perceived level of experience of the hypnotist, and both found subjects to be less responsive with "inexperienced" hypnotists. Greenberg and Land (1970) also found that subjects' self-reports of hypnosis favored "experienced" hypnotists, although objective responding was not greater. Systematically varying cue properties of the hypnotist may be related to interesting differences in subjects' responses.

Congruence of Self and Role

For some time, common sense and clinical evidence have indicated the importance of motivational variables in hypnosis. Subjects who say they are afraid of being hypnotized are not as likely to participate in hypnotic suggestions or to be as cooperative with the induction. Thus, there appear to be perceived requirements of the hypnotic role that subjects match with their view of themselves, and thus enhance or deter their responsiveness.

Relating scores on standard personality tests to hypnotizability has not been very successful in discovering what types of subjects will be responsive to hypnosis (see, e.g., Barber, 1969, p. 93). However, the importance of self–role congruence has been shown in studies measuring special self-characteristics (Andersen, 1963; As, 1963; Coe & Sarbin, 1966; Shor, Orne, & O'Connell, 1962; Tellegen, 1978; Tellegen & Atkinson, 1974). Questionnaires have been constructed on the rational basis that certain self-characteristics are similar to the requirements made of hypnotic subjects. Some items inquire directly about subjects' motivations for hypnosis, such as "There are things that would worry me about being hypnotized." Other items try to determine subjects' abilities to become absorbed in a role, and others ask about subjects' acceptance of strange or unusual experiences. Significant positive correlations in the neighborhood of .30 to .40 between hypnotic performance and the responses to such questionnaires have been found. J. R. Hilgard (1979) also presented evidence from interviews that supported the importance of self-characteristics in the hypnotic role, especially characteristics that lead to involvement in imagining.

More recently, Nash and Spindler (1989) investigated the relationship of "archaic involvement" (AI) to hypnotic responsiveness. The AI concept, introduced by Shor (1962), refers to a motivated involvement to comply with the intent of the hypnotist. Nash and Spindler constructed a face-valid questionnaire to clarify the dimensions of the concept, finding a somewhat complicated relationship with hypnotic responsiveness. Subjects scoring *below* the hypnosis mean showed a strong positive relationship between their AI scores and hypnotic responsiveness. However, subjects scoring *above* the mean showed no clear relationship between AI and hypnosis. Nevertheless, the mean AI score of the highly responsive hypnotic subjects was significantly higher than that of the less responsive hypnotic subjects. Thus, the way in which subjects view the hypnotist may be important in affecting their responsiveness. For highly responsive subjects, their view of the hypnotist is a distinctive feature of their experience, but it is not equivalent to their degree of responsiveness to hypnosis. Whatever the final interpretation, such research indicates that matching self-characteristics to the hypnotic context may provide important information.

Role Expectations

In the process of socialization, we learn the kinds of behaviors that are expected for different positions. "Role expectations" are collections of beliefs, subjective probabilities, and bits of knowledge that specify the appropriate conduct for persons occupying particular positions. They can also be provided concurrently by the occupants of reciprocal positions. Thus, subjects bring with them preconceived expectations about how hypnotized persons act, and the hypnotist and setting provide further expectations during the session. In fact, Andersen (1963) demonstrated a good deal of agreement about the expectations for the hypnotic role among persons who had never been hypnotized or witnessed a hypnotic performance.

Orne (1959) illustrated the way expectations can function. He demonstrated hypnosis to two college classes. In front of one class, but not the other, a confederate acting as a subject showed "spontaneous" catalepsy of the dominant hand during the induction. Orne casually remarked that such a spontaneous catalepsy was usual while entering hypnosis. Volunteers from both classes were subsequently hypnotized by an associate who was not informed about the antecedent conditions. Students who had witnessed the catalepsy-of-the-dominant-hand phenomenon tended to show it; students from the other class did not. Other earlier work has also supported the potential importance of role expectations (e.g., Coe & Sarbin, 1966; Barber, Dalal, & Calverley, 1968).

More recently, the research of Spanos and his colleagues has demonstrated the crucial role that expectations can play in determining the quality and quantity of hypnotic responsiveness (e.g., Spanos, 1982; Spanos & Chaves, 1989). The studies are far too many to review here, but suffice it to say that manipulating instructions has caused the validities of many previously accepted so-called hypnotic phenomena to be seriously called into question (e.g., the hidden observer, disrupted retrieval in posthypnotic amnesia, source amnesia, trance logic, and hypnotic analgesia, among others). Spanos's work suggests that subjects' expectations during hypnosis may turn out to be one of the most crucial variables within the hypnotic context.

Kirsch and his colleagues have also focused on subjects' expectations (e.g., Council, Kirsch, & Hafner, 1986; Kirsch, 1985; Kirsch, Council, & Vickery, 1984). Their interest, however, has been in the subjects' "response expectancies," defined as "expectancies of the occurrence of nonvolitional responses, either as a function of behavior—or as a function of specific stimuli" (Kirsch, 1985, p. 1189). Nonvolitional responses are those that appear to occur automatically (e.g., fear, sadness, elation, sexual arousal, etc.). Such responses can have positive or negative reinforcement value, and therefore their expectancy can affect the probability of particular voluntary behaviors. What subjects expect and what they act on are not necessarily the same; the crucial aspect is their conclusion that their voluntary actions hold the potential for positive, nonvolitional responses.

In relation to hypnotic conduct, Kirsch (1985) arrived at five conclusions:

1. The important common element across a variety of methods meant to enhance suggestibility, including hypnotic inductions, is whether or not subjects view them as part of a context that is appropriate for that sort of behavior.

2. Subjects behave as they *expect* hypnotized persons to behave, including their reports on their "trance" experiences.

3. Hypnotic inductions enhance responsiveness by altering response expectancies.

4. Procedures designed to modify subjects' expectancies about hypnotic responding affect their responses.

5. High test–retest correlations, taken to indicate a relatively stable trait of hypnotizability, may instead actually reflect the imparting of stable response expectancies. Finally, "It is possible that, with sufficiently strong response expectancies, *all* individuals would show high levels of hypnotic response" (Kirsch, 1985, p. 1196; italics in original).

Role Skills

The efficiency with which people enact specific roles depends in part on the degree to which they possess the skills relevant to that role. A good deal of research has focused on understanding the abilities of good hypnotic subjects. For example, Hilgard, although committed to an altered-state view of hypnosis, has emphasized the ability of subjects to "dissociate" (e.g., E. R. Hilgard, 1974, 1977a, 1977b, 1979). Spanos and Barber (1974) have shown how investigators representing different theoretical viewpoints are converging on the importance of imaginal skills in hypnosis. Although other skills, such as attention focusing, have been of interest (see, e.g., Sarbin & Coe, 1972), the role played by imaginative skills and skills related to creative activities has been of primary interest. Space does not allow a review of these studies, but the reader will find excellent summaries in Sheehan (1979) on imagination, and P. G. Bowers & K. S. Bowers (1979) on creativity.

The classical suggestion effect, in which subjects report a loss of agency ("It happened to me"), is a candidate for a role skill investigation. When subjects utter statements that are clearly counterfactual (e.g., "I am floating") and convince the hypnotist that they "believe" their reports, it is incumbent upon us to account for such observations. The concept of role skills may help.

Sarbin (1980) described the hypnotic situation in terms of the skills of the two participants in using and interpreting implied metaphors. The hypnotist and the subject, if they are to maintain an ongoing relationship (clinical or research), must have at least minimal skill in translating metaphorical statements. Hypnotists' statements such as "You are drifting away," or "You are now a child of 5," and subjects' statements such as "Yes, I am floating," or "I see my kindergarten teacher, Mrs. Jones," must be recognized as tacit metaphors.

Other skills may influence the fine-tuning of the hypnotic perform-ance (Sarbin, 1981). The talent for maintaining a consistent self-narrative—a story about one's self to one's self—is potentially important. Persons who are able to spell out certain aspects of experience, but at the same time cannot spell out others, are able to maintain a consistency in what they tell themselves about themselves, even though their experience appears counterfactual. For example, subjects who are convinced that they cannot remember during posthypnotic amnesia must be capable of attending to material that is allowable for recall, such as how relaxed they felt; at the same time, they must be able *not* to focus on the material to be forgotten or cues that help them remember it.

The utility and the expansion of the role skills concept can be seen in a current controversy over the nature of posthypnotic amnesia. On one side are those theorists who view posthypnotic amnesia as the product of an altered state that acts to reduce subjects' ability to retrieve information (e.g., Evans & Kihlstrom, 1973; Kihlstrom, 1977, 1978; Kihlstrom & Shor, 1978). On the other side are theorists who view posthypnotic amnesia as the product of subjects' skills in not remembering—abilities they can use to deceive others and sometimes even themselves (e.g., Coe, 1978, 1980b, 1989; Coe, Basden, Basden, & Graham, 1976; Howard & Coe, 1980; Schuyler & Coe, 1981, 1989; Spanos & Radtke-Bodorik, 1980; Spanos, Radtke-Bodorik, & Stam, 1980; St. Jean & Coe, 1981). (More is said about posthypnotic amnesia in a later section.)

Role Demands

The *demands of the situation* must be considered in the hypnotic context. Such demands are often overriding and have been described in other contexts, such as the recognition of mores (Sarbin & Allen, 1968).

Orne (1959, 1969) determined, through postexperimental inquiry, that subjects who had accurately perceived the purpose of the experiment responded according to their interpretation of the experimenter's expectations. He speculated that the demand characteristics of the experiment may have aroused in the subjects the norm of "cooperation in the name of science." It made no difference whether subjects were simulating hypnosis or were "real" hypnotic subjects. Orne treats demand characteristics as artifacts; we view them as important determinants in the context.

Orne's simulator design was meant to separate behaviors conforming to implicit demands from those of "real" hypnotic responding (Orne, 1959). A good deal of research has shown that the design does in fact separate simulators from "real" subjects (e.g., the "real" subjects demonstrate trance logic, source amnesia, and other phenomena). However, the design has also been shown to be flawed, in that the demands on simulators are *not* the same as the demands on real subjects. Simulators are acting under the pressure of not being caught faking, and therefore probably become overly cautious and *too* responsive. "Real" subjects, not being under such pressure, are free to be more open and honest about their experiences. For example, Stanley, Lynn, and Nash (1986) demonstrated that one of Orne's trance logic phenomena, the subject's report of a transparent hypnotic hallucination, had "little to do with a heightened tolerance for logical incongruity, but simply reflect[ed] accurate reports of hypnotized subjects' imperfect hallucinatory experience" (p. 452).

It is clear that direct manipulation of demand characteristics affects hypnotic responsiveness (Coe, 1966), and that the wording and style of presenting instructions can change demands (Spanos, 1982; Wagstaff, 1981; Wedemeyer & Coe, 1981).

Reinforcing Properties of the Audience

The effect of the audience in the hypnotic context has not been evaluated with any rigor. One of our experiments suggested possible effects of an audience (Coe, 1966). One group of subjects was told they were being observed through a one-way mirror by clinical psychology graduate students, another group was told nothing (no mirror). Only one of the subjects in the "being observed" sample scored higher on a hypnosis scale than the matched partner in the control sample. A plausible explanation could be that the "observed" subjects reacted to being observed, or "analyzed," by clinical psychology students, and modified their responses in order not to appear poorly adjusted.

In stage hypnosis the audience is an important, if not *the* most important, feature of the context (Meeker & Barber, 1971). The feedback from the audience encourages more and more responsiveness for some subjects, and the stage hypnotist uses the audience purposely to maximize the entertaining quality of the performance.

In other social encounters, audiences are significant features of the total context. The psychology of impression management is not put aside when a person adopts the hypnosis role.

RESEARCH AND APPRAISAL

We now turn to empirical findings as they relate to our theoretical position. However, empirical findings, as reported in scientific journals, tell only a part of the modern story of hypnosis. Other, "nonscientific" influences must be identified, such as the sometimes unrecognized purposes guiding a particular theorist or researcher.

We have selected two phenomena that have claimed to demonstrate hypnosis-specific conduct and thereby to support the position that theoretical concepts specific to hypnosis are necessary. Our position makes the counterclaim that concepts drawn from social psychology are sufficient.

Source Amnesia

The operations defining source amnesia are as follows: (1) Hypnotized subjects are taught a little-known fact while hypnotized (e.g., the color of a heated amethyst). (2) They are given a posthypnotic suggestion that they will be amnesic for the entire hypnotic episode. (3) Posthypnotic amnesia is tested after they are awakened, including specific questions about things they have learned (e.g., "What is the color of a heated amethyst?"). (4) Some subjects give the correct response to the direct questions, but when asked *where* they had learned the answer(s), they say they don't know. That is, they appear to be amnesic for the *source* of their learning.

As we might expect, the investigators who "discovered" source amnesia already favored a view of hypnosis as a mental state (Cooper, 1966, 1972; Evans, 1979a, 1979b; Evans & Thorne, 1966). Being in support of a nonstate position, one of us was quite interested in evaluating critically how they arrived at their conclusions (Coe, 1978, 1989). It was not too surprising to find that Evans and Thorne (1966) made a questionable interpretation of the 6-point rating scale they used to measure source amnesia. According to their scale, they concluded that 10% of their hypnotized subjects, compared to 2% of their waking subjects, showed posthypnotic source amnesia. In the hypnotized 10%, however, they included subjects who actually reported hypnosis as the source of their learning, but the authors somehow decided that these subjects were only "guessing or deducing" the source. (No reliabilities were reported for the scale.) As a special phenomenon of hypnosis, source amnesia evaporated when these questionable subjects were removed as being source-amnesic (hypnotized, 4%; waking, 2%).

Evans and Thorne (1966) also made the surprising statement that recall amnesia and source amnesia were probably independent phenomena arising from different mechanisms. The surprising part of their statement was that they reported four positive correlations (ranging from .37 to .42, all P's .01) between recall amnesia and source amnesia. The "usual" interpretation of such relationships would have been in support of the two's being related, not for their being independent.

The subjects' stories are of potential interest as well. What were they telling themselves about the situation? Most of the high-scoring real subjects, and most of the simulators, did not answer the posthypnotic question correctly in the first place. They said they did not know the answer, and were therefore not faced with deciding how to respond if they had been asked how they knew. But subjects who answered correctly, whether because they reported honestly or because they were not sure what to say, then had to decide what to say about how they knew the correct answer. Subjects who were unsure were faced with an especially ambiguous test situation. Most subjects who answered correctly (at least 90%) simply said that they had learned the answer while they were hypnotized. However, a small percentage showed "source amnesia", that is, they said they did not know how they had learned the answer, or perhaps they reported some other source. The question then becomes this: Were these subjects really amnesic? Or did they simply give an answer that they believed appropriate under the circumstances?

A gap is left in the narrative, but fortunately some recent studies have helped to fill it. Spanos, Gwynn, Della Malva, and Bertrand (1988), in a series of three studies, narrowed down the possibilities that subjects would choose the source amnesia alternative. Their results indicated that under such circumstances source amnesia was simply one of several possible strategies for dealing with an ambiguous test situation. Hypnotic subjects who demonstrate source amnesia are probably not really amnesic after all. They are probably answering in a way that they believe is the most appropriate one at the time, given the conditions. Thus, they employ the strategy of secrets to keep intact their self-narratives.

Breaching Posthypnotic Amnesia

"Breaching posthypnotic amnesia" means that subjects who are presumably amnesic when posthypnotic amnesia is tested will then remember more before the reversal cue if external demands are placed on them to do so. The results of breaching studies have strong implications for theories of posthypnotic amnesia (and hypnosis). The characters in the breaching story are familiar. Investigators favoring a special-state view of hypnosis postulate that subjects will not breach amnesia, and investigators favoring a social-psychological view of hypnosis postulate that they will. If, for example, subjects are experiencing a special, dissociated state that blocks critical material from consciousness, then they should not be able to recall before the prearranged cue is administered, no matter how hard they try (Cooper, 1972; E. R. Hilgard, 1974, 1977a, 1977b; Kihlstrom, 1977, 1978, 1983). On the other hand, if subjects are viewed as employing strategies to deceive the hypnotist and/or themselves, they will be able to recall when external events favor it (Coe, 1978, 1980a, 1980b, 1989; Coe & Sarbin, 1977; Sarbin & Coe, 1972, 1979; Spanos, 1981, 1982, 1986).

The special-state investigators set the stage with two studies, which they interpreted as supporting the hypothesis that posthypnotic amnesia cannot be breached (K. S. Bowers, 1966; Kihlstrom, Evans, Orne, & Orne, 1980). A critical review of posthypnotic amnesia (Coe, 1978) questioned their conclusions, pointing out that in both studies about 50% of their initially amnesic subjects had breached, and that the results could as easily be interpreted in favor of breaching as in opposition to it. Kihlstrom wrote a rebuttal to the critique, interpreting the additional recall of the 50% as a natural remission over time, "at least in inexperienced subjects" (Kihlstrom, 1978, p. 258).

Coe suggested that the strength of the demands to breach was the critical factor in determining the extent of breaching. Kihlstrom did not disagree, but he wrote that until someone provided positive evidence with stronger demands, posthypnotic amnesia remained robust in the face of demands for honesty and extra effort to recall (the breaching conditions in the two studies cited above).

At the time, both Kihlstrom and Coe probably appreciated the professional exposure from the controversy. Even so, it stimulated further research. Following the proposition that stronger demands to breach would lead to more breaching, Coe and associates carried out a series of studies evaluating various types of breaching circumstances.

They begin by comparing independent samples across different breaching conditions, including a control sample that was only asked to recall a second time before the reversal cue (Coe & Sluis, 1989; Coe & Tucibat, 1988; Coe & Yashinski, 1985; Howard & Coe, 1980; Schuyler & Coe, 1981, 1989). In the early studies a "lie detector" condition was used (sometimes subjects were only told the machine worked like a lie detector; sometimes they were told it indicated they were telling a lie), an "honesty" condition (sometimes they were told they were telling the truth), and a no-pressure condition (control). In general, except for the "truth" condition, it was shown that subjects in the breaching conditions recalled more than the controls; that is, they showed significant breaching.

But of more interest was an unexpected finding: Subjects' ratings of their initial, amnesic recall on a simple 4-point rating scale of "volition over remembering" were systematically related to their breaching. Most of the subjects who did *not* breach under pressure also rated their initial recall as either "mostly out of their control" or "completely out of their control" (i.e., as "involuntary"). The findings in the control samples were even clearer. About one-half of the control subjects did breach, but almost all of them rated their initial recall as "voluntary" ("mostly" or "completely" under their control). Thus, subjects' ratings of their control over remembering were seemingly important for making sense of breaching posthypnotic amnesia.

The Coe and Sluis (1989) study considerably increased the demands on subjects to breach. After their initial testing for posthypnotic amnesia, they were given, *in order*, the following conditions: (1) an "honesty" recall; (2) a "you're lying" recall; (3) a recall after viewing a videotape of themselves during the session (see McConkey & Sheehan, 1981; McConkey, Sheehan, & Cross, 1980); and (4) the recall after the cue lifting posthypnotic amnesia. The recall-testing period lasted about 50 minutes. Control subjects sat for the same amount of time, but were only asked whether they remembered more at the times that corresponded to those of the three breaching conditions. The result was that all but 1 of the 19 breaching subjects breached almost entirely before amnesia was lifted, *even* those who rated their recall as "involuntary." Coe and Sluis believed they had made their point—namely, that with enough pressure all subjects would probably breach. Also, there was no natural remission of amnesia over time (as Kihlstrom had postulated) for the involuntary, control subjects. Although the "voluntary" subjects in the control sample breached, the "involuntary" counterparts did not.

Some parts of the breaching narrative appear to be satisfactorily complete at this point; other parts still have some obvious gaps. Kihlstrom's suggestion that posthypnotic amnesia will remain robust in the face of increasing demands to breach has not been supported. It appears highly probable that all subjects are likely to breach as external demands to do so increase. Subjects who rate their amnesia as "voluntary" are likely to breach over time with only additional recall requests, whereas special pressures may well be necessary to cause breaching in subjects who rate their amnesia as "involuntary."

Kihlstrom's theory that posthypnotic amnesia can be expected to dissipate naturally over time still requires further evaluation. We do not know whether "voluntaries" will tell us more if they simply sit for 50 minutes and are then again asked to recall, without recall requests in between. "Involuntaries" will almost certainly not show dissipation over the 50-minute time period if they are not asked to recall until the period is over. But what about a day later, a week later, and so on? The story goes on, awaiting investigators who are interested enough to fill in the empty pages.

CONCLUSION

The version of role theory we presented earlier is still defensible, but because the focus of interest in recent years has been on the subject's phenomenology (or, more accurately, on the subject's self-report), we have expanded the theory. Taking amnesia as a prime exemplar of self-reports, we offered an analysis that added such concepts as secrets, metaphors, deception, and self-deception (Sarbin & Coe, 1979). Subsequently, Sarbin introduced the narrational principle—a principle that views human actions as storied. Instead of accepting self-reports of hallucination, analgesia, and amnesia as reflections of happenings inside some postulated mental apparatus, we take the position that such paradoxical utterances are not happenings in the mind, but doings (i.e., actions of performing persons). These actions are neither random nor mechanical; they are intentional and continuous with the person's self-narrative.

Implicit in the concept of role is the wider conception that any role is enacted in a context, a narrative, involving other persons. And because people have the power of imagination (i.e., silently acting as if), they can construct stories about themselves. Thus, to understand the self-reports of hypnosis subjects, we find the concept of self-narrative indispensable. When subjects enter the laboratory (or clients the consulting room), they do not leave their self-narratives in the outer office as they do their books and raincoats. As they listen to the hypnotic induction, they enter a problem-solving situation—one of how to make sense of the content, much of which (if interpreted literally) could be classified as nonsense. Some people assign literal meanings to the utterances, and we call them nonhypnotizable. Others, however, grasp the concealed intent of the induction: "Please participate in a miniature drama" (Sarbin, 1980, 1986). Having accepted the implied invitation, subjects play out the drama within the constraints of their imaginative and rhetorical skills.

The enactment will usually proceed smoothly, unless what is asked is contrary to important value elements in the subject's self-narrative. But a problematic situation arises when subjects are asked to provide self-reports of their experiences. Take amnesia, for example. In well-disposed subjects, the self-reports imply "I don't remember" or "I don't know." However, we know that under moderate pressures for veridical reporting, about half the subjects breach amnesia and tell us more (e.g., Howard & Coe, 1980). And these are the same subjects who tend to report that they have been "doing" something in order not to remember. It would be correct to conclude that such subjects have been engaging in deception. It could be added that their admission of deception, morally untainted of course, is acceptable to their ongoing self-narratives. In short, they have reasons for accepting the hypnosis role, first claiming amnesia, and then ultimately disclaiming it. As pressures to breach are increased, even subjects who claim they are *not* doing something to maintain amnesia also eventually breach (Coe & Sluis, 1989). Others, however, who are only asked whether they can recall more over the same time period without extra pressures, maintain their claim of being unable to remember. And they tend also to claim that they are *not* doing anything to remain amnesic. These subjects, and those who are under moderate pressures to breach but who do not, may be thought of as self-deceived.

Self-deception is not an occult process, although it is less familiar than repression, rationalization, and the other "mechanisms of defense." Fingarette (1971) has made it clear that people have reasons for wanting to conceal things about themselves from themselves and that they employ various skills to do so.

It is also important to add that self-deception is not necessarily permanent. Freud, for one, wrote convincing narratives about patients who were able to disclose the secrets that they had been hiding from others and from themselves. And, as we have seen, hypnosis subjects under coercive conditions will disclose the secrets they have imposed on the experimental context.

Our conclusion is straightforward: Self-reports are not reflections of mysterious mental states, but can be located in the wider context of self-narratives—where subjects are seen as the agents of their actions, as doers, as performers. Their actions are not prompted by unknowable forces, but are performed for *reasons*. To locate the reasons for paradoxical, counterexpectational behavior, one must look beyond the immediate situation and consider the subjects' self-narratives.

Such a departure from the usual paradigm of rigorous experimentation requires no new methodology. The clinical reports of Josephine Hilgard (J. R. Hilgard, 1979) provide appropriate models. Clinical interviews, a procedure for eliciting self-narratives, support her claim that hypnotizability is related to imaginative involvement ("organismic involvement," in role theory). The wealth of storied information in her book would not have been gathered in the typical laboratory experiment.

In sum, we have tried to show how role theory can be used as a guide for filling in the gaps in our knowledge. Its concepts direct attention to different aspects of persons and situations in the hypnotic context. Its supposition is that conduct cannot be understood accurately in isolation from the environments in which it occurs, and that interactions among situational and personal characteristics must be considered. The metaphors of a contextual view should help to clear away the mystical and the occult associations with hypnosis, which are being kept alive by using opaque concepts such as "trance" and "state" (Sarbin, 1977).

Like all stories, ours has a moral for the next generation of scientists: When faced with a paradox, avoid occult and mentalistic explanations. Instead, look upon hypnotic subjects as the authors of their actions, including what they do and what they say about what they do.

REFERENCES

Andersen, M. L. (1963). *Correlates of hypnotic performance: An historical and role theoretical analysis.* Unpublished doctoral dissertation, University of California, Berkeley.

As, A. (1963). Hypnotizability as a function of nonhypnotic experiences. *Journal of Abnormal and Social Psychology, 66,* 142–150.

Balaschak, B., Blocker, K., Rossiter, T., & Perin, C. T. (1970). Influence of race and expressed experience of the hypnotist on hypnotic susceptibility. *Proceedings of the 78th Annual Convention of the American Psychological Association, 5.*

Barber, T. X. (1965). Measuring "hypnotic-like" suggestibility with and without "hypnotic induction": Psychometric properties, norms and variables influencing response to the Barber Suggestibility Scale (BSS). *Psychological Reports, 16,* 809–844.

Barber, T. X. (1969). *Hypnosis: A scientific approach.* New York: Van Nostrand Reinhold.

Barber, T. X., Dalal, A. S., & Calverley, D. S. (1968). The subjective reports of hypnotic subjects. *American Journal of Clinical Hypnosis, 11,* 74–88.

Barber, T. X., & Wilson, S. C. (1977). Hypnosis, suggestions and altered states of consciousness: Experimental evaluation of the new cognitive–behavioral theory and the traditional trance-state theory of "hypnosis." *Annals of the New York Academy of Sciences, 296,* 34–47.

Bowers, K. S. (1966). Hypnotic behavior: The differentiation of trance and demand characteristic variables. *Journal of Abnormal Psychology, 71*, 42–51.

Bowers, P. G., & Bowers, K. S. (1979). Hypnosis and creativity: A theoretical & empirical rapprochement. In E. Fromm & R. E. Shor (Eds.), *Hypnosis: Developments in research and new perspectives* (2nd ed.). Chicago: Aldine.

Coe, W. C. (1966). Hypnosis as role enactment: The role demand variable. *American Journal of Clinical Hypnosis, 8*, 189–191.

Coe, W. C. (1978). The creditability of posthypnotic amnesia: A contextualist's view. *International Journal of Clinical and Experimental Hypnosis, 26*(4), 218–245.

Coe, W. C. (1980a). On defining altered states of consciousness in hypnosis. *Hypnosis: The Bulletin of the British Society of Experimental and Clinical Hypnosis*, (3), 8–10.

Coe, W. C. (1980b). Posthypnotic amnesia. In R. H. Woody (Ed.)., *Encyclopedia of clinical assessment* (pp. 942–954). San Francisco: Jossey-Bass.

Coe, W. C. (1989). Posthypnotic amnesia: Theory and research. In N. P. Spanos & J. F. Chaves (Eds.), *Hypnosis: The cognitive–behavioral perspective* (pp. 110–148). Buffalo, NY: Prometheus Books.

Coe, W. C., Bailey, J. R., Hall, J. C., Howard, M. L., Jonda, R. L., Kobayashi, K., & Parker, M. D. (1970). Hypnosis as role enactment: The role location variable. In *Proceedings of the 79th Annual Convention of the American Psychological Association, 5*.

Coe, W. C., Basden, B., Basden, D., & Graham, C. (1976). Posthypnotic amnesia: Suggestions of an active process in dissociative phenomena. *Journal of Abnormal Psychology, 85*, 455–458.

Coe. W. C., & Sarbin, T. R. (1966). An experimental demonstration of hypnosis as role enactment. *Journal of Abnormal Psychology, 71*, 400–416.

Coe, W. C., & Sarbin, T. R. (1977). Hypnosis from the standpoint of a contextualist. *Annals of the New York Academy of Sciences, 296*, 2–13.

Coe, W. C., & Sluis, A. (1989). Increasing contextual pressures to breach posthypnotic amnesia. *Journal of Personality and Social Psychology, 57*, 885–894.

Coe, W. C., & Tucibat, M. (1988). *The relationship between volition and the breaching of posthypnotic amnesia.* Paper presented at the meeting of the American Psychological Association, New Orleans, Aug. 1989.

Coe, W. C., & Yashinski, E. (1985). Volitional experiences associated with breaching posthypnotic amnesia. *Journal of Personality and Social Psychology, 48*, 716–722.

Cooper, L. M. (1966). Spontaneous and suggested posthypnotic source amnesia. *Intrnational Journal of Clinical and Experimental Hypnosis, 2*, 180–192.

Cooper, L. M. (1972). Hypnotic amnesia. In E. Fromm & R. E. Shor (Eds.), *Hypnosis: Research developments and perspectives* (pp. 217–252). Chicago: Aldine-Atherton.

Council, J. R., Kirsch, I., & Hafner, L. P. (1986). Expectancy vs. absorption in the prediction of hypnotic responding. *Journal of Personality and Social Psychology, 50*(1), 182–189.

Evans, F. J. (1979a). Contextual forgetting: Posthypnotic source amnesia. *Journal of Abnormal Psychology, 88*, 556–563.

Evans, F. J. (1979b). Hot amethysts, eleven fingers and the Oriental Express. In G. D. Burrows, D. R. Colhson, & L. Dennerstein (Eds.), *Hypnosis 1979*. Amsterdam: Elsevier/North Holland.

Evans, F. J., & Kihlstrom, J. F. (1973). Posthypnotic amnesia as disrupted retrieval. *Journal of Abnormal Psychology, 82*, 317–323.

Evans, F. J., & Thorne, W. A. (1966). Two types of posthypnotic amnesia: Recall amnesia and source amnesia. *International Journal of Clinical and Experimental Hypnosis, 2,* 162–179.

Fingarette, H. (1971). *Self-deception.* London: Routledge & Kegan Paul.

Greenberg, R. P., & Land, J. M. (1970). Influence of some hypnotist and subject variables on hypnotic susceptibility. *Journal of Consulting and Clinical Psychology, 37*(1), 111–115.

Hilgard, E. R. (1974). Toward a neodissocation theory: Multiple cognitive controls in human functioning. *Perspectives in Biology and Medicine, 17,* 301–316.

Hilgard, E. R. (1977a). *Divided consciousness: Multiple controls in human thought and action.* New York: Wiley.

Hilgard, E. R. (1977b). The problem of divided consciousness: A neodissociation interpretation. *Annals of the New York Academy of Sciences, 296,* 48–59.

Hilgard, E. R. (1979). Divided consciousness in hypnosis: The implications of the hidden observer. In E. Fromm & R. E. Shor (Eds.), *Hypnosis: Developments in research and new perspectives* (2nd ed., pp. 45–79). Chicago: Aldine.

Hilgard, E. R., & Crawford, H. J. (1979). The Stanford Hypnotic Arm Levitation Induction and Test (SHALIT): A six-minute hypnotic induction and measurement scale. *International Journal of Clinical and Experimental Hypnosis, 27,* 111–124.

Hilgard, J. R. (1979). *Personality and hypnosis: A study of imaginative involvement* (2nd ed.). Chicago: University of Chicago Press.

Howard, M. L., & Coe, W. C. (1980). The effects of context and subjects' perceived control in breaching posthypnotic amnesia. *Journal of Personality, 48*(3), 342–359.

Kihlstrom, J. F. (1977). Models of posthypnotic amnesia. *Annals of the New York Academy of Sciences, 296,* 284–301.

Kihlstrom, J. F. (1978). Context and cognition in posthypnotic phenomena. *International Journal of Clinical and Experimental Hypnosis, 26,* 246–267.

Kihlstrom, J. F. (1983). Instructed forgetting: Hypnotic and nonhypnotic. *Journal of Experimental Psychology: General, 112,* 73–79.

Kihlstrom, J. F., Evans, F. J., Orne, M. T., & Orne, E. C. (1980). Attempting to breach posthypnotic amnesia. *Journal of Abnormal Psychology, 89,* 603–616.

Kihlstrom, J. F., & Shor, R. E. (1978). Recall and recognition during posthypnotic amnesia. *International Journal of Clinical and Experimental Hypnosis, 26*(4), 330–349.

Kirsch, I. (1985). Response expectancy as a determinate of experience and behavior. *American Psychologist, 40*(11), 1189–1202.

Kirsch, I., Council, J. R., & Vickery, A. R. (1984). The role of expectancy in eliciting hypnotic responses as a function of type of induction. *Journal of Consulting and Clinical Psychology, 52,* 708–709.

London, P. (1962). *Children's Hypnotic Susceptibility Scale.* Palo Alto, CA: Consulting Psychologists Press.

McConkey, K. M., & Sheehan, P. W. (1981). The impact of videotape playback of hypnotic events on posthypnotic amnesia. *Journal of Abnormal Psychology, 90,* 46–54.

McConkey, K. M., Sheehan, P. W., & Cross, D. G. (1980). Posthypnotic amnesia:

Seeing is not remembering. *British Journal of Social and Clinical Psychology, 19,* 99–107.

Meeker, W. B., & Barber, T. X. (1971). Toward an explanation of stage hypnosis. *Journal of Abnormal Psychology, 77,* 61–70.

Morgan, A. H., & Hilgard, J. R. (1979a). The Stanford Hypnotic Clinical Scale for Adults. *American Journal of Clinical Hypnosis, 21,* 134–147.

Morgan, A. H., & Hilgard, J. R. (1979b). The Stanford Hypnotic Clinical Scale for Children. *American Journal of Clinical Hypnosis, 21,* 148–169.

Nash, M. R., & Spindler, D. (1989). Hypnosis and transference: A measure of archaic involvement. *International Journal of Clinical and Experimental Hypnosis, 37,* 129–144.

Orne, M. T. (1959). The nature of hypnosis: Artifact and essence. *Journal of Abnormal and Social Psychology, 58,* 277–299.

Orne, M. T. (1969). Demand characteristics and the concept of quasi-controls. In R. Rosenthal & R. Rosnow (Eds.), *Artifact in behavioral research* (pp. 143–179). New York: Academic Press.

Orne, M. T., & O'Connell, D. N. (1967). Diagnostic ratings of hypnotizability. *International Journal of Clinical and Experimental Hypnosis, 15,* 125–133.

St. Jean, R., & Coe, W. C. (1981). Recall and recognition memory during posthypnotic amnesia: A failure to confirm the disrupted-search hypothesis and the memory disorganization hypothesis. *Journal of Abnormal Psychology, 90*(3), 231–241.

Sarbin, T. R. (1950). Contributions to role-taking theory: I. Hypnotic behavior. *Psychological Review, 57,* 255–270.

Sarbin, T. R. (1956). Physiological effect of hypnotic stimulation. In R. M. Dorcus (Ed.), *Hypnosis and its therapeutic applications.* New York: McGraw-Hill.

Sarbin, T. R. (1977). Contextualism: A world view for modern psychology. In A. Landfield (Ed.), *Nebraska Symposium on Motivation.* Lincoln: University of Nebraska Press.

Sarbin, T. R. (1980). Hypnosis: Metaphorical encounters of the fourth kind. *Semiotica, 30,* 195–209.

Sarbin, T. R. (1981). On self-deception. *Annals of the New York Academy of Sciences, 364,* 220–235.

Sarbin, T. R. (Ed.). (1986). *Narrative psychology: The storied nature of human conduct.* New York: Praeger.

Sarbin, T. R., & Allen, V. L. (1968). Role theory. In G. Lindzey & E. Aronson (Eds.), *Handbook of social psychology* (Vol. 1). Boston, MA: Addison-Wesley.

Sarbin, T. R., & Coe, W. C. (1972). *Hypnosis: A social psychological analysis of influence communication.* New York: Holt, Rinehart & Winston.

Sarbin, T. R., & Coe, W. C. (1979). Psychopathology and hypnosis: Replacing old myths with fresh metaphors. *Journal of Abnormal Psychology, 88*(5), 506–526.

Schuyler, B. A., & Coe, W. C. (1981). A physiological investigation of volitional and nonvolitional experience during posthypnotic amnesia. *Journal of Personality and Social Psychology, 40*(5), 1160–1169.

Schuyler, B. A., & Coe, W. C. (1989). Volitional and nonvolitional experiences during posthypnotic amnesia. *International Journal of Clinical and Experimental Hypnosis, 28,* 320–331.

Sheehan, P. W. (1979). Hypnosis and the process of imagination. In E. Fromm & R. E. Shor (Eds.) *Hypnosis: Developments in research and new perspectives* (pp. 381–411). Chicago: Aldine.

Shor, R. E. (1962). Three dimensions of hypnotic depth. *International Journal of Clinical and Experimental Hypnosis. 10*, 23–28.

Shor, R. E., & Orne, E. C. (1962). *The Harvard Group Scale of Hypnotic Susceptibility, Form A.* Palo Alto, CA: Consulting Psychologists Press.

Shor, R. E., Orne, M. T., & O'Connell, D. N. (1962). Validation and cross-validation of a scale of self-reported personal experiences which predict hypnotizability. *Journal of Psychology, 53,* 55–75.

Spanos, N. P. (1981). Hypnotic responding: Automatic dissociation or situation relevant cognizing? In. E. Klinger (Ed.), *Imagery: Concepts, results and applications.* New York: Plenum Press.

Spanos, N. P. (1982). A social psychological approach to hypnotic behavior. In G. Weary & H. L. Mirels (Eds.), *Integrations of clinical and social psychology* (pp. 231–271). New York: Oxford University Press.

Spanos, N. P. (1986). Hypnotic behavior: A social psychological interpretation of amnesia, analgesia, and "trance logic." *Behavioral and Brain Sciences, 9,* 449–467.

Spanos, N. P., & Barber, T. X. (1974). Toward a convergence in hypnosis research. *American Psychologist, 29,* 500–511.

Spanos, N. P., & Chaves, J. F. (Eds.). (1989). *Hypnosis: The cognitive–behavioral perspective.* Buffalo, NY: Prometheus Books.

Spanos, N. P., Gwynn, M. I., Della Malva, C. L., & Bertrand, L. D. (1988). Social psychological factors in the genesis of posthypnotic source amnesia. *Journal of Abnormal Psychology, 97,* 322–329.

Spanos, N. P., & Radtke-Bodorik, H. L. (1980). Integrating hypnotic phenomena with cognitive psychology: An illustration using suggested amnesia. *Bulletin of the British Society of Experimental and Clinical Hypnosis, 3,* 4–7.

Spanos, N. P., Radtke-Bodorik, H. L., & Stam, H. J. (1980). disorganized recall during suggested amnesia: Fact not artifact. *Journal of Abnormal Psychology, 89(1),* 1–19.

Spanos, N. P., Radtke, H. L., Hodgins, D. C., Stam, H. J., & Bertrand, L. D. (1983). The Carleton University Responsiveness to Suggestion Scale: Normative data and psychometric properties. *Psychological Reports, 53,* 523–535.

Stanley, S., Lynn, S. J., & Nash, M. R. (1986). Trance logic, susceptibility screening, and the transparency response. *Journal of Personality and Social Psychology, 50,* 447–454.

Tart, C. T. (1979). Measuring the depth of an altered state of consciousness, with particular reference to self-report scales of hypnotic depth. In E. Fromm & R. E. Shor (Eds.), *Hypnosis: Developments in research and new perspectives* (2nd ed.). Chicago: Aldine.

Tellegen, A. (1978). *Differential Personality Questionnaire.* Minneapolis: University of Minnesota.

Tellegen, A., & Atkinson, G. (1974). Openness to absorption and self-altering experiences ("absorption"), a trait related to hypnotic susceptibility. *Journal of Abnormal Psychology, 83,* 268–277.

Wagstaff, G. F. (1981). *Hypnosis, compliance and belief.* New York: St. Martin's Press.

Wedemeyer, C., & Coe, W. C. (1981). Hypnotic state reports: Contextual variation and phenomenological criteria. *Journal of Mental Imagery*, 5(2), 107–118.

Weitzenhoffer, A. M., & Hilgard, E. R. (1959). *Stanford Hypnotic Susceptibility Scale, Forms A and B*. Palo Alto, CA: Consulting Psychologists Press.

Weitzenhoffer, A. M., & Hilgard, E. R. (1962). *Stanford Hypnotic Susceptibility Scale, Form C*. Palo Alto, CA: Consulting Psychologists Press.

Weitzenhoffer, A. M., & Hilgard, E. R. (1967). *Revised Stanford Profile Scales of Hypnotic Susceptibility: Forms I and II*. Palo Alto, CA: Consulting Psychologists Press.

A Sociocognitive Approach to Hypnosis

NICHOLAS P. SPANOS
Carlton University

INTRODUCTION

Since the late 18th century, the topic of hypnosis (initially labeled "mesmerism") has been associated with a wide range of nonordinary behaviors. Historically, attempts to provide a scientific account of hypnotic phenomena have often taken the nonordinary behavior of hypnotic subjects at face value. These accounts (i.e., "special-process theories") have been grounded on the assumption that hypnotic behavior differs fundamentally from nonhypnotic responding, and , for this reason, hypnotic responding requires special or nonordinary explanations. Typically, these traditional accounts have held that hypnotic procedures produce an altered state of consciousness (a hypnotic trance state) in predisposed (i.e., highly hypnotizable) individuals, and that this altered state in turn produces or facilitates the automatic occurrence of response to suggestions (Sarbin, 1962; Spanos & Gottlieb, 1979).

The sociocognitive account of hypnotic responding that I describe herein challenges the assumptions that underlie traditional views of hypnosis. According to my account, hypnotic behaviors, despite their nonordinary appearance, are fundamentally similar to other more mundane forms of social action and can be accounted for without recourse to special psychological states or processes. Rather than viewing hypnotic subjects as "entranced" or "dissociated," I view them as agents who are attuned to contextual demands and who guide their behavior in terms of their understandings of situational contingencies and in terms of the goals they wish to achieve (Spanos, 1982, 1986a, 1986b, 1986c, 1989). Thus, from my perspective, successful hypnotic responding to suggestions for age regression, analgesia, amnesia, and the like reflects goal-directed actions by subjects who, in coordinated fashion, generate experiences and enact behaviors in order to meet what they tacitly understand to be the requirements of the test situation.

My sociocognitive formulation is strongly related to formulations proffered by Barber (1969), Coe (1978, 1989), Sarbin (1950, 1989; Sarbin & Coe, 1972) and Wagstaff (1981, 1986), as well as other investigators (see Spanos & Chaves, 1989). All of these formulations have as their modern precursor the work of Robert White (1941). Although White (1941) believed that hypnotic responding involved an altered state of consciousness, he also conceptualized such behavior as determined by subjects' implicit expectations and guided by their attempts to present themselves in terms of what they believed the hypnotist was looking for. Thus, for White (1941), hypnotic behavior was motivated, goal-directed, and interpersonal. Hypnotic subjects used the information transmitted to them by the hypnotist to continually refine their image of what constituted "being hypnotized." Such subjects were seen as motivated to present themselves in terms of the conception that they and the hypnotist shared concerning what constituted hypnotic behavior.

The most important theoretical extension of White's (1941) work has been provided by T. R. Sarbin (1950, 1962, 1989). Sarbin (1950) built on White's (1941) notion that hypnotic responding is goal-directed action, and was the first modern theorist to explicitly reject the notion that hypnotic responding requires an explanation in terms of altered states of consciousness. Sarbin (1950) was heavily influenced by the symbolic interactionist tradition in social psychology. This tradition (Biddle & Thomas, 1966; Stryker, 1981) draws many of its metaphors from the theater and conceptualizes people as actors whose interactions are guided by the information they possess about one another's social roles.

Resistance to Sarbin's (1950) role theory formulation was maintained, in part, by the persistent belief that hypnotic procedures produced at least some highly unusual responses that transcended the capacities of "nonhypnotized" subjects. Beginning in the late 1950s, however, this issue was made central to the research program initiated by T. X. Barber (1969). Barber's (1969) research aim was to delineate the social-psychological antecedents of hypnotic behavior. To this end, he and his associates experimentally examined a wide range of suggested behaviors (for reviews, see Barber, 1969; Barber, Spanos, & Chaves, 1974). The results of these studies demonstrated the following: (1) Control subjects, who were administered no special preliminary procedures of any kind, regularly enacted the criterion responses called for by suggestions for age regression, hallucination, pain reduction, amnesia, and so on. (2) The administration of a hypnotic procedure produced only a small increment

in responsiveness to suggestions above control levels. (3) Task-motivational instructions given to nonhypnotic subjects produced as large an
increment in responsiveness to suggestion as did hypnotic induction
procedures.

Barber's (1969) repeated demonstrations that hypnotic responses
were not extraordinary and could be easily matched by the behavior or
nonhypnotic subjects have provided empirical legitimation for the view
that hypnotic responding is goal-directed action. My own sociocognitive
view of hypnosis has been built on the frameworks provided by the work
of Sarbin and Barber.

THEORETICAL CONCEPTS AND PRINCIPLES

The sociocognitive view of hypnotic responding is premised on the notion
that people are sentient agents continually involved in organizing sensory
inputs into meaningful categories or schemas that are used to guide
actions. People negotiate their environments in terms of their implicit
understandings. Interaction between individuals usually proceeds
smoothly, because the interacting parties share similar understandings of
their common situation and of the reciprocal roles they are to play within
the confines of their shared definition of the situation (Stryker, 1981).

Interaction proceeds through mutually negotiated self-presentations
and reciprocal role validation. Role enactment is rule-governed and
involves the tacit understandings of the actors concerning (1) the way in
which the situation is defined, and (2) the behaviors that are considered
appropriate to that definition of the situation. From this perspective,
hypnotic responding is viewed as role enactment. The term "hypnosis" is
seen as referring not to a "state" or condition of the person, but to the
historically rooted conceptions of hypnotic responding that are held by the
participants in the minidrama that is labeled the "hypnotic situation".
Hypnotic responding is conceptualized as context-dependent and as
determined by subjects' willingness to adopt the hypnotic role; by their
understandings of what is expected in that role; by how their understandings of role requirements change as the situation unfolds;by how they
interpret the ambiguous communications that constitute hypnotic test
suggestions; by their abilities to generate the imaginal and other
experiences called for by the suggestions; and by how feedback from the
hypnotist and from their own responding influences the definitions they
hold of themselves as hypnotic subjects. Thus, according to the sociocognitive formulation, hypnotic behavior appears to be unusual not because it
has unusual causes, but because the hypnotic role calls for (and the
hypnotic situation legitimates) unusual behavioral enactments. In the

remainder of this chapter, I examine the implications of this view for an understanding of several of the phenomena considered central to the topic of hypnosis.

RESEARCH AND APPRAISAL

Reports of Responding Involuntarily

Hypnotic subjects sometimes report that their responses to suggestions occur effortlessly and involuntarily. Special-process theorists have used such reports as evidence that hypnotic subjects have lost control over their own responding—for example, "one of the most striking findings of hypnosis is the loss of control over actions normally voluntary" (Hilgard, 1977a, p. 115). My sociocognitive position suggests instead that hypnotic subjects retain control of their behavior, but sometimes come to interpret their goal-directed responses as involuntary occurrences (Spanos, Rivers, & Ross, 1977; Spanos, 1986b; Spanos, Salas, Bertrand, & Johnston, 1989).

People in our culture hold relatively well-developed schemas concerning what it means to by "hypnotized." Central to these schemas is the belief that the responses to suggestions made by "hypnotized" subjects are involuntary occurrences (London, 1961; McConkey, 1986; Spanos, Salas, et al., 1989). Subjects who participate in hypnosis experiments hold the same preconceptions about hypnotic behavior as individuals in the culture at large. Moreover, the procedures to which these subjects are exposed in the hypnotic test situation usually reinforce the notion that hypnotic responses are involuntary happenings rather than self-initiated actions. The most important aspect of the hypnotic test situation in this regard is probably the wording of test suggestions (Spanos, 1986b).

Hypnotic suggestions do *not* explicitly instruct subjects to carry out overt behaviors. Instead, suggestions are worded in the passive voice and inform subjects that certain events are happening *to* them. For instance, suggestions inform subjects that an outstretched arm feels light and is rising in the air; that they are unable, despite their efforts, to stand up from the chair; and so on. In short, suggestions invite subjects to adopt and temporarily treat as veridical an imaginary or counterfactual definition of the situation—namely, that their own actions are no longer self-initiated or goal-directed.

A number of studies indicate that the passive wording of suggestions is a particularly important determinant of subjects' reports that their responses have occurred involuntarily (Miller & Bowers, 1986; Spanos & Barber, 1972; Spanos & de Groh, 1983; Spanos & Katsanis, 1989; Weitzenhoffer, 1974). For example, (Spanos & Gorassini, 1984) administered three suggestions calling for motoric responses (e.g., arm lowering) under one condition, and direct instructions calling for the same behaviors under a second condition. The instructions and suggestions were equal in length but differed in their designation of the target behavior as either a voluntary action (e.g., "Raise you arm") or an involuntary happening (e.g., "Your arm is rising"). Subjects almost always made the overt movements when given the instructions, but they frequently failed to do so when given the suggestions. On the other hand, subjects rated their movements as more involuntary when given the suggestions as opposed to the instructions.

Of particular importance is the finding of several studies that hypnotic and nonhypnotic subjects gave equivalently high ratings of involuntariness when administered suggestions and equivalently low ratings when administered instructions (Spanos & Gorassini, 1984; Spanos & Katsanis, 1989). For example, we (Spanos & Katsanis, 1989) extended work by Miller and Bowers (1986) on the relationship between hypnotic procedures and reports of involuntary pain reduction. Miller and Bowers (1986) found that hypnotic subjects given a passively worded suggestion were more likely to indicate that their pain reductions occurred without cognitive effort than were nonhypnotic subjects who had been explicitly instructed to use cognitive strategies actively to reduce their pain. Miller and Bowers (1986) concluded that pain reduction in hypnosis occurs as a result of an unconscious dissociation process, whereas nonhypnotic analgesia is mediated by the use of cognitive strategies.

We (Spanos & Katsanis, 1989) suggested instead that hypnotic and nonhypnotic subjects are equally likely to use cognitive strategies, and, furthermore, that the extent to which subjects define their pain reductions and their use of coping strategies as effortful or effortless is more closely tied to the wording of instructions and suggestions than to the definition of the situation as hypnotic or nonhypnotic. We administered hypnotic suggestions for analgesia to some highly hypnotizable subjects and nonhypnotic analgesia suggestions to others. Half of the subjects in each group were informed that pain reduction would occur effortlessly and involuntarily (e.g., "Simply let everything that is suggested happen to you"). The remaining hypnotic and nonhypnotic subjects were informed that analgesia required them to direct their thoughts and images actively. The suggestion administered to all four groups called for subjects to imagine their test hand as protected by a heavy glove.

Subjects in the two hypnotic treatments defined themselves as being more deeply hypnotized than did those in the nonhypnotic treatments. Nevertheless, subjects in the four groups reported equivalent reductions in pain and equivalent use of coping imagery. Most importantly, hypnotic *and* nonhypnotic subjects who received passively worded suggestions tended to rate their pain reductions and coping strategies as occurring automatically and without active effort, whereas hypnotic *and* nonhypnotic subjects who received actively worded suggestions tended to rate their pain reductions and strategies as requiring active cognitive effort.

Our failure (Spanos & Katsanis, 1989) to find differences between hypnotic and nonhypnotic subjects in ratings of involuntariness even when the hypnotic subjects defined themselves as much more deeply hypnotized than the nonhypnotic subjects runs contrary to the assertion of Miller and Bowers (1986) that highly hypnotizable hypnotic subjects experience their pain reductions as occurring more effortlessly and involuntarily than do nonhypnotic subjects. These findings (along with others reviewed later) are also difficult to reconcile with the notion that reports of involuntariness reflect a hypnosis-facilitated dissociation in cognitive controls (Hilgard, 1977a; Miller & Bowers, 1986). On the other hand, these findings are consistent with the hypothesis that both hypnotic and nonhypnotic analgesia result from the goal-directed cognizing of active agents, as well as the hypothesis that reports of involuntary analgesia are not intrinsic to hypnotic responding, but instead reflect schema-based interpretations of goal-directed action.

Suggestion wording is not the only variable that influences the involuntariness reports of hypnotic subjects, and the role of other factors in this regard has been reviewed in detail elsewhere (Lynn, Rhue, & Weeks, 1989; Spanos, 1986c).

Individual Differences

It is well known that people show wide individual differences in response to hypnotic suggestions and that these individual differences tend to remain stable across different hypnotizability scales and after even long temporal intervals (Hilgard, 1987). Relatedly, in the 1960s and 1970s, a number of experiments aimed at enhancing hypnotic responsiveness obtained only small and sometimes nonsignificant increments (Perry, 1977). Taken together, the long-term stability of hypnotizability, its cross-scale consistency, and its apparent resistance to modification have led to the hypothesis that hypnotizability reflects a stable and relatively unchangeable trait-like psychological capacity (Bowers, 1976; Hilgard, 1977a; Perry, 1977).

Unlike trait formulations, a sociocognitive approach emphasizes that stable individual differences in hypnotizability reflect, to a substantial degree, stability in the attitudes, expectations, and interpretations that subjects bring to or develop in the hypnotic test situation (Diamond, 1977; Spanos, 1986a). The sociocognitive approach does not deny that stable differences in imaginal propensities or in other cognitive abilities may play an important role in hypnotizability. However, stable cognitive abilities are likely to exert their effects only in interaction with the situation-specific attitudes and interpretations that constitute subjects' understandings of task demands and subjects' motivations to align their experiences and behaviors in terms of those demands (Spanos, 1986a).

The important role of context-specific variable in influencing the cross-test stability of hypnotic responsiveness was recently illustrated by varying the definition of the situation in which subjects were tested for responsiveness to suggestions. We (Spanos, Gabora, Jarrett, & Gwynn, 1989) tested subjects on two different hypnotizability scales. For half the subjects both scales were defined as tests of hypnosis; under these circumstances, a high correlation was obtained between scores on the two scales. For the remaining subjects only the first scale was defined as a test of hypnosis. After responding to this scale, subjects were recruited for what they believed was a different experiment on creative imagination. When the second scale was administered, the hypnotic induction was replaced by short instructions informing subjects that the scale assessed their ability to be imaginatively creative. Under these circumstances, the correlation between the two scales was significantly and substantially lower than it was when both scales were defined in terms of hypnosis. Furthermore, subjects exhibited higher responsiveness on the second scale when it was defined in terms of imagination as opposed to hypnosis. More specifically, subjects who scored high on the first scale (always defined as a test of hypnosis) also tended to score high on the second scale, regardless of how the latter was defined. However, subjects who scored low on the first scale scored much higher on the second scale when it was defined as a test of imagination rather than one of hypnosis.

These findings indicate that much of the stability in hypnotic responding that is usually attributed to a trait may instead reflect stability in subjects' understandings and interpretations of hypnosis. When subjects' understandings about the test situation change, their responses may also change. Furthermore, defining the situation as hypnosis may often suppress rather than facilitate the responses of many subjects.

Attitudinal and Imaginal Correlates. Many studies have reported significant correlations between degree of positive attitudes toward hypnosis and hypnotizability (see de Groh, 1989, for a review). However, in many cases the correlations between these variables were quite low. When evaluating these results, one should keep in mind that the statistical procedures employed in these studies usually assessed only linear relationships.

We (Spanos, Brett, Menary, & Cross, 1987) plotted attitude-toward-hypnosis scores against hypnotizability scores and found that the relationship between these variables was fan-shaped rather than linear. Subjects with strong negative attitudes toward hypnosis never obtained high hypnotizability scores. As attitudes became increasingly positive, hypnotizability scores increased. Nevertheless, even when attitudes were highly positive, substantial numbers of subjects continued to score low in hypnotizability. We (Katsanis, Barnard, & Spanos, 1988) found a similar fan-shaped relationship when plotting subjects' expectancies of hypnotic responding against their hypnotizability scores.

These findings suggest that negative attitudes and low expectations suppress hypnotizability, whereas positive attitudes and expectations allow subjects to attain high hypnotizability scores. However, positive attitudes and expectations, in and of themselves, do not engender high hypnotizability. Relatively positive attitudes and expectations may be important, but they are not sufficient requirements for the attainment of high hypnotizability (Spanos & Barber, 1974).

Work conducted in several laboratories (reviewed by de Groh, 1989) suggests that at least moderate levels of imaginal propensity (e.g., imagery vividness, absorption, fantasy proneness) may also be helpful but not sufficient for the attainment of high hypnotizability. More specifically, de Groh's (1989) review indicates that subjects who report very low levels of imaginal propensity almost always score low in hypnotizability, whereas those who report moderate to high levels may achieve all levels of hypnotizability. de Groh's (1989) review further indicates that even in combination, attitudes, expectations, and imaginal propensities do a relatively poor job of predicting high hypnotizability. A substantial number of subjects who hold positive attitudes and expectations and who report relatively strong imaginal propensities continue to score low on hypnotizability. Some recent work from my laboratory suggests that the low hypnotizability scores attained by such subjects may be related to their tacit interpretations during the administration of test suggestions.

Interpretation of Suggested Demands

As indicated earlier, hypnotic test suggestions are worded in the passive voice and do not explicitly instruct subjects to enact target responses. Because of such passive wording, suggestions are ambiguous communications that are open to varied interpretations. For example, subjects may interpret a suggestion for arm levitation in several different ways. First, they may de-emphasize the implication that the response should be defined as involuntary, and simply raise an arm. This pattern of responding is not uncommon. For instance, we (Spanos, Radtke, Hodgins, Stam, & Bertrand, 1983) found that hypnotic subjects who made the behavioral responses required by suggestions defined those responses as feeling more voluntary than involuntary about half the time.

Second, subjects may interpret the suggestion as a literal request to wait passively for the are to "go up by itself." These subjects may hold positive attitudes and expectations and may be able to form vivid images. However, they have failed to understand that they must initiate the movements that are to be defined as *not* self-initiated (i.e., as involuntary). Waiting passively is by far the most common interpretation made of suggestions (Katsanis et al., 1988), and is probably among the more important reasons for the fact that most hypnotic subjects fail most of the suggestions administered to them.

A third pattern of responding involves enacting the requisite behavioral response while simultaneously defining that response as an involuntary occurrence. Subjects may do this by initiating the requisite action (e.g., slowly raising the arm) while simultaneously attending to the passive wording of the suggestion and to the images of involuntary responding (e.g., helium being pumped into the hollow arm) directly or indirectly cued by the suggestion (Angelini & Stanford, 1987; Spanos et al., 1977). In short, these subjects tacitly understand that they must carry out actions, but at the same time they interpret their actions as involuntary occurrences (i.e., active interpretation).

We (Katsanis et al, 1988) examined these ideas by giving subjects brief descriptions of the suggestions they would receive during hypno-tizability testing. Subjects were then asked to predict their forthcoming response to each suggestion. Following hypnotizability testing, subjects were given another description of each suggestion and were asked to choose which of several response alternatives best described the interpretation that they had adopted during the suggestion period. For instance, one alternative described attempting to resist suggested effects; another described a passive interpretation; and still another described an active interpretation (i.e., enacting a response while imaging events that would help to define it as involuntary). A separate score for each interpretation was obtained by summing the number of suggestions on which subjects adopted each interpretation. We found that subjects with uniformly high expectations showed substantial variability in their hypnotizability scores. However, this residual variability was related to the manner in which they interpreted suggestions: Those with high expectations plus an active interpretation attained significantly higher scores on subjective and behavioral dimensions of hypnotizability than those with high expecta-tions plus passive interpretation.

In a second study, we (Katsanis et al., 1988) divided subjects into those with high and low imagery ability. Subjects with poor imagery appeared to be unable to generate the imaginary events called for by the hypnotic test suggestions, regardless of their expectations and interpreta-tions. However, among subjects with the requisite imaginal ability, hypnotizability was in large measure determined by the extent to which they adopted an active interpretational set that enabled them to translate their imaginal abilities into subjectively convincing hypnotic enactments.

Modifying Hypnotizability

I have argued up to this point that hypnotizability can be usefully conceptualized in terms of subjects' attitudes, expectations, interpretations of test demands, and imaginal propensities. Consequently, it should be possible to enhance hypnotizability by maximizing the standing of subjects on these antecedent variables. Numerous studies (reviewed by Diamond, 1977, 1982; Perry, 1977; Spanos, 1986a) that used a wide range of treatment interventions (e.g., electroencephalographic [EEG] biofeedback, meditation training) failed to achieve large hypnotizability gains. However, most of these studies were based on the special-process view that high hypnotizability requires a "trance state," and therefore employed treatment interventions that were designed to facilitate alterations in consciousness (e.g., sensory isolation). From a sociocognitive perspective, there is little reason to expect that such interventions should enhance hypnotizability.

A few early studies approached the modifiability of hypnotizability from a social learning perspective rather than from a special-process perspective, and several of these studies obtained substantial hypnotizability gains (Diamond, 1972; Kinney & Sachs, 1974; Sachs & Anderson, 1967; Springer, Sachs & Morrow, 1977). In these studies subjects were administered training that was designed to change their attitudes and interpretations about hypnotic responding and to foster the subjective changes called for by test suggestions.

More recently, a series of experiments from my laboratory has addressed this issue by exposing subjects low in hypnotizability to a three-component cognitive skills training package aimed at enhancing hypnotizability. The components are as follows: (1) providing information that enhances subjects' attitudes and expectations concerning hypnosis; (2) teaching subjects to become absorbed in the use of imagery strategies as an aid to experiencing their suggested responses as involuntary; and (3) informing subjects that hypnotic responses do not "just happen" but must be enacted, and that enacted responses can be made to feel involuntary through appropriate imagining.

A number of studies from my laboratory that used this three-component training package (the Carleton Skills Training Program, or CSTP) found large gains on both behavioral and subjective indices of hypnotizability. Such gains with the CSTP have now been replicated in laboratories other than my own (Bertrand, Stam & Radtke, 1990; Gfeller, Lynn, & Pribble, 1987). Moreover, several studies also indicate taht CSTP-induced gains generalize to novel and difficult suggestions and are maintained even after long intervals of time (Gfeller et al., 1987; Spanos, de Groh, & de Groot, 1987; Spanos, Cross, Menary, & Smith, 1988; Spanos, Lush, & Gwynn, 1989).

Recently, Bates, Miller, Cross, and Brigham (1988) failed to obtain large gains in hypnotizability when using the CSTP. However, the trainers in that study made no attempt to establish rapport with their subjects. Bates et al. (1988) argued that the large CSTP hynotizability gains achieved in studies other than their own may have stemmed from behavioral compliance induced by high levels of subject–trainer rapport. More specifically, this hypothesis (Bates et al., 1988) appears to imply the following: (1) Subjects administered the CSTP do *not* learn to have the subjective experiences called for by suggestions; (2) these subjects make the overt responses required by suggestions and then misdescribe their subjective experiences in order to please their trainers; and (3) subjects wish to please their trainers because they have developed a strong sense of rapport with the trainers during CSTP administration. This compliance hypothesis assumes that subject–trainer rapport coupled with demands for enhanced hypnotizability are sufficient for producing large hypnotizability gains. From this perspective, the information provided by skill training is irrelevent. Any training procedure that produces high levels of rapport and contains strong and clear demands should be as effective as skill training at enhancing hypnotizability.

To test these ideas, we (Spanos, Flynn, & Niles, 1990) administered the CTSP to one group of subjects low in hypnotizability and relaxation/imagery training to a second group. The relaxation/imagery training was designed to foster high levels of rapport, and informed subjects repeatedly that their training would substantially enhance their hypnotizability. However, the relaxation/imagery training did not teach subjects to adopt an active interpretation of suggested demands or to apply their imagery skills to the requirements of suggestions. Subjects in the relaxation/imagery and CTSP groups attained equivalent levels of rapport with their trainers. Nevertheless, only those administered the CTSP exhibited enhancements in hypnotizability.

In a second experiment (Spanos, Flynn, & Niles, 1990, Experiment 2), subjects in one condition were administered the CSTP by a warm, pleawsant trainer who fostered high rapport. Those in a second group were administered the CSTP by a cold, aloof, apparently uninterested trainer. Only those subjects trained under conditions of high rapport exhibited hypnotizability gains. Relatedly, two other studies (Cross & Spanos, 1988; Gfeller et al., 1987) found that the extent to which skill-trained subjects rated themselves as liking and feeling in rapport with their trainers correlated with their degree of post-training hypnotizability gain.

Taken together, the findings of these studies suggest that subjects who like and feel in rapport with their trainers are more likely than those who do not feel in rapport to learn and to implement the skills, attitudes, and interpretations conveyed by skill training. On the other hand, high rapport and strong demands, in the absence of information about how to bring about the combination of subjective and behavioral effects called for, do not produce large hypnotizability increments.

Although skill training substantially enhances hypnotizability, skill-trained subjects still exhibit wide variability in posttraining hypno- tizability levels. One reason for this residual variability stems from the fact that subjects differ in their openness to training information aimed at changing their attitudes. For instance, we (Spanos, Cross, Menary, Brett, & de Groh, 1987) found that subjects who, despite skill training, continued to hold relatively negative attitudes about hypnosis exhibited smaller posttreatment hypnotizability gains than those who developed relatively more positive attitudes about hypnosis.

Recall our (Katsanis et al, 1988) finding that subjects who (without benefit of training) adopted an active interpretation toward suggested demands *and* reported relatively good imagery attained relatively high hypnotizability scores. On the other hand, subjects with poor imagery tended to score relatively low in hypnotizability, regardless of their interpretational set toward suggestions. These findings suggest that some subjects with positive attitudes and appropriate interpretations of hypnosis may benefit relatively little from skill training because they do not possess the imaginal abilities required to generate the subjective experiences called for by suggestions. In support of this hypothesis, two studies (Spanos, Cross, et al., 1987; Cross & Spanos, 1988) found that subjects low in hypnotizability who obtained low scores on a questionnaire measure of imagery vividness attained lower behavioral and subjective hypnotizability scores following administration of the CSTP than did lows who obtained relatively high imagery vividness scores.

In summary, the available data contradict the hypothesis that hypnotizability is an unmodifiable trait or capacity. On the contrary, subjects exhibit dramatic changes in their responsiveness to suggestions as a a function of how the test situation is defined to them (Spanos, Gabora, et al., 1989). Moreover, substantial numbers of lows exhibit large and enduring gains in hypnotizability following skill training. Not surpris- ingly, relevant skills are learned more effectively when the trainer is warm, friendly, and likable as opposed to cold and uninterested. However, warmth and high trainer–subject rapport in and of themselves do not appear to induce large hypnotizability gain. The extent to which subjects exhibit training-induced gains in hypnotizability is influenced by the success of the training at fostering positive attitudes and interpretations, as well as by subjects' level of imagery skill. These findings are consistent with the sociocognitive view that performance on hypnotizability scales reflects the operation of interrelated sets of modifiable attitudes, interpretations, motivations, and expectations in interaction with imaginal propensities (Diamond, 1974, 1977; Sachs, 1971; Spanos, 1986a). The sociocognitive view acknowledges that compliance with situational demands may play a role in the hypnotizability gains produced by skill training. There is, in fact, strong evidence that compliance is an integral part of hypnotic responding and that "natural highs" (i.e., subjects who attain high hypnotizability without benefit of training) exaggerate and misrepresent their experiences to varying degrees in order to meet the demands of suggestions (Spanos, Flynn, & Gabora, 1989; Spanos, Perlini, Patrick, Bell, & Gwynn, 1990; Spanos, Burgess, & Perlini, 1990; Wagstaff, 1981, 1986). Given that such behavior is characteristic of natural highs in hypnotic settings it would be surprising if "created highs" (i.e., those who score high in hypnotizability after skill training) did not also exhibit some compliance. However, the available data also suggest that compliance, in and of itself, cannot account adequately for hypnotic behavior in either natural highs or created highs (Spanos, 1986a, 1991).

To date, very little work has examined the consistency of skill-training-induced gains across different testing contexts. However, it is important to keep in mind that the responsiveness to suggestions of natural highs can vary quite dramatically as a function of how the definition of the context in which they are tested varies (Spanos, Gabora, et al., 1989, Experiment 2). Therefore, with respect to the cross-situational consistency of gains from skill training, the relevant research issue should not be whether such gains are cross-situationally maintained; instead, it should be a delineation of the conditions under which they are and are not maintained.

Compliance, Reinterpretation, and Suggestions for Reduced Sensitivity

In everyday social life, people regularly misrepresent their private experiences. In many situations such misrepresentation is carried out in order to reduce strain and facilitate smooth interaction. Maintaining a demeanor of sorrowful respect, despite private feelings of loathing, at the funeral of a despised colleague is an example. Misrepresentation of this kind is routinely expected in a wide range of social situations, and in these situations it is often awarded positive labels (e.g., "tact," "kindness," "interpersonal sensitivity"). Such normatively induced misdescriptions of private experience are labeled "compliance" (Kiesler & Kiesler, 1970).

Hypnosis experiments are normatively governed social situations, and subjects typically view such experiments as important scientific endeavors that require their serious cooperation. Consequently, subjects are often motivated to generate the behavioral and subjective responses called for by suggestions. However, scientific endeavors also include norms for honest and accurate reporting, and subjects are implicitly aware that behavioral responses to suggestions that are unaccompanied by the requisite subjective experiences are defined as cheating.

Many subjects who are unable to generate the subjective experiences called for fail suggestions, instead of compliantly enacting the requisite behavioral responses. On the other hand, subjects probably differ in the criteria they set concerning the magnitude of the subjective response needed to legitimate the requisite behavioral responses. Moreover, subjects who make a behavioral response but are uncertain that their subjective response has been of sufficient magnitude may be motivated to exaggerate their subjective response when reporting it. Subjects may also differ from one another in the extent to which they become invested in enacting the "good subject" role. For example, subjects who have previously passed most suggestions and come to define themselves as "highs" may be particularly tempted to misdescribe and exaggerate their experience in order to maintain a self-presentation as deeply hypnotizable.

Misdescription of Private Experience. To examine these ideas, we (Spanos, Flynn, & Gabora, 1989) gave highly hypnotizable hypnotic subjects the negative hallucination suggestion that when they opened their eyes, they would see a blank piece of paper. On the paper, however, was drawn a large and easily visible number 8. When they opened their eyes and looked at the paper, 15 of these 45 highs stated repeatedly that the paper was blank and that they could see nothing on it. Following termination of hypnosis, these 15 subjects were interviewed about their experiences by a second experimenter. In order to pressure subjects into reporting what they had actually seen, the interviewer stated that she was not interested in distinguishing the performance of deeply hypnotized subjects from that of fakers. According to the interviewer, fakers insist that they never see anything on the paper, whereas deeply hypnotized subjects initially see a figure on the paper that gradually fades from view. The interviewer then asked subjects to draw what they had seen on the paper at different intervals, so that she could determine how the figure had faded from view over time. The interviewer never told subjects the figure that had been on the paper. Nevertheless, 14 out of the 15 subjects who originally claimed that the paper was blank correctly drew a number 8 when prompted by the interviewer to draw what they had seen.

These findings indicate that subjects were being less than forthright when they initially stated that they could see nothing on the paper. Obviously, these subjects had seen the number 8, but had denied doing so in order to fulfill what they perceived to be the role demands of the experimental situation. During the interview the role demands changed when reports of "seeing nothing" were defined as "faking." Under these circumstances, these subjects acknowledged by their drawings that they had in fact seen the number 8 on the paper.

The findings of this study (Spanos, Flynn, & Gabora, 1989) do not preclude the possibility that at least some subjects may have achieved some level of perceptual distortion during the suggestion period by using such strategies as defocusing their eyes, crossing their eyes, looking away from the number, or generating visual images in an attempt to occlude the number. However, subjects' drawings made it clear that any such attempts were less than completely successful, and that subjects' initial statements that they saw nothing on the page were at best exaggerations and at worst out-and-out misdescriptions of their private experiences.

Exaggeration and misdescription of private experience are not restricted to negative hallucination responding. For example, we (Spanos & Bodorik, 1977) obtained postexperimental testimony from subjects who had been administered an hypnotic amnesia suggestion. Half of the subjects who displayed total amnesia (i.e., who recalled none of the target items during the suggestion period) later reported that they had purposely withheld (rather than forgotten) at least some of the target items. As Coe (1989) pointed out, one can only wonder at the proportion of amnesics who withheld target information but did not confess during the postexperimental interview.

In replicating a study by Laurence and Perry (1983), we (Spanos & McLean, 1986) "age-regressed" subjects back to a previous night during which they had slept soundly. (It had been previously determined that subjects had not awakened on the night in question.) During the regression procedure, subjects were asked whether they had heard noises that awakened them. At this point some subjects stated that they did hear such noises. Later, during a posthypnotic interview, some of these subjects insisted that they really had been awakened by noises on the night in question, and that this was not something that they simply imagined in response to a suggestion by the hypnotist. Laurence and Perry (1983) had obtained similar results and interpreted their findings to mean that their subjects were unable to distinguish suggestion-induced imaginary noises from what had actually transpired on the night in question. We (Spanos & McLean, 1986) suggested instead that the subjects' failure to distinguish fantasy from reality reflected a reporting bias induced by the demands of the experimental situation.

To examine this hypothesis, we (Spanos & McLean, 1986) "rehypno- tized" subjects and exposed them to a "hidden-observer" procedure, which tacitly defined good hypnotic performance as the ability (rather than the inability) to distinguish imaginings from reality. Under these circum- stances, almost all of the subjects who earlier stated that they had actually been awakened by noises on the night in question not indicated that the noises had been imaginings suggested by the hypnotist. Thus, the subjects' initial reports that they had been awakened by noises were suggestion-induced misdescriptions aimed at fostering the impression that they were unable to distinguish hypnotically induced fantasy from reality. In short, the findings of numerous studies provide strong support for Wagstaff's (1981, 1986) contention that compliance is an integral component of hypnotic responding.

Deception or Reinterpretation? To further examine the issue of compliance, we (Spanos, Perlini, et al., 1990) tested subjects on three trials of painful stimulation. On the first trial (trial 1), subjects received the pain stimulus for 60 seconds without any preceding instruction. Fifteen seconds after termination of the pain stimulus, subjects rated the intensity of the pain they had experienced at the 60-second point. Next, subjects were administered either hypnotic or nonhypnotic suggestions for pain reduction. At the end of the suggestion, subjects were again administered the 60-second pain stimulus and again waited 15 seconds after termination of the stimulus to rate pain intensity (trial 2). Following the pain rating, the suggestion was canceled, and the subjects were then administered their third and final 60-second pain trial (trial 3). For half of the subjects (controls), trial 3 was the same as trial 1; these subjects simply underwent the 60 seconds of painful stimulation and 15 seconds later rated their level of pain. For the other half of the subjects, trial 3 also consisted of 60 seconds of painful stimulation. However, in the 15 seconds between the termination of the stimulus and their reporting of the pain, these subjects were administered a statement designed to induce compliance. For instance, during this interval subjects who had been administered hypnotic analgesia suggestions on trial 2 were told that highly hypnotizable subjects like themselves often slipped spontaneously into hypnosis when exposed to repeated pain trials, and that for this reason, they probably had felt very little pain on trial 3. It is important to keep in mind that control subjects and subjects given the compliance instruction were treated in the same way before and during the trial 3 pain stimulation. Consequently, any reduction in reported pain for the compliance subjects relative to the controls on trial 3 could not reflect actual differences in the amount of pain experienced on trial 3. Instead, such a difference in reported pain could only reflect a reporting bias induced by the compliance instruction.

Among hypnotic subjects, we (Spanos, Perlini, et al., 1990) found that highs reported almost as much pain reduction following the compliance instruction (trial 3) as following the hypnotic analgesia suggestion (trial 2). Highs who did not receive the compliance instruction reported high levels of pain on trial 3. In other words, among highs the compliance instruction induced a substantial reporting bias: Highs given this instruction reported substantially less pain than they actually experienced in trial 3.

Lows among the hypnotic subjects in this experiment did not report pain reductions following either the hypnotic analgesia suggestion (trial 2) or the compliance instruction (trial 3). Among subjects who received the compliance instruction, the correlation between reported pain decrements on trial 2 and trial 3 was substantial. In other words, the subjects who reported high levels of suggested analgesia on trial 2 tended to be the same people who exhibited large reporting biases on trial 3. Furthermore, for hypnotic subjects the magnitude of the correlation between hypnotizability scores and trial 3 reporting bias scores did not differ significantly from the correlation between hypnotizability and trial 2 hypnotic analgesia reports.

We (Spanos, Perlini, et al., 1990) also tested nonhypnotic subjects. As in previous studies (e.g., Spanos, Kennedy, & Gwynn, 1984), we found that lows who had been administered an analgesia suggestion without a prior hypnotic induction procedure reported as much pain reduction (on trial 2) as highs, and greater pain reduction than lows among the hypnotic subjects. Importantly, both low and high nonhypnotic subjects exhibited a reporting bias following the trial 3 compliance instruction. The fact that lows exhibited a reporting bias when they had been previously administered a nonhypnotic analgesia suggestion, but no reporting bias when they had been previously administered an hypnotic suggestion, indicates that the tendency of subjects to exhibit such a bias cannot be explained simply in dispositional terms. Instead, the extent to which subjects exhibited a reporting bias appears to have been dependent on the extent to which they became invested in the role of responsive experimental subject. When the situation was defined as hypnosis, investment in the "responsive subject" role was restricted to highs. Only these subjects reported significant pain reductions on trial 2 (hypnotic analgesia), and therefore only these subjects were exposed to pressure that required them to report low trial 3 pain scores in order to maintain the responsive subject role.

Recently, we (Spanos, et. al., 1990) replicated the Spanos, Perlini, et al. (1990) findings after replacing the pain reduction task with a suggested deafness task. In this replication, we found that subjects who reported hearing loss following a deafness suggestion on trial 2 also exhibited a strong reporting bias following the trial 3 compliance instruction. Once again, hypnotic highs reported more trial 2 deafness and exhibited more trial 3 reporting bias than hypnotic lows. Nonhypnotic highs and lows reported equivalent levels of deafness and exhibited equivalent reporting bias on trial 3.

At least two hypotheses can account for the findings of the Spanos, Perlini, et al. (1990) and Spanos et al. (1990) experiments. Both hypotheses are premised on the notion that subjects who responded to the compliance instruction were invested in the "good subject" role and were motivated to present themselves in a manner consistent with that role. The first hypothesis suggests that subjects who exhibited a reporting bias were deceptive when reporting the level of pain or the degree of loudness they experienced on trial 3. The second hypothesis suggests that the compliance instruction led motivated subjects to reinterpret or reclassify their remembered experiences as less intense than they initially believed. This latter hypothesis does not imply that subjects were deceptive. Instead, it suggests that subjects' memory for their trial 3 experience was altered by the process of motivated reinterpretation induced by the compliance instruction.

The deception and reinterpretation hypotheses are not mutually exclusive: Not only may both processes have occurred, but both may have occurred in the same subject. For example, some subjects who initially lied by reporting less pain than they believed they actually felt may, as they reflected longer on the situation, have convinced themselves that "maybe it didn't hurt that much after all." Such a change in conviction may have been brought about by several factors, including assuaging the guilt of having defined themselves as cheating, and observing the unquestioned acceptance by the experimenter of their low ratings.

Reinterpretation of sensory experience, as opposed to reduction in the intensity of sensory experience, may be the primary mechanism through which standard suggestions (as well as compliance instructions) for pain reduction and deafness normally operate (Spanos, 1982, 1989; Jones & Spanos, 1982). Standard suggestions differ from the compliance instructions we used (Spanos, Perlini, et al., 1990) in two important respects. Suggestions precede rather than follow stimulus presentation, and suggestions usually provide a cognitive strategy (e.g., "Imagine your hand is numb and insensitive," "imagine cotton wads stuffed in your ears"). One common interpretation of suggested effects holds that strategy-induced attentional shifts away from sensory stimulation reduce sensory discriminability (e.g., McCaul & Malott, 1984). Although this position is intuitively reasonable, the evidence for it is not strong. For instance, several studies indicate that the discriminability of both painful stimuli (Jones, Spanos, & Anuza, 1987) and auditory stimuli (Spanos, Jones, & Malfara, 1982) can remain unchanged despite suggestion-induced reports of reduced pain and reduced hearing. These findings may indicate that suggestions for reduced sensitivity produce their effects by inducing subjects to reinterpret (rather than to "block out") sensory activity (e.g., in pain experiments subjects may interpret the noxious stimulation as relatively more throbbing and tingling than painful). From this perspective, the cognitive strategy activity induced by suggestions may serve more to facilitate and reinforce reinterpretation of sensory events than to reduce discriminability (Spanos, 1982, 1989). For instance, subjects who observe themselves relaxing and imagining pleasant events during painful stimulation may employ these observations as evidence that they are successfully coping, and therefore that "it can't hurt all that much" (Spanos, 1982).

Of course, an explanation of suggestion-induced sensory effects in terms of deception is also possible (Wagstaff, 1981). To a degree that is not yet specified, subjects may knowingly report lower levels of sensation than they experience, and may exaggerate the extent to which they employed cognitive strategies, in order to meet suggested demands. However, recent findings (Spanos, Perlini, & Robertson, 1989) indicate that a deception hypothesis in and of itself cannot account adequately for the reduced pain reports that accompany suggested analgesia. In that study, subjects who received hypnotic or nonhypnotic suggestions for analgesia, and subjects who received a placebo, reported equivalent expectations for pain reduction. Nevertheless, subjects who received the suggestions reported greater pain reduction than those who received the placebo. Given that the suggestion and placebo procedures generated equivalent demands for reporting reduced pain (as indicated by the equivalent expectations for pain reduction in suggestion and placebo groups), the heightened pain reduction reported by subjects in the suggestion treatment becomes difficult to explain in terms of description alone.

In summary, data from a number of different experiments support the hypothesis that compliance is an important component of hypnotic responding. Subjects who become invested in the role of hypnotic subject (i.e., those high in hypnotizability) sometimes exaggerate and purposefully misdescribe their experiences in order to fulfill suggested demands. Although the extent to which compliance influences hypnotic responding remains unclear, the contribution of this factor is likely to be substantial. Recent findings on suggested analgesia and deafness indicate that reporting bias rather than reduction in sensory experience may account for much of so-called "hypnotic analgesia" and "hypnotic deafness." Although the occurrence of reporting bias may indicate that subjects are consciously faking their responses, such bias may also indicate that they nondeceptively reinterpret their experiences. In either case, the findings of these studies support the hypothesis that hypnotic behavior is motivated, goal-directed action.

High Hypnotizability and Special Processes

As pointed out by Coe (1989), it is sometimes argued by special-process theorists that the behavior of the large majority of hypnotic subjects can be accounted by adequately as motivated, context-supported, goal-directed action, but that the behavior of very highly hypnotizable subjects requires the positing of special psychological processes. Below I review research concerning the performance of highs with respect to three phenomena that are central to contemporary hypnosis research. In each case, it has been argued that the phenomena in question requires the positing of special psychological processes. I argue instead that these phenomena can be better understood from a sociocognitive perspective.

Breaching of Hypnotic Amnesia

Comprehensive views of the hypnotic amnesia of literature that underscore the goal-directed nature of amnesia responding are provided elsewhere (Coe, 1978, 1989; Spanos, 1986b; Spanos & Radtke, 1982). Here I focus on only one aspect of hypnotic amnesia: the supposed inability (as opposed to unwillingness) of highly hypnotizable amnesic subjects to recall the information covered by an amnesia suggestion.

Highly hypnotizable hypnotic subjects who are administered a suggestion to forget previously learned material frequently claim that they are unable to recall much or any of the material. Nevertheless, when the suggestion is canceled by a prearranged cue, these subjects easily remember the "forgotten" material (Spanos & Radtke, 1982). Special-process theorists have traditionally argued that the recall deficits of these subjects reflect a temporary inability (as opposed to unwillingness) to recall the target material (Cooper, 1972). Kihlstrom, Evans, Orne, and Orne (1980) attempted to buttress this contention by demonstrating that such amnesia is impervious to instructional demands. Following an amnesia suggestion, Kihlstrom et al. (1980) gave subjects two trials on which to try to recall target items. Between these two trials, experimental subjects were exposed to various instructions designed to "breach" (i.e., to break down) amnesia. For instance, those in one condition were instructed to be honest on the uncoming second trial, whereas those in another condition were urged to try their best to recall on the second trial. Control subjects were administered the two trials without intervening instructions. Subjects in all conditions (including the controls) recalled more on the second trial than on the first. However, subjects in the various breaching instruction conditions did not recall more on the second trial than did controls.

On the basis of these findings, Kihlstrom et al. (1980) argued that at least some hypnotic subjects lose control over memory retrieval processes, and therefore are unable to recall efficiently. According to this hypothesis, forgotten memories become dissociated from consciousness; therefore, they cannot be retrieved despite the enhanced efforts induced by instructions to be honest, try harder, and so forth. However, the "amnesic barrier" that separates the dissociated memory from consciousness tends to "wear down" with time, and for this reason control subjects as well as those given the breaching instructions tend to recall some of the "forgotten memories" with the passage of time.

Following the Kihlstrom et al. (1980) investigation, a number of studies strengthened the breaching manipulations administered to subjects. Along with exhortations to be honest, these manipulations included attaching subjects to a "lie detector," providing expectations for increased recall, and furnishing videotaped feedback of subjects' own amnesia responding (Coe & Sluis, 1989; Coe & Yashinski, 1985; Dubreuil, Spanos, & Bertrand, 1983; Howard & Coe, 1981; McConkey & Sheehan, 1981; Schuyler & Coe, 1981). Many of the breaching manipulations used in these studies were more effective than the instructions used by Kihlstrom et al. (1980), and led to significantly less amnesia (i.e., more breaching) in experimental subjects than in controls. For instance, Coe and Sluis (1989) induced strong social pressure to breach by administering both honesty instructions and "lie detector feedback" that informed highly hypnotizable amnesic subjects that they were not telling all they knew. Under these circumstances, all but one subject exhibited substantial breaching of amnesia. In short, when social pressure is made strong enough, almost all hypnotically amnesic subjects recall much of the supposedly forgotten material.

Why do hypnotically amnesic subjects often fail to breach amnesia when instructed to be honest or to try their best to recall? My colleagues and I (Spanos, Radtke, & Bertrand, 1984) suggested that highly hypnotizable subjects are often intent on presenting themselves as deeply hypnotized during the test session. For this reason they tend to ignore or reinterpret instructions that, if followed, would compromise their self-presentation. The complete reversal of hypnotic amnesia following exhortations to be honest or to try harder would violate the role requirements for presenting as deeply hypnotized, and would also call into question the legitimacy of subjects' previous failures to recall. In short, amnesic subjects have a vested interest in not recalling despite exhortations to the contrary. For this reason, many of them fail to breach unless they can be fooled into believing (e.g., via a lie detection manipulation) that the experimenter can accurately determine the validity of their response.

If amnesic subjects were really unable to recall, then they would be unable to reverse their amnesia even if they wished to do so. On the other hand, if highly hypnotized hypnotic subjects retain control over their memory processes, then it should be possible to induce them to breach amnesia easily and completely by convincing them that breaching (rather than continued nonrecall) is congruent with their role as deeply hypnotized.

We (Spanos, Radtke, & Bertrand, 1984) examined these ideas by testing eight very highly hypnotizable subjects who in previous testing had consistently described their responses to suggestions as involuntary, and who failed repeatedly to breach amnesia despite exhortations to report honestly. Following a procedure modified from Hilgard (1979), these subjects were informed that during hypnosis hidden parts of their minds remained aware of things that they could no longer consciously remember. Specifically, these subjects were told that one hidden part remained aware of everything that occurred in their right hemisphere, while a different hidden part remained aware of everything in their left hemisphere. Subjects learned a list that contained both abstract and concrete words. Half were told that abstract words were stored by their right hemisphere and that concrete words were stored by their left. The remaining subjects were given the opposite information concerning storage location. Following a suggestion to forget the words, all subjects showed high levels of amnesia. Before canceling the suggestion, however, the experimenter successively contacted each subject's right and left "hidden parts." All subjects recalled all of their "right-hemisphere" words but none of their "left-hemisphere" words when contact was made with their "right hidden part." All exhibited the opposite pattern of recall when contact was made with their "left hidden part." In other words, every one of these highly hypnotizable hypnotic subjects breached amnesia easily and completely when doing so supported their self-presentation as deeply hypnotized. In a related experiment, Silva and Kirsch (1987) also demonstrated that highly hypnotizable hypnotic subjects breached amnesia when they were led to believe that breaching was the response expected from excellent hypnotic subjects.

The findings of breaching studies indicate quite clearly that even very highly hypnotizable hynotically amnesic subjects do not lose voluntary control over their memory processes. To describe these subjects as unable to remember is simply inaccurate. Instead, these subjects are skilled at conveying the impression that they have lost control over their memories by successively recalling and failing to recall as the situation demands. The findings of the breaching studies do not necessarily mean that amnesic subjects are simply lying; at least some of these subjects may retrospectively interpret their recall failures as involuntary occurrences. In short, some hypnotically amnesic subjects may succeed in convincing themselves as well as their audience that they "really couldn't remember."

Posthypnotic Responding

Posthypnotic suggestions inform subjects that, after awakening, they will respond to some predetermined cue but will not remember having been given the suggestion to do so (e.g., "Whenever I remove my glasses you will touch your ear, but you will not remember my having told you to do this"). Subjects who carry out posthypnotic responses give the appearance of being automata; they carry out seemingly meaningless responses in an apparently automatic fashion, and they claim not to know why they respond as they do.

Special-process theorists have usually argued that the posthypnotic responses of at least some highly hypnotizable subjects are, in fact, the automatic occurrences that they appear to be (Erickson & Erickson, 1941; LeCron & Bordeaux, 1947; Nace & Orne, 1970; Orne, Sheehan, & Evans, 1968; Weitzenhoffer, 1953). Alternatively, the sociocognitive perspective conceptualizes posthypnotic responding as goal-directed action aimed at fulfilling hypnotic role demands (Barber, 1962; Coe, 1973, 1976; Spanos, Menary, Brett,Cross, & Ahmed, 1987; Wagstaff, 1981).

Special-process theorists who view posthypnotic responding as automatic also hold that it occurs outside of the experimental context, when subjects no longer associate the eliciting cue with their role as hypnotic subjects (Orne, 1979; Orne et al., 1968). In an important study, Fisher (1954) tested this hypothesis by giving 13 highly responsive hypnotic subjects the suggestion to posthypnotically touch their ear whenever they heard the word "psychology." Immediately after termination of the hypnotic procedure, the cue word was presented. All 13 subjects touched their ears. Fisher then subtly redefined the situation to imply that the experiment had ended; under these circumstances, only 2 of the subjects continued to respond to the cue word. In the final phase of the study, Fisher (1954) again redefined the situation to imply that the experiment was still in progress, and 11 subjects gave the posthypnotic response on cue. In a related study, St. Jean (1978) reported that almost all subjects stopped responding posthypnotically to a prerecorded auditory stimulus when the experimenter hurriedly left the room to attend to an emergency.

The fact that the majority of subjects in the Fisher (1954) and St. Jean (1978) experiments did not continue responding posthypnotically when they believed that the experiment was over provides support for the sociocognitive view. Nevertheless, a few of the subjects in both of these experiments continued to respond posthypnotically, despite the redefinition of the situation. Speical-process theorists can interpret these findings to mean that posthypnotic responding occurred automatically in at least a few subjects. On the other hand, sociocognitive theorists can argue that a few perceptive subjects realized that they were being surreptitiously tested, and therefore maintained their role-appropriate posthypnotic enactments.

Orne et al. (1968) claimed strong support for special-process theories in an experiment that compared highly hypnotizable hypnotic subjects with subjects low in hypnotizability who were explicitly instructed to fake hypnosis (i.e., simulators). All of Orne et al.'s (1968) subjects were tested in two sessions spaced 2 days apart. In the first session subjects were told that they would touch their ears whenever they heard the word "experiment," and would continue to respond in this manner until the suggestion was canceled by the hypnotist in their second session. Both hypnotic subjects and simulators exhibited high levels of posthypnotic responding when they were formally tested by the hypnotist in their first and second sessions. Following their first sessions, subjects were sent to another room to be scheduled by the secretary for their next appointment. As a natural part of the scheduling procedure, the secretary used the cue word "experiment" and noted subjects' responses. When subjects arrived for their next appointment, they were again met and surreptitiously tested by the secretary. Orne et al. (1968) found that 5 out of 17 of the hypnotic subjects, but none of the simulators, responded to the secretary's presentation of the cue word on both test days.

In the Orne et al. (1968) study, the hypnotic subjects and the simulators were exposed to the same hypnotic test procedures. Furthermore, the hypnotist was blind to subjects' hypnosis–simulation status. Because of these similarities in their testing situations, Orne et al. (1968) contended that hypnotic subjects and simulators were exposed to the same experimental demands and developed the same expectations concerning what constituted role-appropriate hypnotic behavior. For this reason, the failure of any simulators to respond posthypnotically to the secretary's cue was taken to mean that the experimental situation had not engendered expectations for such responding in *either* the hypnotic or the simulating subjects. Therefore, a factor other than experimentally induced expectations was posited to explain the behavior or the five hypnotic subjects who responded to the secretary's cue. Orne et al. (1968) argued that, in at least a few subjects, "hypnosis is able to produce an enduring response which is automatically instigated by an appropriate signal" (p. 195).

Although the Orne et al. (1968) findings are often cited as strong evidence against sociocognitive formulations (Bowers, 1976; Orne, 1979; Sheehan & Orne, 1968), methodological limitations in the design of that study preclude such a conclusion. The most important limitation stems from Orne et al.'s (1968) assumption that hypnotic and simulating subjects were exposed to the same experimental demands. Findings from numerous studies (reviewed by de Groot & Gwynn, 1989) now call this assumption into serious question and indicate instead that hypnotic and simulating subjects are exposed to very different demands. In other words, it may be differences in expectations, rather than psychological processes unique to hypnotic subjects, that account of differences between hypnotic and simulating subjects.

The simulation instructions administered to subjects in Orne's (1979) laboratory emphasize that simulators are to fool the *hypnotist*. In the

Orne et al. (1968) study, such an emphasis on fooling the hypnotist may have deflected the attention of simulators away from cues that were associated with the secretary. The fact that only a minority of hypnotic subjects responded to the secretary indicates that her presentations of the cue word were relatively subtle. Therefore, these cues may not have been noticed or may have been considered irrelevant by the simulators, who (unlike the hypnotic subjects) had been explicitly informed that their only task was to fool the hypnotist (Wagstaff, 1981).

In order to examine the automaticity hypothesis more thoroughly, my colleagues and I (Spanos, Menary, et al., 1987) presented posthypnotic cues to subjects in a context that was further removed from the experimental situation than had been the case in the Orne et al. (1968) study. In an initial session, subjects with high hypnotizability were given the posthypnotic suggestion to cough whenever they heard the word "psychology," and were informed that they would continue to make this response until they returned to the laboratory a week later to be tested once again. On the day of the retest, subjects were exposed to the cue word "psychology" on three different informal test occasions that were associated with increasing closeness to the experiment. The first and most important informal test occurred in a corridor completely outside the laboratory area. Each subject was approached by a confederate whom the subject had never previously met. The confederate posed as a lost student and asked subjects for directions to the *psychology* department (this department is located two floors above the hypnosis laboratory). After finishing with this confederate, subjects proceeded to the laboratory entrance where they were met by a second confederate, a graduate student whom they had never met. The graduate student administered the second informal test by casually asking subjects whether they were here for a *psychology* experiment. Subjects were then escorted to the hypnotist, who commented while walking with them to the experimental room, "I'm glad that you could make it in for today's *psychology* experiment."

The Spanos, Menary, et al., (1987) experiment also included two groups of low-hypnotizability simulators. Those in the standard-simulation group were given faking instructions emphasizing that they were to fool the hypnotist, as in the Orne et al. (1968) study. Those in a modified-simulation group were given instructions emphasizing that they were to try and fool not only the hypnotist, but also anyone else who might be connected with the experiment.

All of the subjects in the Spanos, Menary, et al., (1987) study made the requisite posthypnotic response when formally tested by the hypnotist both in their initial session and a week later in their retest session. For this reason, any failure on the part of subjects to make this response during the informal tests cannot be explained away by arguing that the tendency to respond posthypnotically had simply decayed with time between the two formal sessions. None of the high subjects, and also none of the low subjects in either simulation group, made the posthypnotic response to the cue given by the first confederate. Furthermore, none of the highs and only one simulator (from the modified-simulation group) made the posthypnotic response to the cue of the second confederate. About half of the subjects in each group made the posthypnotic response when informally tested by the hypnotist while walking to the experimental test room.

The findings of the Spanos, Menary, et al., (1987) study very clearly contradict the special-process notion that posthypnotic responding is an involuntary occurrence elicited automatically outside the experimental context. Instead, posthypnotic responding, like hypnotic amnesia, appears to be best conceptualized as goal-directed action aimed at fulfilling the role expectations associated with "being hypnotized" (Barber, 1969; Coe, 1976; Fisher, 1954; Spanos, 1986; Wagstaff, 1981).

Hypnotic Analgesia and the Hidden Observer

Hilgard (1977a, 1979) has developed an influential special-process theory of hypnosis that revolves around the notion of dissociation. According to this view, hypnotic responding occurs when the "part" of the person that responds to suggestions is partially split off from the "part" associated with consciousness. This splitting of cognitive subsystems implies that incoming perceptual information is processed in parallel by the two subsystems. Moreover, an amnesic barrier constructed between the subsystems prevents the "conscious part" of the person from gaining access to the information in the dissociated subsystem.

According to Hilgard (1977a), many subjects experience dissociation to only a slight degree (if at all), and such people remain unresponsive to hypnotic procedures and to suggestions that call for reality distortion (e.g., amnesia, pain reduction). On the other hand, in subjects with the requisite capacity, dissociation is supposedly facilitated by the administration of hypnotic induction procedures. Highly hypnotizable subjects are supposedly capable of profound dissociation, and for this reason they respond easily to a wide range of suggestions. However, subjects low in hypnotizability supposedly have little capacity foe dissociation, and therefore they are purportedly unable to respond at high levels to suggestions that require this capacity (e.g., suggestions for pain reduction).

In sociocognitive approaches, suggested analgesia is viewed more as an achievement brought about by sentient individuals than as a happening that occurs when subjects passively "dissociate" (Barber et al., 1974; Coe & Sarbin, 1977; Spanos, 1986b). According to this formulation, hypnotic procedures are no more intrinsically effective at facilitating pain reduction than are other procedures that enhance subjects' motivations and expectations of success. This formulation further suggests that highs and lows can generate equivalent reductions in pain. Thus, the usual correlation between hypnotizability and degree of hypnotic analgesia is thought to reflect not so much differences in the pain-reducing abilities of highs and lows as differences in the attitudes, motivations, expectations, and interpretations with which the two groups approach the analgesia test situation.

When applied to hypnotic analgesia, Hilgard's (1977a, 1979) dissociation formulation makes a number of relatively specific predictions. For example, the following should hold true, according to Hilgard (1977a, 1977b, 1979): (1) Other things being equal, hypnotic suggestions for analgesia should be more effective at reducing pain than nonhypnotic analgesia suggestions should be; and (2) among hypnotic subjects, lows should be unable to reduce pain to the same extent as highs. The empirical findings that relate to each of these hypotheses have been reviewed in detail elsewhere (Spanos, 1986b, 1989); therefore, I summarize them only briefly here. Contrary to Hilgard's (1977a, 1977b) theorizing, the large majority of available studies (reviewed by Spanos, 1989) indicate that analgesia suggestions alone and analgesia suggestions preceded by an hypnotic induction procedure are equally effective at reducing reported pain and enhancing pain tolerance. This conclusion holds not only for samples of unselected subjects, but also for samples that include only highly hypnotizable subjects. Moreover, this conclusion holds not only for the results of studies on laboratory-induced pain, but also for the results of clinical studies where hypnotic and nonhypnotic suggestions were compared in the treatment of various pain syndromes (for reviews, see Chaves, 1989; Spanos, 1991).

Hilgard's (1977a, 1977b) notion that highs are intrinsically better than lows at reducing pain with suggestion is also contradicted by the available empirical data. When lows are motivated to engage in cognitive pain-reducing strategies in contexts that they do not associate with hypnosis or with their earlier hypnotizability test sessions, then these subjects exhibit reductions in reported pain and increments in pain tolerance that are as large as those exhibited by highs (e.g., Spanos, Kennedy, & Gwynn, 1984; Spanos, Perlini, & Robertson, 1989). In other words, these findings indicate that, for some subjects, exposure to hypnotic procedures engenders unhelpful attitudes and expectations that interfere with responsiveness to analgesia suggestions. Relatedly, the knowledge that one has previously scored low on hypnotizability appears to engender negative performance expectations, which carry over into those analgesia test situations that are viewed as connected to hypnosis or suggestibility. In short, the relationship between suggestion-induced analgesia and hypnotizability appears to be context-specific and easily disrupted. Thus, this relationship appears to have little to do with a stable capacity for dissociation, but much to do with subjects' situation-specific attitudes, motivations, and interpretations of test demands.

The Hidden-Observer Phenomenon. The findings cited most often in support of Hilgard's (1979) dissociation formulation came from a series of so-called "hidden-observer" experiments (for reviews, see Hilgard, 1979; Spanos, 1989). Most of these experiments used only highly hypnotizable subjects. Typically, these subjects were exposed to a baseline pain simulation trial (e.g., immersion of a hand in ice-cold water for 60 seconds). At set intervals during the trial, subjects gave verbal ratings of pain intensity. Afterwards, subjects were given an hypnotic procedure and instructions implying that a hidden part of them would remain aware of pain and other experiences that their "hypnotically analgesic part" would be unaware of. Later, during hypnotic analgesia testing, these subjects were instructed to give overt (verbal) reports that indicated the degree of pain experienced by their "conscious, hypnotized part" and hidden reports (numbers tapped out in a previously taught key-pressing code) that supposedly reflected the pain felt by their "hidden part." Many of the highs exposed to this paradigm exhibited hypnotic analgesia by reporting low levels of overt pain. Frequently, however, these same subjects also reported (via key pressing) high levels of hidden pain.

According to Hilgard (1979), hidden-pain reports do *not* result from suggestion or from experimental demands. Instead, Hilgard (1979) assumes that hypnotically analgesic subjects experience high levels of hidden pain, regardless of whether or not they are instructed to access hidden pain. However, this hidden pain remains separated by an amnesic barrier unless and until the experimenter obtains hidden reports. Thus, according to Hilgard (1979), explicit hidden-observer instructions do *not* provide subjects with the idea that they have a hidden part or with the idea that hidden reports and overt reports should be different. Instead, Hilgard (1979) argues that these instructions simply provide a structured setting that allows pre-existing hidden pain to come more easily to light.

A sociocognitive alternative to dissociation theory suggests that ratings of hidden pain and reports of experiencing a "hidden part" stem from the interpretations that subjects place on the instructions used in hidden-observer experiments (Coe & Sarbin, 1977; Spanos, 1982; Spanos & Hewitt, 1980; Wagstaff, 1981). Two experiments from my laboratory (Spanos, Gwynn, & Stam, 1983; Spanos & Hewitt, 1980) garnered support for these ideas by demonstrating that the direction of hidden reports varied with the expectations conveyed by hidden-observer instructions.

In the first experiment (Spanos & Hewitt, 1980), we exposed highly hypnotizable subjects in one condition to the procedures used by Hilgard, Morgan, and Macdonald (1975) for eliciting hidden reports. The instructions given to these subjects implied that a hidden part of them would continue to feel high levels of pain while their hypnotized part experienced reduced pain (i.e., "more aware" instructions). Highs in a second condition were exposed to similar procedures but were informed that their hidden pain was so deeply hidden that it would be even less aware of what had been experienced than was their hypnotized part. Subjects in the two conditions showed "hidden observers" with opposite characteristics. Those exposed to Hilgard's standard "more aware" hidden-observer procedures reported higher levels of hidden than overt pain. However, those given "less aware" instructions reported lower levels of hidden than overt pain.

The Spanos and Hewitt (1980) findings strongly indicate that hidden-observer responding is goal-directed action that is shaped by the demands conveyed in hidden-observer instructions. For instance, subjects may meet demands for reporting both relatively high and relatively low levels of pain by shifting attention away from and back to the noxious stimulation when instructed to give both overt- and hidden-pain reports, respectively. The oscillating pain experience produced by such contextually cued attentional shifts might then be interpreted as emanating from different "parts" or levels of consciousness.

In the second experiment, (Spanos, Gwynn & Stam, 1983), we replicated and extended the Spanos and Hewitt (1980) findings by again informing hypnotically analgesic subjects that they possessed a hidden part that could report on its level of pain. Initially, however, these subjects were not provided with information concerning whether hidden reports should indicate higher levels, lower levels, or the same level of pain as overt reports (i.e., "low-cue" condition). If hidden-observer instructions simply access a pre-existing cognitive subsystem that "holds" high levels of dissociated pain, then such information should be unnecessary. When accessed, the "hidden part" should simply report the high levels of pain that "it" experiences.

Contrary to the dissociation hypothesis, subjects reported no significant differences between overt and hidden pain when given the low-cue instructions. Later, these same subjects reported significantly less hidden than overt pain and more hidden than overt pain as they were sequentially exposed to instructional demands that called for each of these patterns of responding.

In short, the Spanos and Hewitt (1980) and Spanos, Gwynn, and Stam (1983) studies provide strong evidence for a sociocognitive account of hidden-observer responding. Hypnotically analgesic subjects failed to exhibit higher hidden than over pain, depending upon the expectations conveyed by their instructions.

Criticisms of the Sociocognitive View of Hidden-Observer Responding. Although Hilgard (1987; Hilgard & Hilgard, 1983) is aware of my criticisms of his hidden-observer work, his only response has been to cite two experiments (Nogrady, McConkey, Laurence, & Perry, 1983; Zamansky &Bartis, 1985) that he believes have effectively rebutted these criticisms. Therefore, I briefly examine these two studies.

Nogrady et al. (1983) compared highly hypnotizable subjects against low-hypnotizability subjects explicitly instructed to fake hypnosis. Subjects in both groups were administered ambiguous hidden-observer instructions that hinted, but did not explicitly indicate, that reports of higher hidden than overt pain were called for. A minority of the hypnotic subjects, but none of the simulators, reported higher hidden than overt pain. The Nogrady et al. (1983) study was premised on the assumption that hypnotic subjects and simulators were exposed to the same situational demand characteristics. Consequently, these investigators concluded that the higher rate of hidden-observer responding in hypnotic subjects than in simulators could *not* be explained in terms of situational demands.

As indicated in a previous section, the available evidence now indicates that hypnotic subjects and simulators are *not* exposed to the same situational demands. For instance, when exposed to ambiguous test situations, simulators often respond more conservatively than hypnotic subjects in order to avoid being "found out" by the experimenter (Sheehan, 1970). The differences found by Nogrady et al. (1983) may simply indicate that simulators responded to the ambiguous hidden-observer instructions used in that study somewhat more conservatively than the hypnotic subjects. Because those instructions did not make clear that higher hidden than overt pain was the "correct" response, simulators may have been less likely than hypnotic subjects to experiment with a response option that could risk their exposure as fakers.

Nogrady et al.'s (1983) most interesting finding was not their uninterpretable difference between hypnotic subjects and simulators, but the fact that well over half of their hypnotic subjects failed to exhibit a hidden-observer effect when the cues calling for this pattern of responding were subtle. Along the same lines, recall that we (Spanos, Gwynn, & Stam, 1983) practically eliminated hidden-observer responding by eliminating even subtle cues that called for its occurrence. Taken together, the results of these two studies (Nogrady et al., 1983; Spanos, Gwynn, & Stam, 1983) are inconsistent with Hilgard's hypothesis that a nonsuggested subsystem that "holds" high levels of pain invariably accompanies hypnotic analgesia.

Zamansky and Bartis (1985) conducted an experiment that they claimed reduced the impact of situational demands on hidden-observer responding. Because hidden-observer responding continued to occur in what they described as a low-demand experimental situation, Zamansky and Bartis (1985) concluded that their findings helped "to place the notion of the hidden observer on a substantially more secure footing" (p. 246).

These investigators used suggestions for a negative hallucination rather than for analgesia. For example, on one suggestion task, subjects were told that when they opened their eyes they would see only a blank page. However, the page actually had on it a clearly visible number. Hypnotic subjects "passed" this suggestion if they reported seeing nothing on the page. The page was then removed from view, and subjects were given explicit hidden-observer instructions informing them that their "hidden part" was aware of all they had experienced during the suggestion. When their "hidden part" was instructed to respond, all of these subjects correctly reported the number that had been on the page. Zamansky and Bartis (1985) argued that these subjects had not consciously seen the number on the page, but that their hidden part had unconsciously seen and stored this information. Supposedly, this hidden part was not influenced by situational demands. Instead, "it" simply reported what "it" had seen when instructed to do so.

On the basis of their results, Zamansky and Bartis (1985) concluded that "the interpretation that the hidden observer report is simply a creation of experimental demands becomes much less tenable" (p. 244). How Zamansky and Bartis (1985) could arrive at this conclusion on the basis of their data is difficult to see. They provided no evidence whatsoever in support of the contention that their experimental procedures minimized or controlled for the impact of contextual demands. On the contrary, their use of explicitly worded hidden-observer instructions made relevant contextual demands highly salient.

We (Spanos, Flynn, & Gwynn, 1988) examined these issues by modifying the Zamansky and Bartis paradigm. We gave highly hypnotizable hypnotic subjects a suggestion for a negative hallucination and then showed them a page with the number 18 printed on it. Half of the subjects who reported that the page was blank were given standard hidden-observer instructions implying that their "hidden part" knew the number that had been on the page. The remaining half of these subjects were told that their "hidden part" reversed everything that it saw. Because the page with the number had been removed before administration of the hidden-observer instructions, subjects in the reversal condition could give the correct response only by knowing that the page contained an 18, knowing that the reverse of 18 is 81, and responding to demands for the reversed number. All of the subjects in the standard condition reported having seen an 18, while all of those in the reversal condition reported having seen an 81. In short, the hidden reports of subjects in the Zamansky and Bartis (1985) paradigm, like the hidden reports proffered in Hilgard's (1979) paradigm, are very clearly influenced by instructional demands. Rather than reflecting "hidden" information that cannot be consciously accessed, these reports reflect subjects' use of unfolding contextual information to generate enactments that are congruent with their beliefs concerning what is expected from them in the experimental situation.

CONCLUSIONS

The sociocognitive perspective is premised on the idea that the suggested phenomena tied most closely to the concept of hypnosis are historically rooted social actions that are fundamentally similar to other, more mundane forms of social behavior. According to this view, the traditional conceptualization of hypnosis as a "trance state" that is induced by certain rituals (hypnotic induction procedures), and that in turn produces unusual behavior, is misleading. Instead, hypnotic induction procedures are seen as the historical remnants of misguided 19th-century attempts to conceptualize the behaviors associated with this topic as somehow connected with sleep. From a sociocognitive perspective, "hypnotic behaviors" are social artifacts (Radtke, 1989; Spanos & Chaves, 1989). These behaviors do not reflect the essential characteristics of an invariant "trance state." Instead, they are rule-governed, context-dependent social actions that reflect the conceptions of hypnosis shared by subjects and hypnotists in particular historical circumstances. Thus, from a sociocognitive perspective, the goal of research is not to isolate a hypnotic essence, but instead to integrate hypnotic responding into a more general theory of social action.

Acknowledgments. Work on this chapter was supported by grants from the Natural Sciences and Engineering Council of Canada and from the Social Sciences and Humanities Research Council of Canada.

REFERENCES

Angelini, R. F., & Stanford, R. G. (1987, August–September). *Perceived involuntariness: The interaction of incongruent proprioception and supplied imagery.* Paper presented at the 95th Annual Convention of the American Psychological Association, New York.

Barber, T. X. (1962). Hypnotic age regression: A critical review. *Psychosomatic Medicine, 24,* 286–299.

Barber, T. X. (1969). *Hypnosis: A scientific approach.* NY: Van Nostrand Reinhold.

Barber, T. X. (1979). Suggested ("hypnotic") behavior: The trance paradigm versus an alternative paradigm. In E. Fromm & R. E. Shor (Eds.), *Hypnosis: Developments in research and new perspectives* (2nd ed., pp. 217–271). Chicago: Aldine.

Barber, T. X., Spanos, N. P., & Chaves, J. F. (1974). *Hypnosis, imagination and human potentialities.* Elmsford, NY: Pergamon Press.

Bates, B. L., Miller, R. J., Cross, J. J., & Brigham, T. A. (1988)Modifying hypnotic suggestibility with the Carleton Skills Training Program. *Journal of Personality and Social Psychology, 55*, 120–127.

Bertrand, L. D., Stam, H. J., & Radtke, H. L. (1990). *The Carleton skill training package for modifying hypnotic susceptibility: A replication and extention.* Unpublished manuscript, University of Calgary.

Biddle, B. J., & Thomas, E. J. (Eds.). (1966) *Role theory: Concepts and research.* NY: Wiley.

Bowers, K. S. (1976). *Hypnosis for the seriously curious.* Monterey, CA: Brooks/Cole.

Chaves, J. F. (1989). Hypnotic control of clinical pain. In N. P. Spanos & J. F. Chaves (Eds.), *Hypnosis: The cognitive-behavioral perspective* (pp. 242–272). Buffalo, NY: Prometheus.

Coe, W. C. (1973). A further evaluation of responses to an uncompleted posthypnotic suggestion. *American Journal of Clinical Hypnosis, 15*, 223–228.

Coe, W. C. (1976). The elusive nature of completing an uncompleted posthypnotic suggestion. *American Journal of Clinical Hypnosis, 18*, 263–271.

Coe, W. C. (1978). The credibility of posthypnotic amnesia: A contextualist's view. *International Journal of Clinical and Experimental Hypnosis, 26*, 218–245.

Coe, W. C. (1989). Posthypnotic amnesia: Theory and Research. In N. P. Spanos & J. F. Chaves (Eds.), Hypnosis: The cognitive–behavioral perspective (pp. 110–148). Buffalo, NY: Prometheus Books.

Coe, W. C., & Sarbin T. R. (1977). Hypnosis from the standpoint of a contextualist. Annals of the New York Academy of Sciences, 295, 2–13.

Coe, W. C., & Sluis, A. S. E. (1989). INcreasing contextual pressures to breach posthypnotic amnesia. *Journal of Personality and Social Psychology, 57*, 885–894.

Coe, W. C., & Yashinski, E. (1985). Volitional experiences associated with breaching posthypnotic amnesia. *Journal of Personality and Social Psychology, 48*, 716–722.

Cooper, L. M. (1972). Hypnotic amnesia. In E. Fromm & R. E. Shor (Eds.), *Hypnosis: Research developments and perspectives* (pp. 217–252). Chicago: Aldine-Atherton.

Cross, W., & Spanos, N. P. (1988). The effects of imagery vividness and receptivity on skill training induced enhancements in hypnotic susceptibility. *Imagination, Cognition and Personality, 8*, 89–103.

de Groh, M. (1989). Correlates of hypnotic susceptibility. In N. P. Spanos & J. F. Chaves (Eds.), *Hypnosis: The cognitive–behavioral perspective* (pp. 32–63). Buffalo, NY: Prometheus Books.

de Groot, H. P., & Gwynn, M. I. (1989). Trance logic, duality and hidden observer responding. In N. P. Spanos & J. F. Chaves (Eds.), *Hypnosis: The cognitive–behavioral perspective* (pp. 187–205). Buffalo, NY: Prometheus Books.

Diamond, M. J. (1972). The use of observationally-presented information to modify hypnotic susceptibility. *Journal of Abnormal Psychology, 79*, 174–180.

Diamond, M. J. (1974). Modification of hypnotizability: A review. *Psychological Bulletin, 81*, 180–198.

Diamond, M. J. (1977). Hypnotizability is modifiable. *International Journal of Clinical and Experimental Hypnosis, 25*, 147–165.

Diamond, M. J. (1982). Modifying hypnotic experience by means of indirect hypnosis and hypnotic skill training: An update. *Research Communications in Psychology, Psychiatry and Behavior, 7*, 233–239.

Dubreuil, D. L., Spanos, N. P., & Bertrand, L. D. (1983). Does hypnotic amnesia dissipate with time? *Imagination, Cognition and Personality*, *2*, 103–113.

Erickson, M. H., Erickson, E. M. (1941). Concerning the nature and character of post-hypnotic behavior. *Journal of General Psychology*, *24*, 95–113.

Fisher, S. (1954). The role of expectancy in the performance of posthypnotic behavior. *Journal of Abnormal and Social Psychology*, *49*, 503–507.

Gfeller, J., Lynn, S. J., & Pribble, W. (1987). Enhancing hypnotic susceptibility: Interpersonal and rapport factors. *Journal of Personality and Social Psychology*, *52*, 586–595.

Hilgard, E. R. (1977a). *Divided consciousness: Multiple controls in human thought and action.* NY: Wiley.

Hilgard, E. R. (1977b). The problem of divided consciousness: A neodissociation interpretation. *Annals of the New York Academy of Sciences*, *296*, 48–59.

Hilgard, E. R. (1979). Divided consciousness in hypnosis: The implications of the hidden observer. In E. Fromm & R. E. Shor (Eds.), *Hypnosis: Developments in research and new perspectives* (2nd ed., pp. 45–79). Chicago: Aldine.

Hilgard, E. R. (1987). Research advances in hypnosis: Issues and methods. *International Journal of Clinical and Experimental Hypnosis*, *35*, 248–264.

Hilgard, E. R., & Hilgard, J. R. (1983). *Hypnosis in the relief of pain* (2nd ed.). Los Altos, CA: William Kaufmann.

Hilgard, E. R., Morgan, A. H., & Macdonald, H. (1975). Pain and dissociation in the cold pressor test: A study of hypnotic analgesia with "hidden reports" through automatic key-pressing and automatic talking. *Journal of Abnormal Psychology*, *84*, 280–289.

Howard, M. L., & Coe, W. C. (1980). The effects of context and subjects' perceived control in breaching posthypnotic amnesia. *Journal of Personality*, *48*, 342–359.

Jones, B., & Spanos, N. P. (1982). Suggestions for altered auditory sensitivity, the negative subject effect and hypnotic susceptibility: A signal detection analysis. *Journal of Personality and Social Psychology*, *43*, 637–647.

Jones, B., & Spanos, N. P., & Anuza, T. (1987). *Functional measurement analysis of suggestions for hypnotic analgesia.* Unpublished manuscript, Carleton University.

Katsanis, J., Barnard, J., & Spanos, N. P. (1988). Self-predictions, interpretational set and imagery vividness as determinants of hypnotic responding. *Imagination, Cognition and Personality*, *8*, 63–77.

Kiesler, C. A., & Kiesler, S. B. (1970). *Conformity.* Reading, MA: Addison-Wesley.

Kihlstrom, J. F., Evans, F. J., Orne, E. C., & Orne, M. T. (1980). Attempting to breach posthypnotic amnesia. *Journal of Abnormal Psychology*, *89*, 603–616.

Kinney, J. M., & Sachs, L. B. (1974). Increasing hypnotic susceptibility. *Journal of Abnormal Psychology*, *83*, 145–150.

Laurence, J. R., & Perry, C. W. (1983). Hypnotically created memory among high hypnotizable subjects. *Science*, *222*, 523–524.

LeCron, L., & Bordeaux, J. (1947). *Hypnotism today.* NY: Grune & Stratton.

London, P. (1962). Subject characteristics in hypnosis research: I. A survey of experience, interest and opinion. *International Journal of Clinical and Experimental Hypnosis*, *9*, 151–166.

Lynn, S. J., Rhue, J. W., & Weeks, J. R. (1989). Hypnosis and experienced nonvolition: A sociocognitive integrative model. In N. P. Spanos & J. F.

Chaves (Eds.), *Hypnosis: The cognitive-behavioral perspective* (pp. 78–109). Buffalo, NY: Prometheus Books.

McCaul, K. D., & Malott, J. M. (1984). Distraction and coping with pain. *Psychological Bulletin, 95*, 516–533.

McConkey, K. M. (1986). Opinions about hypnosis and self-hypnosis before and after hypnotic testing. *International Journal of Clinical and Experimental Hypnosis, 34*, 311–319.

McConkey, K. M., & Sheehan, P. W. (1981). The impact of videotape playback of hypnotic events on posthypnotic amnesia. *Journal of Abnormal Psychology, 90*, 46–54.

Miller, M. E., & Bowers, K. S. (1986). Hypnotic analgesia and stress inoculation in the reduction of pain. *Journal of Abnormal Psychology, 95*, 6–14.

Nace, E. P., & Orne, M. T. (1970). Fate of an uncompleted posthypnotic suggestion. *Journal of Abnormal Psychology, 75*, 278–285.

Nogrady, H., McConkey, K. M., Laurence, J. R., & Perry, C. W. (1983). Dissociation, duality, and demand characteristics in hypnosis. *Journal of Abnormal Psychology, 92*, 223–235.

Orne, M. T. (1979). On the simulating subject as a quasi-control group in hypnosis research: What, why and how? In E. Fromm & R. E. Shor (Eds.), *Hypnosis: Developments in research and new perspectives* (2nd ed., pp. 519–565). Chicago: Aldine.

Orne, M. T., Sheehan, P. W., & Evans, F. J. (1968). The occurrence of posthypnotic behavior outside the experimental setting. *Journal of Personality and Social Psychology, 26*, 217–221.

Perry, C. W. (1977). Is hypnotizability modifiable? *International Journal of Clinical and Experimental Hypnosis, 25*, 125–146.

Radtke, H. L. (1989). Hypnotic depth as social artifact. In N. P. Spanos & J. F. Chaves (Eds.), *Hypnosis: The cognitive-behavioral perspective* (pp. 64–75). Buffalo, NY: Prometheus Books.

Sachs, L. B. (1971). Construing hypnosis as modifiable behavior. In A. Jacobs & K. B. Sachs (Eds.), *Psychology of private events* (pp. 65–71). NY: Academic Press.

Sachs, L. B., & Anderson, W. L. (1967). Modification of hypnotic susceptibility. *International Journal of Clinical and Experimental Hypnosis, 15*, 172–180.

St. Jean, R. (1978). Posthypnotic behavior as a function of experimental surveillance. *American Journal of Clinical Hypnosis, 20*, 250–255.

Sarbin, T. R. (1950). Contributions to role-taking theory: I. Hypnotic behavior. *Psychological Review, 57*, 255–270.

Sarbin, T. R. (1962). Attempts to understand hypnotic phenomena. In L. Postman (Ed.), *Psychology in the making* (pp. 745–785).

Sarbin, T. R. (1989). The construction and reconstruction of hypnosis. In N. P. Spanos & J. F. Chaves (Eds.), *Hypnosis: The cognitive-behavioral perspective* (pp. 400–416). Buffalo, NY: Prometheus Books.

Sarbin, T. R. & Coe, W. C. (1972). *Hypnosis: A social psychological analysis of influence communication.* NY: Holt, Rienhart & Winston.

Schuyler, B. A., & Coe, W. C. (1981). A physiological investigation of volitional and nonvolitional experience during posthypnotic amnesia. *Journal of Personality and Social Psychology, 40*, 1060–1069.

Sheehan, P. W. (1970). Analysis of the treatment effects of simulation instructions in the application of the real–simulating model of hypnosis. *Journal of Abnormal Psychology, 75*, 98–103.

Sheehan, P. W., & Orne, M. T. (1968). Some comments on the nature of posthypnotic responding. *Journal of Nervous and Mental Disease, 146*, 209–220.

Silva, C. E., & Kirsch, I. (1987). Breaching hypnotic amnesia by manipulating expectancy. *Journal of Abnormal Psychology, 96*, 325–329.

Spanos, N. P. (1982). A social psychological approach to hypnotic behavior. In G. Weary & H. L. Mirels (Eds.), *Integrations of clinical and social psychology* (pp. 231–271). NY: Oxford University Press.

Spanos, N. P. (1983). The hidden observer as an experimental creation. *Journal of Personality and Social Psychology, 44*, 170–176.

Spanos, N. P. (1986a). Hypnosis and the modification of hypnotic susceptibility: A social psychological perspective. In P. L. N. Naish (Ed.), *What is hypnosis?* (pp. 85–120). Philadelphia: Open University Press.

Spanos, N. P. (1986b). Hypnotic behavior: A social psychological interpretation of amnesia, analgesia and "trance logic." *Behavioral and Brain Sciences, 9*, 489–497.

Spanos, N. P. (1986c). Hypnosis, nonvolitional responding and multiple personality: A social psychological perspective. In B. Maher & W. Maher (Eds.), *Progress in experimental personality research*. (Vol. 14, pp. 1–62). NY: Academic Press.

Spanos, N. P. (1989). Experimental research on hypnotic analgesia. In N. P. Spanos & J. F. Chaves (Eds.), *Hypnosis: The cognitive-behavioral perspective* (pp. 206–240). Buffalo, NY: Prometheus Books.

Spanos, N. P. (1991). Hypnosis, hypnotizability and hypnotherapy. In C. R. Snyder (Ed.), *Handbook of social and clinical psychology*. Elmsford, NY: Pergamon Press.

Spanos, N. P., & Barber, T. X. (1972). Cognitive activity during "hypnotic" suggestibility: Goal-directed fantasy and the experience of nonvolition. *Journal of Personality, 40*, 510–524.

Spanos, N. P., & Barber, T. X. (1974). Toward a convergence in hypnosis research. *American Psychologist, 29*, 500–511.

Spanos, N. P., & Bodorik, H. L. (1977). Suggested amnesia and disorganized recall in hypnotic and task-motivated subjects. *Journal of Abnormal Psychology, 86*, 295–305.

Spanos, N. P., Brett, P. J., Menary, E. P., & Cross, W. P. (1987). A measure of attitudes toward hypnosis: Relationships with absorption and hypnotic susceptibility. *American Journal of Clinical Hypnosis, 30*, 139–150.

Spanos, N. P., Burgess, C. A., & Perlini, A. H. (1990). *Compliance and suggested deafness in hypnotic and nonhypnotic subjects*. Unpublished manuscript, Carleton University.

Spanos, N. P., & Chaves, J. F. (1989). The cognitive–behavioral alternative in hypnosis research. In N. P. Spanos & J. F. Chaves (Eds.), *Hypnosis: The cognitive-behavioral perspective* (pp. 9–16). Buffalo, NY: Prometheus Books.

Spanos, N. P., Cross, W. P., Menary, E. P., Brett, P. J., & de Groh, M. (1987). Attitudinal and imaginal ability predictors of social cognitive skill-training enhancements in hypnotic susceptibility. *Personality and Social Psychology Bulletin, 13*, 379–398.

Spanos, N. P., Cross, W. P., Menary, E. P., & Smith, J. (1988). Long term effects of cognitive skill training for the enhancement of hypnotic susceptibility. *British Journal of Experimental and Clinical Hypnosis, 5*, 73–78.

Spanos, N. P., & de Groh, M. (1983). Structure of communication and reports of involuntariness by hypnotic and nonhypnotic subjects. *Perceptual and Motor Skills, 57*, 1179–1186.

Spanos, N. P., de Groh, M., & de Groot, H. P. (1987). Skill training for enhancing hypnotic susceptibility and word list amnesia. *British Journal of Experimental and Clinical Hypnosis, 4*, 15–23.

Spanos, N. P., Flynn, D. M., & Gabora, N. J. (1989). Suggested negative visual hallucinations in hypnotic subjects: When no means yes. *British Journal of Experimental and Clinical Hypnosis, 6*, 63–67.

Spanos, N. P., Flynn, D. M., & Gwynn, M. I. (1988). Contextual demands, negative hallucinations, and hidden observer responding: Three hidden observers observed. *British Journal of Experimental and Clinical Hypnosis, 5*, 5–10.

Spanos, N. P., Flynn, D. M., & Niles, J. (1990). Rapport and cognitive skill training in the enhancement of hypnotizability. *Imagination, Cognition and Personality, 9*, 245–262.

Spanos, N. P., Gabora, N. J., Jarrett, L. E., & Gwynn, M. I. (1989). Contextual determinants of hypnotizability and of relationships between hypnotizability scales. *Journal of Personality and Social Psychology, 57*, 271–278.

Spanos, N. P., Y Gorassini, D. M. (1984). Structure of hypnotic test suggestions and attributions of responding involuntarily. *Journal of Personality and Social Psychology, 46*, 688–696.

Spanos, N. P., & Gottlieb, J. (1979). Demonic possession, mesmerism and hysteria: A social psychological perspective on their historical interrelationships. *Journal of Abnormal Psychology, 88*, 527–546.

Spanos, N. P., Gwynn, M. I., & Stam, H. J. (1983). Instructional demands and ratings of overt and hidden pain during hypnotic analgesia. *Journal of Abnormal Psychology, 92*, 479–488.

Spanos, N. P., & Hewitt, E. C. (1980). The hidden observer in hypnotic analgesia: Discovery or experimental creation? *Journal of Personality and Social Psychology, 39*, 1201–1214.

Spanos, N. P., Jones, B., & Malfara, A. (1982). Hypnotic deafness: Now you hear it—now you still hear it. *Journal of Abnormal Psychology, 90*, 75–77.

Spanos, N. P., & Katsanis, J. (1989). Effects of instructional set on attributions of nonvolition during hypnotic and nonhypnotic analgesia. *Journal of Personality and Social Psychology, 56*, 182–188.

Spanos, N. P., Kennedy, S. K., & Gwynn, M. I. (1984). The moderating effects of contextual variables on the relationship between hypnotic susceptibility and suggested analgesia. *Journal of Abnormal Psychology, 93*, 285–294.

Spanos, N. P., Lush, N. I., & Gwynn, M. I. (1989). Cognitive skill training enhancement of hypnotizability: Generalization effects and trance logic responding. *Journal of Personality and Social Psychology, 56*, 795–804.

Spanos, N. P., & McLain, J. M. (1986). Hypnotically created pseudomemories: Memory distortions or reporting biases? *British Journal of Experimental and Clinical Hypnosis, 3*, 155–159.

Spanos, N. P., Menary, E. P., Brett, P. J., Cross, W. P., & Ahmed, Q. (1987). Failure of posthypnotic responding to occur outside the experimental setting. *Journal of Abnormal Psychology, 96*, 52–57.

Spanos, N. P., Perlini, A. H., Patrick, L., Bell, S., & Gwynn, M. I. (1990). The role of compliance in hypnotic and nonhypnotic analgesia. *Journal of Research in Personality, 24,* 433–453.

Spanos, N. P., Perlini, A. H., & Robertson, L. A. (1989). Hypnosis, suggestion and placebo in the reduction of experimental pain. *Journal of Abnormal Psychology, 98*, 285–293.

Spanos, N. P., & Radtke, H. L. (1982). Hypnotic amnesia as strategic enactment: A cognitive social-psychological perspective. *Research Communications in Psychology, Psychiatry and Behavior, 7*, 215–231.

Spanos, N. P., Radtke, H. L., & Bertrand, L. D. (1984). Hypnotic amnesia as a strategic enactment: Breaching amnesia in highly susceptible subjects. *Journal of Personality and Social Psychology, 47*, 1155–1169.

Spanos, N. P., Radtke, H. L., Hodgins, D. C., Stam, H. J., & Bertrand, L. D. (1983). The Carleton University Responsiveness to Suggestion Scale: Normative data and psychometric properties. *Psychological Reports, 53*, 523–535.

Spanos, N. P., Rivers, S. M., & Ross, S. (1977). Experienced involuntariness and response to hypnotic suggestions. *Annals of the New York Academy of Sciences, 296*, 208–221.

Spanos, N. P., Salas, J., Bertrand, L. D., & Johnston, J. (1989). Occurrence schemas, context ambiguity and hypnotic responding. *Imagination, Cognition and Personality, 8*, 235–247.

Springer, C. J., Sachs, L. B, & Morrow, J. E. (1977). Group methods of increasing hypnotic susceptibility. *International Journal of Clinical and Experimental Hypnosis, 25*, 184–191.

Stryker, S. (1981). Symbolic interactionism: Themes and variations. In M. Rosenber & R. H. Turner (Eds.), *Social psychology: Sociological perspectives* (pp. 3–29). NY: Basic Books.

Wagstaff, G. F. (1981). *Hypnosis, compliance and belief.* NY: St. Martin's Press.

Wagstaff, G. F. (1986). Hypnosis as compliance and belief: A sociocognitive view. In P. L. N. Naish (Ed.), *What is hypnosis?* (pp. 59–84). Philadelphia: Open University Press.

Weitzenhoffer, A. M. (1953). *Hypnotism: An objective study in suggestibility.* NY: Wiley.

Weitzenhoffer, A. M. (1974). When is an "instruction" an "institution"? *International Journal of Clinical and Experimental Hypnosis, 22* 258–269.

White, R. W. (1941). A preface to a theory of hypnotism. *Journal of Abnormal and Social Psychology, 36*, 477–505.

Zamansky, H. S., & Bartis, S. P. (1985). The dissociation of an experience: The hidden observer observed. *Journal of Abnormal Psychology, 94*, 243–248.

CHAPTER 12

Compliance, Belief, and Semantics in Hypnosis: A Nonstate, Sociocognitive Perspective

GRAHAM F. WAGSTAFF
University of Liverpool

INTRODUCTION

The phenomena associated with hypnosis have been with us for well over 200 years, yet many academics and clinicians seem resistant to the idea that hypnotic phenomena can be explained in terms of knowledge that is readily available. However, if I were to summarize my position on hypnosis in one sentence, it would be as follows: If we have not been able to find *the* explanation for hypnotic phenomena, it is not because we lack the technology; it is because there *is* no single explanation for all hypnotic phenomena (Wagstaff, 1981c, 1982a, 1983a, 1983b, 1986a).

Hypnotic phenomena only become enigmatic when we erroneously generalize from one to another, and forge links where no link exists. For example, when given a particular suggestion for amnesia, some subjects may report that they cannot remember their own names. One explanation for this would be that these subjects are simply complying with expectations of the hypnotist and lying to give the appearance of being "amnesic." But a common argument against this explanation is that this cannot be the case, because patients can endure surgery with hypnosis, and *they* are not lying or shamming. Thus, for instance, Marcuse (1976) says, "The problem of shamming or conscious simulation is most clearly answered in this question of anaesthesia" (p. 49). However, this argument assumes that hypnotic subjects failing to recall their names and hypnotic subjects enduring surgery are behaving in these ways for the same reason—perhaps because they are in the same "state," or because amnesia and anesthesia are linked by a common "hypnotic process." But as soon as one rejects this assumption, it becomes obvious that such a generalization is logically flawed. Translated into a syllogism, the argument goes as follows: "Hypnotic anesthesia is a hypnotic phenomenon. Hypnotic anesthesia is not faked. Therefore, hypnotic phenomena are not faked." This actually makes as much sense as "Rover is black. Rover is a dog. Therefore, dogs are black."

In my opinion, the concept singly most responsible for holding back progress in understanding the nature of hypnotic phenomena is the notion of hypnosis as a "state." For as soon as we start talking about this "state," whether it be metaphorical, literal, physiological, or psychological, the implication seems to be that there is some common element binding hypnotic phenomena together, and that in seeking this element we will somehow discover what "it" is that explains the remarkable things we associate with hypnosis. As I hope to make clear shortly, I reject the notion of a hypnotic state for a number of reasons; however, one of the most important of these is that I think it deflects our attention away from the disparate sorts more mundane concepts and processes we need to account for the phenomena we associate with hypnosis (Wagstaff, 1981c, 1986a).

In many respects my perspective coincides with the ideas advanced by Sarbin, and later theorists such as Barber, Coe, and Spanos; as such, my approach could be variously described as "nonstate," "social-psychologi-cal," "cognitive-social," or "role enactment." My personal preference is for the rather ugly label "nonstate, sociocognitive," because I reject the utility of the term "hypnotic state," and I emphasize mainly (but certainly not exclusively) social and cognitive factors in my approach (Wagstaff, 1986a). There are obvious points of overlap between my approach and the approaches of these other "nonstatists," and they have provided me with a rich source of ideas and experiments I can use to develop and illustrate my case. However, if I had to identify a single figure who has had the most influence on my thinking, I would definitely choose Martin Orne, even though Orne and I may think rather differently about different aspects of hypnotic phenomena. Orne's work indicated to me that all too often so-called "hard" scientists and experienced clinicians approach their investigations with a disturbing naiveté about the social character of the phenomena they may produce (Orne, 1962, 1969, 1970). Equally importantly, his work seemed to imply that to make sense of the extraordinary we do not need to look to the extraordinary; we do not necessarily need bizarre theories and mechanisms to account for apparently bizarre phenomena.

In some respects one could trace the historical antecedents of my view to the skepticism that greeted the claims of the later 17th-century and early 18th-century practitioners of animal magnetism, and their successors, the hypnotists. However, I would dissociate myself from many of these skeptics for a number of reasons. For example, the Franklin commission of 1784 attempted to explain the phenomena associated with animal magnetism mainly by reference to "imagination," and also concluded that if animal magnetism did not exist it could not be useful. In 1837, another commission also dismissed the magnetists' claims, but by this time the tendency was to argue that magnetism was "fraudulent" (Sheehan & Perry, 1976). However, in my view any attempt to dismiss hypnotic phenomena as *all* fraud, or *all* imagination, or *all* anything, is overly simplistic and doomed to failure. Moreover, the fact that a particular theory is rejected does not mean that the techniques associated with it are necessarily therapeutically ineffective. For example, instructions that facilitate relaxation or coping skills may still be beneficial in therapy, regardless of whether we postulate magnetic fluid or a hypnotic state as the mechanism involved.

Consequently, I think the spirit of my view is better illustrated by reference to Hull's classic work *Hypnosis and Suggestibility: An Experimental Approach*, published in 1933. Hull did not set out to determine whether hypnosis was all faked or useless; rather his rationale was "to divest hypnosis of the air of mystery which usually surrounds it, by showing it to be entirely of a piece with everyday human nature" (p. 41). However, it seems to me that, regardless of the method of investigation we use, any attempt to "divest hypnosis of the air of mystery which usually surrounds it" is ultimately going to end up with an appeal to parsimony, or "Occam's razor"; thus, it is with this principle that I begin to describe the general rationale behind my position.

Applying Occam's Razor to Hypnosis

When attempting to provide an account of any particular phenomenon, scientists often apply the principle attributed to the 14th-century English philosopher William of Occam, known as "Occam's razor." The principle is that "entities are not to be multiplied without necessity" (Jones & Dixon, 1985, p. 629). The assumption is that before we can accept that a particular phenomenon requires the postulation of an extra unknown, unlikely, or complex factor x, in addition to other established factors (a, b, c, and d), we need first to demonstrate that the phenomenon cannot be understood or explained in terms of factors a, b, c and d alone. It is not scientists alone who make use of this principle; it is very much a part of everyday life. For example, most people in Western culture now doubt the existence of witches and leprechauns, but their doubts are not based on the fact that science has conclusively proved that witches and leprechauns do *not* exist; rather they are based on the assumption that the postulation of witches and leprechauns is not useful in explaining the phenomena that might be used as evidence for their existence. We cannot prove that witches and leprechauns do *not* exist; they certainly exist figuratively in dictionaries and story books, and some people apparently believe in them. Nevertheless, most people would reject them as literal entities.

In my opinion, there is much evidence to suggest that if we apply the principle of Occam's razor to the area of hypnosis, there is little point in holding onto the traditional idea that there exists *a* particular brain state or *an* "altered state of consciousness" we can label "hypnosis," which is somehow important in accounting for the phenomena we call "hypnotic." Moreover, although science has not proved, and never can prove that no such state exists, I would nevertheless consider the concept of "hypnotic state" (along with all its derivatives, such as "hypnotic depth," "trance experience," and "hypnotic vs. waking suggestibility") to be unnecessary and misleading anachronisms—leftovers from a mainly 19th-century paradigm that has long outlived its usefulness. In contrast with the traditional state terminology, I would suggest that a more appropriate vocabulary for dealing with the phenomena we usually term "hypnotic" would include terms such as "conformity," "compliance," "belief," "attitudes," "expectations," "attention," "concentration," "relaxation," "distraction," "role enactment," and "imagination."

I should make it clear, however, that the emphasis on this kind of vocabulary (and the concepts and processes implied by it) is not simply a piece of superficial semantic juggling; it has important implications for how we go about the task of investigating and accounting for the phenomena that are usually connected with the term "hypnosis." For example, in questioning the utility for a theory of hypnosis of postulating a hypnotic state, I would not necessarily wish to deny that some subjects believe they are having or have had a "hypnotic trance experience," because they may find this an appropriate way of labeling their experiences (Wagstaff, 1981c). Neither would I necessarily deny that for a few people it may even be therapeutically useful for them to believe this (Wagstaff, 1987b, 1987c). But I consider there to be a crucial distinction between the notion of *believing* that one is in a hypnotic state, and actually *being* in one.

Let us suppose, for instance, that a man commits a crime, but then in his defense alleges that he was "hypnotized" when he did it, and was therefore not responsible for his actions. According to my view, it would be very relevant from a legal perspective to know, for instance, whether he was lying and using this explanation as an excuse for his behavior, or whether he really believed he was "hypnotized." But it would be as inappropriate to attempt to establish whether or not he had been in a hypnotic state as it would be to establish whether he had been taken over by a leprechaun. Moreover, we would no more bring in experts on "the hypnotic state" to test whether or not he is capable of showing the "signs" that characterize this "state" than we would bring in experts on leprechauns to test a man's claim that he was possessed by a leprechaun. Indeed, one could honestly believe that one was "hypnotized" without showing any conventional "signs," if one's expectations were unconventional.

Also, there seems to be a crucial difference between the proposal that a hypnotic subject is in an "altered state of consciousness" because he or she is, for example, "relaxed" or "concentrating," and the idea that there is *an* altered state of consciousness we can label "hypnosis." Benson and Klipper (1976) have noted that when some people relax and concentrate, they indeed report what could be called an altered state of consciousness. This state could even be labeled a "trance," and Edmonston (1977) has suggested that this response may underlie what he calls "neutral hypnosis." However, the evidence suggests that one does not need to be relaxed to respond to hypnotic suggestions (Bányai & Hilgard, 1976; Malott, 1984), and the relationship between hypnotic responsiveness and concentration or absorption has also been questioned (Reilley & Rodolfa, 1981; Zamansky, 1977). Given these considerations, the description of hypnosis as an altered state because of what it shares with relaxation and concentration seems rather misleading.

The Need for a Change in Terminology

I would argue that the need for a change of orientation and language in the way we attempt to account for the phenomena subsumed under the term "hypnosis" is particularly important now, as many of the traditional concepts and terms have begun to take on a sort of ambiguous "double life": they are neither totally figural nor literal, neither extraordinary nor ordinary, and not mysterious yet enigmatic nevertheless. For example, in the early days of hypnosis and its predecessor, animal magnetism, most proponents seemed in no doubt as to the reality of the concepts they were using to explain the phenomena they observed. Mesmer did not appear to use "magnetic fluid" only as a metaphor; Puységur, Braid and Charcot apparently really did seem to believe there was *an* altered state of consciousness that was an important concomitant of the kinds of phenomena they observed, such as amnesia, hallucinations, and analgesia (Wagstaff, 1981c; Sheehan & Perry, 1976). In modern times, many of those who continue to use much of the vocabulary of the state view of hypnosis seem a good deal more cautious, but the caution is confusingly mixed with fragments from the older tradition. Thus, for instance, we are told that hypnosis is probably not a single state, but nevertheless "the" hypnotic state has certain defining characteristics (E. R. Hilgard, 1986, pp. 163–165 and 183). We are also told that although few now claim that hypnosis enables one to transcend waking capacities (Sheehan, 1983), hypnotic analgesia is more profound than waking analgesia (E. R. Hilgard & Hilgard, 1983).

It is important to note that the difficulty in ridding hypnosis of its enigmatic quality continues with the recent re-emergence of dissociation (Bowers, 1983; E. R. Hilgard, 1974, 1978, 1986). For example, E. R. Hilgard and Hilgard (1983) claim that hypnotic analgesia is more effective than waking analgesia, because when subjects "enter hypnosis" they dissociate. But we still need to know why it is this that subjects who are capable of dissociation dissociate more in the "hypnotic" than in the "waking" state. "Dissociation" cannot be readily used as a *synonym* for "hypnosis"; if it were, we would label anyone dissociating as "hypnotized." This would seem to make little sense, since according to E. R. Hilgard (1978) examples of "dissociation" can be found in split-brain patients (patients whose hemispheres have been largely surgically separated) and in cases of anorexia nervosa (a condition in which, he claims, patients' bodily needs and appetites have become "dissociated"). There is surely little to be gained from labeling split-brain patients and anorexics as "hypnotized." Indeed, Hilgard proposes that in cases of multiple personality (which he alleges is also due to dissociation), one can sometimes *only* reveal the dissociation when the person is in "a trance-like state" (1978, p. 34). In other words, being in a "hypnotic state" is not simply another way of saying "being dissociated." Rather, hypnosis is postulated as something through which hypnotic subjects or patients are able to *reveal* their dissociations, and also presumably to manipulate and inhibit them, if hypnotherapy is effective. Consequently, even if we accept the validity of the phenomena alleged to illustrate dissociation, we are still left with an enigmatic hypnotic factor, which not only is supposed to be indexed by the appearance of a "trancelike-state," but now somehow enables hypnotic subjects to reveal, release, or inhibit the dissociative capacities that reside within them. So just as we had "waking suggestion" and "hypnotic suggestion," we now seem to have "waking dissociation" and "hypnotic dissociation."

However, as I have pointed out at the beginning of this chapter, I believe that the many conceptual and semantic difficulties involved in defining some enigmatic "hypnotic factor" that either is itself, or is attached to a "hypnotic state" are avoidable, because there is actually no need to postulate one. The need only arises when the question "What is hypnosis?" is interpreted in the same way as it was construed by Braid and Charcot, and assumes the existence of some "thing"—some physiological or psychological process, mechanism, or condition in the brain. I would suggest that this orientation is inappropriate because, as Sarbin has been arguing for over 40 years, hypnosis is more appropriately seen as a *social invention* (Sarbin, 1989). Seen as a social invention, hypnosis is not a creature of biological evolution, genetically transmitted; it is a human creation, culturally transmitted. Once we view hypnosis as a social invention or construction, it becomes obvious that we are very unlikely ever to be able to link all the phenomena connected with it to some psychological or physiological process. Different phenomena may require different kinds of explanations. Moreover, not only may different hypnotic phenomena require different kinds of explanations, but also a range of processes may interact to give rise to individual phenomena, and the interactions between these processes may differ from situation to situation and from person to person. Consequently, asking such questions as "Is hypnosis faked?" or "Is hypnosis relaxation?" is rather like asking "Do doctors wear dark suits?"

I therefore suggest that if we are to progress in understanding the nature of hypnotic phenomena, we would do better just to disregard all the standard references to "trances," "altered states," "alternate states," "waking states," and so on, and then to look at each hypnotic situation simply for what it is. For example, in a typical hypnosis situation, one person, labeled a "hypnotist," performs a ritual on another, labeled a "subject" or "patient." The aim of the ritual is to inform or suggest to the subject that if he or she listens to the ritual and carries out the instructions or responds to suggestions, he or she will enter a sort of state in which interesting, important, and perhaps unusual things will happen. The ritual is then followed by further instructions and suggestions. Now to understand why such a situation should apparently be able to evoke such remarkable phenomena as reports of amnesia, hallucinations, and analgesia, we should perhaps look outside the traditional domain of hypnosis and examine other contexts that may share commonalities with this kind of situation.

In the next section, I endeavor to describe some of the concepts and processes which I think are particularly useful in linking hypnotic situations with others. I also attempt to show how I think some of the apparently more unusual aspects of hypnotic behavior may be explained in terms from mainstream psychology, without the necessity of postulating unusual and complex mechanisms and processes. However, before I do this, I need to clarify an issue that has an important bearing on my approach to explaining hypnotic phenomena. The issue is that of what we should and should not expect of a theory of hypnosis.

Expectations of a Theory of Hypnosis

What we should expect of an adequate theory of hypnosis is presumably an intelligible account of the behavior we observe in situations defined as "hypnotic" or as "hypnosis." However, we should not expect a theory of hypnosis to detail what accounts for a behavior that can occur in any situation, whether hypnotic or not. For example, the fact that a person is able to digest food is very interesting, but we do not expect a theory of *hypnosis* to explain how it is that hypnotic subjects can digest food, because they could do it whether they were "hypnotized" or not. On the other hand, if a person were able to digest food three times as fast in a hypnotic situation as he or she would in any other situation, we would expect a theory of hypnosis to give us some insight into how this could happen. This would all seem rather obvious, but consider the implications.

Let us take a more relevant example. One of the most impressive demonstrations by stage hypnotists is the "human plank feat." A hypnotic subject (usually male) is suspended between two chairs, and a volunteer stands on the chest of the subject. The members of the audience are impressed, and they may assume that the subject would not be able to perform this feat without the aid of "hypnosis." Any adequate theory of hypnosis must explain this phenomenon; the sort of explanatory hypothesis I would offer, in common with most theorists, would be that the subject could probably perform this feat regardless of whether or not he was in a situation defined as "hypnosis"; the people in the audience are only impressed because they do not know this. It actually *is* the case that without hypnotic induction, a normal man can support at least 300 pounds on his chest in this position with little discomfort (Barber, 1969). Consequently, I would suggest that my hypothesis is an adequate parsimonious explanation for this phenomenon.

But let us suppose that someone then says, "I agree that you do not need to be hypnotized to do this feat, but you haven't *explained* it, have you? What I want to know is this: *how* is it that a man can support 300 pounds on his chest in this position?" My answer to such a person would be that even if I have not a clue how a man can support 300 pounds on his chest, this in no way impugns the explanatory power of my theory of *hypnosis*; indeed, it is irrelevant to my theory. I no more need to answer this question than I need to explain how hypnotic subjects are able to digest food or see in color. A corollary of this is that it makes no logical sense to say that hypnosis is inexplicable, simply because hypnotic subjects sometimes do things that are in themselves inexplicable. For example, we have not yet devised a definitive theory of color vision, but we would not say that hypnosis is "inexplicable" because hypnotic subjects can see in color. The only fact relevant to a theory of hypnosis is that most people can see in color, whether they are "hypnotized" or not. On the other hand, if only hypnotic subjects could be persuaded to see in monochrome, there would indeed be something to explain. This is a crucial point, because I believe it establishes the legitimate boundaries of what one can reasonably expect from a theory of hypnosis, as distinct from a theory of the whole of human functioning; it is within such boundaries that my particular approach functions. It also draws attention to the fact that any theory of hypnosis claiming that there are important differences between behavior in hypnotic behavior in and nonhypnotic situations, but that we as yet do not know what could possibly cause them, is not actually *explaining* anything at all.

In view of my general approach, it should be noted that when I now use terms such as "hypnosis" and "hypnotic," I am using the terms purely operationally. A hypnotic subject is in a situation or context defined as "hypnosis"; a "hypnotized" person is one who responds in some way to the procedures designated as "hypnotic"; and so on. When I use these terms, I am not referring to or implying the existence of a brain state or psychological process called "hypnosis" (Wagstaff, 1981c).

THEORETICAL CONCEPTS AND PRINCIPLES

The two main concepts in my approach are "compliance" and "belief" (Wagstaff, 1979, 1981c, 1986a). I emphasize these concepts because I think they orient us toward the examination of hypnotic phenomena in a particularly useful way.

Within social psychology, the term "compliance" refers to a special form of conformity (Kiesler & Kiesler, 1970; Tedeschi, Linskold, & Rosenfeld, 1985). It normally refers to overt behavior that becomes like the behavior that others show or expect,and is most usually applied to conforming responses that tend to run counter to private convictions. For example, in a set of classic studies, Asch (1956) demonstrated that many subjects were prepared to make incorrect judgments of the lengths of lines when confronted by the erroneous judgments of others who had previously been briefed by the experimenter to make incorrect judgments. Importantly, however, most commentators have assumed that the subjects in Asch's studies did know that their responses were incorrect, but that they conformed to the majority nevertheless. That is, it is assumed that Asch's subjects exhibited compliance, saying one thing to conform to the majority, but not privately accepting the judgments they had made.

As Orne (1966) has pointed out, when a hypnotic subject responds to a hypnotic suggestion by simply deliberately performing some action, without an appropriate hypnotic experience (such as the experience of nonvolition), then the response can also be described as one of compliance. Accordingly, taking Orne's lead, I have identified two categories of responses to hypnotic suggestions that would normally constitute examples of "compliance only." The first type of response is that in which a volitional act is supposed to reflect an underlying subjective experience, but this is not the case; for example, in response to a pain stimulus subjects say they are not feeling pain when privately pain is felt, or they move their hands as if brushing away a "hallucinated" fly but do not experience a hallucinated fly at all. The second type of response is that in which an act is supposed (explicitly or implicitly) to be performed nonvolitionally, but the subject performs the act consciously or deliberately. For example, a subject may deliberately raise an arm in response to an arm levitation suggestion without feeling that the arm "rises by itself." It should be noted that if compliance does play an important part in hypnotic responding, the responses given by subjects will depend very much on their perception of what is *expected* of them. And what hypnotic subjects expect in a particular hypnotic situation will depend on an interplay of preconceptions held before the immediate context, and cues (both explicit and implicit) in the immediate context (Wagstaff, 1981c).

However, although I consider compliance to be a pivotal concept in understanding hypnotic phenomena, we also need a concept to deal with veridical reports and experiences of hypnotic suggestions. The term "belief" may be useful for this purpose (Wagstaff, 1981c). The standard dictionary definitions of "belief" appear to indicate that the term is very appropriate in this role; it means, for example, "acceptance of a thing as true; trust (in) (Oxford); faith (Chambers)". Belief is a useful concept because it enables us to distinguish between compliant and "honest" reporting in hypnotic situations without assuming that a subject's response must coincide with some preconceived traditional idea of what constitutes a "true" or "genuine" hypnotic response. In this respect, expectations would seem to play a crucial role again, for whether subjects honestly believe that their responses correspond with "being hypnotized" or are "genuine" responses to suggestions will depend on their expectations of what is appropriate.

For example, if subjects expect hypnotic induction to result in some profound experience of an altered state, but it does not, they may not believe they are "hypnotized" (though they may still comply with what they think is expected of them). On the other hand, if subjects expect hypnosis to be nothing more than a feeling of being relaxed and comfortable, and this is what they experience, they may honestly believe they are "hypnotized" (even though no profound alteration in consciousness is experienced). Similarly, if in response to a hallucination suggestion subjects describe an object, although not privately experiencing some full-blown hallucination, it does not necessarily mean that they are just complying or "faking." They may simply be "imagining" the object in their "mind's eye," as it were. Whether they *believe* their reports to be false or genuine will depend on their expectations of what is required of them. Are they *expected* to report only a full-blown hallucination, or will the exercise of simple imagination do (Wagstaff, 1981c, 1983a, 1985c, 1986a)?

Support for Compliance in the Social-Psychological Literature

At first, the idea that hypnotic subjects might be faking their responses to comply with expectations may seem absurd. Indeed, the tendency either to play down or even to ridicule this possibility is common. One way to play down compliance is to point to phenomena that seem to be inconsistent with compliance, such as surgery (see, e.g., Marcuse, 1976). But as I have already been pointed out, unless one makes the very big assumption that patients undergoing surgery are able to do so for the same reason that others display apparent phenomena such as negative hallucinations, automatic writing, or age regression, then the argument is logically flawed. Another approach is simply to dismiss compliance out of hand, as though it were an established fact that it is not significant. Thus, for example, E. R. Hilgard and Hilgard (1983) claim that "deliberate 'faking' . . . is very rare and not important" (p. 16). Another tactic is to introduce a negative stereotype of a compliant subject—for example, as someone trying to fool the hypnotist as a joke (Esdaile, cited by Marcuse, 1976), or as a "notorious liar" (Zamansky, 1989). However, in contrast, the social-psychological literature presents a rather different picture of compliance.

In addition to the studies by Asch (1956) mentioned earlier, many other studies outside the area of hypnosis indicate the importance of compliance in social behavior. Some of the best known are those of Milgram (1974), who demonstrated that over 60% of his sample of ordinary people were prepared to administer large doses of electric shock to a screaming "victim" when ordered to do so by the experimenter. The shocks were not actually real; indeed, Orne and Holland (1968) have suggested that the subjects may actually have perceived that the situation was safe. Nevertheless, inasmuch that subjects were at least prepared to give the impression that they were more or less torturing someone, this would still seem to be a fairly convincing demonstration of compliance. Perhaps even more persuasive was a follow-up by Sheridan and King (1972), who replaced the human actor with a *real* victim, a puppy, which was given *real* electric shocks; however, subjects in this study still obeyed and shocked the puppy with maximum shock. Of particular interest in the Milgram obedience studies was that when Milgram described his experimental setup to a mixed group of students, psychiatrists, and middle-class adults, not one said that he or she would obey the experimenter, and another sample predicted that only a pathological fringe of 1–2% would respond (Milgram, 1974). Thus there was a vast discrepancy between how people thought they would respond and what actually happened—a finding that is probably very relevant to studies of hypnosis.

However, the motive for compliant behavior does not have to derive from explicit instructions or demands. Orne (1962) has emphasized that in experimental situations subjects often perceive their task as being to fulfill the experimenter's expectations and to behave as "good" subjects. Orne has pointed out that people will carry out quite ridiculous requests if the context is appropriate. In one example, by Menaker (cited in Orne, 1962), subjects were asked to perform serial additions on sheets; on each sheet were 224 additions, and each subject was given 2,000 sheets. Each subject's watch was removed, and the instruction was "Continue to work; I will return eventually." The result was that, 5 1/2 hours later, the *experimenter* gave up! Orne (1962) regards Menaker's observations as similar to those of Frank (1944), who also found that experimental subjects were quite prepared to carry out disagreeable and nonsensical tasks. Orne also emphasizes that subjects often pick up subtle cues as to how to behave from a variety of sources, and he has coined the term "demand characteristics" to refer to those cues that can influence the subject's behavior so that it accords with the role of a "good" subject. Furthermore, Orne points out that the tendency for subjects to try to be "good" subjects and fulfill the experimenter's expectations has been known for a long time. Thus, in 1908, Pierce commented:

> It is to the highest degree probable that the subject's . . . general attitude of mind is that of ready complacency and a cheerful willingness to assist the investigator in every possible way by reporting to him those very things he is most eager to find, and that the very questions of the experimenter . . . suggest the shade of reply expected. (Cited in Orne, 1962, p. 472)

An obvious question, however, is this: why do people behave in this way? One view is that important social rules govern experimental situations and equivalent situations. Experimenters, like clinicians, have a specified role in a social situation, and this creates a moral demand to be treated and valued in a certain way; to disobey an experimenter and ruin an experiment is to commit a severe social impropriety (Milgram, 1974). Thus, Frank (1944) argues that when subjects enter an experimental situation, they are unwilling to break the tacit agreement made when they volunteered to take part—that is, to do whatever the experiment requires of them. Nevertheless, the wish to please the experimenter does not necessarily have to stem from a desire to avoid hurting or embarrassing the experimenter. Subjects in experimental situations may also develop "evaluation apprehension" (Weber & Cook, 1972) and want to be seen in a good light, as helpful, cooperative individuals. They may therefore also comply as a device to promote their self-image, to gain attention, and so on. Moreover, the motivation to comply does not necessarily have to stem from a desire to gain or maintain approval or to avoid embarrassment or hurt to others; it could also occur as a species of "informational conformity." That is, people may comply as a means of gaining information, as an exploratory device.

However, no matter what the cause, it seems that once people have complied with the demand characteristics of an experiment, it is no mean feat trying to make them "own up," especially if an admission would be personally embarrassing and/or hurtful to others. This point is well illustrated in a classic study by Levy (1967), which involved asking subjects to perform a verbal learning task. Before the experiment, some of the subjects were told surreptitiously by a confederate about the experimental hypothesis. This was very significant, as the experiment would only be valid if the subjects did *not* know the experimental hypothesis. However, Levy found that *not one* of these subjects volunteered that they had this knowledge during the experiment. Moreover, on questioning, only 1 subject out of 16 "owned up" to having been told about the experiment, and 75% denied any prior knowledge of the experiment at all! Levy concludes that "to rely upon the subject as an expert witness would be to betray as much naivete of the experimenter as that which he hopes exists in his subject" (p. 48). Such evidence indicates that attempts to make subjects provide accurate reports by simply asking them what "really" happened, or asking them to be "honest," are not likely to be particularly effective.

The social influence processes that can induce compliance are thus very powerful. Moreover (and importantly), to be compliant in an experimental or any other social situation, one does not have to be a swindler, a gullible fool, a trickster, or a "notorious liar," but an ordinary socialized individual who reponds to social expectations or obligations. Furthermore, one does not need to be physically coerced (or even mildly intimidated) to be compliant; and when one recognizes the social factors that may give rise to compliance, such as the wish to cooperate, to be helpful, and to achieve the goals of the interaction, the branding of compliant subjects as "jokers" or "notorious liars" seems rather inappropriate. Of course, people can have somewhat less honorable motives for complying. People can comply because they seek attention or want to have fun, and there are interesting examples in the scientific literature (see, e.g., Hansel, 1966). The point I wish to establish here, however, is that it is also perfectly possible to label a piece of behavior as "compliant" without in any way questioning the integrity of the person producing it. Indeed, it is not difficult for experimenters, quite unwittingly, to put their subjects in a genuine moral dilemma.

In view of these considerations, it seems reasonable to argue on *a priori* grounds that compliance is a likely rather than an unlikely factor in hypnotic responding. In fact, the hypnotic situation is ripe for this kind of response. It is not only a situation in which one person attempts to influence another, and in which the roles and statuses are clearly defined, but also a situation in which people are invited to experience interesting and unusual events. Consequently, normative considerations will dictate what responses are required so that subjects will appear helpful and cooperative, and informational considerations will invite subjects to deliberately carry out suggestions on the understanding that little is likely to happen if they do not *do* anything. Indeed, I would argue that the main reasons why people start to respond to hypnotic procedures stem from one or the other (or both) of these factors: the desire to cooperate, and the desire to find out what will happen (Wagstaff, 1981c). In therapeutic situations, these factors will be complemented by an important additional desire to do anything that will be therapeutically beneficial.

A THREE-STAGE PROCESS: EXPECTATION, STRATEGY, COMPLIANCE

However, although there are strong motives to comply in hypnotic situations, compliance brings disadvantages. Compliant subjects may feel deceitful; their self-image may be threatened; they may feel very disappointed. Accordingly, there are also strong pressures for subjects to want to *believe* that their overt motor responses and verbal reports actually correspond to the private experiences expected of them. Hypnotic subjects may therefore be highly motivated to carry out suggestions so that they are not only publicly, but also privately, acceptable. The factors that give rise to compliance and belief thus may interact, and I have found it useful to conceive of this interaction as part of a three-stage process, which I call the "ESC" (expectation, strategy, compliance) process (Wagstaff, 1983a, 1986a; Wagstaff & Benson, 1987). Thus when subjects enter a hypnotic situation, they do the following:

1. They work out what is appropriate to the role.
2. They apply "normal" cognitive strategies or activities to make the experiences veridical or "believable," in line with expectations and what is explicitly or implicitly demanded in the suggestions.
3. If the application of "normal" strategies fails, is not possible, or is

deemed inappropriate in the context, they behaviorally comply or "sham."

Importantly, stages 2 and 3 are not to be seen as necessarily occurring in numerical sequence; indeed, for reasons I have stated above, some subjects may actually employ compliance (stage 3) in the hope that actions and experiences will eventually become congruent. Others may go straight to stage 3 and comply, without attempting any particular strategy to make overt behavior and private experience congruent; thus, they skip stage 2 altogether. Others may attempt stage 2, fail to produce congruent actions and experiences, and stop at this point. Also, the way in which the ESC process operates may differ not only between subjects, but also *within* subjects in different suggestions. It may be much easier to make overt behavior and private experience coincide in response to, for example, a suggestion for body swaying or arm lowering than to a hallucination suggestion. Nevertheless, according to this scheme, compliance will operate to the greatest extent when social pressures and susceptibility to them are greatest, and when the strategies in stage 2 have failed to produce congruent subjective and behavioral responses.

The kinds of strategies employed in stage 2 of the ESC process may vary from subject to subject and from suggestion to suggestion. The sorts of activities I have in mind have been detailed by myself and other nonstate theorists elsewhere (see, e.g., Barber, Spanos, & Chaves, 1974; Lynn, Rhue, & Weekes, 1989; Spanos, Rivers, & Ross, 1977; Wagstaff, 1981c), and they include such activities as the following. In response to an ideomotor suggestion such as arm lowering, subjects may try hard to imagine that their arms are heavy. In nonhypnotic situations many people seem to have no difficulty passing this suggestion (i.e., experiencing the movement as "involuntary") as long as they "think along with the suggestion" and do not just "wait for something to happen." To respond to a challenge suggestion, all that is required is to obey the instructions. For example, if it is suggested to a subject that an arm is stiff, then so long as the subject keeps the arm stiff, he or she will not be able to bend it (this is akin to trying to stand up and sit down at the same time). In response to an amnesia suggestion, the subject may try some inattention strategy to avoid thinking about the target material. To respond to an analgesia suggestion, subjects may try hard to distract themselves, or to keep calm and tolerate the pain, or even to concentrate on the pain. To respond to a hallucination suggestion, subjects may try hard to *imagine* the suggested object. Most people can picture and describe an object in "their mind's eye," as it were.

Nevertheless, the range of phenomena achievable by these strategies will obviously be limited, and this leads me to doubt the validity of certain hypnotic effects that appear to lie outside the capacities of these strategies. It should be remembered that no matter how interesting and inexplicable we may find the behaviors of people with clinical problems, the subjects who participate in most laboratory studies on hypnosis are not brain-damaged, or classified as psychotic or as suffering from any other psychological disorder. Consequently, I think it highly improbable, for example, that hypnotic subjects can perform a writing task posthypnotically, without being aware of it (Stevenson, 1976), or that they can fail selectively to see material that is placed before their open eyes, only to "see" it when another level or part of the mind is contacted (Zamansky & Bartis, 1985). In fact, though I do not doubt that some people who are ill or on drugs may find themselves hallucinating "as real as real," I remain to be convinced that a normal healthy hypnotic subject (or a nonhypnotic subject, for that matter) can actually hallucinate "as real as real" on command or in response to suggestion. I am also dubious of the claim that anyone who attempts to carry out an amnesia suggestion is engaged in an active but futile attempt to remember (Kihlstrom, 1978; Bowers, 1983). I would argue that, if anything, the hypnotically amnesic subject is actively trying *not* to remember. Neither am I convinced that it is possible for someone with a normal visual system to "see," rather than simply to imagine, people walking around a room without their heads and feet; nor do I accept that it is possible to contact and talk to different parts of a person's consciousness in such a way that the different parts of consciousness are not aware of each other (E. R. Hilgard, 1986; E. R. Hilgard & Hilgard, 1983). I suspect that the most parsimonious explanations of these phenomena can be couched in terms of compliance and the overinterpretation of subjects' verbal reports. I elaborate on the latter point shortly.

Areas of Ambiguity

However, according to my view, there are important areas of ambiguity at the interface of expectation, strategy, and compliance. For example, a number of "normal" psychological phenomena that are sometimes employed in hypnotic situations, because of their ambiguous status, can be used by subjects as evidence of being "hypnotized"; these include relaxation effects, eye fixation, gravity, and imagery (Barber, 1969; Barber et al., 1974; Kidder, 1973; Skemp, 1972; Wagstaff, 1981c). Even one's own compliance may be a source of surprise and disbelief and may require rationalization (Wagstaff, 1981c). Attributions based on these factors will be mediated by expectations. Compliance occurs when,in accordance with role expectations, overt behavior and private conviction diverge. Consequently, as previously mentioned, one person's compliance may be another person's "believed-in" response, depending on expectations.

For example, subjects who pretend not to be able to see something that they actually can see as clear as day are exhibiting pure compliance. But if in response to an amnesia suggestion subjects successfully employ a distraction strategy so that they cannot remember, say, a word list, this could be interpreted in different ways. For subjects who think they are really supposed to find that the list has "disappeared from mind" and will not return despite active efforts to recall it, the use of an inattention or distraction strategy will be likely to be construed as an act of compliance. On the other hand, for subjects who think it is perfectly legitimate to interpret the amnesia suggestion as an invitation to attend away from the target material, then, as long as the inattention strategy is effective, they can honestly claim they have "forgotten." Again, however, I doubt very much whether any inattention strategy would enable normal healthy individuals to forget their own names, the number 7, or anything at all that they had known or seen a few seconds previously. Such claims I would tend to put down to compliance (Wagstaff, 1986a).

However, even a subject who is very compliant in hypnotic situations will not necessarily need to comply to produce certain responses. One must not assume that compliance will necessarily be all-or-none *within* subjects. Whether a subject actually needs to comply on a particular suggestion in order to give the appearance of passing it will depend on that subject's expectations as to what is appropriate as a response. For example, as I have mentioned, many (probably most) people are capable of passing an arm-lowering suggestion without "faking it" as long as they involve themselves in the suggestion, do not resist, and accept that this kind of deliberate involvement is a legitimate strategy. But it does not follow that because people can pass an arm lowering suggestion in this way, they will *not* go on to "fake" a negative hallucination suggestion. According to the ESC process, a person playing the role of a highly susceptible subject only needs to exhibit behavioral compliance when the strategies do not "work" within the criteria set by expectations.

One of the most striking illustrations I have come across of the possibility that compliance is unlikely to be all-or-none within subjects in hypnotic situations comes from the report of a woman, T. L., who contacted me following a talk I had given on hypnosis. T. L. told me that she had undergone major surgery with hypnosis and she had a videotape of the operation. Hypnosis had been chosen because she had a chest condition that precluded the use of a general anesthetic. However, she said that while the surgery itself was a success, the preoperative hypnotic induction ritual and suggestions for age regression were not at all successful; in fact, she had simply "gone along" and complied with the suggestions without feeling at all "hypnotized." T. L.'s testimony would tend to endorse the proposal that the success of so-called "hypnotic" surgery is related to factors not specific to hypnosis, such as the use of suggestions for the attenuation of pain; the reduction of anxiety by careful provision of detailed information; the encouragement of coping strategies, such as distraction and positive self-statements; the fostering of belief in the capacity to cope with the situation; and, in some cases, the use of local anesthetics (Barber et al., 1974; Chaves, 1989; Spanos, 1989; Wagstaff, 1981c). It could be argued that T. L. had slipped into a hypnotic state without being aware of it, but I would consider such an explanation to be unparsimonious and unnecessary.

The kinds of strategies I envisage as operating in the ESC process are predominantly *deliberate*. That is, they are conscious, effortful attempts to bring about the suggested effects. This raises the knotty question of conscious and unconscious processes. Some doubt our abilities to report on our everyday mental activities (Nisbett & Wilson, 1977), so it is a moot point whether many of our most mundane everyday activities could be truly described as "deliberate." However, using the logic I have put forward with regard to the legitimate requirements of a theory of hypnosis, I would argue that hypnotic phenomena are only unconscious to the extent that nonhypnotic equivalents can be described as unconscious. For example, regardless of whether they occur in hypnotic or nonhypnotic contexts, certain phenomena have a reputation for being undeliberate or automatic; these include suggested skin irritation (itching), suggested or imitated coughing, and the body sway response (Hull, 1933; Wagstaff, 1981c). It seems manifestly the case that if one suggests to people for long enough that they are moving backward or forward, or their heads are itching, or their throats are dry, that some seem to end up swaying, scratching their heads, and clearing their throats. Such phenomena have been categorized under various headings, such as "imitation" or "mimicry," "ideomotor action," and "empathy," and are familiar in everyday life.

However, although a theory of suggestibility per se would need to explain these are interesting phenomena, as far as my theory of hypnosis is concerned I need go no further than to propose that the explanation for why they may occur in hypnotic situations would be no different from the explanation for why they may occur in nonhypnotic situations, and "hypnosis" is an irrelevant consideration. On the other hand, I am dubious of claims that hypnosis can be used to manipulate the conscious–unconscious barrier in some remarkable way. For example, Bowers (1966, 1983) claims it is possible for a hypnotic subject to forget on command a set of suggestions, and then posthypnotically to respond "unconsciously" to these previously delivered suggestions, to the extent of beginning sentences with the words "he" and "they" while remaining unaware of doing so. According to my view, this finding is more parsimoniously explicable in terms of compliance. Consequently, even allowing for the fact that none of us may be particularly good at articulating the processes that give rise to our behavior, I would argue (as many other nonstate theorists do) that hypnotic subjects are best conceived as conscious, decision-making, cognizing agents actively trying to fulfill role demands; they are just as aware of what they are doing as any of us in nonhypnotic situations. They have not "entered" or "slipped into" a state in which the unconscious–conscious barrier can be manipulated in some special way.

Individual Differences in Hypnotic Responding

One fairly obvious implication of all this is that I would predict substantial individual differences in responsiveness to hypnotic procedures, for a number of reasons. For instance, even if responsiveness to hypnotic suggestions were totally due to compliance, it would not follow that everyone would respond to everything. Subjects can choose to be a little susceptible, somewhat susceptible, or highly susceptible; they can decide that no one would pass certain suggestions, and that some suggestions are more credible than others (Wagstaff, 1977b). Asch's (1956) subjects varied considerably in the degree of compliance they showed, and some did not comply at all; also, in Milgram's (1974) studies, not everyone responded to the instructions. This does not mean, however, that there would necessarily be strong correlations between hypnotic responsiveness and compliance in other situations, because there are a number of factors counteracting such a trend.

First, conformity in general tends to be situation-specific and difficult to predict across situations (McGuire, 1968; Wagstaff, 1981c, 1983b). Second, as I have pointed out, hypnotic responding is likely to be influenced by informational conformity—that is, the tendency to comply with suggestions as a device to "see what will happen." This may result in what social psychologists call the "foot-in-the-door effect" (Freedman & Fraser, 1966). Having unwittingly committed themselves, some subjects may find it easier to continue complying than to pull out. Thus a subject who ends up complying with various hypnotic suggestions may not necessarily be a "compliant" person at all (inasmuch as one exists). He or she may just as easily be someone who tries out suggestions and then finds it difficult to extricate himself or herself from the situation (Wagstaff, 1981c). Moreover, some people may find play-acting suggestions quite rewarding, especially when reinforced by positive comments from the hypnotist or experimenter. And this leads to another point: It cannot be assumed that a person who complies on a few or all suggestions would be unwilling to repeat the experience on a future occasion. As any experimental psychologist knows, many subjects will return again and again to perform the most boring, arduous, and sometimes painful tasks. There is no reason to suspect that compliant responding in hypnotic situations would be unstable or unreliable. The question of why people return to do further experiments, especially when renumeration is poor or nonexistent and when the experiments are dull or even downright distressing, is an interesting one, but one not limited to studies of hypnosis. In therapy, however, the contingencies governing return may be rather more straight-forward: The patient may really have little alternative but to "keep trying," and the therapist may still provide comfort, good advice, and attention, even if the patient is just complying.

Another reason why a sociocognitive approach to hypnosis would predict substantial individual differences would be that subjects differ in their expectations of and attitudes to hypnosis (Wagstaff, 1988c), and in their willingness to carry out suggestions. Some may feel negative and worried, whereas others may feel positive and enthusiastic; some may feel that something very unusual will happen, whereas others may feel that nothing particularly extraordinary will occur; some may feel incapable of or embarrassed about acting out suggestions, whereas others may revel in the opportunity; some may assume that things are supposed to happen to them, whereas others assume that they have to make things happen; and so on. All these factors will combine and interact to create a complex balance of what one of my colleagues in my early days at Liverpool, Sonja Hunt, calls, "strain" and "binding" factors (Hunt, 1979). Binding factors include the desire to appear cooperative, the wish not to fail to fulfill the purposes of the encounter, and the wish to gain knowledge and have unusual experiences. By contrast, strain factors include perceiving the task as trivial, embarrassing, difficult to perform, dangerous, or counter to expectations. Consequently, how a particular subject responds in any hypnotic situation will depend upon how these strain and binding factors are weighted, and they will inevitably be weighted differently for different subjects. Nevertheless, again, there is no reason to predict that in the absence of any attempt to manipulate them, responses will necessarily be unstable or unreliable on repeated testing.

RESEARCH AND APPRAISAL

A steady stream of research continues to support two basic predictions from my approach. First, there is as yet no definitive physiological evidence for the existence of a unique "hypnotic state." Some continue to allege that there are important physiological correlates of hypnosis (Gruzelier, 1988); however, as their studies lack adequate control procedures to account for the effects of equivalent suggestions given independently in nonhypnotic contexts, their results may reflect nothing more than hypnotic subjects' mundane strategies for enacting the hypnotic role. Most evidence supports the view that the physiological responses of subjects given hypnotic induction procedures are no different from those of nonhypnotic subjects given similar suggestions (Sarbin & Slagle, 1979; Wagstaff, 1981c; Wagstaff, Hearne, & Jackson, 1980).

Second, there is as yet no conclusive evidence that hypnotic subjects can transcend their normal capacities. Typically, studies claiming transcendence have been methodologically flawed, either because they have failed to supply appropriate motivating instructions to their control groups, or because they have used within-subject designs (i.e., subjects have acted as their own controls). This latter type of design is inappropriate in hypnosis experiments, because the evidence suggests that subjects tend to suppress their performance in the "waking control" condition, in order to give a spurious boost to their performance in the hypnotic condition (Wagstaff, 1981c, 1983d). When adequate controls are applied, hypnotic subjects do not transcend nonhypnotic performance on measures of hypnotic deafness, blindness, color blindness, visual acuity, objective measures of the ability to hallucinate, memory (including forensic analogues), physical endurance, age regression, and so on (Barber, 1969; Barber et al., 1974; O'Connell, Shor, & Orne, 1970; Wagstaff, 1981a, 1981c, 1982d, 1982e, 1983c, 1984, 1985b, 1985d, 1988a, 1989; Wagstaff & Sykes, 1984; Wagstaff & Ovenden, 1979; Wagstaff, Traverse, & Milner, 1982). Studies of pain remain controversial, but simulators can successfully imitate the overt responses of hypnotically susceptible subjects given suggestions for pain relief in the laboratory, and a number of studies indicate that suggestions given without hypnotic induction are as effective as hypnotic suggestions for analgesia (Spanos, 1986b, 1989; Wagstaff, 1981c). Moreover, attempts to find physiological correlates of hypnotic analgesia have been inconclusive (Wagstaff, 1981c). I have already mentioned some of the factors that are most likely responsible for the ability to tolerate or attenuate clinical pain (see Chaves, 1989), none of which requires the necessity of inducing a "hypnotic state."

Studies on the clinical uses of hypnosis tend to point again to the operation of factors that are not unique to the hypnosis situation in accounting for "success" in hypnotherapy—that is, factors such as social support, covert modeling, relaxation, and placebo effects. Moreover, in some cases the influence of compliance cannot be ruled out (Wagstaff, 1981c, 1985e, 1986a, 1987b, 1987c). I would certainly not wish to deny, though, that for some patients there may actually be unique advantages to defining a context as "hypnosis"; for example, "hypnotic amnesia," if only pretended, is a potentially useful device not only for saving face, but also for providing a legitimate context for controlling the vivid remembering of traumatic experiences.

However, it is not the claim of transcendence that seems to dominate most modern academic debate on hypnosis; rather, the controversies tend to center round some rather more subtle phenomena related to verbal reports of hallucinations, amnesia, and analgesia (Wagstaff, 1987a, 1988d). The literature on these issues is voluminous; I could not possibly discuss every phenomenon and how I would explain it in this short chapter. What I intend to do instead, therefore, is to present a scheme onto which the reader can map any studies he or she comes across.

Three Categories of Hypnotic Phenomena

The first part of the scheme involves conceptualizing hypnotic phenomena as falling into three main categories, A, B, and C, as follows:

A. *Attributable to simulation*. These are phenomena attributable to compliance. The behaviors are overtly performed, but there is no congruent private experience.

B. *Not simulated, but attributable to processes not specific to hypnosis*. These are phenomena that are not perceived as simulated, but do not require the postulation of some specialized hypnotic process to account for them. They can include the effects of deliberate strategies aimed to bring about suggested responses (e.g., such as thinking along with suggestions, the use of imagination, and the use of distraction and inattention), as well as phenomena associated with relaxation and placebo effects. It should be noted that some of these phenomena will not necessarily *always* belong in this category. If a subject perceives that the phenomenon is not congruent with expectations, it will fall into category A, simulation; one person's compliance may be another person's "believed-in" or genuine response, depending on expectations.

C. *Attributable to an hypnosis specific process*. Included here are phenomena that require the postulation of some hypnosis-specific process such as hypnotic dissociation (E. R. Hilgard, 1986); thus, phenomena in this category allegedly take on a special quality because the subject has "entered" or "slipped into" a "state of hypnosis." The crucial difference between the phenomena in this category and those in A and B is that those in A and B are "waking phenomena," whereas those in C are "hypnotic phenomena." For instance, "waking suggestibility" would belong in B, whereas "hypnotic suggestibility" would belong in C; "hypnotic analgesia" would belong in C, but "waking analgesia" would belong in B.

Now, according to a nonstate sociocognitive perspective, category C is redundant. Indeed, the assignment of any phenomenon to category C can be viewed as a category error—an error produced by a failure to perceive that phenomena can actually be accommodated by the use of categories A and B, either singly or in combination. Indeed, I would argue that sometimes category errors in assigning hypnotic phenomena are similar to the sort of conceptual error identified by Ryle (1973). For example, if people are shown a right glove and then a left glove, but then they say "I've seen the right glove and the left glove, but where's the pair of gloves?," they have committed a category error. A pair of gloves is indeed more than a right glove and more than a left glove, but it is not more than a right and left glove in *combination*. In the same way, to say hypnosis is more than compliance, and more than strategic enactment or suggestion, or more than a placebo, does not mean it is something else *other* than all these things.

Six Possible Sources of Error

The second part of the scheme involves the identification of six possible sources of error that could give rise to the assumption that the special hypnosis-specific category (C) is necessary to account for hypnotic phenomena. The first source of error involves prematurely rejecting a phenomenon from the compliance category (A), without actually adequately testing whether it can be attributed to simulation or compliance. For example, Kihlstrom, Evans, Orne and Orne (1980) found that some highly susceptible subjects continued to show hypnotic amnesia, in spite of explicit instructions to actively try to remember and to be honest. Kihlstrom et al. interpreted this to mean that hypnotic amnesia is more than compliance and more than deliberate inattention. However, given the previous discussion of the phenomenon of compliance, and particularly Levy's (1967) findings on how difficult it is to get subjects to "own up," it would seem very unlikely that honesty demands or demands to remember would be effective on someone fully committed to complying with the hypnotic role.

What is needed to test fully for whether amnesia can be breached is a face-saving device. One such device would be to allow subjects to describe themselves as having "role-played" rather than as having been in a "trance," and to do this *after* they have been given an amnesia suggestion but *before* amnesia is tested. I found that this procedure did indeed eliminate reports of amnesia, whereas subjects who were not allowed to say they were role-playing displayed amnesia in the usual way (Wagstaff, 1977a). Interestingly, in this latter study some of those allowed to say they were role-playing still reported "feeling hypnotized," which can be seen as attesting to my thesis that compliance is unlikely to be all-or-none within subjects. A number of other studies and considerations indicate that other hypnotic amnesia phenomena (e.g., disorganized retrieval in partial amnesia, source amnesia) are also readily explicable in terms of compliance (Wagstaff, 1977c, 1981b, 1981d, 1981e, 1982b, 1982c; Wagstaff & Carroll, 1987).

A second source of error involves assigning a phenomenon to the special hypnosis category (C) because it does not fit in the simulation or compliance category (A), without considering that it could belong in the nonspecific-to-hypnosis, nonsimulation category (B). Take, for example, the finding reported by Orne (1959) that whereas a control group of simulators instructed to fake hypnosis tended to report opaque hallucinations in response to a hallucination suggestion, some "real" hypnotic subjects reported transparent hallucinations. According to Orne (1959) and Bowers (1983), the reporting of transparent hallucinations is an example of "trance logic"—a form of illogical reasoning—and attests to the reality of hypnotic phenomena. In fact, according to Bowers (1983), "trance logic" is an example of "hypnotic dissociation" (i.e., it belongs in category C). However, others have found that asking subjects simply to *imagine* an object is all that is necessary to evoke a report of a transparent hallucination (Johnson, Maher, & Barber, 1972).

It could therefore be the case that a report of a transparent hallucination is simply a way of saying "I imagined it"; that is, though it may not belong in A, it may belong in B. Reports of differences between simulators and "real" hypnotic subjects on this response tend to be confounded by the fact that simulators are usually selected because they are not hypnotically susceptible, and there is evidence that when high-susceptibility simulators are used, even the simulators will report transparency. It may be the case, therefore, that some transparency responses do belong in category A (see Wagstaff, 1981c, 1981d); nevertheless, we can at least allow the possibility that some belong in B, and in either case there seems no need to assign them to C. I should emphasize, however, that Orne himself does *not* argue that his experiments support the view that certain responses are unique to hypnosis; he argues only that they are not attributable to simulation. Nevertheless, others have been less cautious in interpreting his studies, so that is why I have mentioned them here.

A third source of error derives from manipulating a strategy that might allow one to assign a phenomenon to B, but when the strategy fails, assigning the phenomenon in question to C, when it actually belongs to A. For example, Zamansky (1977) investigated the hypothesis that genuine responsiveness to hypnotic suggestions is accomplished by actively imagining the suggested effects while ignoring conflicting information. To test this he gave subjects hypnotic suggestions such as arm catalepsy ("you cannot bend your arms") and finger lock ("your fingers are stuck together"), but at the same time he asked them to imagine that they *could* perform the acts of bending their arms and separating their fingers. The results indicated that the subjects carried out the suggestions. They failed to bend their arms and separate their fingers, despite the conflicting images.

Zamansky's explanation for this was couched in terms of dissociation; he hypothesized that the part of the mind responding to the suggestion was dissociated from the part involved in the imaginings. In other words, he concluded that this phenomenon belongs in C. However, I would argue that it is more parsimonious to assign it to A. Indeed, what Zamansky may have demonstrated is the utmost significance of compliance in hypnotic responding, because if subjects are deprived of what is necessary to perform a category B phenomenon, then all that is left for them to do is to comply overtly, if they are still to repond. Indeed, Zamansky's finding can be interpreted as a fairly dramatic example of the operation of the ESC process I have identified earlier in the chapter. When subjects are stripped of their rationale for categorizing their responses as "genuine," all they are left with is compliance.

A very similar, perhaps even more obvious example is provided by Gill and Brenman (1959). They report:

> First we would induce hypnosis in someone previously established as a "good'" subject; then we would ask him how he knew he was in hypnosis. . . . He might reply he felt relaxed. Now we would suggest that the relaxation would disappear but he would remain in hypnosis. Then we would ask again how he knew he was in hypnosis. He might say because his arm "feels numb"—so again, we would suggest the disappearance of this sensation. We continued in this way until we finally obtained the reply, "I know I am in hypnosis because I *know* I will do what you tell me." This was repeated with several subjects, with the same results. (p.36)

Such a result also clearly seems to go against the idea that responsiveness to hypnotic suggestions is determined by thinking along with suggestions, or by absorption or involvement in imaginings. However, according to my interpretation, this is another very clear demonstration that if subjects are stripped of what is needed to attribute their experiences to "hypnosis," or to experience their responses are genuine, all that remains are subjects' quite blatant admissions that they will comply with whatever the hypnotist says.

A fourth source of error comes from "reading too much" into an honest report belonging to category B and unparsimoniously assigning it to C. For example, Sheehan and McConkey (1982) cite a number of examples of subjects' reports, which the authors claim reflect "experiences of trance." However, to me, many of these "experiences of trance" look simply like reports of subjects involved in feelings of relaxation and using mundane imagination. For instance, in one case, while the authors are talking about deepening one subject's "trance," the subject concerned is talking about "becoming more and more relaxed" (p. 112).

One of the difficulties with hypnosis research is that once a hypnotist starts communicating with a subject using the language of suggestions, the possibility exists that the subject will start to talk back in metaphors. Indeed, the reporting of perfectly mundane experiences in the form of metaphors not only may exacerbate the fourth sort of error, but may also lead to a fifth. The fifth error is to fail to recognize when a subject is actually trying to admit that he or she has complied with the demand characteristics of the situation—that is, to "read too much" into an honest report of a phenomenon that belongs in category A and unparsimoniously assume that it belongs in C. For example, E. R. Hilgard (1986) claims that when a hypnotic subject is given an analgesia suggestion, two levels of pain can be experienced: first, the profound analgesia due to hypnotic dissociation, and second, the "hidden pain" reported by a "hidden observer" contacted "under hypnosis.' Thus, the classic "hidden-observer effect" in hypnotic analgesia is that the hidden observer reports *more* pain than the hypnotized part. But consider the following reports by some subjects of their experiences of the hidden observer: "The hidden observer is more aware and *reported honestly* what was there"; "The hidden observer is like *the way things really are*"; "When the hidden observer was called up, the hypnotized part had to step back for a minute and let the hidden part *tell the truth*" (Knox, Morgan, E. R. Hilgard, 1974, pp. 845-846); "I'm not sure if the hypnotized part may have known it was there but *didn't say it*" (E. R. Hilgard, Morgan, & Macdonald, 1975, p. 286). (My italics in all cases.)

These may look like instances of dissociated cognitive subsystems to some; to me they look like reports from subjects trying to say that they actually felt pain but reported otherwise. It is as though the metaphor of the hidden observer enabled them to report honestly and tell the truth, while saving face. It is relevant to note here that the hidden observer phenomenon is easily produced by subjects instructed to "fake" hypnosis, so what is expected or required is quite obvious (Wagstaff, 1980). However, I should stress again that I am *not* claiming *all* reports of hypnotic analgesia are "faked." Although some subjects may pretend they feel less pain than they do, others may be applying the sorts of deliberate strategies outlined by Spanos (1986b, 1989) and gaining some relief; some reports may reflect both. However, it is surely important to recognize when subjects may actually try to admit to compliance, albeit in a way that is as face-saving as possible for all concerned.

Another possible example of this kind of error is to be found in some interpretations of a study by Pattie (1935). In this study, a woman who claimed hypnotic uniocular blindness was eventually found not to be blind. Subsequently, she admitted that she had employed tricks or devices to give the appearance of being blind, including practicing being blind at home with a friend! However, she was only able to recall all this while "under hypnosis." Her admission that she had done this was very distressing for her, and given that she was only trying to perform the role of a "good subject," it would seem uncharitable in the extreme to brand her a "cheat" or "prankster." But Bowers (1983) goes further and suggests that because she would only make the admission while "hypnotized," she was displaying "unconscious cooperation" and not "purposeful deception" (p. 12). In contrast, however, I would suggest that instead of assuming the woman had amnesia and could only remember "under hypnosis," it makes more sense to argue that she was using amnesia as a face-saving device. In fact, it would be difficult to find a clearer example of compliance. The idea that a woman would "unconsciously" go home and practice being blind with a friend seems unlikely to me unless she was suffering from some severe psychological disorder. Finally, perhaps the most blatant example of this kind of error is to be found in Wolberg's claim that "Generally, the subject will deny having been in a hypnotic state, even when he has achieved the deepest somnambulistic trance" (1972, p. 49). Of course, Wolberg could be correct, but I would reject his interpretation on grounds of parsimony.

A sixth and final source of error is claiming that something belongs in category C, and not in categories A or B, when it is an irrelevant consideration. For example, Bowers and Davidson (1986) claim that sociocognitive views of hypnosis cannot cope with the fact that there are stable individual differences in hypnotic responding. However, there is no need to assume that even if hypnosis were a "state," susceptibility to it would be stable. The hypnotic "state" could be influenced by all sorts of fluctuating factors. Moreover, nonstate theorists such as Sarbin have long been interested in individual differences (Sarbin & Coe, 1972), and many correlates of hypnotic susceptibility have been found that are perfectly compatible with a sociocognitive view.

For example, hypnotic susceptibility has been reported to correlate to some degree with a number of variables, including conformity in the Asch paradigm (Shames, 1981); self-reports of imaginative or fantasy involvement (J. R. Hilgard, 1970; Tellegen & Atkinson, 1974; Wilson & Barber, 1983); the ability to act out a pantomime and the ability to simulate items on a hypnosis scale (Sarbin & Coe, 1972); and influencibility and positive attitudes to hypnosis (Moore, 1964; Spanos, 1986a). Equally significantly, attempts to relate hypnotic susceptibility to skills less obviously related to a sociocognitive view, such as the ability to concentrate and focus attention, have proved negative (Reilley & Rodolfa, 1981), have been difficult to replicate (Spanos, 1982), or leave significant numbers of people low in these skills still able to perform high on scales of hypnotic susceptibility (Wagstaff, 1985a). However, my point here is not that a sociocognitive view is more able to cope with individual differences than a state view; rather, it is that the findings that people respond differently on hypnosis tests, and that hypnosis tests are reliable, are actually *irrelevant* to whether hypnotic phenomena belong in category A, B or C. There is no reason why there should not be reliable individual differences in responses to phenomena in any of these categories.

Nevertheless, one implication of my position is that if hypnotic responding is determined by the ESC process—in particular, if "genuine" or "believed-in" responsiveness is determined by whether or not subjects have appropriate expectations and use the deliberate strategies necessary to bring about suggested effects—then by manipulating the expectations in the first part of the ESC process and instructing subjects in how to apply the strategies in the second part of the ESC process, it may be possible to modify hypnotic susceptibility. Spanos and his associates appear to have done exactly this (Spanos, 1986a; Bertrand, 1989). By inculcating appropriate expectancies of and positive attitudes toward hypnosis, and teaching subjects a variety of deliberate strategies, Spanos and colleagues have turned previously low-susceptibility subjects into highly susceptible subjects.

However, of considerable interest to me is the criticism by some state theorists of Spanos that his modification procedures have simply encouraged compliance. This is interesting not only because it seems somewhat ironical that compliance can be so readily dismissed one moment, only to become as all-important the next, but also because the kind of scenario Spanos and associates have created for their subjects is actually likely to *minimize* compliance in the hypnotic situation. Indeed, Spanos and colleagues have created what I consider to be the exact conditions that encourage "genuine," "believed in," or noncompliant responding. That is, they have created a situation in which strategy and expectation are congruent. For example, a deliberate inattention strategy that produces "forgetting" is only a compliant response if the expectations of the subject rule out the use of such a strategy in a hypnotic situation. However, if such a strategy is legitimated by bringing a subject's expectations into line, then it is *not* a compliant response. It is a genuine category B phenomenon. Consequently, although I would not expect Spanos and colleagues to have totally eliminated compliance, I would argue that their subjects are probably *less* likely to be compliant than their "natural" counterparts.

CONCLUSIONS

I would draw three main conclusions from my analysis, which have implications for the directions in which future research should proceed. First, I think we have reached a methodological and conceptual impasse in making sense of subjects "experiences of hypnosis," and I am dubious about whether there is much future in attempting to introduce more and more elaborate designs to tease out the finer details of "the experience of hypnosis." Hypnotic "experiences" seem often to be a *product* of experimental procedures, rather than something measured *by* them (see Spanos,

1986a), and we are rapidly approaching the stage where Occam's razor is the only device we can use to decide between competing paradigms (Wagstaff, 1986b, 1988b). Second, and more importantly, studies of hypnosis have drawn our attention to a number of mundane yet fascinating phenomena that do beg for explanations, even though, as I have pointed out, a theory of hypnosis per se does not need to provide such explanations. For example, we need to know how a placebo works; how suggestions can affect dermatological responses; how imagination can produce the experience of a dry mouth, an itch, or nausea; how coping strategies can affect the experience of pain; and so on. However, I would consider these phenomena to be best investigated without any reference at all to "hypnosis," because placing them in a context called "hypnosis" probably serves only to confound them with extra demand characteristics. Nevertheless, third, I still think there is a very important place for the study of hypnosis per se—not hypnosis as a "state" or brain process, but hypnosis as a label for a context or situation. For example, what are the advantages and disadvantages of telling people or leading them to believe that they are in a hypnotic state? Is allowing clinical patients to pretend they are "hypnotized" a particularly useful way of enabling them to talk about difficult problems with the minimum of embarrassment? What, if anything, is lost or gained by telling subjects that hypnosis is compliance with imagination? It may yet be found that, for some people at least, defining a situation or experience as "hypnosis" may have unique advantages. If so, however, we can best capitalize on these advantages if, as theorists, we adopt a common language familiar to mainstream psychology, rather than an ambiguous language of metaphors left over from a bygone era.

REFERENCES

Asch, S. E. (1956). Studies of independence and conformity: A minority of one against a unanimous majority. *Psychological Monographs*, 70 (9, Whole No. 416).

Bányai, E. I., & Hilgard, E. R. (1976). A comparison of active alert hypnotic induction and traditional relaxation induction. *Journal of Abnormal Psychology*, 85, 218–224.

Barber, T. X. (1969). *Hypnosis: A scientific approach*. New York: Van Nostrand Reinhold.

Barber, T. X., Spanos, N. P., & Chaves, J. F. (1974). *Hypnosis, imagination, and human potentialities*. Elmsford, NY: Pergamon Press.

Benson, H., & Klipper, M. Z. (1976). *The relaxation response*. London: Collins.

Bertrand, L. D. (1989). The assessment and modification of hypnotic susceptibility. In N. P. Spanos & J. F. Chaves (Eds.), *Hypnosis: The cognitive–behavioral perspective* (pp. 18–31). Buffalo: Prometheus Books.

Bowers, K. S. (1966). Hypnotic behavior: The differentiation of trance and demand characteristic variables. *Journal of Abnormal Psychology, 71*, 42–41.

Bowers, K. S. (1983). *Hypnosis for the seriously curious.* New York: Norton.

Bowers, K. S., & Davidson, T. M. (1986). On the importance of individual differences in hypnotic ability. *Behavioral and Brain Sciences, 9*(4), 468–469.

Chaves, J. F. (1989). Hypnotic control of clinical pain. In N. P. Spanos & J. F. Chaves (Eds.), *Hypnosis: The cognitive–behavioral perspective* (pp. 242–272). Buffalo: Prometheus Books.

Edmonston, W. E., Jr. (1977). Neutral hypnosis as relaxation. *American Journal of Clinical Hypnosis, 30*, 69–75.

Frank, D. P. (1944). Experimental studies of personal pressure and resistance: 1. Experimental production of resistance. *Journal of General Psychology, 30*, 23–41.

Freedman, J. L., & Fraser, S. C. (1966). Compliance without pressure: The foot-in-the-door technique. *Journal of Personality and Social Psychology, 7*, 117–124.

Gill, M. M., & Brenman, M. (1959). *Hypnosis and related states.* New York: International University Press.

Gruzelier, J. (1988). The neuropsychology of hypnosis. In M. Heap (Ed.), *Hypnosis: Current clinical, experimental and forensic practices.* London: Croom Helm.

Hansel, C. E. M. (1966). *ESP: A scientific evaluation.* London: MacGibbon & Key.

Hilgard, E. R. (1974). Toward a neo-dissociation theory: Multiple cognitive controls in human functioning. *Perspectives in Biology and Medicine, 17*, 301–316.

Hilgard, E. R. (1978). States of consciousness in hypnosis: Divisions or levels? In F. H. Frankel & H. S. Zamansky (Eds), *Hypnosis at its bicentennial: Selected papers* (pp.15–36). New York: Plenum.

Hilgard, E. R. (1986). *Divided consciousness: Multiple controls in human thought and action* (expanded ed.). New York: Wiley.

Hilgard, E. R., & Hilgard, J. R. (1983). *Hypnosis in the relief of pain.* Los Altos, CA: William Kaufmann.

Hilgard, E. R., Morgan, A. H., & Macdonald, H. (1975). Pain and dissociation in the cold pressor test: A study of hypnotic analgesia with "hidden reports" through automatic key-pressing and automatic talking. *Journal of Abnormal Psychology, 84*, 280–289.

Hilgard, J. R. (1970). *Personality and hypnosis: A study of imaginative involvement.* Chicago: University of Chicago Press.

Hull, C. L. (1933). *Hypnosis and suggestibility: An experimental approach.* New York: Appleton-Century-Crofts.

Hunt, S. M. (1979). Hypnosis as obedience behavior. *British Journal of Social and Clinical Psychology, 18*, 21–27.

Kiesler, C. A., & Kiesler, S. B. (1970). *Conformity.* Reading, MA: Addison-Wesley.

Johnson, R. F., Maher, B. A., & Barber, T. X. (1972). Artifact in the "essence of hypnosis": An evaluation of trance logic. *Journal of Abnormal Psychology, 79*, 212–220.

Jones, B., & Dixon, M. V. (1985). *The Macmillan dictionary of biography.* London: Papermac.

Kidder, L. H. (1973). On becoming hypnotized: How skeptics become convinced. A case of attitude change? *American Journal of Clinical Hypnosis, 16*, 1–8.

Kihlstrom, J. F. (1978). Context and cognition in posthypnotic amnesia. *International*

Journal of Clinical and Experimental Hypnosis, 26, 246–267.

Kihlstrom, J. F., Evans, F. J., Orne, E. C., & Orne, M. T. (1980). Attempting to breach hypnotic amnesia. *Journal of Abnormal Psychology, 89,* 603–616.

Knox, J. V., Morgan, A. H., & Hilgard, E. R. (1974). Pain and suffering in ischemia: The paradox of hypnotically suggested anesthesia as contradicted by reports from the "hidden observer." *Archives of General Psychiatry, 30,* 840–847.

Levy, L. H. (1967). Awareness learning and the beneficent subject as expert witness. *Journal of Personality and Social Psychology, 6,* 365–370.

Lynn, S. J., Rhue, J. W., & Weekes, J. R. (1989). Hypnosis and experienced nonvolition: A social cognitive integrative model. In N. P. Spanos & J. F. Chaves (Eds.), *Hypnosis: The cognitive–behavioral perspective* (pp. 78–109). Buffalo: Prometheus Books.

Malott, J. M. (1984). Active–alert hypnosis: Replication and extension of previous research. *Journal of Abnormal Psychology, 93,* 246.

Marcuse, F. L. (1976). *Hypnosis: Fact and fiction.* Harmondsworth, England: Penguin Books.

McGuire, W. J. (1968). Personality and susceptibility to social influence. In E. F. Borgatta & W. W. Lambert (Eds.), *Handbook of personality theory and research* (pp. 1130–1187). Chicago: Rand McNally.

Milgram, S. (1974). *Obedience to authority.* London: Tavistock.

Moore, R. K. (1964). Susceptibility to hypnosis and susceptibility to social influence. *Journal of Abnormal and Social Psychology, 68,* 282–294.

Nisbett, R., & Wilson, T. D. (1977). Telling more than we can know: Verbal reports on mental processes. *Psychological Review, 84,* 231–259.

O'Connell, D. N., Shor, R. E., & Orne, M. T. (1970). Hypnotic age-regression: An empirical and methodological analysis. *The Journal of Abnormal Psychology Monograph Supplement, 76,* 3(part 2,) 1–32.

Orne, M. (1959). The nature of hypnosis: Artifact and essence. *Journal of Abnormal Psychology, 58,* 277–299.

Orne, M. T. (1962). On the social psychology of the psychological experiment: With particular reference to demand characteristics and their implications. *American Psychologist, 17,* 776–783.

Orne, M. T. (1966).Hypnosis, motivation and compliance. *American Journal of Psychiatry, 122,* 721–726.

Orne, M. T. (1969). Demand characteristics and the concept of quasi-controls. In R. Rosenthal & R.L. Rosnow (Eds.), *Artifact in behavioral research* (pp. 143–179). New York: Academic Press.

Orne, M. T. (1970). Hypnosis, motivation and the ecological validity of the psychological experiment. In W. J. Arnold & M. M. Page (Eds), (Vol. ___, pp. 187–265). *Nebraska Symposium on Motivation.* Lincoln: University of Nebraska Press, .

Orne, M. T., & Holland, C. C. (1968). On the ecological validity of laboratory deceptions. *International Journal of Psychiatry, 6,* 282–293.

Pattie, F. A. (1935). A report of attempts to produce uniocular blindness by hypnotic suggestion. *British Journal of Medical Psychology, 15,* 230–241.

Reilley, R. R., & Rodolfa, E. R. (1981). Concentration, attention and hypnosis. *Psychological Reports, 48,* 811–814.

Ryle, G. (1973). *The concept of mind.* Harmondsworth, England: Penguin Books.

Sarbin, T. R. (1989). The construction and reconstruction of hypnosis. In N. P. Spanos & J. F. Chaves (Eds.), *Hypnosis: The cognitive–behavioral perspective* (pp.400–416). Buffalo: Prometheus Books.

Sarbin, T. R., & Coe, W. C. (1972). *Hypnotic behavior: The psychology of influence communication.* New York: Holt, Rinehart & Winston.

Sarbin, T. R., & Slagle, R. W. (1979). Hypnosis and psychophysiological outcomes. In E. Fromm & R. E. Shor (Eds.), *Hypnosis: Developments in research and new perspectives* (2nd ed., p. 273–303). Chicago: Aldine.

Shames, M. L. (1981). Hypnotic susceptibility and conformity: on the mediational mechanism of suggestibility. *Psychological Reports, 49,* 563–565.

Sheehan, P. W. (1983). [Review of *Hypnosis, compliance and belief* by G. F. Wagstaff]. *Bulletin of the British Society of Experimental and Clinical Hypnosis, 6,* 39–43.

Sheehan, P. W., & McConkey, K. M.(1982). *Hypnosis and experience: The exploration of phenomena and process.* Hillsdale, NJ: Erlbaum.

Sheehan, P. W., & Perry, C. W. (1976). *Methodologies of hypnosis: critical appraisal of contemporary paradigms of hypnosis.* Hillsdale, NJ: Erlbaum.

Sheridan, C. L., & King, R. G. (1972). Obedience to authority with an authentic victim. *Proceedings of the 80th Annual Convention of the American Psychological Association, 7,* 165–166.

Skemp, R. R. (1972). Hypnosis and hypnotherapy considered as cybernetic processes. *British Journal of Clinical Hypnosis, 3,* 97–107.

Spanos, N. P. (1982). A social psychological approach to hypnotic behavior. In G. Weary & H. L. Mirels, (Eds), *Integrations of clinical and social psychology* (pp. 231–271). Oxford: Oxford University Press.

Spanos, N. P. (1986a). Hypnosis and the modifications of hypnotic susceptibility. A social psychological perspective. In P. L. N. Naish (Ed.), *What is hypnosis? Current theories and research* (pp. 85–120). Milton Keynes, England: Open University Press.

Spanos, N. P. (1986b). Hypnotic behavior: A social psychological interpretation of amnesia, analgesia and "trance logic." *Behavioral and Brain Sciences, 9,* 449–502.

Spanos, N. P. (1989). Experimental research on hypnotic analgesia. In: N. P. Spanos & J. F. Chaves (Eds.), *Hypnosis: The cognitive–behavioral perspective* (pp. 206–240). Buffalo: Prometheus Books.

Spanos, N. P., Rivers, S. M., & Ross, S. (1977). Experienced involuntariness and response to hypnotic suggestions. *Annals of the New York Academy of Sciences, 296,* 208–221.

Stevenson, J. H. (1976). The effect of post-hypnotic dissociation on the performance of interfering tasks. *Journal of Abnormal Psychology, 85,* 398–407.

Tedeschi, J. T., Lindskold, S., & Rosenfeld, P. (1985). *Introduction to social psychology.* St. Paul, MN: West.

Tellegen, A., & Atkinson, G. (1974). Openness to absorbing and self-altering experiences ("absorption") a trait related to hypnotic susceptibility. *Journal of Abnormal Psychology, 83,* 268–277.

Wagstaff, G. F. (1977a). An experimental study of compliance and post-hypnotic amnesia. *British Journal of Social and Clinical Psychology, 16,* 225–228.

Wagstaff, G. F. (1977b). Goal-directed fantasy, the experience of nonvolition and compliance. *Social Behavior and Personality*, 5, 389–393.

Wagstaff, G. F. (1977c). Post-hypnotic amnesia as disrupted retrieval: A role-playing paradigm. *Quarterly Journal of Experimental Psychology*, 29, 499–504.

Wagstaff, G. F. (1979). The problem of compliance in hypnosis: A social psychological viewpoint. *Bulletin of the British Society of Experimental and Clinical Hypnosis*, 2, 3–5.

Wagstaff, G. F. (1980). *Dissociation and compliance: Or how "hidden" is the "hidden-observer"?* Unpublished manuscript, University of Liverpool.

Wagstaff, G. F. (1981a, October). Forensic hypnosis: Fact and fallacy. *Police Review*, pp. 2116–2117.

Wagstaff, G. F. (1981b). Hypnotic amnesia and compliance. *Bulletin of the British Society of Experimental and Clinical Hypnosis*, 4, 17–18.

Wagstaff, G. F. (1981c). *Hypnosis, compliance and belief*, Brighton, England: Harvester.

Wagstaff, G. F. (1981d). Source amnesia and trance logic: Artifacts in the essence of hypnosis? *Bulletin of the British Society of Experimental and Clinical Hypnosis*, 4, 3–5.

Wagstaff, G. F. (1981e). Suggested amnesia, compliance and inattention encoding specificity. *Bulletin of the British Society of Experimental and Clinical Hypnosis*, 4, 14–15.

Wagstaff, G. F. (1982a). [A comment on Gibbon's "Hypnosis as a trance state: The future of a shared delusion"]. *Bulletin of the British Society of Experimental and Clinical Hypnosis*, 5, 5–7.

Wagstaff, G. F. (1982b). Amnesia, compliance and men of straw: A tailpiece. *Bulletin of the British Society of Experimental and Clinical Hypnosis*, 5, 42–45.

Wagstaff, G. F. (1982c). Disorganized recall, suggested amnesia and compliance. *Psychological Reports*, 51, 1255–1258. c.

Wagstaff, G. F. (1982d).Hypnosis and recognition of a face. *Perceptual and Motor Skills*, 55, 816–818.

Wagstaff, G. F. (1982e). Recall of witnesses under hypnosis. *Journal of the Forensic Science Society*, 22, 33–39.

Wagstaff, G. F. (1983a). [A comment on McConkey's "Challenging hypnotic effects: The impact of conflicting influences on response to hypnotic suggestion"]. *British Journal of Experimental and Clinical Hypnosis*, 1, 11–15.

Wagstaff, G. F. (1983b). [A reply to Fellows's and Sheehan's reviews of *Hypnosis, compliance and belief*]. *Bulletin of the British Society of Experimental and Clinical Hypnosis*, 6, 45–50.

Wagstaff, G. F. (1983c, March). Hypnosis and the law: A critical review of some recent proposals. *Criminal Law Review*, pp. 152–157.

Wagstaff, G. F. (1983d). Suggested improvement of visual acuity: A statistical re-evaluation. *International Journal of Clinical and Experimental Hypnosis*, 31, 239.

Wagstaff, G. F. (1984). The enhancement of witness memory by "hypnosis": A review and methodological critique of the experimental literature. *British Journal of Experimental and Clinical Hypnosis*, 2, 3–12.

Wagstaff, G. F. (1985a). [A comment on "Attentional concomitants of hypnotic susceptibility" by A. Sigman, K. C. Phillips, and B. Clifford]. *British Journal of Experimental and Clinical Hypnosis*, 2, 76–80.

Wagstaff, G. F. (1985b). [A reply to Perry and Nogrady's "Use of hypnosis by the police in the investigation of crime: Is guided memory a safe substitute?"]. *British Journal of Experimental and Clinical Hypnosis*, *3*, 39–42.

Wagstaff, G. F. (1985c). [Discussion commentary on Gibson's "Experiencing hypnosis versus pretending to be hypnotized: Observations on hypnosis training workshops"]. *British Journal of Experimental and Clinical Hypnosis*, *2*, 114–117.

Wagstaff, G. F. (1985d). Hypnosis and the law: The role of induction in witness recall. In D. Waxman, P. C. Misra, M. Gibson, & M. A. Basker (Eds.), *Modern trends in hypnosis*. New York: Plenum.

Wagstaff, G. F. (1985e). Is hypnotherapy a placebo? in M. Heap (Ed.), *Proceedings of the First Annual Conference of the British Society of Experimental and Clinical Hypnosis* (pp. 132–143). 132–143. Chatham, England: British Society of Experimental and Clinical Hypnosis.

Wagstaff, G. F. (1986a). Hypnosis as compliance and belief: A sociocognitive view. In P. L. N. Naish (Ed.), *What is hypnosis? Current theories and research* (pp. 59–84). Milton Keynes, England: Open University Press.

Wagstaff, G. F. (1986b). State versus nonstate paradigms of hypnosis: A real or a false dichotomy? *Behavioral and Brain Sciences*, *9*, 486–487.

Wagstaff, G. F. (1987a). Hypnosis. In H. Beloff & A. Colman (Eds.), *Psychology survey* (Vol. 6, pp 234–254). Leicester: British Psychological Society.

Wagstaff, G. F. (1987b). Hypnotic induction, hypnotherapy and the placebo effect. *British Journal of Experimental and Clinical Hypnosis*, *4*, 168–170.

Wagstaff, G. F. (1987c). Is hypnotherapy a placebo? *British Journal of Experimental and Clinical Hypnosis*, *4*, 135–140.

Wagstaff, G. F. (1988a). Comments on the 1987 Home Office Draft Circular: A response to the comments of Gibson, Haward and Orne. *British Journal of Experimental and Clinical Hypnosis*, *5*, 145–149.

Wagstaff, G. F. (1988b). Critical evaluation of the ethogenic analysis of hypnotic pain. *New Ideas in Psychology*, *6*, 75–86.

Wagstaff, G. F. (1988c). Public conceptions of forensic hypnosis: Implications for education and practice. In M. Heap (Ed.), *Hypnosis: Current clinical, experimental and forensic practices* (pp. 395–403). London: Croom Helm.

Wagstaff, G. F. (1988d). Theoretical and experimental issues. In M. Heap (Ed.), *Hypnosis: Current clinical, experimental and forensic practices* (pp. 25–39). London: Croom Helm.

Wagstaff, G. F. (1989). Forensic aspects of hypnosis. In N. P. Spanos & J. F. Chaves (Eds.), *Hypnosis: The cognitive–behavioral perspective* (pp. 340–357). Buffalo: Prometheus Books.

Wagstaff, G. F., & Benson, D. (1987). Exploring hypnotic processes with the cognitive-simulator comparison group. *British Journal of Experimental and Clinical Hypnosis*, *4*, 83–91.

Wagstaff, G. F., & Carroll, R. (1987). The cognitive-simulation of hypnotic amnesia and disorganized recall. *Medical Science Research*, *15*, 85–86.

Wagstaff, G. F., Hearne, K. M. T., & Jackson, B. (1980). Post-hypnotically suggested dreams and the sleep cycle: An experimental re-evaluation. *IRCS Medical Science*, *8*, 240–241.

Wagstaff, G. F., & Ovenden, M. (1979). Hypnotic time distortion and free-recall learning: An attempted replication. *Psychological Research*, *40*, 291–298.

Wagstaff, G. F., & Sykes, C. T. (1984). Hypnosis and the recall of emotionally toned material. *IRCS Medical Science, 12*, 137–138.

Wagstaff, G. F., Traverse, J., & Milner, S. (1982). Hypnosis and eyewitness memory: Two experimental analogues. *IRCS Medical Science, 10*, 894–895.

Weber, S. J., & Cook, T. D. (1972). Subject effects in laboratory research: An examination of subject notes, demand characteristics and valid inference. *Psychological Bulletin, 77*, 273–295.

Wilson, S. C., & Barber, T. X. (1983). The fantasy-prone personality: Implications for understanding imagery, hypnosis and parapsychological phenomena. In A. A. Sheikh (Ed.), *Imagery: current theory, research and application.* (pp. 340–387). New York: Wiley.

Wolberg, L. R. (1972). *Hypnosis: Is it you?* New York: Harcourt Brace Jovanovich.

Zamansky, H. S. (1977). Suggestion and countersuggestion in hypnotic behavior. *Journal of Abnormal Psychology, 86*, 346–351.

Zamansky, H. S. (1989). Suggested negative hallucinations in hypnotic subjects: When no means yes. *British Journal of Experimental and Clinical Hypnosis, 6*, 68–70.

Zamansky, H. S., & Bartis, S. P. (1985). The dissociation of an experience: The hidden observer observed. *Journal of Abnormal Psychology, 94*, 243–248.

An Integrative Model of Hypnosis

STEVEN JAY LYNN and JUDITH W. RHUE
Ohio University

INTRODUCTION

Sarah is curious, even excited, about the prospect of being hypnotized. She is willing and ready to "let go," to experience the modifications of consciousness called for by the hypnotist. She is able to adopt an experiential set based on a readiness to undergo hypnotic events that are suggested—a set in which experiences have a "quality of effortlessness, as if they happened by themselves" (Tellegen, 1981, p. 222). Sarah feels comfortable with the hypnotist; she is ready to trust her, even to please her by being a cooperative subject; and she fully expects to enjoy the experience of responding to suggestions.

When Sarah receives the first suggestion for her outstretched hand to feel heavy and drop to her leg, as if there were a weight attached to it, she intends to experience heaviness in the hand; she wishes to have the experience of a weight pulling her hand down; and she actively creates a vivid imaginal and sensory representation of the hand being pulled down by the imaginary weight. For the most part, her imaginings flow effortlessly with the suggestion. After her attention is momentarily diverted, she recreates images and feelings that are consistent with suggested events. Rather than thinking of the heaviness and movement of her hand as the result of holding it outstretched past the point of comfort, Sarah perceives the downward movement of her hand as involuntary; that is, she adopts the passive wording for her hand to move downward by itself as a way of interpreting and understanding her behavior. She also views her successful response as a product of the direct effects of suggestions, of the hypnotist's abilities and efforts, and of an altered state of consciousness. Her positive response provides Sarah with a sense of confidence, reinforces her feelings of security in the hypnotic situation, and confirms the belief that she is hypnotized. Not surprisingly, she passes many suggestions.

Alan too is curious about hypnosis, yet he feels threatened by the prospect of being hypnotized. He is reluctant to respond fully to the hypnotist's suggestions; to do so would be an admission of passivity and weakness. Alan's agenda is to resist rather than respond to hypnotic suggestions. Because Alan views hypnosis as a contest of wills, he feels tense, ready to do battle rather than cooperate with the hypnotist.

In response to the suggestion for his hand to feel heavy and drop to his leg, Alan stubbornly holds it up, despite the feeling of heaviness that develops. Just to "play the game," Alan makes a half-hearted attempt to imagine that his arm is heavy. His imaginings, however, do not flow with or reflect the suggested events; rather, his thought stream is punctuated with such ideas as "This is silly" and "This will never work." Arm heaviness does develop, but Alan believes that it has nothing to do with the suggestion; rather, he interprets it as the inevitable result of the force of gravity. At the end of the suggestion, Alan concludes that he was not hypnotized. Alan's attitude can best be described as "cynical"; he makes no overt response to the suggestions that follow.

Sarah, a so-called hypnotic "virtuoso," and Alan, an "oppositional" subject, score at the high and low extremes of hypnotizability scales, respectively. Their prehypnotic attitudes, beliefs, and expectancies about hypnosis are markedly different. So too are their intentions, their feelings about the hypnotist, their stream of behaviors and thoughts, and their appraisal and interpretations of suggested activities and the broader hypnotic situation. Sarah's and Alan's hypnotic performances reflect their individuality—their unique abilities, sensitivities, needs, and goals. Their very different responses to even a single hypnotic suggestion represent the confluence of cognitive, affective, and behavioral events and processes that have personal and interpersonal meaning and ramifications.

What these contrasting examples suggest is that hypnotic action and experience are the end results of what subjects think and believe about hypnosis, what they imagine or fail to imagine, what they attend to or do not attend to, what they wish to do or not to do, and how they perceive hypnotic communications and come to evaluate their experience. Hypnotized persons, just like nonhypnotized persons, act in terms of their aims, according to their point of view, and in relation to their interpretation of appropriate behavior and feelings (Lynn, Rhue, & Weekes, 1989, 1990; Shapiro, 1985). Furthermore, hypnotized subjects do not relinquish control of their actions during hypnosis. In fact, hypnotic performances and subjective experiences are shaped by the same sorts of personal strivings and needs that affect subjects' responses outside the hypnotic context: to optimize affect and minimize conflict, and to maintain a sense of personal control, self-esteem, and the regard of others (Lynn, Rhue, & Weekes, 1989).

For these reasons, and the fact that we do not invoke exotic or unusual processes, mechanisms, or mental states to understand hypnotic experience and conduct, our analysis can be thought of as a "common-sense" approach to a complex and puzzling set of phenomena. The same processes and mechanisms that can account for hypnotic behavior can account for even the most mundane actions that are performed on an everyday basis. For example, we contend that what have been referred to as "dissociative" and "nonvolitional" aspects of hypnosis can be explained in terms of subjects' expectancies about hypnosis, operating in conjunction with features of the hypnotic context to discourage awareness of the personal and situational factors that influence hypnotic behavior and to foster the perception that behavior is automatic and involuntary.

At the focal point of our analysis are the broad demands that emanate from the hypnotic context, and the subject's willingness and ability to adopt the roles and related experiences called for by diverse suggestions. Our model is indebted to the seminal theorizing of Martin Orne (1959), who highlighted the importance of demands that define the parameters of hypnotic conduct and perceptions. Hypnotic responding reflects subjects' sensitivity to explicit and implicit role demands that unfold in the context of the transactions between the hypnotist and subject. Our analysis is also influenced by sociocognitive (e.g., Barber, Spanos, & Chaves, 1974; Sarbin & Coe, 1972; Spanos, 1986; Spanos, Salas, Bertrand, & Johnston, 1989) and interactive–phenomenological (Sheehan & McConkey, 1982) theorists, who view hypnotizable subjects as active cognizers who are invested in meeting the requirements of hypnotic behavior and actively strive to fulfill the perceived requirements of the hypnotic situation.

Our examples at the outset also suggest that hypnotic responding cannot be reduced to a solitary ability, trait, or mechanism. It is, rather, an amalgam of social and cognitive processes and abilities. This way of thinking about hypnosis was set forth in T. X. Barber's (1969) functional or "scientific" account of hypnosis. Barber's goal was to identify social, cognitive, and contextual variables functionally related to hypnotized subjects' behavior and subjective experience. In so doing, Barber called particular attention to the subjects' attitudes, beliefs, and motivation, and to the characteristics of hypnotic procedures and suggestions. Like Barber, we contend that hypnotic conduct is ultimately the product of many variables that interact in complex ways.

For more than a decade, our research has been devoted to examining "candidate variables" (e.g., imagination, rapport, expectancies) that theory and research suggest are prominent determinants of hypnotized subjects' responses. For example, researchers with a sociocognitive orientation have informed our analysis by highlighting the impact of the following variables on the subjects' construction of hypnosis: preconceptions about hypnosis (e.g., Spanos, Cobb, & Gorassini, 1985; Spanos, Brett, Menary, & Cross, 1987), the structure and wording of test suggestions (e.g., Spanos & Gorassini, 1984), patterns of imaginative activity that accompany responses to many test suggestions (e.g., Spanos & Barber, 1972), context-generated expectancies (e.g., Kirsch, 1985), and self-observation of hypnotic responses (e.g., Wedemeyer & Coe, 1981).

We believe that the multilayered richness, diversity, and complexity of hypnotic performances can best be captured and understood by examining the role of situational, intrapersonal, and interpersonal variables in accounting for individual differences in hypnotic responses. It is no less important to understand the affect-laden, interpersonal dimension of hypnosis than it is to understand subjects' ability to create subjectively compelling images of suggested events. Our approach thus stands in contrast to models that give primary weight to single determinants of hypnotizability, such as relaxation, dissociation, or psychological regression.

In acknowledging the many possible interactions among candidate variables that influence hypnotic responsiveness, our analysis has much in common with the interactional theories described in this book. We recognize that it is often difficult, if not impossible, to isolate single variables in the flow of hypnotic experience and unfolding action. Imaginings, goal-directed strivings, attitudes, representations of the hypnotist, and expectancies, for example, are viewed as mutually interacting and perhaps inseparable facets of subjects' behavioral and experiential stream. To the degree that performance and experience match implicit and explicit standards for successful responding, subjects will experience hypnotic events as flowing and spontaneous. Ultimately, the transformations in consciousness and behavior allied with hypnotic suggestions must be understood in light of their dynamic, fluid quality, rather than in static terms of a single ability, state of mind, or achievement of the hypnotist.

Because of the importance we attach to understanding this dynamic mix of social and cognitive determinants and constructs derived from social and cognitive psychology, we have characterized our analysis as an "integrative" approach. We use the term "integrative" in another sense: to capture our view of the hypnotizable subject as a creative agent who successfully seeks and integrates information from an array of situational, intrapersonal, and interpersonal sources.

Relative to other sociocognitive analyses of hypnosis, ours devotes greater attention to affect and interpersonal factors, performance standards, the dynamic and highly personal nature of subjects' intentions and information processing during hypnosis, and the features of the hypnotic context that discourage awareness and analysis of the personal and situational factors that influence hypnotic behavior. At the same time, relative to other sociocognitive theorists, we place less emphasis on concepts such as compliance and conformity (e.g., Spanos, Wagstaff) and self-presentation, role enactment, and role playing (e.g., Coe and Sarbin, Spanos). Our concern is instead focused on the general human capacity for creating psychological situations that engender desired experiences.

THEORETICAL CONCEPTS AND PRINCIPLES

Hypnosis as Voluntary Social Behavior

In common with sociocognitive theories, one of our pivotal assumptions is that hypnotic behavior is social behavior. Hypnotic behaviors have many parallels with familiar behaviors in cooperative settings characterized by scripted, asymmetric relations among participants (e.g., psychotherapy). Like many other social behaviors, such as conversational behaviors that are experienced as spontaneous in reaction to social stimuli, hypnotic behaviors are neither clearly premeditated nor undertaken in the service of goals clearly defined in advance. As Bargh (1984) has noted, a person lacks awareness of nearly all of his or her cognitive processes, even those that are consciously triggered. At the experiential level, the dichotomy between willed action and total passivity is not descriptive of much complex human behavior. Not infrequently, hypnotic and nonhypnotic behavioral sequences are described by actors as involving a twining of passive and willed elements. Indeed, hypnotized subjects vary in terms of how conscious and aware they are of initiating and performing actions, and how purposeful they feel their thoughts and actions are (Lynn, Rhue, & Weekes, 1990).

Nevertheless, we argue that hypnotic subjects' responses have all of the properties of voluntary action. Their actions are directed toward goals, are regulated in terms of their needs and intentions, and can be progressively changed to realize goals. Their mental activities are not passive happenings; rather, they are purposeful, attuned to personal strivings, and geared toward fulfilling implicit and explicit contextual demands. According to Heckhausen and Beckmann (1990), actions are controlled by intentions that can be thought of as "goals pictured in the mind's eye" (p. 36). In this sense, the imagined suggested experience is a goal in itself. Hypnotized subjects' behavior is "goal-directed," insofar as successful hypnotic behaviors often have clear-cut direction along lines implied by the suggestion (see Hyland, 1988, for a similar definition of goal-directed behavior). Yet hypnotized subjects' cognitive activities demonstrate their active attempts to fulfill the role requirements of hypnotic suggestions; these attempts sometimes include ingenious elaborations of suggestions (see Sheehan & McConkey, 1982). Also, hypnotized subjects retain the ability to initiate and terminate their behaviors and cognitive activities, as well as to resist or oppose the hypnotist. In short, hypnotized subjects can be said to exhibit control (see Uleman, 1987) over their actions and imaginings (Lynn, Rhue, & Weekes, 1990).

The stream of hypnotized subjects' experiences is not fundamentally different from everyday life: It can be described as a flow of images, feelings, personal associations, and self-evaluations that may be represented verbally and visually, and in tandem with suggestion-related sensations. In this "experiential stream," concrete and abstract thinking, and reality-based and fantasy-based thinking, coexist (Lynn, Rhue, & Weekes, 1990; Sheehan and McConkey, 1982).

Because hypnotizable subjects often maintain that their behavior feels involuntary, the theorist's challenge is to provide an account not only of hypnotized subjects' behavioral responses but also of their experience of nonvolition. To meet this challenge, it is neccessessary to understand how subjects construct their perceptions of hypnotic behavior and suggested experiences. This construction can be understood, in part, as a product of situational and self-representations.

Prehypnotic Factors: Schemas and Appraisals

"Scripts" or "schemas" can be thought of as knowledge structures about the nature and appropriate sequence of events, persons, or tasks in situations. These representations play a guiding role in social interactions (Abelson, 1981; Schank & Abelson, 1977; Tomkins, 1979) and correspond roughly to roles and role perceptions as discussed by role theorists (e.g., Coe, 1987; Sarbin & Coe, 1972). Simply defining the situation as hypnosis activates social and cultural schemas. These include stereotypic attributes, behaviors, and experiences of hypnotizable individuals: that hypnosis is an altered state of consciousness, that the hypnotist is a powerful figure, that hypnotizable subjects are passive and receptive, and that hypnotic suggestions are carried out automatically or effortlessly (McConkey, 1986; McCord, 1961; L. Wilson, Greene, & Loftus, 1986).

Our appraisals of hypnotic conduct are no different from our appraisals of mundane events, at least insofar as we are inclined to construct our perceptions by way of culturally based schemas or attributional categories. An example relevant to our discussion would be the schemas or categories of "actions" and "occurrences" (Kruglanski, 1975). An action is commonly assumed to be determined by the actor's will, whereas an occurrence is largely independent of the will and is caused by factors other than the self (Kruglanski, 1975). Actions are deemed voluntary, whereas occurrences are not. As sociocognitive theorists (Coe, 1978; Sarbin & Coe, 1979; Spanos, Brett et al., 1987) have pointed out, people do not accept direct responsibility for "occurrences" or "happenings." The tactic of disclaiming responsibility is expressed in these sorts of statements about everyday actions: "It just happened to me," "I couldn't help it," and "I couldn't stop myself." Hypnotic conduct, then, which is frequently perceived as involuntary, automatic, and effortless, is not so far removed from other spheres of life.

The attributional process itself, and many of subjects' assumptions about hypnosis, are not fully articulated, elaborated, or subject to conscious inspection. Nonetheless, identifying the situation as "hypnosis" has important consequences. It increases subjects' readiness to attribute suggestion-related hypnotic actions to an altered state of consciousness, to the hypnotist's ability and efforts, and to automatic "happenings." In short, defining the situation as "hypnosis" primes the attributional category of "occurrences."

Anticipations and Agendas

Anticipations are important if not central aspects of motivation (Shapiro, 1985). We use the term "agenda" to describe the constellation of personal anticipations and goals (i.e., plans, intentions, wishes, and expectancies) related to hypnotic responses and experiences. Yet the broad agenda—to "be hypnotized"—more often than not reflects diverse motives. For example, some subjects wish to experience hypnotic events just to "see what will happen," or in order to achieve a hypnotic "state" that is a desirable end in itself. Some subjects exhibit a particular wish to please the hypnotist that echos back to earlier meaningful relationships. This motivated cognitive commitment or preparedness to respond to the hypnotist can be seen in subjects' exquisite sensitivity to the hypnotist's behavior and communications (Sheehan & McConkey, 1982; Sheehan, 1980). Still other subjects wish to pass many suggestions in order to feel a sense of mastery that derives from succeeding at the task at hand. These motives are not mutually exclusive; in fact, most subjects probably have multiple motives for wishing to "be hypnotized." Regardless of the agenda, it is like other motives or intentions in that once it is formed or engaged, it no longer requires much conscious control to proceed forward (Beckmann, 1987; Heckhausen & Beckmann, 1990).

Agendas are shaped by the personal connotations that hypnosis has for a particular subject. These connotations are related to subjects' learning history and self-perceptions; to how subjects would like to be and not to be (see Markus & Nurius, 1986); and to how subjects wish to be perceived by others. The agenda mirrors the self-image and the social image; both are reflected in hypnotic conduct. For example, hypnosis has positive connotations for subjects whose beliefs about the attributes of a "good" hypnotic subject are consistent with prized attributes (e.g., cooperativeness, imaginativeness, flexibility, creativity). These subjects are more likely to exhibit rapport with the hypnotist and a readiness to undergo experiential events that are suggested; to access fantasies, imaginings, and memories that facilitate responding to suggestions such as age regression; and to interpret their suggestion-congruent sensations and responses as evidence that they are "hypnotized."

Rapport

The image that we present to ourselves and others is affected by the social context. Because one of the most salient features of the hypnotic situation is the relationship between the hypnotist and the subject (Diamond, 1984), the interpersonal dimension of hypnosis is particularly important. The typical hypnotic ritual involves the subject's closing his or her eyes and assuming a receptive role with a person who speaks in a quiet yet authoritative way. Depending on the associations and affect evoked by this situation, the hypnotic scenario may be inviting or threatening. A subject who is uncomfortable with or does not trust the hypnotist may wish to appear strong and assertive rather than docile and passive. Certain subjects' agenda is to maintain control in the hypnotic situation and to monitor the self. Such vigilance deters imaginative involvement and primes behavior that is experienced as effortful, planned, and voluntary.

This recalcitrant stance is much more common among low- than among high-hypnotizable subjects. In fact, below, we review evidence indicating that highly hypnotizable subjects continue to respond to the hypnotist despite the establishment of suboptimum rapport. Rapport seems to be a particularly important response determinant for low-hypnotizable subjects. Differences between relatively unhypnotizable and high hypnotizable subjects have traditionally been ascribed to the latter subjects' cognitive characteristics or to a "special process." These differences, however, may be attributable in part to unhypnotizable subjects' poor rapport with the hypnotist, oppositionality, and negative attitudes elicited by the hypnotic situation.

Conflict and Ambivalence

Our discussion might imply that agendas are conflict-free, stable, and clear-cut. Yet this is not the case. Conflict is a prominent feature of hypnotic experience (McConkey, 1983). Not infrequently, the desire to experience alterations of consciousness conflicts with concerns about remaining "in control" and independent of another's influence. The demands for cooperation inherent in a treatment or scientific endeavor, curiosity, and the desire to please the hypnotist incline subjects to have hypnosis-related experiences. However, negative preconceptions and fears can produce an internal dialogue of fears of losing control of mental and bodily functions, and can heighten concerns about appearing passive, weak, and gullible. Feelings of competitiveness and resentments against authority figures (i.e., the hypnotist) may also contribute to the conflict. Also, subjects' imaginings, memories, and associations in response to certain suggestions (e.g., for age regression and hypnotic dreaming), may evoke anxiety and even negative hypnotic aftereffects in rare instances (see Brentar & Lynn, 1989). Given cultural stereotypes and misconceptions about hypnosis, along with the importance certain subjects place on rational, reality-bound thinking, it is not surprising that some subjects resolve hypnotic conflict about responding either by not responding or by voluntarily complying with suggestions in the absence of accompanying subjective experiences.

As task involvement, affect, and rapport with the hypnotist ebb and flow, the agenda is subject to change. Shifts in anticipations and intentions, in turn, effect involvement, affect, and rapport in a recursive fashion. For example, any thought or feeling that disrupts the sense of safety and security about being hypnotized may simultaneously compromise rapport with the hypnotist; defocus attention to suggestions; interrupt the free-flowing, spontaneous, involuntary quality of responding; and diminish subjects' enthusiasm and willingness to be hypnotized. When this occurs, subjects may label themselves as "poor subjects," focus on task-irrelevant thoughts, and generate negative response expectancies that further dampen rapport and performance. What this suggests is that many subjects are neither clearly resistant nor totally receptive to hypnosis. Not only do some subjects lack a schema for the hypnotic experience, but they also are ambivalent about experiencing hypnotic effects.

Hypnotic Communications

An important determinant of the unfolding agenda is the subject's response to the hypnotist and the communications contained in the hypnotic induction. Initial hypnotic communications provide an introduction to hypnosis and are designed to promote rapport with the subject. They are also aimed at correcting misconceptions about hypnosis and instilling positive attitudes about hypnosis. Some subjects who are initially reluctant to be hypnotized feel comforted by the relaxation suggestions contained in the induction. The induction, which starts with "easy" suggestions (e.g., eye closure), that many subjects pass, can provide a success experience that contradicts initial skepticism about the ability to be hypnotized. This can bolster confidence and perhaps can increase the likelihood of responding to subsequent suggestions.

A number of mechanisms can account for how hypnotic communications affect subjects. Typical hypnotic inductions orient the subject to reduce vigilance and relax physically and mentally; to focus attention directly on subjective experience and on the hypnotist's communications; and to give free rein to fantasy and imagination in line with suggested events (Field, 1965; Lynn, Rhue, & Weekes, 1989). Hypnotic communications contain cues, demands, and explicit instructions for focusing attention and imagining in line with the aims of suggestions. This informs subjects about what constitutes an appropriate attentional, behavioral, and experiential response. Hypnotic communications also inform subjects that various effects are "happening" to them (e.g., "Your hand is rising by itself"; Spanos, 1982a), which fosters perceptions of suggestion-related involuntariness.

We believe that responsive subjects associate words in the induction with features of hypnosis by way of a process of analogy. For example, a hypnotizable subject who receives repeated suggestions to "sleep" may be inclined to respond "as if" hypnosis were sleep. Of course few subjects literally fall asleep during hypnosis, because situational demands to remain attentive to the hypnotist contradict this behavior. Yet it is easy for subjects to discern the implication that one is relatively passive (e.g., eyes closed, limited bodily movements) and does not consciously control one's actions, as in sleep. Receptive subjects grasp this analogy and adopt this way of framing their experiences.

The focus on sensations of relaxation and sleepiness also discourages the subject from adopting an analytical attitude and searching for causes of behavior outside the hypnosis framework. The suggested imagery and passive wording of suggestions (Spanos & Katsanis, 1989) promote a receptive mode of experiencing (Deikman, 1966) versus analytic attending (Spanos, Gottlieb, & Rivers, 1980). Alterations in information processing, such as a tendency to engage in primary-process thinking (Fromm, Oberlander, & Gruenwald, 1970; Hammer, Walker, & Diment, 1978; Popham & Bowers, 1988) and a tendency toward the imagistic rather than the conceptual, may also occur. Although M. E. Miller and Bowers (1986) attribute these alterations to dissociative processes, they may instead be attributable to suggestions for eye closure, mental and physical relaxation, and attention to imagery and fantasy.

Widespread beliefs that hypnosis produces alterations in consciousness, along with direct suggestions for alterations in subjective experience, also contribute to modifications of attention and information processing, as well as to changes in the subjects' internal state. Internal states and their determinants, however, often are ambiguous and poorly understood. There are at least three reasons for this ambiguity. First, our vocabulary for bodily feelings and sensations is meager; somatic feelings often are nebulous and defy adequate description (Sarbin & Coe, 1979). Second, hypnotic behavior is influenced by subtle contextual cues (e.g, wording of suggestions) that go undetected as the actual determinants of feelings and actions. Third, subjects' cognitive processes are at times unavailable to conscious scrutiny. In short, subjects have imperfect access not only to their mental states (T. Wilson, 1985), but also to their bodily states.

When internal states are ambiguous or poorly understood, subjects are particularly likely to adopt the hypnotist's language (e.g., "Responses occur effortlessly") as a way of coming to understand their experience. If sensations or bodily cues are ambiguous, the context in which the cues are embedded can also affect the labeling and understanding of their meaning (Trope, 1986). For instance, relaxation in the hypnotic context is likely to be attributed to an altered state of consciousness, whereas relaxation before bedtime is more likely to be ascribed to tiredness. In summary, hypnotic communications provide guidelines for behavioral and imaginative activities while they promote the perception of alterations of consciousness and of action as involuntary and dissociative.

The Subject as "Information Seeker"

An important assumption of our model is that subjects are "information seekers." Well-motivated subjects are attuned to the hypnotist and his or her communications for information about how to respond. Subjects often are successful in integrating complex and even conflicting role and situational demands. Yet subjects often lack the sense that this process is deliberate and that conscious effort or choice accompanies response to suggestion.

The absence of perceived effort derives in part from the fact that many individuals experience imagery and fantasy as spontaneous, freeflowing, and automatic. The absence of perception of conscious choice stems from the fact that the direction for action is supplied by the hypnotist along lines scripted by the hypnotic communications. So long as suggested demands are clear and subjects have the requisite abilities and willingness to have convincing subjective experiences, they need not make conscious, effortful judgments about how to respond. Furthermore, the fact that the hypnotized subject responds *after* the hypnotist's suggestions may promote the perception that hypnotic phenomena arise from the hypnotist's efforts or abilities. Indeed, if subjects uniquely or consistently associate hypnotic effects with the hypnotist or the hypnotist's suggestions, rather than with their own efforts or to features of the hypnotic context, they are likely to identify their suggestion-related responses as involuntary (Lynn, Rhue, & Weekes, 1990).

Performance Standards

Although subjects approach hypnosis with very different agendas, even subjects who are motivated to experience hypnotic events adopt different standards for deeming their hypnotic experience satisfactory. Because subjects do not routinely benefit from direct response feedback from the hypnotist, and because of the inherent ambiguity in evaluating response adequacy, subjects must come to their own conclusions about whether they have responded successfully. So by their very nature, performance standards are criteria that are personal, subjective, and relativistic.

A great deal of human behavior reflects a process of feedback control (Carver, 1979; Carver & Scheier, 1981, 1982, 1990; Norman, 1981; Powers, 1973). Like any other goal-directed behavior (Carver, 1979; G. A. Miller, Galanter, & Pribram, 1960), hypnotic conduct is in part accomplished by assessments of its effectiveness in achieving personal standards and goals. Hypnotizable subjects ordinarily do not engage in a great deal of conscious self-analysis or self-monitoring of their actions or experience in relation to performance standards. Unless derailed, the free-flowing quality of hypnotic experience is maintained, and subjects are not likely to question that they are hypnotized or responding adequately. Subjects' tacit understanding that they are "good subjects" confirms response expectancies and perpetuates the perception of hypnotic action as effortless.

Yet this process can be undermined. For instance, subjects may lack requisite imaginal abilities. No matter how hard they attempt to access memories and events of childhood, for example, they may nevertheless be unable to have a personally compelling experience of age regression. Another possibility is that subjects may adopt performance standards that are so difficult to meet that they are dissatisfied and frustrated with their response. For instance, a subject who expects to experience immediate and profound changes in consciousness may be daunted by his or her inability to achieve this goal. Under these circumstances, the subject may attend to the objective reality of the situation; may have task-irrelevant, self-denigrating, and distracting thoughts; and may analyze his or her hypnotic actions as the by-products of naturally occurring phenomena (e.g., may wonder whether his or her hand was heavy because it was outstretched). Any one of these outcomes would be expected to suppress subsequent responding and to short-circuit feelings of involuntariness.

In contrast, successfully imagining and experiencing a suggestion bolsters motivation, perceptions of successful responding, and response expectancies (see also Kirsch, 1985, 1990). What our discussion suggests is that the standards subjects adopt to evaluate their experience and performance may be as important as their imaginative ability (see Sheehan & McConkey, 1982). Subjects vary in their abilities to represent suggested events imaginatively, yet it may be primarily those subjects who adopt a stringent criterion for evaluating the reality of the event who denigrate their experience/performance and engage in a spiral of negative cognitions and affect that hampers their performance. In summary, subjects' interpretation of hypnotic behavior is dependent not only on their abilities to experience hypnotic events, but also on the criteria they use to evaluate their responses and experiences.

Before we conclude this section, it is worthwhile to note that hypnotizability may be a mosaic of abilities or personal qualities of the subject. For example, subjects may differ in their attentional, fantasy, and imaginative abilities. They may also differ in their ability to detect, interpret, and respond appropriately to subtle messages and cues inherent in communications and interpersonal behaviors, across a range of hypnotic and nonhypnotic situations. Furthermore, individual differences may exist in the ability to translate suggestions into sensations (e.g., feeling "wet" while imagining oneself swimming); this ability may be independent to some extent of imagery vividness or fantasy proneness in general. And finally, the ability to participate fully in a cooperative relationship in which the role of the "good subject" is enacted is undoubtedly important. At any rate, we doubt that a single hypnotic ability will be isolated that accounts satisfactorily for individual differences in hypnotic performance.

RESEARCH AND APPRAISAL

One of our primary hypotheses is that hypnotic behavior is social behavior that is influenced by the same processes that influence mundane behaviors. One stream of our research involves the examination of claims that hypnosis evokes a particular state of consciousness with definable properties. We have targeted four phenomena for study—literalism of responding, loss of reality testing during hypnosis, trance logic, and involuntariness of responding— that have enjoyed appeal to proponents of the view that hypnosis is a state of consciousness with identifiable properties. In addition to studying these phenomena, we have conducted research examining the effects of manipulating subjects' performance standards, and we have pursued a decade-long research program on the fantasy-prone person. One particular focus of the latter research program has been on elucidating the relation between long-standing fantasy and imaginative interests and abilities and hypnotizability.

Is Hypnosis an Altered State of Consciousness?
A Study of Four Phenomena

Literalism of Response

For more than four decades, literalism of response has been regarded as a marker of the hypnotic state. Theoreticians such as White (1941), Pattie (1956), Weitzenhoffer (1957), and more recently Shor (1962), have all noted that literalism is a sign of hypnotized subjects' behavior or of the hypnotic state. Yet it was Milton Erickson (Erickson, Hershman, & Secter, 1961) who most forcefully argued that literalism is one of the key indicators of the presence of "trance." According to Erickson, literalism involves an exact reception of ideas without an elaboration of them in terms of implied or associated meanings.

Over a 25-year period, Erickson (1980) assessed literalness of responding in 1,800 hypnotized subjects' responses and 3,000 responses of waking subjects. To test literalism, Erickson asked mundane questions such as "Do you mind telling me your name?" The results reported were nothing short of astonishing: 95% of the subjects in the waking state—whether friends, acquaintances, or even total strangers—acquiesced to the implication of the question (e.g., by actually stating their names). In contrast, 80% of the subjects in a "light trance" uttered "No" or exhibited a negative shaking of the head, and 90% of subjects in a "medium trance" and 97% of subjects in a "deep trance" behaved in this manner. Unfortunately, the series of informal trials comprising this experiment would be impossible to replicate exactly.

To evaluate these dramatic claims more formally, we conducted two studies in our laboratory (Green, et al., 1990; Lynn, Green, et al., 1990) after we learned of McCue and McCue's (1988) research that failed to corroborate the high rate of literalism reported by Erickson. Unfortunately, McCue and McCue's procedures were not well standardized. To provide a more controlled and more carefully standardized investigation, we (Green et al., 1990) contrasted high hypnotizable hypnotic subjects' and relatively unhypnotizable simulating subjects' responses to questions of the type used by Erickson. Our hypnotic "virtuosos" had extremely high scores (11–12) on both the Harvard Group Scale of Hypnotic Susceptibility, Form A (HGSHS:A; Shor & Orne, 1962), and the Stanford Hypnotic Susceptibility Scale, Form C (SHSS:C; Weitzenhoffer & Hilgard, 1962). Simulators exhibited a greater rate of literalism (58.3%) than "virtuosos" (29.2%).

We also tested nonhypnotized subjects for literalism in a naturalistic setting (Green et al., 1990). We found that hypnotized subjects and subjects approached in or outside the campus library responded comparably. The fact that more than a fifth of the library sample's responses were literal (21.78%) refutes Erickson's assertion that literalism is rarely exhibited by awake subjects. The fact that simulators were more literal than hypnotized subjects raises the possibility that Erickson's subjects' literal responses were products of demands that encouraged literal responding.

Our second study (Lynn, Green, et al., 1990) was designed to contrast "literal" versus "nonliteral" responding in hypnotized and task-motivated (Barber, 1969) subjects preselected for high hypnotizability. Task-motivated subjects received instructions that instilled a high level of motivation to imagine and respond to experimental tasks. We found no evidence to support Erickson's assertions: 87.5% of hypnotizable subjects' responses were nonliteral. Hypnotic and task-motivated subjects did not differ in their literal responding. What can account for the small number of literal responses among hypnotic and nonhypnotic subjects? We found evidence that literal responses were associated with subjects' perceptions about what constituted appropriate behavior and with their feeling passive in the situation. That is, hypnotized subjects who responded "Yes" or "No" to a question felt more passive than subjects who enacted a behavioral response to the question that tested literalism. In conclusion, our studies of literalism, along with McCue and McCue's (1988) research, suggest that Erickson's (1980) claims are highly misleading. Compliance with task demands and feelings of passivity, rather than a particular altered state or condition of the person, are sufficient to account for literalism during hypnosis.

Hypnosis and Reality Testing

One of the assumptions of our analysis is that hypnotized subjects do not relinquish their ability to monitor everyday events. Freud (1916–1917/ 1963) addressed the question of whether hypnosis affects reality monitoring. He asserted that hypnosis has the potential to alter ego functions, resulting in a diminution of reality testing. More recently, Shor (1959, 1962, 1970) contended that hypnotized subjects experience a fading of the generalized reality orientation that typifies the everyday waking frame of reference. E. R. Hilgard (1977) noted that when subjects are deeply involved in hypnosis, the reality-oriented part of the monitoring function of the personality may recede into the background of consciousness, failing to subject hypnotic experience to everyday "reality tests."

According to Sheehan and McConkey (1982), contemporary hypnosis theorists have tended to underplay the extent to which reality features of the environment are processed by the hypnotized subject. Sheehan and McConkey (1982) provided numerous examples of hypnotized subjects' ability to process reality features of the environment outside the context of suggestion, while retaining the ability to respond successfully to suggestions.

We (Lynn, Weekes, & Milano, 1989) were curious about whether subjects retained an ability to discriminate objective events from suggested sources of input when they were required to identify whether a telephone ring and conversation was a "real" event or was suggested. We assigned hypnotizable and simulating subjects to one of four conditions: heard a phone ring and conversation; received a suggestion to hear a phone ring and conversation; received a suggestion and heard a phone ring and conversation; or neither heard a phone ring nor received a suggestion.

Hypnotizable subjects who indicated that they were deeply hypnotized evidenced no impairment in their ability to discriminate whether an event actually occurred during hypnosis. With few exceptions, the hypnotizable subjects who listened to an actual phone ring stated that the phone rang. Simulators behaved comparably. Subjects apparently do not believe that the hypnotized subject loses touch with the environment: Hypnotizable subjects exhibited an awareness of detail incidental to the framework of suggestion. Indeed, many of the hypnotized subjects recalled the conversation almost word for word. Simulators failed to mimic the hypnotizable subjects' detailed recall of the conversation and suggestion wording. Hypnotized subjects are apparently even more in contact with the environment than unhypnotizable role-playing subjects believe them to be. When subjects received a suggestion to hear a phone ring, only 11.5% indicated it rang in reality in their open-ended reports; in response to a forced-choice question, none did so. In spontaneous reports, none of the hypnotizable subjects who heard a phone ring indicated it was suggested; only one did so in response to a forced-choice item, as opposed to two simulators.

In summary, hypnotizable subjects retain the ability to monitor reality. Although hypnotic suggestions are associated with shifts in awareness and attention, subjects are not deluded by suggestions into confusing fantasy with reality. Instead, they remain attuned to their environment and successfully discriminate suggestions and external events. Our research underscores the hypnotized subject's sensitivity to the total context of the hypnotic proceedings—a sensitivity that encompasses the ability to represent "objective reality" accurately.

Trance Logic

In his classic 1959 paper on the nature of hypnosis, Orne concluded that one of the principal features of the hypnotic state is the ability to tolerate logical inconsistencies that would be disturbing in the waking state (p. 297). Orne defined trance logic as the "ability of the subject to mix freely his perceptions derived from reality with those that stem from imagination and are perceived as hallucinations" (p. 259). He argued that "These perceptions are fused in a manner that ignores everyday logic" (p. 295).

The most consistent support for trance logic has been marshalled using an index termed "image transparency." Orne (1959) reported that some hypnotizable subjects asked to hallucinate an experimental assistant not only "saw" the assistant, but could see *through* the assistant at the same time. In contrast, simulating subjects never ascribed transparent qualities to hallucinated images in their spontaneous reports of their hallucinations. Orne (1959) offers the following example of a hypnotizable subject's account of "transparency": "This is very peculiar; I can see Joe sitting in the chair and I can see the chair through him" (p. 295). It would seem that the subject simultaneously acknowledges the reality of the hallucinated image, yet reports it as transparent. Reports of image transparency have distinguished hypnotizable and unhypnotizable simulating subjects in many studies (McDonald & Smith, 1975; Orne, 1959; Peters, 1973; Sheehan, Obstoj, & McConkey, 1976; Stanley, Lynn, & Nash, 1986; Spanos, Bridgeman, Stam, Gwynn, & Saad, 1983; Spanos, de Groot, Tiller, Weekes, & Bertrand, 1985). Furthermore, no simulating subject has ever spontaneously reported transparency.

Yet there is reason to question whether transparency reports represent a special feature of hypnosis and signify logical incongruity. First, a number of studies (e.g., Rhue & Lynn, 1987; Spanos, Churchill, & McPeake, 1976; Spanos, Mullens, & Rivers, 1979; Spanos et al., 1989; Spanos & Radtke, 1981) have shown that image transparency is reported by imagining as well as hypnotic subjects. Second, image transparency is not "illogical" (Stanley et al., 1986; Lynn, Weekes, & Rhue, 1990; Spanos, 1986). Rather, a parsimonious hypothesis is that transparency reports simply reflect the fact that the subject is unable to maintain a solid, visually compelling image of the assistant or object for the duration of the suggestion (see Spanos, de Groot, & Gwynn, 1987; Stanley et al., 1986). The following transparency reports are representative of those reported in the literature, and illustrate this point nicely. Regarding a cup Stanley et al. (1986, p. 450): (1)"Sometimes, like right when I blink, it looks transparent"; (2)"It looks transparent when it fades"; (3)"It goes from transparent to white, in and out." Regarding a person: (1)"I could get flashes . . . but the middle was real foggy"; (2)"almost as if it were a ghost . . . I thought that I could go right through her and she wouldn't be there at all" (Peters, 1973, p. 46); (3)"He looks like air" (McDonald & Smith, 1975, p. 86); (4)"faint outline"; (5)"an outline, not as distinct"; (6)"a shadowy figure"; (7)"I see bits of him." And finally, regarding a decorative, elaborate Easter tree (Sheehan et al., 1976, p. 466): "It was hazy, kind of translucent". Note that very few of these responses specifically identify the hallucinated image as transparent. In fact, in the entire trance logic literature, the word "transparent" is mentioned by the subject in only 10% of the responses coded as "transparent." Notably, as in the examples above, each response so coded makes reference to the lack of solidity of the image or to the failure to perceive the image as realistic in some way.

The hypothesis that transparency reports represent hypnotizable subjects' descriptions of their active yet unsuccessful attempts to maintain compelling hallucinations is supported by research demonstrating that hypnotic and nonhypnotic subjects who report transparent imagery also rate the image as less realistic or vivid than subjects who report a solid or lifelike image. That is, hypnotizable subjects frequently report that hallucinated images are vague, incomplete, and evanescent (Ham & Spanos, 1974; Rhue & Lynn, 1987; Sheehan et al., 1976; Spanos et al., 1983; Spanos, Ham, & Barber, 1973; Stanley et al., 1986; Spanos et al., 1979).

There is nothing "illogical" about honestly reporting one's incomplete or less than compelling suggestion-related experiences. This is illustrated by a study that we recently conducted (Lynn, Weekes, & Rhue, 1990). In response to the question "Was there anything that was illogical or didn't make sense to you about the way you responded to one or more of the suggestions?", only 1 of 29 highly hypnotizable subjects who reported that they were able to hallucinate the image of a coexperimenter, indicated that anything associated with their perception of the hallucinated image was "illogical." The experiences of certain hypnotizable subjects appear incongruous only from the perspective of the observer evaluating behavior outside the field of the subject's phenomenal world and the framework of the target suggestion (for a related argument, see Sheehan & McConkey, 1982; Lynn, Weekes, Milano, Brentar, & Green, 1988).

Nor is it necessary to explain real–simulating differences in terms of the unique cognitive capacity of the deeply hypnotized subject to tolerate a heightened sense of logical incongruity. An alternative account of real–simulating differences on trance logic measures (e.g., Stanley et al., 1986; Spanos, 1986; Spanos, de Groot, et al., 1985; Spanos, de Groot, & Gwynn, 1987; Spanos & Radtke, 1981; Wagstaff, 1981) emphasizes the divergent instructional sets and task demands that real versus simulating subjects encounter. Unlike hypnotizable subjects, simulators' verbal reports reflect not their actual experience, but their goal of avoiding detection as role-playing subjects. Never having experienced hypnosis, simulators have no reason to believe that even talented hypnotic subjects are unable to have subjectively compelling, complete hallucinatory experiences. Equating an "excellent" response with a complete response, simulators assume that hypnotized subjects have a compelling, lifelike experience of the to-be-hallucinated object or person. In short, hypnotizable subjects' honest report of their incomplete experiences, combined with simulators' "complete" responding, provides a plausible account of real–simulator differences (see Lynn et al., 1988; Spanos, 1986).

Research on trance logic provides an interesting illustration of how an understanding of individual differences in subjects' report criteria may account for hypnotic phenomena. Just as variability exists in hypnotizable subjects' ability to imagine persons and objects with lifelike properties (see Rhue & Lynn, 1987), so too does variability exist in terms of subjects' willingness to state that they "see" a hallucinated image that is suggested. Certain subjects report that they can see a hallucinated image of the assistant only if the image appears solid and lifelike. Assuming that they are capable of generating the requisite imagery, when tested for image transparency they say that they "see" the hallucinated image, and also report that it appears solid. In so doing, they fail the test of "trance logic." Other subjects, however, report that they see the hallucinated assistant's image, even though its appearance is neither solid nor lifelike. These hypnotizable subjects report image transparency, and therefore pass the "trance logic" test.

In addition to image transparency, the seemingly incongruous behavior of some age-regressed subjects has been taken as evidence of trance logic. The incongruous behavior most frequently examined is that of the regressed subject's correctly spelling words that are beyond the cognitive abilities of a normal child at the target age. In a typical study, subjects first receive a suggestion to regress to age 5, for example, and then are asked to spell a complex sentence such as "I am participating in a psychological experiment." Subjects who spell one or more of the "adult" words correctly are said to exhibit "trance logic." Whereas a number of investigations (Perry & Walsh, 1978; Nogrady, McConkey, Laurence, & Perry, 1983; Spanos, de Groot, et al., 1985) have reported significant differences between hypnotizable and simulating subjects on this task, other investigations (Peters, 1973; Stanley, et al., 1986) have not reported significantly more incongruous writing for hypnotic "reals" than for simulators. Furthermore, McConkey and Sheehan (1980) were unable to differentiate real and simulating subjects under some cue conditions, especially those emphasizing the illogical response (i.e., to spell correctly).

Just as incomplete involvement or absorption in a hallucinated image is associated with image transparency, the correct spelling of words during age regression is associated with incomplete absorption in the role of being a child (see Spanos, 1986; Stanley et al., 1986). According to this hypothesis (see Spanos, 1986), subjects who are able to think, feel, and act like children consistently during the writing task would exhibit the least "trance logic" (i.e., correct "adult" spelling). Consistent with this hypothesis, measures of subjects' belief in the reality of the suggested situation have been found to correlate negatively with incongruous writing during age regression (Spanos, de Groot, & Gwynn, 1987). These findings are clearly at odds with what we term the "trance logic hypothesis," which holds that subjects who are able to have the most compelling "childlike" response to the task would evidence the most incongruous behavior

We hold that "trance logic" responding can also be understood in terms of hypnotizable subjects' tacit interpretations of the complex demands of the trance logic paradigm. The request to write a complex sentence during age regression constitutes a suggestion nested within the more encompassing suggestion to regress to an earlier age. Those subjects who spell in a "childlike" manner—who fail to exhibit "trance logic"—behave in a manner congruent with the "childlike" role implied by the suggestion. So, if subjects adopt the role called for by the suggestion, while construing the request to write as a validation of their "childlike" status, they are unlikely to spell in an "adult" manner.

In contrast, we hypothesize that subjects who exhibit "trance logic" interpret the hypnotist's forceful request to spell the "adult" words as an indication that such behavior is appropriate, if not imperative. Spelling in an "adult" fashion may be legitimated by the failure to have a compelling age regression experience—to "be a child." For some hypnotized subjects, the presentation of the sentence "I am participating in a psychological experiment," combined with the request to spell it, focuses their attention more on the present than the past and interferes with involvement in the experience of "being a child" (Stanley et al., 1986), as in the following postexperimental report: "I felt myself to be a child—up until writing— especially the sentence" (Stanley et al., 1986, p. 452). Thus, the cue properties of the words and the task demands of spelling may engender incomplete involvement and conflict about whether to respond "as a child" (in line with the demand inherent in the age regression suggestion), or to write as an adult (in line with the direct request to spell the "adult" words). So whether or not hypnotizable subjects evidence "trance logic" may depend on how they integrate and resolve conflicting situational demands.

It stands to reason that if the test context minimizes conflict about responding like an adult, then a higher rate of trance logic should be expected. In dreams, subjects can experience a merger of fantasy and reality and can behave in a manner that is not strictly logical. With this in mind, we administered suggestions for subjects to spell "adult" words when asked to have a hypnotic dream about when they were 7 years old, and compared their rate of incongruous spelling with that of subjects who received standard age regression suggestions (Lynn et al., 1988). As we predicted, when the request to spell was embedded in the hypnotic dream context, which fostered a melding of fantasy and reality, hypnotizable subjects were more likely to spell "adult" words correctly (i.e., to exhibit trance logic) than when the standard suggestion context reinforced a more literal "childlike" regression to childhood.

We also found that none of the subjects who met our most stringent criterion for responding to the age regression suggestion, as gauged by primitive, childlike handwriting, spelled the word "psychological" correctly. Thus, subjects who fully adopted the role of "child" did not exhibit trance logic. Furthermore, a high correlation between incomplete responding to the age regression suggestion (adult-like handwriting) and correct spelling was secured. Thus, the subjects who evinced the most compelling experiences of age regression, and who according to the incongruity hypothesis would be expected to evince the most incongruous or childlike behavior during age regression, were in fact the least likely to spell "adult" words correctly. Taken together, our results provide strong support for the "common-sense" hypothesis that trance logic behavior is associated with incomplete responding, and that subjects behave in a manner consistent with the role they adopt vis-à-vis the age regression suggestion.

Is Hypnotic Behavior Involuntary?

The experience of involuntariness is one of the hallmarks of hypnosis. It has variously been attributed to an exaltation of ideomotor reflex excitability (Bernheim, 1880/1906), to a state of enhanced concerted attention upon a single idea (Braid, 1846/1970; Bramwell, 1903/1956), and more recently to dissociation (E. R. Hilgard, 1977). The research described below reinforces a recurrent theme in this chapter: Even the most dramatic reports of alterations of consciousness and experience can be accounted for in rather mundane terms; they do not reflect a true loss of behavioral control. Instead, our research suggests that involuntariness reports are shaped by multiple determinants, including subjects' preconceptions (e.g., occurrence schemas), self-representations, and agendas; their expectancies and suggestion-related imaginings; their rapport with the hypnotist; and the tactics they use to resolve conflicting situational demands.

Prehypnotic Factors: Occurrence Schemas. One tenet of our analysis is that prehypnotic expectancies and occurrence schemas have a bearing on subjects' responses and experience of involuntariness. Research conducted in our laboratory (Lynn, Nash, Rhue, Frauman, & Sweeney, 1984) has shown that when highly hypnotizable subjects are provided with prehypnotic information indicating that involuntary experiences are normative, subjects' perception of involuntariness is enhanced relative to when they are provided with prehypnotic information indicating that voluntary control over action is normative. Research by Spanos and his colleagues (Spanos, Brett, et al., 1987; Spanos et al., 1989) indicates that subjects generally believe that individuals who are hypnotized respond to suggestions involuntarily. This latter finding suggests that culturally based expectancies about hypnosis are associated with the belief that hypnotic actions are involuntary occurrences.

"Occurrence schemas" are culturally based ideas associated with the perception of hypnosis and involuntariness. One such idea is that the hypnotized subject's response is a product of the hypnotist's ability and effort. In support of the hypothesis that occurrence schemas are associated with involuntariness reports, we found that subjects' ratings of involuntariness were associated with the belief that hypnotic behavior is a function of the hypnotist's ability and effort (Lynn, Snodgrass, Hardaway, & Lenz, 1984; Lynn, Snodgrass, Rhue, Nash, & Frauman, 1987). In the first study (Lynn, Snodgrass, et al., 1984), subjects' posthypnotic attributions of response causality to the hypnotist's ability and effort were found to be associated with posthypnotic ratings of involuntariness. In a second study (Lynn, Snodgrass, Hardaway, & Lenz, 1987), subjects' prehypnotic ratings (i.e., expectancies) of the hypnotist's ability and effort correlated positively with involuntariness ratings (R's = .44 and .34, respectively) *after* hypnosis, even with hypnotizability statistically partialed out of the analysis.

In a third study, we (Lynn, Jacquith, Jothirathnam, & Rhue, 1987) tested the hypothesis that dominant Western cultural beliefs about hypnosis (e.g., occurrence schemas) prime subjects to label their sugges-tion-related sensations and movements as involuntary. We administered a hypnotizability scale and measures of imagination, waking suggestion, and involuntariness to English-speaking students at the University of Malaysia. We compared their performance with Malaysian students at Ohio University who had been residents of the United States for at least 6 months (average stay 2.5 years), and with native U.S. citizens who were students at Ohio University. We found that the mean scores on the measures of hypnosis, imagination, and waking suggestion were virtually identical across all three samples. However, in the sample of Malaysian students tested in Malaysia, where subjects were unfamiliar with Western ideas about hypnosis, none of the correlations among the measures were statistically significant. Although a measure of involuntariness failed to correlate with hypnotizability in the sample of Malaysian students tested in Malaysia, a significant correlation between involuntariness and hypno-tizability was obtained in the sample of Malaysian students tested at Ohio University. Furthermore, in the sample of Malaysian students tested at Ohio University, all of the measures intercorrelated in a manner comparable to that of the native U.S. sample.

Self-Representations and Rapport. According to our account, subjects' self-representations and agendas are important determinants not only of affect and action, but also of the need to retain control during hypnosis. As we have noted earlier, whereas some subjects have a positive, expectant attitude about experiencing hypnosis, others exhibit considerable appre-hension and fear. Not only is the clinical literature (Baker, 1986; Levitan & Jevne, 1986; Murray-Jobsis, 1986) replete with examples of resistant clients who are fearful of relinquishing control in the hypnotic situation, but empirical research has also shown that some subjects resist or oppose hypnotic suggestions in order to maintain their sense of freedom, to appear nongullible, and to seem "in control" (Jones & Spanos, 1982; Spanos & Bodorik, 1977).

We (Lynn et al., 1986) recently examined high- and low-hypnotiza-ble subjects' ability to oppose motoric suggestions. Compared to high-hypnotizable subjects, those with low-hypnotizability acted in opposition to more suggestions, experienced less suggestion-related involuntariness, and reported much less conflict about opposing the hypnotist. In fact, many unhypnotizable subjects appeared to take great pleasure in opposing the hypnotist. Relative to the highly hypnotizable group, they rated their rapport as poor and expressed less liking for the hypnotist. When subjects received a plausible paradoxical communication that linked demonstrating control with responding to the hypnotist, low-hypnotizable subjects who received the paradoxical message responded to more suggestions than did low-hypnotizable subjects who were not so instructed.

Perhaps even more interesting was the finding that nearly a quarter of the unhypnotizable subjects who were instructed that control could be demonstrated by moving in response to suggestion demonstrated their control by moving in the direction opposite that called for by the suggestion. No high hypnotizable subject responded in this manner. Combined, our results underscore the point that many unhypnotizable subjects are not simply passive, uninvolved responders; rather, they are motivated to assert their independence from the hypnotist's influence, actively and purposefully (Lynn, Rhue, & Weekes, 1990).

Because low-hypnotizable subjects appear to be particularly resistant to responding to the hypnotist, we (Lynn, Weekes, et al., in press) recently hypothesized that increasing rapport with the hypnotist might optimize their responding and increase their perceptions of involuntariness. We tested high- and low-hypnotizable subjects in conditions designed to establish a positive rapport or to establish a distant, aloof, and "scientific" relationship with the subject. In support of our hypothesis, we found that the relatively unhypnotizable subjects were more responsive to the hypnotist and rated their responses as more involuntary following procedures that optimized rapport. However, rapport was not sufficient to account for hypnotizability differences. That is, even when the less hypnotizable subjects were tested under optimum interpersonal conditions, they were not as responsive as highly hypnotizable subjects tested under less than optimum conditions. Nevertheless, facilitating rapport with the hypnotist increased responsivity to suggestions and enhanced feelings of involuntariness.

The findings pertinent to high-hypnotizable subjects were equally informative. Their behavior was stable across testing contexts. Even in the face of suboptimum rapport with the hypnotist, they maintained high levels of responding (see Lynn, Rhue, & Weekes, 1990). High-hypnotizable subjects' preparedness to respond thus transcends variations in the structure of the hypnotic relationship. Their motivated commitment, along with a proclivity to adopt an experiential set based on a readiness to undergo whatever experiential events are suggested (Tellegen, 1981), may account for why hypnotizable subjects exhibit a sensitivity to prehypnotic expectancies (Lynn, Nash, et al., 1984), to minor variations in the wording of suggestions (see Spanos, 1986), and to subtle alterations in the test context (Spanos, 1986).

In summary, hypnotizable and unhypnotizable subjects have very different agendas. Responsive subjects are attuned to the hypnotist and features of the test setting for cues that optimize performance and maximize the involuntary quality of experience. In contrast, in the absence of special efforts to improve rapport with the hypnotist, unhypnotizable subjects maintain a guarded, vigilant, and ultimately nonresponsive set that precludes experiencing the free-flowing, spontaneous, involuntary quality of suggestion-related responses.

The Ability to Resist Suggestions. Perhaps the acid test of whether hypnotic behavior is involuntary is whether subjects are truly unable to resist suggestions. A number of studies (Baker & Levitt, in press; E. R. Hilgard, 1963; Levitt, 1986; Levitt & Baker, 1983; Levitt & Henderson, 1980; Wells, 1940; Young, 1927, 1928) that examined subjects' ability to resist suggestions when specifically instructed to do so have yielded contradictory or inconclusive data.

To examine the determinants of subjects' perceptions of involuntariness, we conducted a series of studies. In these studies, hypnotic subjects were first hypnotized and then instructed to vividly imagine and experience motoric suggestions that were to follow, but to resist engaging in movements. We found that high-hypnotizable subjects, when asked to resist suggested responses, often failed to do so, and afterward stated that their movements occurred despite their best efforts to counter or prevent them. In this context, movements may be thought of as a behavioral index of nonvolition. Hypnotized subjects, as opposed to imagining subjects (Lynn, Nash, Rhue, Frauman, & Stanley, 1983) and simulating subjects (Lynn, Nash, et al., 1985), moved in response to countersuggestion (i.e., "Imagine but resist moving") and defined their suggestion-related responses as involuntary. Contrary to Arnold's (1946) ideomotor action hypothesis that sustained imagining is related to involuntary responding, hypnotizable imagining subjects reported feeling as absorbed and involved in imaginings as did hypnotic subjects, but resisted responding to suggestions.

The real–simulating differences obtained in our earlier research could be interpreted as supporting a neodissociation account of involuntariness. However, other findings (Lynn et al., 1984) suggest that the responses of both real and simulating subjects are expectancy-based. Simulating subjects, relative to hypnotizable subjects, moved less and tended to report that other "good" subjects were less likely to move in response to countersuggestion. Thus, real and simulating subjects may have responded differently because they had different expectancies about how hypnotizable subjects behave in the experimental context. This is not surprising. As we have indicated in our discussion of trance logic, real–simulator differences may reflect between-group differences in expectancies arising from divergent demands associated with the task of simulation (Sheehan, 1971b; Spanos, et al., 1983). Furthermore, simulators may have adopted a conservative response set, and "not moved" when in doubt as to how to respond.

In a second study (Lynn, Nash, et al., 1984), we tested the hypothesis that hypnotizable subjects are responsive to the broad expectational context in which the experiment is conducted. The reader will recall that one assumption of our model is that prehypnotic expectancies shape subjects' perceptions of their ongoing hypnotic experience. Because many hypnotized subjects do not experience their hypnotic actions as either completely voluntary or completely involuntary, prehypnotic normative information would be expected to have a substantial impact on subjects' perceptions of involuntariness. Prior to hypnosis, and prior to being instructed to resist suggestions, an experimental assistant informed subjects either that other "good" hypnotic subjects successfully resist suggestions and retain control over their movements, or that other "good" subjects fail to resist suggestions and experience loss of voluntary control over their actions during hypnosis. This information had a strong effect on subjects' ability to resist the hypnotist, and tended to affect subjects' reports of suggestion-related involuntariness in line with induced expectancies about appropriate responding.

This study also demonstrated that rapport plays a role in subjects' experience of involuntariness. Hypnotizable subjects with highly positive rapport resolved hypnotic conflict by achieving a compromise between meeting normative expectations (e.g., to respond) and complying with the hypnotist's counterdemand (i.e., to resist). Hypnotizable subjects with less positive rapport responded primarily in accordance with the normative expectations. This research is consistent with other research demonstrating that involuntariness reports are associated with ratings of rapport with the hypnotist (Lynn, Nash, et al., 1984; Lynn, Snodgrass, et al., 1987; Lynn et al., 1988), and with the view, propounded by Sheehan and his colleagues (e.g., Dolby & Sheehan, 1977; McConkey, 1979; Sheehan, 1971a, 1980), that some hypnotizable subjects may be specially motivated to be highly responsive to the hypnotist.

Another assumption of our model is that hypnotizable subjects use a variety of tactics to achieve suggestion-related effects and to minimize conflicting role demands. We assume that when hypnotized subjects are instructed to resist a suggestion, many experience conflict about responding versus resisting. Hypnotizable subjects may be pulled in the direction of responding to the suggestion while wishing to resist the suggestion, in keeping with the explicit instructions to do so. In this case, how can conflicting role demands be resolved? One way is by giving priority to the repeated suggestions to move, rather than the instruction to resist the suggestion's pull. Subjects are particularly likely to resolve conflict in this manner when the experimenter defines "involuntary" responding as the hallmark of a "good" hypnotic subject.

Subjects can successfully meet both experimental demands—that is, to "sincerely wish" to resist the suggestion yet fail to do so—by engaging in strategic behaviors. An example would be focusing attention on suggestion-related sensations and interpreting these sensations as indicative of the compelling power of the suggestion based on tacit understandings shaped by perceiving the situation as "hypnotic." When subjects do this, the hypnotic suggestion's "power" overcomes the "wish to resist." Indeed, the subjects' conviction that they "sincerely wish" to resist the pull of the suggestion, while they fail to resist responding, constitutes powerful affirmation that they are indeed "good" hypnotic subjects. When subjects are told that hypnotic subjects are able to resist suggestions successfully, we hypothesize that they also use sensation-related sensations as a cue. However, in this case, sensations serve as a cue to remind the subjects to exert sufficient effort to resist the suggestion's "pull" in a manner consistent with hypnotic role demands.

The degree to which subjects are conscious of using the sorts of tactics described above, rather than responding on the basis of their tacit understandings of demands, is unclear. It is clear, however, that very subtle influences can shape subjects' perceptions of their actions in a given context. In conditions in which suggestions are administered in an awake/alert imagining context, there is no reason for subjects to associate responses with the experience of nonvolition. What if imagining subjects came to associate or connect imagined responses to suggestion with "involuntary" responding? Would they then move in response to suggestions, despite instructions to resist, as did hypnotized subjects in our first countersuggestion study (Lynn et al., 1983)?

To address this question, we attempted to forge a contextual connection between imagination and involuntary responding. We assumed that during hypnosis, hypnotizable subjects would experience their responses to suggestions as involuntary. To foster the perception that these "involuntary" responses were associated with imagination (Lynn, Snodgrass, Rhue, & Hardaway, 1987), in the initial hypnosis screening session we informed subjects that hypnosis was actually a "test of imagination." To fortify the link between imagination and involuntariness, we administered the hypnotic induction along with other imagination measures. In a second session, we instructed high- and low-hypnotizable subjects to imagine along with suggestions but to resist responding to motoric suggestions. Subjects received either instructions to use goal-directed fantasies (GDFs) or no facilitative instructions.

GDFs are defined as imagined situations that, if they were to occur in reality, would be expected to lead to the involuntary occurrence of the motor response called for by the suggestion (Spanos, Rivers, & Ross, 1977, p. 211). For instance, subjects who are administered a hand levitation suggestion exhibit a GDFRs (i.e., goal-directed fantasy report) if they report such events as imagining a helium balloon lifting their hand, or a basketball being inflated under their hand. Subjects involved in GDFs attend to their imaginings while ignoring or reinterpreting information that contradicts the "reality" of the imagined events (Spanos et al., 1977). Suggestions worded to stimulate GDFs provide subjects with a cognitive strategy for generating and intensifying feelings of involuntariness (see Spanos, 1971; Spanos & Barber, 1972). Because the imaginative strategies are implicit in the wording of the suggestion, subjects are unlikely to attribute the feelings that ensue from adopting the strategies to their own agency. Studies have indicated that GDFRs are related to subjects' tendency to define their overt response to suggestion as an involuntary occurrence (e.g., Lynn, Snodgrass, Rhue, & Hardaway, 1987; Spanos, 1971; Spanos, Spillane, & McPeake, 1976; Spanos & Barber, 1972; Spanos & Gorassini, 1984; Spanos & McPeake, 1977; Spanos et al., 1977), though not necessarily to their overt response to suggestion per se (Buckner & Coe, 1977; Coe, Allan, Krug, & Wurzman, 1974; Lynn, Snodgrass, Rhue, & Hardaway, 1987; Spanos, 1971; Spanos & Barber, 1972; Spanos & McPeake, 1974; Spanos, Spillane, & McPeake, 1976).

We found that hypnotizable imagining subjects in this study (Lynn, Snodgrass, et al., 1987) exhibited greater responsiveness (i.e., failed to resist suggestions) than did a comparable sample of imagining subjects in our previous countersuggestion study (Lynn et al., 1983) when no attempt was made to foster a connection between imagining and involuntary responding in the initial screening session. Furthermore, the responses of imagining subjects were comparable to those of hypnotized subjects in our earlier countersuggestion research (Lynn et al., 1983). That is, imagining subjects tended to move in response to suggestion, despite being instructed to resist. As in many GDF studies, correlational analyses revealed that GDFs were associated with the experience of involuntariness; however, GDF's were not associated with responding to suggestion. With instructions designed to increase the use of GDFs, low- and high-hypnotizable subjects reported equivalent GDF absorption and frequency of GDFs. However, highly hypnotizable subjects responded more and reported greater involuntariness than less hypnotizable subjects, even when their GDFs were equivalent.

We therefore found no support for the hypothesis that sustained, elaborated suggestion-related imagery mediates response to suggestion (Arnold, 1946). We also failed to find support for Zamansky and Clark's (1986) hypothesis that low-hypnotizable subjects, lacking the capacity to dissociate incompatible cognitions from relevant ones, are able to pass suggestions only when it is possible to become absorbed in them. Even when low- and high-hypnotizable subjects were absorbed in GDFs to a comparable extent, the lows were not as responsive to suggestions as the highs. High and low subjects held very different expectancies about imagining and hypnotic responding: The former believed that imaginative subjects responded to more suggestions, and believed that a greater correspondence existed between imagining and responding. These measures of expectancy predicted both responding and involuntary experience.

The fact that hypnotizable and nonhypnotizable subjects construe the relation between imagining and the occurrence of suggested responses in very different ways suggests the following interpretation of the relation between hypnotizable and involuntariness: When instructed to do so, low-hypnotizable subjects respond to suggestion by engrossing themselves in suggestion-related imagery. However, they fail, for the most part, to perceive or construct a connection between their suggestion-related imaginings and moving in response to suggestion. This suggests that despite being absorbed in imagery, less hypnotizable subjects wait passively for suggested events to occur. Not surprisingly, nothing happens. In contrast, high-hypnotizable subjects take a much more active and constructive approach to the situation. They are successful in creating role-related experiences and behaving as suggested while simultaneously generating imagery of a kind that qualifies their responding as an involuntary happening.

Hypnotizable subjects are so adept at adopting an overarching schema to account for hypnotic responses that they are able to integrate diverse experimental demands and respond in overt opposition to suggestions while defining their responses as involuntary. Spanos, Weekes, and de Groh (1984) informed subjects that deeply hypnotized individuals could imagine an arm movement in one direction while their unconscious caused their arm to move in the opposite direction. Even though subjects so informed moved in the opposite direction, they imagined suggested effects and described their counter suggestion behavior as involuntary.

In summary, the research reviewed here provides strong support for the argument that hypnotic behavior is goal-directed, purposeful, and strategic. Moreover, the studies are consistent with our hypothesis that involuntariness reports are shaped by prehypnotic expectancies and relationship factors.

Hypnosis and Performance Standards

Hypnotists have long been aware of the importance of imparting the belief that patients successfully respond to suggestions (Edmonston, 1986). Hypnotists often use techniques that involve suggesting naturally occurring responses (lowering of an outstretched arm), interpreting observed behavior as evidence of successful hypnotic responding, and preventing or reinterpreting failures to respond to suggestions (see Barber et al., 1974; Edmonston, 1986; Wickless & Kirsch, 1989). That is, hypnotists attempt to ensure that patients believe that they have matched a standard associated with successful performance.

Research supports the wisdom of such stratagems. For instance, Spanos and Gorassini (1984) found that a direct relationship existed between the degree of involuntariness and the congruence between the aim of suggestion and naturally occurring feedback. Suggestions that expose subjects to contradictory sensory information, such as levitation of an outstretched arm, would be difficult to interpret as involuntary. The authors found that subjects who were asked to imagine a force acting on their outstretched arm to make it feel lighter (arm rising) rated their experience as more voluntary than subjects asked to imagine a force acting on their arm to make it feel heavier (arm lowering). Relatedly, Angelini and Stanford (1987) found that subjects who received suggestions for arm levitation rated their responses as more involuntary when the suggestions contained vivid suggestion-relevant imagery. They argued that the imagery served to divert subjects' attention from suggestion-incongruent proprioceptive information, which interferes with a sense of perceived involuntariness. We believe that suggestion-consistent sensations or proprioceptive feedback promotes the perception that responses are successful—that is, that they are consistent with the aims of suggestions, and that they meet or surpass performance standards.

The importance of confirmation of suggested experiences is perhaps most dramatically illustrated in a recent study by Wickless and Kirsch (1989). These researchers provided subjects with experiential confirmation of six hypnotic suggestions by surreptitiously altering the external environment. Subjects also received bogus feedback from personality tests to indicate that they had particular talent for hypnosis. Nearly three-quarters of these subjects scored in the high-hypnotizability range on the SHSS:C; none of the subjects scored in the low-hypnotizability range.

McConkey (1986) found that low- versus medium- and high-hypnotizable subjects had distinctly different prehypnotic expectancies, which suggested that they used different performance standards to evaluate their responses. That is, more than 80% of the low subjects believed that hypnosis was a dramatically altered state of consciousness. In contrast, the medium and high subjects generally believed that hypnosis was a normal state of focused attention. Presumably, the low subjects were unable to achieve the high level of hypnotic performance dictated by their prehypnotic expectancies, and their performance suffered as a result.

Studies based on a social learning/cognitive skill model of hypnotic responsiveness have documented appreciable increases on behavioral and subjective measures of susceptibility following hypnotizability modification training (see Spanos, 1986). Hypnotizability modification research suggests that responsiveness to suggestions is enhanced when people are told that hypnosis is not a dramatically altered state of consciousness (see Kirsch, 1990; Spanos, 1986). On the other hand, when the message conveyed to subjects is that "the people best able to respond hypnotically usually imagine most vividly" (Bates, Miller, Cross, & Brigham, 1988), it appears to suppress hypnotizability gains. Making imagery vividness salient, and relating training success to an ability that many less hypnotizable subjects lack, may diminish the likelihood of securing treatment effects.

Only a few studies have attempted to manipulate subjects' criteria for evaluating their hypnotic performance or their expectation of task difficulty. Barber and Calverley (1964) found that subjects scored higher on behavioral and subjective indices of hypnotizability when they were told that it was easy to respond to suggestions than when they were told that it was difficult to respond. A recent study (Lynn, Jacquith, Gasior, Green, & Maré, 1990) demonstrated that establishing a stringent performance standard suppresses hypnotic responding and feelings of involuntariness. We provided subjects with two very different prehypnotic rationales. To establish a stringent performance standard, we informed subjects that individuals who respond to more than a few suggestions experience an immediate suggestion-related response and imagine suggestions vividly and realistically ("as real as real"). To establish a lenient performance standard, we informed subjects that individuals who respond to more than a few suggestions do not respond to suggestions immediately or imagine suggested events realistically. A group of control subjects who received standard hypnosis instructions contained in the HGSHS:A were included in the design.

As we predicted, when subjects received prehypnotic information designed to establish a stringent performance standard, they responded to fewer suggestions, were less subjectively involved in suggestions, and experienced less suggestion-related involuntariness than no-instruction control subjects. The decrement in responding was impressive: Although uninstructed subjects passed more than 6.5 suggestions, "stringent" subjects passed 4.5 suggestions and postexperimentally indicated that they passed only 2.5 suggestions. In addition, compared to subjects who received the stringent standard, subjects who were informed that responsive subjects do not necessarily respond quickly or perceive hypnotic events "as real as real" experienced greater suggestion-related involvement and involuntariness, believed that they responded to more suggestions, and were more satisfied with their experience of hypnosis.

One of our most interesting findings was that making salient *any* performance standard, even if it was lenient, affected subjects' experience of hypnosis. When prehypnotic information established a lenient standard, they experienced less suggestion-related involuntariness, believed that they responded more slowly, and believed they responded to fewer suggestions than did subjects who received the standard prehypnotic information. Our findings, then, are consistent with the hypothesis that when a performance standard is made salient, subjects compare their hypnotic experience and performance with that standard, and engage in a matching-to-standard process that generates performance-based concerns and attenuates hypnotic involvement.

Hypnotizability and Fantasy Proneness

In a series of articles, S. C. Wilson and T. X. Barber (1981, 1983) described their serendipitous discovery of a group of individuals whom they alternately termed "fantasy addicts," "fantasy-prone personalities," and "fantasizers." Although fantasizers differ in many respects, they share a deep, profound, and long-standing involvement in fantasy and imagination. Wilson and Barber contended that fantasizers' intense imaginal involvements represent manifestations of adaptive fantasy abilities at the high extreme of a continuum of fantasy proneness. They estimated that fantasy proneness is evident in as much as 4% of the population.

Wilson and Barber discovered fantasizers in the context of an intensive interview study of excellent hypnotic subjects. In describing the characteristics of the trait of fantasy proneness, Wilson and Barber noted that their 27 excellent hypnotic subjects reported certain experiences with greater frequency than did the 25 nonexcellent (poor, medium, and medium-high in hypnotizability) hypnotic subjects with whom they were compared. Many fantasizers reported spending at least half of their waking lives fantasizing. They also reported the ability to hallucinate objects and to fully experience what they fantasized ("as real as real"). This included rich and vivid imagery before sleep, vivid recall of personal experiences, the achievement of orgasm in the absence of physical stimulation, and physical reactions, (e.g., anxiety and nausea) to observed violence on television. Wilson and Barber reported that 60% of the women they asked reported that they had had a false pregnancy at least once. Many fantasizers also reported psychic and out-of-body experiences, as well as occasional difficulty in differentiating fantasized events and persons from nonfantasized ones. Finally, fantasizers exhibited a sensitivity to social norms, which resulted in a secret fantasy life that few were privy to.

These descriptions of fantasy-prone persons were so fascinating that we initiated a research program to extend Wilson and Barber's exploratory research. Because Wilson and Barber believed that a close association exists between fantasy proneness and responses to suggestion, we investigated the relation between fantasy proneness and hypnotizability. The concept of "fantasy proneness" is largely derivative of and encompasses the construct of "imaginative involvement," which Josephine Hilgard (1970, 1974,

1979) first elaborated and which is thought to represent a central dimension underlying hypnotic responsiveness. Hilgard found evidence to support her belief that the capacity for imaginative involvement facilitates a temporary absorption in satisfying experiences in which fantasy plays a prominent role. Allied to the concepts of fantasy proneness and imaginative involvement is the construct of "absorption" (Tellegen & Atkinson, 1974). Tellegen and Atkinson (1974) contended that the capacity for absorbed and self-altering attention represents an essential component of hypnotic susceptibility. Studies using scales designed to measure imaginative involvement and absorption (see Lynn & Rhue, 1988) have documented a modest association (R's = .25–.40) between hypnotizability and absorption.

Altogether, five studies (Council & Huff, 1990; Green, Lynn, Rhue, Williams, & Maré, 1989; Lynn & Rhue, 1988; Rhue & Lynn, 1989; Siuta, in press) have examined the relation between hypnotizability and fantasy proneness. A questionnaire adapted from the interview schedule used by S. C. Wilson and T. X. Barber (1981), the Inventory of Childhood Memories and Imaginings, was used to classify subjects. To conform with Wilson and Barber's estimates of the prevalence of hypnosis persons, we selected fantasizers who scored in the upper 2–4% of the population. We contrasted their performance with nonfantasizers who scored in the lower 2–4%. A medium group of subjects scored in the range between the scores of the fantasy-prone subjects and the nonfantasizers. In four of these studies (Council & Huff, 1990; Lynn & Rhue, 1988; Rhue & Lynn, 1989; Siuta, in press), fantasizers were found to be more hypnotizable than nonfantasizers when the HGSHS:A was used as a criterion measure. In one study (Lynn & Rhue, 1988), high fantasizers scored higher than medium and low fantasizers; in the remaining three studies, high and medium fantasizers were equally hypnotizable, yet were more hypnotizable than nonfantasizers. Clearly, fantasy proneness was a less than perfect predictor of hypnotizability. In fact, in each of these studies hypnotizability and fantasy proneness were only modestly correlated (about R = .25).

Wilson and Barber stated that 96% of their high-hypnotizable subjects could be described as fantasy-prone. One reason why they might have secured evidence for an impressive link between hypnotizability and fantasy proneness is that they selected subjects on the basis of their hypnotic talent rather than on the basis of their fantasy proneness. To address this question, we (Green et al., 1989) selected subjects who scored in the upper 5% of hypnotizability; they were required to score 11 and 12 on both the HGSHS:A and on the individually administered SHSS:C. We compared these subjects' scores on our index of fantasy proneness with subjects who scored 11 or 12 on the HGSHS:A but were not screened on the SHSS:C. These subjects scored within the upper 10% of our hypnosis population. These groups were contrasted with subjects who scored in the

9–10 range on the HGSHS:A, with subjects who scored in the 4–8 (medium-hypnotizable) range on the HGSHS:A, and finally, with subjects who scored in the 0–3 (low-hypnotizable) range on the HGSHS:A.

Only 2 of our 12 subjects (16.66%) who were screened with both hypnotizability scales could be classified as fantasizers. Although the majority of high-hypnotizable subjects could not appropriately be described as fantasy-prone, the highly hypnotizable subjects (who passed at least 11 HGSHS:A suggestions), were found to have higher fantasy-proneness scores than low-hypnotizable subjects. However, medium-hypnotizable subjects were no more fantasy-prone than were low-hypnotizable subjects. In summary, we were unsuccessful in approximating Wilson and Barber's finding that there is a close association between hypnotizability and fantasy proneness.

Our results indicate that less correspondence between fantasy proneness and hypnotizability exists than Wilson and Barber's research suggested. This is really not so surprising. It is quite clear that negative attitudes, lack of motivation, atypical interpretation of suggestions, and poor rapport with the hypnotist dampen responding in even highly imaginative subjects. To pass hypnotic suggestions, it is not enough to have a vivid imaginal representation of a suggested event. It is possible to be absorbed in imaginings, yet to lack a sense of subjective conviction that a hallucination, for example, is "real" (Barber, 1969; Spanos & Radtke, 1981). If the imaginal representation falls short of the threshold of conviction, then the subject may "fail" the suggestion.

CONCLUSIONS

Our analysis of hypnotic action suggests that hypnotic responding is not the product of a fundamentally altered, narrowly defined "state of consciousness." As creative agents who shape their experience and direct their actions in terms of their anticipations, agendas, and perceptions of contextual and interpersonal demands, hypnotized subjects are neither passive nor automatic in their behavior. Indeed, there are at least five reasons to reject the hypothesis that hypnotic responding is automatic and involuntary:

1. Hypnotic responses have all of the properties of behavior that is typically defined as voluntary; that is, they are purposeful, are directed toward goals, are regulated in terms of subjects' intentions, and can be progressively changed to achieve goals.
2. Hypnotizable subjects can resist suggestions when resistance is defined as consistent with the role of "good" hypnotized subjects.

3. Hypnotic behaviors are neither reflexes nor manifestations of innate stimulus–response connections.
4. Hypnotic performances consume attentional resources in a manner comparable to that of nonhypnotic performances.
5. Hypnotic subjects' cognitive activities clearly demonstrate their attempts to fulfill the requirements of hypnotic suggestions, which include experiencing suggestion-related effects as involuntary (Lynn, Rhue, & Weeks, 1990).

The entire chain of events of imagining/attending, experiencing, responding, and viewing the response as an involuntary occurrence is goal-directed, even though subjects may not experience the links of the chain in a deliberate, effortful, or even conscious manner (Lynn, Rhue, & Weekes, 1990). In short, hypnotic behavior is "involuntary" only in the sense that subjects perceive it as such.

We do not believe that it is fruitful to continue the search for a single hypnotic ability. Hypnotic activity is multidetermined, multifactorial, and requires variety of "abilities." Hypnotic responsiveness rests on an infrastructure of tacit understandings and assumptions about the nature of hypnosis, aspects of the situation, and the relationship with the hypnotist, which together sculpt the hypnotic proceedings.

To optimize responding, the subject must view hypnotic action through the lens of an occurrence schema, must discern the appropriate implication of hypnotic communications, must be able to generate subjective experiences consistent with expectancies and standards of "good enough" hypnotic conduct, and must establish an adequate rapport with the hypnotist that promotes the free-flowing quality of hypnotic experience. Imaginative abilities are important to the extent that imagery is accessible, spontaneous, and promotes the flow of uninhibited action and experience. However, only a minimal degree of fantasy ability is necessary for many subjects to adopt the definition of the situation called for by many suggestions (Lynn & Rhue, 1988). It may be more important than imaginative abilities for the subjects to adopt a lenient or attainable performance standard; not to dwell or focus on the objective reality of the situation; not to have task-irrelevant thoughts; and not to analyze the causes of their actions.

In this chapter we have attempted to describe what we believe to be the key actions and transactions that describe "hypnosis." And yet we are keenly aware of the limitations of our knowledge about hypnosis and our theory-building efforts. As we have implied, hypnotic conduct and experience are not readily divisible into mutually exclusive categories of "affect," "behavior," and "cognition." Cognitive activity, for example, may be saturated with emotion, and emotions may in turn spur mental associations consistent with expressed affect. Nor is it clear that such constructs as "motivation," "expectancies," "rapport," and "imagination" are necessarily independent. Rather, they seem to us to reflect different ways of understanding persons who in fact function as whole, inherently indivisible organisms. Although we are far from having a coherent picture of the hypnotized person as a unified whole, we believe that this is the most fruitful path for researchers and theoreticians to follow.

REFERENCES

Abelson, R. P. (1981). Script as a psychological concept. *American Psychologist, 36,* 715–729.

Angelini, R. F., & Stanford, R. G. (1987). *Perceived involuntariness: The interaction of incongruent proprioception and supplied imagery.* Paper presented at the meeting of the American Psychological Association, New York.

Arnold, M. B. (1946). On the mechanism of suggestion and hypnosis. *Journal of Abnormal and Social Psychology, 41,* 107–128.

Baker, E. L. (1986). Hypnosis with psychotic and borderline patients. In B. Zilbergeld, M. G. Edelstein, & D. L. Araoz (Eds.), *Hypnosis: Questions and answers.* New York: Norton.

Baker, E. L., & Levitt, E. E. (in press). The hypnotic relationship: An investigation of compliance and resistance. *Int. J. of Clinical and Experimental Hypnosis.*

Barber, T. X. (1969). *Hypnosis: A scientific approach.* New York: Van Nostrand Reinhold.

Barber, T. X., & Calverley, D. S. (1964). The definition of the situation as a variable affecting "hypnotic-like" suggestibility. *Journal of Clinical Psychology, 20,* 438–440.

Barber, T. X., Spanos, N. P., & Chaves, J. (1974). *Hypnosis, imagination, and human potentialities.* Elmsford, NY: Pergamon Press.

Bargh, J. A. (1984). Automatic and conscious processing of social information. In R. S. Wyer & T. K. Srull (Eds.), *Handbook of social cognition* (Vol. 3, pp. 1–43). Hillsdale, NJ: Erlbaum.

Bates, B. L., Miller, R. J., Cross, J. J., & Brigham, T. A. (1988). Modifying hypnotic sugestibility with the Carleton Skills Training Program. *Journal of Personality and Social Psychology, 55,* 120–127.

Beckmann, J. (1987). Metaprocesses and the regulation of behavior. In F. Halisch & J. Kuhl (Eds.), *Motivation, intention and volition* (pp. 371–386). Berlin: Springer-Verlag.

Bernheim, H. (1906). *Suggestive therapeutics.* New York: G. P. Putnam's Sons. (Original work published 1880)

Braid, J. (1970). The power of the mind over the body. In M. M. Tinterow (Ed.), *Foundations of hypnosis: From Mesmer to Freud* (pp. 347–364). Springfield, IL: Charles C. Thomas. (Original work published 1846)

Bramwell, J. M. (1956). *Hypnotism: Its history, practice and theory.* New York: Julian Press. (Original work published 1903)

Brentar, J., & Lynn, S. J. (1989). *Hypnosis and "negative effects": The evidence examined.* Paper presented at the meeting of the American Psychological Association, New Orleans.

Buckner, L. G., & Coe, W. C. (1977). Imaginative skill, wording of suggestions, and hypnotic susceptibility. *International Journal of Clinical and Experimental Hypnosis, 25*, 27–35.

Carver, C. S. (1979). A cybernetic model of self-attention processes. *Journal of Personality and Social Psychology, 50*, 1216–1221.

Carver, C. S., & Scheier, M. F. (1981). *Attention and self-regulation: A control-theory approach to human behavior.* New York: Springer-Verlag.

Carver, C. S., & Scheier, M. F. (1982). Outcome expectancy, locus of attribution for expectancy, and self-directed attention as determinants of evaluations and performance. *Journal of Experimental Social Psychology, 18*, 184–200.

Carver, C. S., & Scheier, M. F. (1990). Origins and functions of positive and negative affect: A control-process view. *Psychological Review, 97*, 19–35.

Coe, W. C. (1978). The credibility of posthypnotic amnesia: A contextualist's view. *International Journal of Clinical and Experimental Hypnosis, 26*, 218–245.

Coe, W. C. (1987). *Hypnosis: Wherefore art thou?* Paper presented at the meeting of the American Psychological Association, New York.

Coe, W. C., Allen, J. L., Krug, W. M., & Wurzman, A. G. (1974). Goal-directed fantasy in hypnotic responsiveness: Skill, item wording, or both? *International Journal of Clinical and Experimental Hypnosis, 22,* 157–166.

Council, J. R., & Huff, K. (1990). Hypnosis, fantasy activity, and reports of paranormal experiences of high, medium, and low fantasizers. *British Journal of Experimental and Clinical Hypnosis, 7*, 9–15.

Deikman, A. J. (1966). Deautomization and the mystic experience. *Archives of General Psychiatry, 29*, 329–343.

Diamond, M. J. (1984). It takes two to tango: Some thoughts on the neglected importance of the hypnotist in an interactive hypnotherapeutic relationship. *American Journal of Clinical Hypnosis, 27*, 3–13.

Dolby, R. M., & Sheehan, P. W. (1977). Cognitive processing and expectancy behavior in hypnosis. *Journal of Abnormal Psychology, 86*, 334–345.

Edmonston, W. E., Jr. (1986). *The induction of hypnosis.* New York: Wiley.

Erickson, M. H. (1980). Literalness: An experimental study. In E. Rossi (Ed.), *The collected papers of Milton H. Erickson on hypnosis*: (Vol. 3, pp. 92–99). *Hypnotic investigation of psychodynamic processes.* New York: Irvington. (Original work published 1960)

Erickson, M. H., Hershman, S., & Sector, I. I. (1961). *The practical application of medical and dental hypnosis.* New York: Julian Press.

Field, P. B. (1965). An inventory scale of hypnotic depth. *International Journal of Clinical and Experimental Hypnosis, 13*, 238–249.

Freud, S. (1963). Introductory lectures on psycho-analysis. In J. Strachey (Ed. and Trans.), *The standard edition of the complete psychological works of Sigmund Freud* (Vol. 15, pp. 1–240; Vol. 16, pp. 241–496). London: Hogarth Press. (Original work published 1916–1917)

Fromm, E., Oberlander, M. I., & Gruenwald, D. (1970). Perceptual and cognitive processes in different states of consciousness: The waking state and hypnosis. *Journal of Projective Techniques and Personality Assessment, 34*, 375–387.

Green, J. P., Lynn, S. J., Rhue, J. W., Williams, B., & Maré, C. (1989). *Fantasy proneness in highly hypnotizable subjects.* Paper presented at the meeting of the American Psychological Association, New Orleans.

Green, J. P., Lynn, S. J., Weekes, J. R., Carlson, B. W., Brentar, J., Latham, L., & Kurtzhals, R. (1990). Literalism as a marker of hypnotic "trance": Disconfirming evidence. *Journal of Abnormal Psychology, 99*, 16–21.

Ham, M. W., & Spanos, N. P. (1974). Suggested auditory and visual hallucination in task-motivated and hypnotic subjects. *American Journal of Clinical Hypnosis, 17*, 94–101.

Hammer, A. G., Walker, W., & Diment, A. D. (1978). A nonsuggested effect of trance induction. In F. Frankel & H. S. Zamansky (Eds.), *Hypnosis at its bicentennial: Selected papers* (pp. 91–100). New York: Plenum.

Heckhausen, H., & Beckman, J. (1990). Intentional action and action slips. *Psychological Review, 97*, 36–48.

Hilgard, E. R. (1963). Ability to resist suggestions within the hypnotic state: Responsiveness to conflicting communications. *Psychological Reports, 12*, 3–13.

Hilgard, E. R. (1977). *Divided consciousness: Multiple controls in human thought and action.* New York: Wiley.

Hilgard, J. R. (1970). *Personality and hypnosis: A study of imaginative involvement.* Chicago: University of Chicago Press.

Hilgard, J. R. (1974). Imaginative involvement: Some characteristics of the highly hypnotizable and nonhypnotizable. *International Journal of Clinical and Experimental Hypnosis, 22*, 138–156.

Hilgard, J. R. (1979). Imaginative and sensory–affective involvements: In everyday life and hypnosis. In E. Fromm & R. Shor (Eds.), *Hypnosis: Developments in research and new perspectives* (2nd ed., pp. 483–518). Chicago: Aldine.

Hyland, M. (1988). Motivational control theory: An integrative framework. *Journal of Personality and Social Psychology, 55*, 642–651.

Jones, B., & Spanos, N. P. (1982). Suggestions for altered auditory sensitivity, the negative subject effect, and hypnotic susceptibility: A signal detection analysis. *Journal of Personality and Social Psychology, 43*, 637–647.

Kirsch, I. (1985). Response expectancy as a determinant of experience and behavior. *American Psychologist, 40*, 1189–1202.

Kirsch, I. (1990). *Changing expectations: A key to effective psychotherapy.* Pacific Grove, CA: Brooks/Cole.

Kruglanski, A. W. (1975). The endogenous–exogenous partition in attribution theory. *Psychological Review, 82*, 387–405.

Levitan, A. A., & Jevne, R. (1986). Patients fearful of hypnosis. In B. Zilbergeld, M. G. Edelstein, & D. L. Araoz (Eds.), *Hypnosis: Questions and answers.* New York: Norton.

Levitt, E. E. (1986). *Coercion, voluntariness, compliance, and resistance: Reflections of the essence of hypnosis.* Paper presented at the meeting of the American Psychological Association, Washington, DC.

Levitt, E. E., & Baker, E. (1983). The hypnotic relationship—Another look at coercion, compliance and resistance: A brief communication. *International Journal of Clinical and Experimental Hypnosis, 23*, 59–76.

Levitt, E. E., & Henderson, G. H. (1980, October). *Voluntary resistance to neutral hypnotic suggestions.* Paper presented at the meeting of the Society for Clinical and Experimental Hypnosis, Chicago.

Lynn, S. J., Green, J. P., Weekes, J. R., Carlson, B. W., Brentar, J., Latham, L., &

Kurzhals, R. (1990). Literalism and hypnosis: Hypnotic versus task-motivated subjects. *American Journal of Clinical Hypnosis, 23,* 113–119.

Lynn, S. J., Jacquith, L., Gasior, D., Green, J., & Maré, C. (1990). *Hypnotizability and performance standards.* Unpublished manuscript, Ohio University.

Lynn, S. J., Jacquith, L., Jothiratnam, & Rhue, J. W. (1987). *Hypnosis and imagination: A multi-cultural comparison.* Unpublished manuscript, Ohio University.

Lynn, S. J., Nash, M. R., Rhue, J. W., Frauman, D. C., & Stanley, S. (1983). Hypnosis and the experience of nonvolition. *International Journal of Clinical and Experimental Hypnosis, 31,* 293–308.

Lynn, S. J., Nash, M. R., Rhue, J. W., Frauman, D. C., & Sweeney, C. (1984). Nonvolition, expectancies, and hypnotic rapport. *Journal of Abnormal Psychology, 93,* 295–303.

Lynn, S. J., & Rhue, J. W. (1988). Fantasy proneness: Hypnosis, developmental antecedents, and psychopathology. *American Psychologist, 43,* 35–44.

Lynn, S. J., Rhue, J. W., & Weekes, J. R. (1989). Hypnosis and the experienced nonvolition: A sociocognitive integrative model. In N. P. Spanos & J. Chaves (Eds.), *Hypnosis: The cognitive–behavioral perspective* (pp. 78–109). Buffalo, NY: Prometheus Books.

Lynn, S. J., Rhue, J. W., & Weekes, J. R. (1990). Hypnotic involuntariness: A social cognitive analysis. *Psychological Review, 97,* 169–184.

Lynn, S. J., Snodgrass, M., Hardaway, R., & Lenz, J. (1984). *Hypnotic susceptibility: Predictions and evaluations of performance and experience.* Paper presented at the meeting of the American Psychological Association, New York.

Lynn, S. J., Snodgrass, M., Rhue, J. W., & Hardaway, R. (1987). Goal-directed fantasy, hypnotic susceptibility, and expectancies. *Journal of Personality and Social Psychology, 53,* 933–938.

Lynn, S. J., Snodgrass, M., Rhue, J. W., Nash, M. R., & Frauman, D. C. (1987). Attributions, involuntariness, and hypnotic rapport. *American Journal of Clinical Hypnosis, 30,* 36–43.

Lynn, S. J., Weekes, J. R., & Milano, M. (1989). Reality versus suggestion: Pseudomemory in hypnotized and simulating subjects. *Journal of Personality and Social Psychology, 98,* 137–144.

Lynn, S. J., Weekes, J. R., Milano, M., Brentar, J., & Green, J. P. (1988). *Hypnotic age regression and "trance logic": Effects of suggestion context and absorption.* Unpublished manuscript, Ohio University.

Lynn, S. J., Weekes, J. R., Neufeld, V., Zivney, O., Brentar, J., & Weiss, F. (in press). Hypnotizability and interpersonal climate. *Journal of Personality and Social Psychology.*

Lynn, S. J., Weekes, J. R., & Rhue, J. W. (1990). *Is trance logic illogical?* Unpublished manuscript, Ohio University.

Lynn, S. J., Weekes, J., Snodgrass, M., Abrams, L., Weiss, F., & Rhue, J. W. (1986). *Control and countercontrol in hypnosis.* Paper presented at the meeting of the American Psychological Association, Anaheim, CA.

Markus, H., & Nurius, P. (1986). Possible selves. *American Psychologist, 41,* 954–969.

McConkey, K. M. (1979). Conflict in hypnosis: Reality versus suggestion. In G. D. Burrows, D. R. Collison, & L. Dennerstein (Eds.), *Hypnosis 1979.* Amsterdam: Elsevier/North-Holland.

McConkey, K. M. (1983). Challenging hypnotic effects: The impact of conflicting influences on responses to hypnotic suggestion. *British Journal of Experimental and Clinical Hypnosis, 1*, 3–10.

McConkey, K. M. (1986). Opinions about hypnosis and self-hypnosis before and after hypnotic testing. *International Journal of Clinical and Experimental Hypnosis, 34*, 311–319.

McConkey, K. M., & Sheehan, P. W. (1980). Inconsistency in hypnotic age regression and cue structure as supplied by the hypnotist. *International Journal of Clinical and Experimental Hypnosis, 28*, 394–408.

McCord, H. (1961). The image of the trance. *International Journal of Clinical and Experimental Hypnosis, 9*, 305–307.

McCue, P. A., & McCue, E. C. (1988). Literalness: An unsuggested (spontaneous) item of hypnotic behavior? *International Journal of Clinical and Experimental Hypnosis, 36*, 192–197.

McDonald, R. D., & Smith, J. R. (1975). Trance logic in tranceable and simulating subjects. *International Journal of Clinical and Experimental Hypnosis, 23*, 80–89.

Miller, G. A., Galanter, E., & Pribram, K. H. (1960). *Plans and the structure of behavior.* New York: Holt, Rinehart & Winston.

Miller, M. E., & Bowers, K. S. (1986). Hypnotic analgesia and stress inoculation in the reduction of pain. *Journal of Abnormal Psychology, 95*, 6–14.

Murray-Jobsis, J.M. (1986). Patients who claim they are not hypnotizable. In B. Zilbergeld, M. G. Edelstein, & D. L. Araoz (Eds.), *Hypnosis: Questions and answers.* New York: Norton.

Norman, D. A. (1981). Categorization of action slips. *Psychological Review, 88*, 1–15.

Nogrady, H., McConkey, K. M., Laurence, J. R., & Perry, C. (1983). Dissociation, duality, and demand characteristics in hypnosis. *Journal of Abnormal Psychology, 92*, 223–235.

Orne, M. T. (1959). The nature of hypnosis: Artifact and essence. *Journal of Abnormal and Social Psychology, 58*, 277–299.

Pattie, F. A. (1956). Methods of induction, susceptibility of subjects, and criteria of hypnosis. In R. M. Dorcus (Ed.), *Hypnosis and its therapeutic applications* (pp. 1–24). New York: McGraw-Hill.

Perry, C., & Walsh, B. (1978). Inconsistencies and anomalies of response as a defining characteristic of hypnosis. *Journal of Abnormal Psychology, 87*, 574–577.

Peters, J. E. (1973). *Trance logic: Artifact or essence of hypnosis?* Unpublished doctoral dissertation, Pennsylvania State University.

Popham, C. E., & Bowers, K. (1988). *Holistic vs. primary processing: Cognitive processing under hypnosis.* Paper presented at the meeting of the Society of Clinical and Experimental Hypnosis, Asheville, North Carolina.

Powers, W. T. (1973). *Behavior: The control of perception.* Chicago: Aldine.

Rhue, J. W. & Lynn, S. J. (1987). Fantasy proneness: The ability to hallucinate "as real as real." *British Journal of Experimental and Clinical Hypnosis, 4*, 173–180.

Rhue, J. W. & Lynn, S. J. (1989). Fantasy proneness, hypnotizability, and absorption: A re-examination. *International Journal of Clinical and Experimental Hypnosis, 37*, 100–106.

Sarbin, T. R., & Coe, W. C. (1972). *Hypnosis: A social psychological analysis of influence communication.* New York: Holt, Rinehart & Winston.

Sarbin, T. R., & Coe, W. C. (1979). Hypnosis and psychopathology: Replacing old myths with fresh metaphors. *Journal of Abnormal Psychology, 88,* 506–526.

Schank, R., & Abelson, R. P. (1977). *Scripts, plans, goals and understanding.* Hillsdale, NJ: Erlbaum.

Shapiro, D. (1985). *Autonomy and rigid character.* New York: Basic Books.

Sheehan, P. W. (1971a). Countering preconceptions about hypnosis: An objective index of involvement with the hypnotist. *Journal of Abnormal Psychology, 78,* 299–322.

Sheehan, P. W. (1971b). Task structure as a limiting condition of the occurrence of the treatment effects of simulating instruction in application of the real–simulating model of hypnosis. *International Journal of Clinical and Experimental Hynosis, 19,* 260–276.

Sheehan, P. W. (1980). Factors influencing rapport in hypnosis. *Journal of Abnormal Psychology, 89,* 263–281.

Sheehan, P. W., Obstoj, I., & McConkey, K. (1976). Trance logic and cue structure as supplied by the hypnotist. *Journal of Abnormal Psychology, 85,* 459–472.

Sheehan, P. W., & McConkey, K. (1982). *Hypnosis and experience: The exploration of phenomena and processes.* Hillsdale, NJ: Erlbaum.

Shor, R. E. (1959). Hypnosis and the concept of the generalized reality-orientation. *American Journal of Psychotherapy, 13,* 582–602.

Shor, R. E. (1962). Three dimensions of hypnotic depth. *International Journal of Clinical and Experimental Hypnosis, 10,* 23–28.

Shor, R. E. (1970). The three-factor theory of hypnosis as applied to the book-reading fantasy and to the concept of suggestion. *International Journal of Clinical and Experimental Hypnosis, 28,* 89–98.

Shor, R. E., & Orne, E. C. (1962). *Harvard Group Scale of Hypnotic Susceptibility.* Palo Alto, CA: Consulting Psychologists press.

Siuta, J. (in press). Hypnotizability and fantasy proneness: Toward cross-cultural comparisons. *British Journal of Experimental and Clinical Hypnosis.*

Spanos, N. P. (1971). Goal-directed fantasy and the performance of hypnotic test suggestions. *Psychiatry, 34,* 86–96.

Spanos, N. P. (1982a). A social psychological approach to hypnotic behavior. In G. Weary & H. Mirels (Eds.), *Integrations of clinical and social psychology* (pp. 331–371). New York: Oxford University Press.

Spanos, N. P. (1982b). Hypnotic behavior: A cognitive, social psychological perspective. *Research Communications in Psychology, Psychiatry, and Behavior, 7,* 199–213.

Spanos, N. P. (1986). Hypnotic behavior: A social psychological interpretation of amnesia, analgesia, and "trance logic." *Behavioral and Brain Sciences, 9,* 449–502.

Spanos, N. P., & Barber, T. X. (1972). Cognitive activity during hypnotic suggestion: Goal-directed fantasy and the experience of non-volition. *Journal of Personality, 40,* 510–524.

Spanos, N. P., & Bodorik, H. L. (1977). Suggested amnesia and disorganized recall in hypnotic and task-motivated subjects. *Journal of Abnormal Psychology, 86,* 295–305.

Spanos, N. P., Brett, N. P., Menary, E. P., & Cross, W. P. (1987). A measure of attitudes toward hypnosis: Relationships with absorption and hypnotic susceptibility. *American Journal of Clinical Hypnosis, 30,* 139–150.

Spanos, N. P., Bridgeman, M., Stam, H. J., Gwynn, M., & Saad, C. L. (1983). When seeing is not believing: The effect of contextual variables on the reports of hypnotic hallucinators. *Imagination, Cognition and Personality, 3*, 195–209.

Spanos, N. P., Churchill, N., & McPeake, J. D. (1976). Experiential response to auditory and visual hallucination suggestion in hypnotic subjects. *Journal of Consulting and Clinical Psychology, 44*, 729–738.

Spanos, N. P., Cobb, P. C., & Gorassini, D. R. (1985). Failing to resist hypnotic test suggestions: A strategy for self-presenting as deeply hypnotized. *Psychiatry, 48*, 282–292.

Spanos, N. P., de Groot, H. P., & Gwynn, M. I. (1987). Trance logic as incomplete responding. *Journal of Personality and Social Psychology, 53*, 911–921.

Spanos, N. P., de Groot, H. P., Tiller, D. K., Weekes, J. R., & Bertrand, L. D. (1985). "Trance" logic, duality, and hidden observer responding in highly hypnotizable and in simulating subjects: A social psychological perspective. *Journal of Abnormal Psychology, 94*, 611–623.

Spanos, N. P., & Gorassini, D. R. (1984). Structure of hypnotic test suggestions and attributions of responding involuntarily. *Journal of Personality and Social Psychology, 46*, 688–696.

Spanos, N. P., Gottlieb, J., & Rivers, S. M. (1980). The effects of short-term meditation training on hypnotic responsivity. *Psychological Record, 30*, 343–348.

Spanos, N. P., Ham, M. W., & Barber, T. X. (1973). Suggested ("hypnotic") visual hallucinations: Experimental and phenomenological data. *Journal of Abnormal Psycholgy, 81*, 96–106.

Spanos, N. P., & Katsanis, J. (1989). Effects of instructional set on attributions of nonvolition during hypnotic and nonhypnotic analgesia. *Journal of Personality and Social Psychology, 56*, 182–188.

Spanos, N. P., & McPeake, J. D. (1977). Cognitive strategies, goal-directed fantasy, and response to suggestions in hypnotic subjects. *American Journal of Clinical Hypnosis, 20*, 114–123.

Spanos, N. P., Mullens, D., & Rivers, S. M. (1979). The effects of suggestion structure and hypnotic vs. task-motivation instructions on response to hallucination suggestions. *Journal of Research in Personality, 13*, 59–70.

Spanos, N. P., & Radtke, H. L. (1981). Hypnotic and visual hallucinations as imaginings: A cognitive–social psychological perspective. *Imagination, Cognition and Personality, 1*, 147–170.

Spanos, N. P., Rivers, S. M., & Ross, S. (1977). Experienced involuntariness and response to hypnotic suggestions. *Annals of the New York Academy of Sciences, 296*, 208–221.

Spanos, N. P., Salas, J., Bertrand, L. D., & Johnston, J. (1989). Occurrence schemas, context ambiguity and hypnotic responding. *Imagination, Cognition and Personality, 8*, 235–247.

Spanos, N. P., Spillane, J., & McPeake, J. C. (1976). Suggestion elaborateness, goal-directed fantasy, and response to suggestion in hypnotic and task-motivated subjects. *American Journal of Clinical Hypnosis, 18*, 254–262.

Spanos, N. P., Weekes, J. R., & deGroh, M. (1984). The "involuntary" countering of suggested requests: A test of the ideomotor hypothesis of hypnotic responsiveness. *British Journal of Experimental and Clinical Hypnosis, 1*, 3–11.

Stanley, S. M., Lynn, S. J., & Nash, M. R. (1986). Trance logic, susceptibility screening, and the transparency response. *Journal of Personality and Social Psychology, 50,* 447–454.

Tellegen, A. (1981). Practicing the two disciplines for relaxation and enlightenment: Comment on "Role of the feedback signal in electromyograph biofeedback: The relevance of attention" by Qualls and Sheehan. *Journal of Experimental Psychology: General, 110,* 217–226.

Tellegen, A., & Atkinson, G. (1974). Openness to absorbing and self-altering experiences ("absorption"), a trait related to hypnotic susceptibility. *Journal of Abnormal Psychology, 83,* 268–277.

Tomkins, S. S. (1979). Script theory: Differential magnification of affects. In H. E. Howe, Jr., & R. A. Diensbier (Eds.), *Nebraska Symposium on Motivation* (Vol. 26). Lincoln: University of Nebraska Press.

Trope, Y. (1986). Identification and inferential processes in dispositional attribution. *Psychological Review, 93,* 239–257.

Uleman, J. S. (1987). Consciousness and control: The case of spontaneous trait inferences. *Personality and Social Psychology Bulletin, 13,* 337–354.

Wagstaff, G. F. (1981). *Hypnosis, compliance and belief.* New York: St. Martin's Press.

Wedemeyer, C., & Coe, W. C. (1981). Hypnotic state reports: Contextual variation and phenomenological criteria. *Journal of Mental Imagery, 5,* 107–118.

Wells, W. R. (1940). Ability to resist artificially induced dissociation. *Journal of Abnormal and Social Psychology, 35,* 261–272.

Weitzenhoffer, A. M. (1953). *Hypnotism: An objective study in suggestibility.* New York: Wiley.

Weitzenhoffer, A. M. (1957). *General techniques of hypnotism.* New York: Grune & Stratton.

Weitzenhoffer, A. M., & Hilgard, E. R. (1962). *Stanford Hypnotic Susceptibility Scale: Form C.* Palo Alto, CA: Consulting Psychologists Press.

White, R. W. (1941). An analysis of motivation in hypnosis. *Journal of General Psychology, 24,* 145–162.

Wickless, C., & Kirsch, I. (1989). The effects of verbal and experiential expectancy manipulation on hypnotic susceptibility. *Journal of Personality and Social Psychology, 57,* 762–768.

Wilson, L., Greene, E., & Loftus, E. F. (1986). Beliefs about forensic hypnosis. *International Journal of Clinical and Experimental Hypnosis, 34,* 110–121.

Wilson, S. C., & Barber, T. X. (1981). Vivid fantasy and hallucinatory abilities in the life histories of excellent hypnotic subjects ("somnambules"): Preliminary report with female subjects. In E. Klinger (Ed.), *Imagery: Concepts, results, and applications* (Vol. 2, pp. 133–152). New York: Plenum Press.

Wilson, T. (1985). Self-deception without repression. In M. W. Martin (Ed.), *Self-deception and self-understanding.* Lawrence: University of Kansas Press.

Young, P.C. (1927). Is rapport an essential characteristic of hypnosis? *Journal of Abnormal and Social Psychology, 22,* 130–139.

Young, P. C. (1928). The nature of hypnosis: As indicated by the presence or absence of posthypnotic amnesia and rapport. *Journal of Abnormal and Social Psychology, 22,* 372–382.

Zamansky, J. S., & Clark, L. E. (1986). Cognitive competition and hypnotic behavior: Whither absorption? *Int. J. of Clinical and Experimental Hypnosis, 34,* 205–214.

The Social Learning Theory of Hypnosis

IRVING KIRSCH
University of Connecticut

INTRODUCTION

Response expectancy theory (Kirsch, 1985, 1990) is an extension of social learning theory. In social learning theory, behavior is predicted by the expectancy that it will lead to particular outcomes and by the value of those outcomes to the individual (Rotter, 1954). Prior to the formulation of response expectancy theory, expected outcomes were assumed to be stimulus events, such as school grades, money, social approval, and the like (Bolles, 1972). Response expectancy theory began with the realization that external stimuli are not the only kinds of outcomes that we anticipate. We also expect to have various reactions to particular stimuli and to our own behavior. For example, we expect to experience pain if a dentist removes a tooth without first administering an anesthetic; we expect to feel more alert after drinking a cup of coffee; and we expect to feel tired the next morning after staying up too late at night. Expected responses of this sort are among the outcomes that people consider in deciding on a course of action.

Response expectancies have an important characteristic that they do not share with most stimulus expectancies: They tend to be self-confirming. We may expect to be paid after working at our jobs, to get wet when walking in the rain, or to win or lose the toss of a coin, but these stimulus expectancies cannot cause those outcomes to occur. In contrast, when we expect to feel anxious, relaxed, joyful, or depressed, our expectations tend to produce those feelings. This observation is the basis for the central thesis of response expectancy theory: Expectancies can generate nonvolitional responses. In response expectancy theory, responses are defined as nonvolitional if they are experienced as occurring without direct volitional effort.[1] Thus, the status of a response as volitional or nonvolitional is dependent solely on the person's subjective experience; no assumption is made about its actual controllability. It is for this reason that I use the term "nonvolitional" instead of the more conventional term "involuntary."

Response expectancy theory is not primarily a theory of hypnosis. It is a theory about one important proximal cause of everyday human experience and behavior. Applications of the theory include the contributions of response expectancies to the etiology and treatment of anxiety disorders, depression, dissociative disorders, and other psychological problems (Kirsch, 1990). However, the subjective experience of nonvolition is widely regarded to be one of the hallmarks of hypnosis, and self-reports of involuntariness are highly correlated with the number of suggestions to which subjects respond behaviorally (Bowers, Laurence, & Hart, 1988). Since response expectancies are capable of generating nonvolitional responses in nonhypnotic settings, it is reasonable to expect that they should do so in hypnotic contexts as well (Kirsch & Council, 1989).

The placebo effect is the prototype of the self-confirming action of response expectancies. Research on placebos has documented a remarkably wide range of expectancy effects, some of which are substantial and long-lasting. Response expectancies have been shown to produce changes in pain perception and tolerance, alertness, tension, relaxation, pulse rate, blood pressure, sexual arousal, aggression, angina, nausea, vomiting, gastric function, agoraphobia, and depression (Kirsch, 1990). In medical research, these effects are regarded as nuisance variables, which are to be controlled for or eliminated. In social learning theory, however, they are a focus of interest. There are not many psychological variables that can lay claim to such a wide range of well-documented effects. Rather than discarding or ignoring them, we ought to be interested in understanding them and exploiting their clinical potential.

In traditional theories of hypnosis, effects that are due to subjects' expectations are regarded as "artifacts," from which the "essence" of hypnosis is to be distinguished (Orne, 1959). A different approach is taken in response expectancy theory. Whether or not a hypnotic response is an artifact depends on whether it reflects a change in subjective experience. Artifacts are responses that are not accompanied by corresponding changes in experience. Conversely, responses that reflect experiential alterations are genuine, regardless of how they were produced. From this point of view, the status of expectancy in hypnosis is an empirical question. When expectancy contributes to a simulation of hypnosis, it is producing an artifact. Conversely, when it contributes to the experience of a hypnotic effect, it is part of the essence of hypnosis.

THEORETICAL CONCEPTS AND PRINCIPLES

A hypnotic response is not the same as the overt behavior by which it is assessed. Indeed, some hypnotic responses (e.g., the "negative hallucination" suggestion on the Stanford Hypnotic Susceptibility Scale, Form C [SHSS:C]) are assessed only via self-report. These self-reports are intentional acts. They are directed at the goal of informing (or misinforming) the hypnotist that one has had the requisite subjective experience. But our interest is not in how words are generated; rather, it is in the subjective experience to which those words refer.

Other behaviors by which hypnotic responsiveness is assessed are frequent occurrences in commonplace nonhypnotic contexts (e.g., raising or lowering an arm). What makes them particularly interesting when they occur in hypnotic contexts are the reported alterations in experience with which they are usually accompanied. In everyday life, one experiences oneself as intentionally raising or lowering an arm. In contrast, hypnotic subjects report that they experience suggested movements as occurring nonvolitionally. Again, our interest is not in how people lift their arms. Rather, it is in the experience of nonvolition that reportedly accompanies this movement. The task for hypnosis scholars is to explain these reported changes in experience.

One possible explanation is that subjects are lying to us when they report these unusual experiences. If hypnotic responses were acts of deliberate deception, aimed at fooling experimenters and hypnotists, then the proper focus of study would be to determine the factors that lead such a large number of people to go to such lengths to deceive others whom they have just met. However, virtually all hypnosis theorists are of the opinion that this is not generally the case, and there are now convincing data in support of that shared opinion. Unlike simulators, highly responsive subjects display hypnotic responses even when there is no one present for them to deceive (Kirsch, Silva, Carone, Johnston, & Simon, 1989). The question, then, is this: How are these changes in experience produced?

Hypnotic Responses: Actions or Outcomes?

In early theories of hypnosis, subjects were viewed as passive automata whose behavior had come under the sway of the hypnotist (see Lynn, Rhue, & Weekes, 1989). That hypothesis is clearly incorrect. Rather than being passive recipients, subjects are active participants in the social interaction that has come to be termed "hypnosis." Hypnotic subjects expend a great deal of effort in order to experience hypnotic responses. They volunteer for hypnosis experiments, ask whether there are other hypnosis experiments in which they can participate, pay fees to be treated by hypnotherapists, and buy tickets to performances by stage hypnotists. During the hypnotic session, they voluntarily comply with various instructions that are a part of hypnotic suggestions, such as holding their arms out in preparation for an arm levitation suggestion. Most importantly, even when not instructed to do so, many (but not all) good hypnotic subjects intentionally generate imagery aimed at producing hypnotic responses (Spanos, 1971; Spanos & Barber, 1972; Lynn, Snodgrass, Rhue, & Hardaway, 1987).

Recognizing the inadequacies of traditional theories, role theorists have proposed that hypnotic responses are voluntary, goal-directed actions, as opposed to "happenings" that occur automatically, with no intentional effort on the part of the subject (Sarbin, 1989; Spanos, 1986). Although this formulation is closer to the mark, it is not precisely on target. Hypnotic subjects emit a variety of goal-directed acts, but their hypnotic responses are neither actions nor happenings. Instead, hypnotic responses are the outcomes or goals toward which subjects' goal-directed actions are aimed. Hypnotic subjects are largely motivated by a desire to experience hypnotic phenomena, and their strategic behavior is aimed primarily at generating those experiences (see Kirsch et al., 1989).

The misidentification of hypnotic responses as actions may be due in part to an assumption that outcomes are stimulus events. However, although some outcomes are external events, others are internal responses (e.g., changes in the experienced painfulness of a stimulus). There are two characteristics of these responses that justify their classification as outcomes or achievements, rather than as simple actions. One of these distinguishing characteristics is people's lack of complete voluntary control over their occurrence. The second is their dependence on intervening actions and cognitions.

People can control their actions, but they do not have full control over the outcomes of those actions. For example, I may decide to shoot an arrow at a target. Because aiming and shooting are completely voluntary, once I decide to do so, the probability that I will shoot the arrow is close to 100%. In contrast, hitting the target is an outcome. If I had full voluntary control over that outcome, the likelihood of the arrow's hitting the target would also be 100%. It is characteristic of outcomes that their probability of occurrence is generally less than 100% and that they can sometimes be quite discrepant from what was intended.

If hypnotic responses were simply voluntary acts, their probability of occurrence would be identical to people's intention to bring them about. But it is not. People can intend to experience a hypnotic response. They can try their best to make it occur. And they can fail! The fact that people often fail to emit intended hypnotic responses indicates that those responses are not fully under their voluntary control. This is one reason for viewing them as outcomes, rather than as actions.

A second characteristic that distinguishes outcomes from actions is that the occurrence of outcomes may depend on various strategic actions or cognitions. Actors who wish to cry, for example, may have to focus their attention on distressing thoughts or memories, and people who want to experience arm levitation may need to imagine circumstances that could produce that experience. In contrast to outcomes, actions do not require the use of intervening strategies for their occurrence. If I merely want to raise my arm, there is no need for me to imagine that it is being pumped up with helium. It is only when I wish to experience that movement as an outcome that the use of some intervening strategy may be required.

How Expectancies Generate Responses

The central hypothesis of social learning theory is that behavior can be predicted by the expectancy that it will lead to particular outcomes and by the value of those outcomes (Rotter, 1954). Thus, the expectancy that one will experience hypnotic responses, and the positive value that is attached to those experiences, lead people to engage in various goal-directed behaviors aimed at generating them. At the most mundane level, this includes seeking out opportunities to be hypnotized and cooperating with the hypnotist's instructions. More importantly, subjects may devise and implement various cognitive strategies aimed at the goal of experiencing hypnotic suggestions (Barber, Spanos, & Chaves, 1974). According to social learning theory, the likelihood of engaging in these strategic actions depends on the expectancy that they will produce hypnotic experiences and on the value that people assign to those experiences. To the extent that the strategies they implement are in fact capable of producing hypnotic experiences, subjects' expectancies will have indirectly affected the probability that the response will occur.

In addition to this indirect effect, response expectancy can have a direct effect on people's responses to hypnosis. According to the theory of reasoned action (Ajzen & Fishbein, 1980), intentions are the immediate determinants of behavioral acts. However, this relation between intention and behavior is explicitly limited to those behaviors that are completely under voluntary control. It does not apply to emotional reactions or to other responses that are experienced as outcomes. According to social learning theory, response expectancies are immediate determinants of nonvolitional responses, in much the same way that intentions are immediate determinants of volitional behavior (Kirsch, 1985, 1990).

Although the role of response expectancies in generating hypnotic responses is similar to the role of intentions in generating voluntary acts, there are also some important differences between the two variables. Both variables are defined as a person's subjective probability that the response

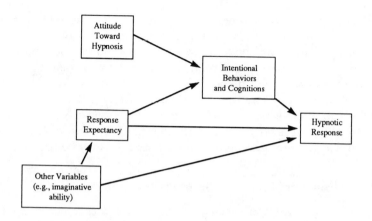

FIGURE 14.1. A social learning model of hypnosis.

will occur, and both are hypothesized to be immediate determinants of the predicted response. However, whereas intentions are the only immediate determinants of voluntary acts, response expectancies are seen as only one of a number of factors that produce nonvolitional responses. For example, although fear can be produced by the expectancy of its occurrence, it can also be elicited by the perception of danger. Similarly, pain perception, tension, nausea, and other responses can be affected by the chemical properties of particular drugs, as well as by placebo-induced expectancies. Furthermore, these two means of having an effect are not mutually exclusive. The chemical properties of a drug and the response expectancies that are activated by one's knowledge about the drug can make independent contributions to the effects of treatment (e.g., Frankenhaeuser, Post, Hagdahl, & Wrangsjoe, 1964). In other words, knowing the intended effects of a medication can enhance its effectiveness.

A similar partitioning of causality applies to hypnotic responses. Any particular variable may have an effect on hypnotic responses that is independent of expectancy, as well as producing an expectancy-mediated effect. In each case, the degree to which the effects of a particular variable are mediated by expectancy must be evaluated experimentally.

The social learning model of hypnosis is illustrated in Figure 14.1. In this model, expectancy and other variables can have both direct and indirect effects on hypnotic responses. In other words, expectancy effects can be immediate, or they can be mediated by various intentional behaviors and cognitions. Conversely, the effects of various person and situation variables may be partially or totally mediated by expectancy. In social learning theory, personality variables are thought of as generalized expectancies, and would be predicted to affect behavior largely via their effects on expectancy (Rotter, 1954; see also Ajzen & Fishbein, 1980). However, in order for a response to occur, it must be within the person's range of capabilities. It is therefore possible that some capacity or ability factor has an impact on hypnotic response that is not mediated by expectancy.

Response Expectancy and Overt Behavior

Finally, we come to the question of how response expectancies influence the overt behavior by means of which responsiveness is measured. Some behaviors are public expressions of subjective states. For example, we grimace when we are in pain, and we tolerate a painful stimulus longer when we experience less pain. This is the nature of many overt hypnotic responses. For example, people may be asked to respond to a hallucinated voice, to report a hypnotically suggested dream, to brush away a hallucinated fly or mosquito, or to tell an experimenter whether they can taste the sourness of an imagined lemon. Since most people do not normally fake hypnotic responses unless asked to do so (Kirsch et al., 1989), most of these actions can be interpreted as voluntary responses that reflect expectancy-induced changes in experience. Others may occur unintentionally, as when a person unthinkingly grimaces at the taste of a vividly imagined lemon. But in either case, they can be regarded as overt expressions of subjective experiences. In principle, they are not different from the verbal self-reports by means of which subjective states are most frequently assessed.

There remain, however, two types of hypnotic response that appear to be somewhat different from simple expressions of subjective states. These are the overt responses to ideomotor (e.g., "Your arm is becoming lighter") and challenge (e.g., "You cannot open your eyes") suggestions. It is possible that these responses are also deliberate expressions of subjective experience. Perhaps people intentionally engage in or inhibit movements that are consistent with their nonvolitional internal experiences. However, most hypnotic subjects report that when responding to ideomotor suggestions, the movements themselves are experienced as involuntary. How are these reports to be explained?

The experienced nonvolitional character of ideomotor responses seems exceptional because we generally regard such gross motor responses as voluntary. However, many of the movements with which we carry out our daily activities occur without an awareness of volition, and this may provide a clue to how ideomotor hypnotic responses can be experienced as nonvolitional. A frequently cited example of this is the phenomenon of having driven to a familiar location while absorbed in thought or conversation, and realizing that one is not aware of the processes of driving there. This phenomenon, which has been referred to as "highway hypnosis," is even more dramatic when a person has intended to go somewhere other than a usual destination, but finds that he or she has unthinkingly and unintentionally gone to the wrong place.

The execution of motor movements without conscious volitional effort is far more common than such exceptional examples as highway hypnosis might suggest. Even when driving with full attention to where we are going, we typically do not think about all the minor adjustments to steering and speed that we make. Similarly, when reading a book, we may turn the pages automatically, without having to think about each page that we turn; we write without thinking of each letter; we eat without being aware of voluntarily lifting the fork each time we do so; when we experience an itch, we may become aware of scratching it only after we have done so; and so on. In most of these cases, the molar acts are intentional and voluntary, but the component movements are experienced as automatic.

There is an important difference between these common automatic movements and hypnotic ideomotor responses. In hypnosis the person's attention is directed toward the movement, whereas nonhypnotic automatic responses most commonly occur when the person's attention is directed elsewhere. However, Lynn et al. (1989) have provided an excellent example of a nonhypnotic situation in which behavioral responses that are normally under voluntary control are emitted involuntarily. In the children's game "Simon Says," one person recites a list of simple instructions (e.g., "Raise your hand"), prefacing each with the phrase "Simon says." Then, without warning, an instruction is given without the prefatory phrase. As Lynn et al. note, "anyone who has played this game knows how difficult it is to inhibit the response when it is not preceded by 'Simon says'" (1989, p. 99).

The degree to which hypnotic responses and automatic movements in nonhypnotic contexts are brought about by a common mechanism remains to be established. But at the very least, nonhypnotic automatic movements may provide people with a sense of what it is like to experience a nonvolitional movement, and this knowledge may make it easier to experience hypnotically suggested movements as nonvolitional.

RESEARCH AND APPRAISAL

How does one determine the degree to which a response is due to expectancy? Separating expectancy effects from those due to other sources is the purpose of including placebo control conditions in medical and psychotherapy research. In these situations, changes in subjects' responses may be due to particular treatment procedures, to changes in expectancy, or to a combination of these two factors. To the degree that response changes covary with the characteristics of treatment and are independent of subjects' beliefs about these treatments, we judge the changes to be due to factors other than expectancy. Conversely, we judge them to be due to expectancy to the extent that they covary with people's beliefs and are independent of specific treatment characteristics.

The logic behind this strategy for separating the effects of expectancy from those of other causal mechanisms can easily be transposed to investigations of hypnosis. To the extent that hypnotic responses are independent of expectancy, they should vary as a function of a variety of situation and person variables (e.g., induction procedures, suggestions, personality characteristics, cognitive strategies, interpretational sets, and hypnotic talent or ability). Conversely, to the extent that hypnotic responses are produced by expectancy, subjects' beliefs about these variables are what should affect their responses. Furthermore, it is not only the occurrence or intensity of the response that may be affected by expectancy, but the qualitative nature of the response as well.

Hypnotic Inductions and Suggestions

The procedures that have been used successfully to elicit hypnotic behavior are sufficiently varied as to have nothing in common except people's belief in their effectiveness. Subjects have been stroked, been poked, been touched with magnets, been given substances to ingest, been instructed to relax, been instructed to stay alert, been connected to bogus machinery, and had lights flashed in their faces. All of these procedures appear to be about equally effective (see Kirsch, 1990).

Some clinicians invest considerable time and money to learn special techniques that have been developed by "masters" of the art. These include permissively worded suggestions, "indirect" suggestions, and inductions that are tailored to individual subjects. One of the most complex of these procedures is the "double induction," which requires the use of two hypnotists, each speaking into a different ear of the subject. To date, research indicates that these special techniques are no more effective than standardized procedures that can be memorized verbatim, read from prepared scripts, or administered via audiotape recordings (Lynn, Neufeld, & Matyi, 1987; Mathews, Kirsch, & Mosher, 1985; Mathews & Mosher, 1988; Spinhoven, Baak, Van Dyck, & Vermeulen, 1988; Van Der Does, Van Dyck, Spinhoven, & Kloosman, 1989).

Although relaxation is stressed in most inductions, Bányai and Hilgard (1976) achieved comparable responsiveness using an induction in which relaxation was prevented by having subjects pedal a stationary bicycle. The effects of standard hypnotic inductions can also be duplicated by administering a placebo pill that is described as a powerful hypnotic drug (Glass & Barber, 1961), as well as by engaging in other credible expectancy manipulations (Council, Kirsch, Vickery, & Carlson, 1983). Clearly, the *sine qua non* of an effective hypnotic induction is the subject's belief in its effectiveness. It follows that hypnotic inductions can best be understood as expectancy modification procedures.

The Nature of Hypnotic Responses

Just as the effectiveness of a hypnotic induction depends on people's expectations, rather than on the component procedures of the induction, so too does the way people behave after being hypnotized. In the 18th century, for example, mesmerized subjects exhibited convulsive seizures during which they laughed, cried, and shrieked. This "crisis," which was believed to be the essence of mesmerism, was at least partly due to the fact that the first mesmerized patient happened to be suffering from a hysterical disorder, the most prominent symptom of which was convulsions. This historical coincidence led to a popular association between mesmerism and convulsions and to the expectancy that convulsive spasms would follow successful magnetization (Kirsch, 1990).

   Currently, hypnotized subjects sit passively with eyes closed, showing little or no spontaneous speech or movement, and speaking slowly and softly in response to questions. Many report experiencing an altered state of consciousness, the most prominent feature of which is relaxation. In fact, relaxation is the only subjective characteristic of the hypnotic "state" that is reported by a majority of hypnotized subjects (Edmonston, 1981). Relaxation has become a prominent component of popular conceptions of hypnosis, and hypnotists generally suggest it explicitly as a part of their induction procedures.

   People differ widely in their reports of other subjective experiences following a hypnotic induction. The occurrence of these less common alterations in consciousness is also related to expectancy. Henry (1985) assessed individual differences in subjects' beliefs about the hypnotic state prior to their first experience of hypnosis, following which they were hypnotized and asked to record what they had actually experienced. Henry reported that the nature of subjects' experiences was largely determined by their expectations. Depending on their prior beliefs, subjects described their "trance" as a state in which time either passed more slowly or more quickly than usual; logical thought was either more or less difficult than normal; the hypnotist's voice sounded closer or farther away than before; sounds were experienced as more muffled or more clear than usual; the subject felt more or less involved than usual; and so on. Hypnotic responsiveness was related to the number of alterations in experience that subjects reported, but not to the nature of those experiences.

These data suggest that there is no particular state of consciousness that can be labeled "trance." Rather, there are a variety of changes in experience that are interpreted as evidence of a trance when they are experienced in a hypnotic context. Some of these are explicitly suggested by the hypnotist; others are generated by subjects' preconceptions about hypnosis. These changes in consciousness lead subjects to believe that they will be able to experience suggested effects—an expectation that is capable of generating those effects (Council, Kirsch, & Hafner, 1986).

In addition to shaping the subjective experience of a trance state, expectancy affects people's responses to hypnotic suggestions. The dependence of particular responses on subjects' expectancies has been demonstrated in a series of studies in which expectancies have been manipulated by the provision of different information to different groups of subjects. In the first of these studies (Orne, 1959), spontaneous arm catalepsy was presented as a characteristic of hypnosis to one group of subjects, but not to another. When subsequently hypnotized and tested for catalepsy, most of those in the first group displayed the response, whereas most subjects in the control group did not. Subsequent studies (reviewed below) have shown that hypnotic amnesia and the apparent inability of highly responsive subjects to resist suggestions are similarly dependent on expectancy.

The spontaneous (i.e., not explicitly suggested) appearance of amnesia for the hypnotic experience is one of great historical importance. It eventually led to the theory of dissociation, which in turn influenced the psychoanalytic concept of the unconscious (Kirsch & Winter, 1983). Nevertheless, the spontaneity of unsuggested amnesia is more apparent than real. Young and Cooper (1972) told one group of subjects that after being awakened, hypnotized subjects would not remember what had happened during hypnosis. A second group was told that this was not true. This information had parallel effects on subjects' expectations and their behavior. In the first group, 48% of the subjects expected to be amnesic and 37% subsequently displayed amnesia. In the second group, 15% expected amnesia and 10% displayed it behaviorally. Thus, most subjects who expected to be amnesic were amnesic, whereas most of those who expected to remember their hypnotic experiences did so.

Popular accounts of hypnosis portray the deeply hypnotized subject as unable to resist the hypnotist's suggestions, and highly suggestible subjects generally behave as if this were true (Levitt, 1986). Nevertheless, there is evidence that this apparent inability to resist depends on subjects' expectations (Lynn, Nash, Rhue, Frauman, & Sweeney, 1984; Spanos, Cobb, & Gorassini, 1985). In these studies, some subjects were told that the ability to resist suggestions was a hallmark of deep hypnosis, whereas other subjects were told the opposite. In both studies, subjects who had been told that successful resistance was an indication of deep hypnosis successfully resisted, whereas those who were told the opposite did not.

Highly responsive subjects who have been given a suggestion to forget certain information act as if their memories are blocked by a powerful amnesic barrier, which they are unable to breach. A colleague and I (Silva & Kirsch, 1987), however, demonstrated that this apparent inability to breach suggested amnesia is dependent on expectancy. We told one group of subjects that when deeply enough hypnotized, people are able to break through amnesic barriers. A second group was told that deeply hypnotized subjects could not overcome suggested amnesia. After a hypnotic induction, subjects were told that they could no longer remember a series of six words that they had memorized. They were then tested for amnesia—a test that all of the subjects passed by failing to recall most of the words. The subjects were then instructed to go even "deeper" into hypnosis, following which they were challenged once again to remember the words. On this second trial, all but two of the subjects who had been told that the ability to breach was a sign of deep hypnosis completely recovered their memory for the list of words. In contrast, none of the subjects who were not given this information breached the hypnotically induced amnesia.

The studies described above demonstrate that a variety of hypnotic responses can be altered by manipulating subjects' expectancies. The real–simulator design developed by Martin Orne (1959) represents another strategy for investigating the role of expectancy in determining the nature of subjects' responses to hypnosis. Although a failure to find differences between "real" subjects and simulators does not mean that a response is due to expectancy, reliable differences may be an indication of responses that are not expected (and therefore not role-played by the simulators).

In developing the real–simulator design, Orne assumed that hypnotic behavior could not be faked well enough to fool an expert (Orne, 1979). However, extensive experimentation using this design has revealed few reliable differences. Those that have emerged are of two types. First, when not aware of being observed, real subjects continue to respond, whereas simulators do not (Kirsch et al., 1989). Second, simulators pretend to be superb subjects, responding to more suggestions and responding more completely to these suggestions than subjects who are not pretending (Spanos, 1986). Rather than indicating unexpected responses, these differences demonstrate that real subjects are not merely faking. They also highlight the fact that hypnotic responses are outcomes, rather than simple actions that can be emitted at will.

In sum, the data on the nature of subjects' responses to hypnosis are similar to those on the effectiveness of hypnotic inductions. Although some subjects are more responsive to hypnosis than others, among responsive subjects the nature of the response is largely determined by expectancy. Typical hypnotic responses can easily be altered by providing subjects with expectancy-altering information. If there are any hypnotic responses that are not consistent with subjects' role expectancies, they remain to be reliably demonstrated.

Personality and Hypnotic Responsiveness

One of the empirically established facts about hypnosis is that hypnotic responsiveness is relatively stable over time (E. R. Hilgard, 1965). This led to the presumption that hypnotizability is a stable trait, and as a consequence investigators began to look for personality correlates of that trait. With one major exception, this search produced largely negative results (Barber, 1964; E. R. Hilgard, 1965). The exception is a personality trait termed "absorption" (Tellegen & Atkinson, 1974) or "imaginative involvement" (J. R. Hilgard, 1979). Measures of this trait have been shown to be moderately but significantly correlated with hypnosis in a relatively large number of studies (see citations in Council et al., 1986), leading many researchers to conclude that a personality correlate of hypnotizability had finally been found.

The initial optimism produced by these studies has since been tempered by the results of a number of studies indicating that the relationship may be an expectancy-mediated artifact. In the first of these studies (Council et al., 1986), the Tellegen and Atkinson absorption scale and a group adaptation of the SHSS:C were administered to two groups of subjects. In one group, the two scales were administered in the usual manner, so that subjects were aware that both were part of the same study. In the second group, the absorption scale was administered in a context that was completely independent of the subsequent test of hypnotic responsiveness. The usual modest correlation between hypnotizability and absorption was found only among those subjects who had been given both scales in the same context.

The effect of context on the relationship between hypnotizability and absorption has now been examined in published studies from four different laboratories (Council et al., 1986; de Groot, Gwynn, & Spanos, 1988; Drake, Cawood, & Nash, 1990/1991; Nadon, Hoyt, Register, & Kihlstrom, 1991). The results of these studies are summarized in Table 14.1. As the table reveals, with context kept completely separate, a significant correlation between absorption and hypnotizability was found in only one study, and even in that study it was only found for the behavioral measure of responsiveness. Although the null hypothesis can never be proved, the sum of these studies suggest that if there is a nonartifactual relation between absorption and hypnotizability, it is likely to be trivial.

TABLE 14.1. Correlations between Absorption and Hypnotic Responsiveness as a Function of Testing Context

	Type of hypnosis measure	
Context	Behavioral	Subjective
Context kept separate		
Council, Kirsch, & Hafner, 1986	.03	.14
de Groot, Gwynn, & Spanos, 1988 (males)	.10	.04
de Groot et al., 1988 (females)	.16	.15
Drake, Cawood, & Nash, in press	.02	
Nadon, Hoyt, Register, & Kihlstrom, 1991 (Study 2)	.18*	.05
Mean correlation	.02	.05
Context established before absorption testing		
Council et al., 1986	.22	.31*
de Groot et al., 1988 (males)	.14	.22
de Groot et al., 1988 (females)	.27*	.31*
Drake et al., 1990/1991 (no delay)	.32*	
Drake et al., 1990/1991 (delay)	.14	
Nadon et al., 1991 (Study 1)	.17*	.22*
Nadon et al., 1991 (Study 2)	.24*	.21*
Mean correlation	.21	.25
Context established after absorption testing		
de Groot et al., 1988 (males)	.14	.13
de Groot et al., 1988 (females)	.32*	.37*
Nadon et al., 1991 (Study 1)	.14*	.19*
Nadon et al., 1991 (Study 2)	.25*	.24*
Mean correlation	.21	.23

*$p < .05$.

The correlations listed at the bottom of Table 14.1 are particularly important because they demonstrate that the administration of the absorption scale in a hypnotic context affects the way people respond to hypnosis, rather than merely altering their responses to the absorption scale. In these samples, subjects were first asked to complete the absorption scale and were then alowed to become aware—either through verbal instructions (de Groot et al., 1988) or through a second administration of the absorption scale (Nadon et al., 1991)—that the experiment concerned the relation between the absorption scale and hypnotizability. Hypnotizability was then assessed. Because the context was not established until after the scale had been completed, it could not have affected the way in which subjects responded to scale items. In this case, the information that the scale might be related to hypnosis could only affect the size of the correlation by altering subjects' responses to hypnotic suggestion. A comparison of these correlations with those at the top of the table suggests that when subjects are aware that the absorption scale they have completed is somehow related to hypnosis, their hypnotic responses are altered in the direction of greater consistency with their responses to the absorption scale.

How does the administration of the absorption scale influence subjects' responsiveness to hypnosis? A clue to the process by which this is accomplished is provided by studies in which subjects were provided with feedback from bogus personality tests (Gregory & Diamond, 1973; Saavedra & Miller, 1983; Wickless & Kirsch, 1989). These studies showed that feedback about subjects' expected levels of hypnotizability significantly affected their subsequent responsiveness to hypnosis. In other words, differences in response expectancy induced by feedback from personality tests can alter hypnotic responsiveness.

It is likely that the context effect on the absorption–hypnotizability relationship is due to a similar mechanism. Measures of imaginative involvement contain items that might easily be recognized by subjects as related to hypnotic responsiveness (e.g., "If I wish, I can imagine that my body is so heavy that I could not move it if I wanted to"). Subjects who find themselves answering "Yes" to many questions on the scale may come to believe that they are more hypnotizable than they had previously thought, whereas those who answer "No" would be likely to draw the opposite conclusion.

More direct evidence that the absorption–hypnotizability relationship is due to response expectancy can be drawn from an earlier study (Council et al., 1983). In that study, we found hypnotic response expectancies, absorption, and hypnotizability to be significantly intercorrelated with each other. However, when variance associated with expectancy was partialed out, the correlation between absorption and hypnotizability was nonsignificant. In fact, it was this finding that led us to design the study in which the context effect was first demonstrated (Council et al., 1986).

Although the relation between absorption and hypnotizability seems to be entirely accounted for by expectancy, fantasy proneness may have a relation to hypnotic responsiveness that is partially independent of expectancy. Fantasy proneness is a construct that is conceptually very similar to absorption. It is assessed on a scale composed primarily of items pertaining to the frequency and intensity with which fantasy was engaged in as a child and as an adult (S. C. Wilson & Barber, 1981). Silva (1990) recently administered a modified version of this scale in a context that was kept separate from subsequent hypnotizability testing.[2] Even with context controlled, fantasy proneness was significantly correlated with behavioral ($r = .29$) and subjective ($r = .32$) measures of hypnotic susceptibility. It was also significantly correlated with response expectancy ($r = .29$), however, which was even more highly correlated with behavioral (r = .38) and subjective (r = .42) hypnotizability scores. Nevertheless, even when expectancy was statistically controlled, the partial correlation of fantasy proneness and subjective responses to suggestion remained significant (r = .21).

Cognitive Strategies

According to Arnold (1946), imagining the occurrence of a movement tends to bring that movement about. On the basis of this hypothesis, Barber et al. (1974) suggested that hypnotic responses are produced when subjects imagine "a situation which, if it actually occurred, would tend to give rise to the behavior that was suggested" (p. 62). In support of this hypothesis, they reviewed a series of studies showing that most subjects who are successful in experiencing hypnotic suggestions spontaneously generate goal-directed fantasies of this sort.

From a social learning perspective, there are three ways in which expectancy and goal-directed fantasy may interact to bring about hypnotic responses. First, it is possible that the effects of expectancies are mediated by subjects' use of imaginative strategies. The expectation that goal-directed fantasies produce hypnotic responses may lead subjects to generate those fantasies, and the fantasies might produce the responses. This is the hypothesis that was proposed by Barber et al. (1974). A second possibility is that the effect of goal-directed fantasy on hypnosis is entirely mediated by response expectancy, so that it is the expectancy rather than the fantasy that is generating the response. Finally, it is possible that goal-directed fantasies generate hypnotic responses and that positive expectancies enhance this effect.

The relations between and among expectancy, goal-directed fantasy, and hypnotizability were investigated most thoroughly in a study reported by Lynn, Snodgrass, et al. (1987). Consistent with the first hypothesis, highly hypnotizable subjects were more likely than subjects low in hypnotizability to believe that imagination could produce involuntary movements, and they were more likely to generate those fantasies spontaneously. On the other hand, when instructed to do so, low-hypnotizability subjects were able to generate just as many fantasies as their highly hypnotizable counterparts, and they were able to become every bit as much involved and absorbed in these fantasies. However, despite the equivalence in their fantasy involvement, less hypnotizable subjects were not as responsive behaviorally to suggestions as the highly hypnotizable subjects. Furthermore, this difference in response despite equivalent levels of imagery was linked to differences in subjects' expectancies. Across groups, the degree to which suggested movements occurred was best predicted by subjects' beliefs that imagination produces movement (r = .64). In contrast, the correlation between fantasy involvement and behavioral response was nonsignificant.

Further evidence of the role of expectancy as a mediator of the relation between imagery and response is provided by two studies in which highly hypnotizable subjects were asked to engage in "counterimagery" while a hypnotic suggestion was being administered (Spanos, Weekes, & de Groh, 1984; Zamansky, 1977). Counterimagery involves imagining events that are inconsistent with suggested responses. For example, during a suggestion for arm heaviness, subjects might be asked to imagine a garden hose with a strong stream of water pushing their hands upward. These studies demonstrated that when given appropriate expectations, people can display hypnotic response while imagining conflicting events.

Finally, my colleagues and I (Kirsch, Council, & Mobayed, 1987) manipulated expectancy information and imagery instructions with a sample of subjects representing a typical range of hypnotizability levels. We told half of the subjects that hypnotic effects were produced by imagination, that goal-directed imagery enhances those effects, and that counterimagery inhibits them. The other subjects were told that hypnotic responses were produced unconsciously, that goal-directed imagery inhibits those responses by keeping the conscious mind focused on the suggestion, and that counterimagery facilitates responsiveness by distracting and confusing the conscious mind. Within these groups, half of the subjects were given hypnotic suggestions in which goal-directed imagery had been embedded, whereas the others were given suggestions containing counterimagery. The results of this study indicated a much stronger effect for expectancy than for imagery. Goal-directed imagery enhanced responding among subjects who had been led to believe that this would be its effect, but inhibited responding when paired with negative expectancy information. Counterimagery inhibited responsiveness when subjects were told that this would be its effect, but had no effect when paired with a response enhancement rationale.

The results of these studies are consistent in showing that the effects of imagery on hypnotic response are at least partially mediated by expectancy. Although subjects who expect that goal-directed fantasies will increase their responsiveness to suggestion are more likely than others to engage in those fantasies, the effect of those fantasies on responses seems to depend largely on subjects' beliefs. Whether imagery also has an effect that is independent of expectancy remains to be determined.

Interpretive Sets

Spanos and his colleagues recently proposed a model of hypnotic responding that is based on a combination of physical compliance and goal-directed imagery (e.g., Gorassini & Spanos, 1986; Katsanis, Barnard,

& Spanos, 1988–1989). According to this model, highly hypnotizable subjects intentionally enact the behavioral component of a hypnotic response, while simultaneously engaging in goal-directed imagery so as to make the response feel involuntary. Two lines of research have been used to test this model. One of these has been to select low-hypnotizability subjects and teach them to generate hypnotic responses in this manner (see Bertrand, 1989, for a review of these studies). A less frequently employed means of testing the model has been to assess people's interpretational sets about hypnotic suggestions and to determine their relationship to levels of responsiveness (Katsanis et al., 1988–1989; Silva, 1990).

These two lines of research have provided mixed support for the interpretational-set model. Teaching people to interpret hypnotic suggestions in this manner produces substantially higher levels of responsiveness (Bertrand, 1989). Among untrained subjects, however, the tendency to endorse an interpretational set involving intentional physical activity appears to be rare. Katsanis et al. (1988–1989) reported that out of seven hypnotic suggestions, the mean number that was interpreted in this manner by untrained subjects was less than one. Silva (1990) found even lower rates of endorsement of a physically active interpretational set. Of 190 subjects, none endorsed this interpretational set for more than three of seven hypnotic responses, and only 21 subjects reported interpreting even one suggestion in this manner. These data suggest that even if subjects can be taught to generate hypnotic experiences by combining intentional compliance with goal-directed imagery, as the modification studies indicate, this is not the typical way in which hypnotic responses are generated among untrained subjects.

Finally, there is some question as to the mechanism by which the effects of the hypnotizability training program are produced. Gearan (1990) administered the Carleton Skills Training Program to a group of low-hypnotizability subjects and then reassessed their levels of responsiveness. In addition, Gearan measured subjects' hypnotic response expectancies both before and after training. Although training produced a significant increase in hypnotic responsiveness, it also produced a corresponding increase in expectancy. Furthermore, when changes in expectancy were partialed out, there was no difference between the responsiveness of trained subjects and that of subjects in the control group.

These data do not establish that the effects of the training program are mediated by expectancy. During the training program, subjects are given an opportunity to practice responding, during which they are able to observe the effects of the program on their own responses. It is quite possible that changes in expectancy are due to changes in responsiveness, rather than the reverse. However, some aspects of Gearan's data argue against this explanation. Posttraining responsiveness scores were more highly correlated with posttraining expectancies than they were with the number of suggestions that subjects were able to pass during the training program. In fact, expectancy significantly predicted response even when within-training behavior was partialed out, whereas the reverse was not true. With expectancy statistically controlled, the relation between prior and subsequent behavior was nonsignificant. These results are rather surprising. From a social learning perspective, asking subjects to comply behaviorally ought to produce effects beyond those that can be attributed to response expectancy.

Self-Predictions of Hypnotic Responsiveness

Although many studies have shown that ratings of expected responding are reliably correlated with responsiveness, the magnitude of association is most often moderate, typically accounting for about 10% of the variance (e.g., Shor, 1971). One way of interpreting these data is that hypnotic responding requires a special talent or ability that is largely independent of expectancy. Expectancy may be the primary determinant of when hypnotic responses will occur and of what those responses will be, but ability may be the primary determinant of the degree to which these responses will occur. Conversely, it is possible that many of the reported correlations are underestimates of the true relation between expectancy and response. In this section, data are reviewed indicating that these moderate correlations are attenuated by problems with how and when hypnotic response expectancies are measured.

Unlike personality traits, expectancies can be quite labile. This is especially true of expectancies about novel situations. It is only with experience that expectancies become more stable and resistant to change. For novice subjects, hypnosis is a situation that is different from other situations in which they have been. In particular, the idea of a "trance" may seem very strange and mysterious to them. As a result, their response predictions are likely to be held with little conviction. For some of these subjects, they amount to guesses rather than expectancies.

The common misconception of hypnosis as an altered state of consciousness makes it even more difficult for subjects to predict their responsiveness to suggestions. For many subjects, hypnotic response expectancies are predicated on achieving this altered state of consciousness. In other words, they may expect to be very responsive, but only if they first experience sufficient changes in their general state of consciousness. Furthermore, what constitutes a "sufficient" change may vary from one person to another. Even before their first experience of hypnosis, people differ in the degree to which they think of it as a state that is very different from normal consciousness. Interestingly, the preconception of hypnosis as an altered state may be associated with lower levels of response to suggestion (McConkey, 1986).

It follows that the initial experience of a hypnotic induction is likely to alter one's expectancies for responding to suggestions. Subjects who experience greater changes in conscious state (feelings of relaxation, numbness, heaviness, etc.) are likely to have heightened expectancies, whereas those experiencing less change are likely to have lowered expectations. In addition, those who think of hypnosis as a drastically altered state of consciousness are likely to be disappointed by the results of the induction, and their response expectancies are likely to be lowered by the experience.

My colleagues and I (Council et al., 1986) tested the hypotheses that hypnotic inductions alter response expectancies and that postinduction expectancies are better predictors of subsequent response. In that study, we assessed expectancy at two different points in time: first immediately prior to a hypnotic induction, and then again immediately after the induction, but prior to the administration of any test suggestions. Both hypotheses were strongly supported. The two measures of expectancy were only moderately correlated ($r = .31$), and postinduction expectancies were significantly better predictors of hypnotic response. In contrast to the typical low but significant correlations that were obtained between preinduction expectancies and response, postinduction expectancies were very highly correlated with both behavioral ($r = .55$) and subjective ($r = .64$) measures of responsiveness.

"Expectancy" is defined as a person's subjective probability, ranging from 0 to 1.00, that some event will occur (Rotter, 1954). In response expectancy theory, the likelihood of a response is hypothesized to be directly related to the subjective probability of its occurrence and inversely related to the difficulty of the response (Kirsch, 1985). In hypnosis research, expectancies of this sort are almost never assessed. Instead of assessing how confident a subject is that a particular response or set of responses will occur, we measure the person's best guess about the number of responses that he or she will be able to experience.

In order to correct for this, my colleagues and I have begun assessing the confidence with which response predictions are held. First we ask subjects to predict whether or not they will be able to experience particular hypnotic suggestions. Then we ask them to rate how confident they are that their predictions are accurate. This yields two independent scores: subjects' best guesses about the number of responses they will experience (their predicted level of response), and the confidence with which these predictions are held. By obtaining both of these ratings at two different points in time (before and after administering the hypnotic induction), we can examine the effect of a hypnotic induction on both expectancy level and confidence. Next, median splits on preinduction and postinduction

TABLE 14.2. **Mean Confidence Ratings and Correlations between Expectancy and Response as a Function of Median Splits on Subjects' Confidence Ratings**

	Preinduction		Postinduction	
	Low confidence (*n* = 87)	High confidence (*n* = 81)	Low confidence (*n* = 75)	High confidence (*n* = 93)
Confidence (mean)[a]	48%	70%	62%	82%
Correlation[b]	.04	.37*	.59*	.84*

[a]Confidence ratings were obtained on a Likert scale with scores ranging from 0 to 5. For ease of interpretation, these have been converted into probabilities ranging from 0% to 100%.
[b]Differences between high confidence and low confidence correlations were significant for both preinduction ($p < .05$) and postinduction ($p < .001$) assessments.
*$p < .001$.

confidence levels allow us to determine whether the correlation between expectancy and response is affected by the degree of confidence with which the expectancies are held.

Preliminary data derived by these methods are presented in Table 14.2. These data indicate that hypnotic inductions alter not only subjects' expectancy ratings, but also their confidence ratings. Besides being more highly correlated with subsequent responsiveness to suggestion, expectancy ratings made after a hypnotic induction (but prior to test suggestions) were held with greater confidence than preinduction expectancies. Furthermore, different levels of confidence were associated with different levels of correlation between expectancy and responsiveness, ranging from a near-zero correlation for low-confidence preinduction expectancies to a correlation accounting for 71% of the variance for highly confident postinduction expectancies. These data indicate that hypnotizability is strongly associated with confidently held response expectancies, but not with mere guesses about one's hypnotizability. People who are convinced that they will be highly responsive succeed in passing many hypnotic suggestions, whereas those who are convinced that they are not hypnotizable achieve low hypnotic response scores.

The failure to include confidence levels in their measure of expectancy may also account for the "fan-shaped" relationship between expectancy and hypnotizability found by Katsanis et al. (1988–1989). They reported that although low-expectancy subjects always obtained low hypnotic response scores, high-expectancy subjects showed much wider variability in responsiveness. Silva (1990) attempted to replicate that finding. However, instead of asking subjects to provide a global prediction of how well they would respond to suggestions, Silva had them indicate their subjective probabilities of passing each suggestion. In contrast to the data reported by Katsanis et al., Silva obtained a scatter plot that was shaped more like a football than a fan. Not only were there few low-expectancy subjects with high hypnotic response scores, but there were equally few high-expectancy subjects with low response scores.

Modifying Hypnotic Response Expectancies

Most efforts at modifying subjects' hypnotic response expectancies have produced only modest effects on responsiveness (Gregory & Diamond, 1973; Saavedra & Miller, 1983; Vickery & Kirsch, in press). However, these efforts relied exclusively on verbal persuasion as the means of changing subjects' expectations. In contrast, D. L. Wilson (1967) reported that an expectancy modification procedure based on direct experience produced substantial effects on waking suggestibility. In Wilson's study, suggestions for altered perceptual experience were surreptitiously confirmed by subtle alterations in environmental conditions. For example, when a suggestion for seeing the color red was given, a faint red tinge was imparted to the room by means of a hidden light bulb.

Cynthia Wickless and I compared the effects of verbal and experiential expectancy manipulations on hypnotic responsiveness (Wickless & Kirsch, 1989). The verbal manipulation consisted of feedback from bogus personality tests. The experiential manipulation was a carefully piloted replication of D. L. Wilson's (1967) procedures. As predicted, the experiential manipulation had a substantially greater impact on hypnotizability scores. However, the highest levels of hypnotizability were found among subjects to whom both expectancy manipulations had been administered. Seventy-three percent of the subjects in this group were found to be highly hypnotizable (SHSS:C scores between 9 and 12), and 27% scored in the moderate range (5–8). There were no low-hypnotizability subjects!

CONCLUSIONS

Two questions can be asked with regard to the roles of expectancy in hypnosis: First, what role does expectancy play in determining hypnotic responsiveness? Second, among responsive subjects, to what extent does expectancy determine when hypnotic responses will be displayed and what those responses will be?

The answer to the second question seems clear. The effectiveness of a hypnotic induction appears to depend entirely on people's beliefs about its effectiveness, and highly hypnotizable subjects respond in accordance with their beliefs about hypnotic responding. In other words, response expectancy may be the sole determinant of the situations in which hypnotic responses occur, and also of the nature of the responses that occur in those situations.

It is worth noting that in a pharmaceutical context, comparable data would be viewed as conclusive evidence that the drug is a placebo. Similarly, these data are sufficient for us to conclude that hypnotic inductions are expectancy modification rituals, and any effects that can be attributed to their use (e.g., increased responsiveness to suggestion) can therefore be interpreted as expectancy effects. Thus, the capacity of people's beliefs and expectations to bring about changes in experience may be the "essence" of hypnosis, and attempts to eliminate expectancy as an "artifact" may be doomed to failure. Once expectancy effects are eliminated, there may be nothing left.

The value of a drug depends on its chemical properties. Therefore, when the effects of a drug are found to be due to expectancy (or to any other psychological factor), the drug is declared to be worthless and it is taken off the market. But these conclusions do not apply to psychological procedures (Kirsch, 1978). The value of a psychological procedure (e.g., hypnosis or psychotherapy) depends on its psychological properties, one of which may be its impact on people's expectancies. Expectancy is a psychological variable. Its effects are no less real or important than effects due to other psychological variables, and there is no reason to treat it as any less legitimate than other psychological mechanisms. Thus, the discovery that the effects of hypnotic inductions and suggestions are due to expectancy in no way diminishes their importance, either clinically or as a focus of research.

There remains the question of individual differences in responsiveness. Here too, the data indicate that expectancy plays a more important role than previously assumed. Confidently held expectations about one's level of response are highly correlated with actual responsiveness, and convincing expectancy manipulations are capable of producing high levels of hypnotizability. Nevertheless, questions about individual differences in responsiveness remain. First, although most of the effects of goal-directed strategies and interpretational sets appear to be mediated by expectancy, it would not be surprising if these variables had independent effects on responsiveness as well. Imagining an experience ought to help bring it about, as should performing movements that are consistent with the experience.

I would also expect there to be a personal factor that is not entirely determined by expectancy, and I find it surprising that measures of such abilities as absorption and imagery vividness generally add so little to the prediction of suggestibility. Differences in ability would provide the most simple explanation for the stability of hypnotic responsivenss. It is also possible, however, that the stability of hypnotizability is a function of expectancies that have been stabilized by testing. Each test of hypnosis confirms the subjects' response expectancies and makes them more resistant to change.

In sum, the data on hypnotizability leave room for the operation of variables other than expectancy. The question that needs to be asked about these variables is whether they can be shown to produce effects that are independent of subjects' expectations, as seems true of fantasy proneness, or whether their effects are entirely mediated by response expectancy, as appears to be the case with absorption. Despite mistaken readings to the contrary, both types of influence are entirely consistent with response expectancy theory (cf. Kirsch, 1985, 1990).

NOTES

1. The qualification "direct" pertains to the fact that a person may engage in a variety of voluntary, goal-directed acts aimed at affecting a nonvolitional response. For example, an insomniac may count sheep, relax muscles, or imagine pleasant events in order to fall asleep. The counting, relaxing, and imagining may be experienced as volitional, whereas the falling asleep is experienced as a nonvolitional consequence that has been automatically produced by those voluntary behaviors.

2. The modification consisted of elimination of two test items that pertained to subjects' attitudes and expectancies about hypnosis. Inclusion of these items might have contaminated the results by allowing subjects to become aware that the scale is thought to be related to hypnosis.

REFERENCES

Ajzen, I., & Fishbein, M. (1980). *Understanding attitudes and predicting social behavior.* Englewood Cliffs, NJ: Prentice-Hall.

Arnold, M. B. (1946). On the mechanism of suggestion and hypnosis. *Journal of Abnormal and Social Psychology, 41,* 107–128.

Bányai, E., & Hilgard, E. R. (1976). A comparison of active–alert hypnotic induction with traditional relaxation induction. *Journal of Abnormal Psychology, 85,* 218–224.

Barber, T. X. (1964). Hypnotizability, suggestibility, and personality: V. A critical review of research findings. *Psychological Reports, 14,* 299–320.

Barber, T. X., Spanos, N. P., & Chaves, J. F. (1974). *Hypnosis, imagination, and human potentialities.* Elmsford, NY: Pergamon Press.

Bertrand, L. D. (1989). The assessment and modification of hypnotic susceptibility. In N. P. Spanos & J. F. Chaves (Eds.), *Hypnosis: The cognitive–behavioral perspective* (pp. 18–31). Buffalo, NY: Prometheus Books.

Bolles, R. C. (1972). Reinforcement, expectancy, and learning. *Psychological Review, 79,* 394–409.

Bowers, P., Laurence, J., & Hart, D. (1988). The experience of hypnotic suggestions. *International Journal of Clinical and Experimental Hypnosis, 36,* 336–349.

Council, J. R., Kirsch, I., & Hafner, L. P. (1986). Expectancy versus absorption in the prediction of hypnotic responding. *Journal of Personality and Social Psychology, 50*, 182–189.

Council, J., Kirsch, I., Vickery, A. R., & Carlson, D. (1983). "Trance" vs. "skill" hypnotic inductions: The effects of credibility, expectancy, and experimenter modeling. *Journal of Consulting and Clinical Psychology, 51*, 432–440.

de Groot, H. P., Gwynn, M. I., & Spanos, N. P. (1988). The effects of contextual information and gender on the prediction of hypnotic susceptibility. *Journal of Personality and Social Psychology, 54*, 1049–1053.

Drake, S. D., Cawood, G. N., & Nash, M. R. (1990/1991). Imaginative involvement and hypnotic susceptibility: A re-examination of the relationship. *Imagination, Cognition and Personality* (Vol. 10, pp. 141–155).

Edmonston, W. E., Jr. (1981). *Hypnosis and relaxation: Modern verification of an old equation.* New York: Wiley.

Frankenhaeuser, M., Post, B., Hagdahl, R., & Wrangsjoe, B. (1964). Effects of a depressant drug as modified experimentally-induced expectation. *Perceptual and Motor Skills, 18*, 513–522.

Gearan, P. (1990). Expectancy change as a mediator of hypnotizability enhancement. In I. Kirsch (Chair), *Hypnotizability and interpretational sets: Conflicting evidence.* Symposium conducted at the meeting of the American Psychological Association, Boston.

Glass, L. B., & Barber, T. X. (1961). A note on hypnotic behavior, the definition of the situation, and the placebo effect. *Journal of Nervous and Mental Disease, 132*, 539–541.

Gorassini, D. P., & Spanos, N. P. (1986). A sociocognitive skills approach to the successful modification of hypnotic susceptibility. *Journal of Personality and Social Psychology, 50*, 1004–1012.

Gregory, J., & Diamond, M. J. (1973). Increasing hypnotic susceptibility by means of positive expectancies and written instructions. *Journal of Abnormal Psychology, 82*, 385–389.

Henry, D. (1985). *Subjects' expectancies and subjective experience of hypnosis.* Unpublished doctoral dissertation, University of Connecticut.

Hilgard, E. R. (1965). *Hypnotic susceptibility.* New York: Harcourt, Brace & World.

Hilgard, J. R. (1979). *Personality and hypnosis: A study of imaginative involvement* (2nd ed.). Chicago: University of Chicago Press.

Katsanis, J., Barnard, J., & Spanos, N. P. (1988–1989). Self-predictions, interpretational set and imagery vividness as determinants of hypnotic responding. *Imagination, Cognition and Personality, 8*, 63–77.

Kirsch, I. (1978). The placebo effect and the cognitive–behavioral revolution. *Cognitive Therapy and Research, 2*, 255–264.

Kirsch, I. (1985). Response expectancy as a determinant of experience and behavior. *American Psychologist, 40*, 1189–1202.

Kirsch, I. (1990). *Changing expectations: A key to effective psychotherapy.* Pacific Grove, CA: Brooks/Cole.

Kirsch, I., & Council, J. R. (1989). Response expectancy as a determinant of hypnotic behavior. In N. P. Spanos & J. F. Chaves (Eds.), *Hypnosis: The cognitive-behavioral perspective* (pp. 360–379). Buffalo, NY: Prometheus Books.

Kirsch, I., Council, J. R., & Mobayed, C. (1987). Imagery and response expectancy as determinants of hypnotic behavior. *British Journal of Experimental and Clinical Hypnosis, 4*, 25–31.

Kirsch, I., Silva, C. E., Carone, J. E., Johnston, J. D., & Simon, B. (1989). The surreptitious observation design: An experimental paradigm for distinguishing artifact from essence in hypnosis. *Journal of Abnormal Psychology, 98*, 132–136.

Kirsch, I., & Winter, C. (1983). A history of clinical psychology. In E. Walker (Ed.), *Handbook of clinical psychology* (pp. 3–30). Homewood, IL: Dorsey Press.

Levitt, E. E. (1986, August). *Compliance, voluntariness, and resistance: Reflections of the essence of hypnosis.* Paper presented at the meeting of the American Psychological Association, Washington, DC.

Lynn, S. J., Nash, M. R., Rhue, J. W., Frauman, D. C., & Sweeney, C. A. (1984). Nonvolition, expectancies, and hypnotic rapport. *Journal of Abnormal Psychology, 93*, 295–303.

Lynn, S. J., Neufeld, V., & Matyi, C. L. (1987). Inductions versus suggestions: Effects of direct and indirect wording on hypnotic responding and experience. *Journal of Abnormal Psychology, 96*, 76–79.

Lynn, S. J., Rhue, J. W., & Weekes, J. R. (1989). Hypnosis and experienced nonvolition: A social-cognitive integrative model. In N. P. Spanos & J. F. Chaves (Eds.), *Hypnosis: The cognitive–behavioral perspective* (pp. 78–109). Buffalo, NY: Prometheus Books.

Lynn, S. J., Snodgrass, M., Rhue, J. W., & Hardaway, R. (1987). Goal-directed fantasy, hypnotic susceptibility, and expectancies. *Journal of Personality and Social Psychology, 53*, 933–938.

Mathews, W. J., Kirsch, I., & Mosher, D. (1985). The "double" hypnotic induction: An initial empirical test. *Journal of Abnormal Psychology, 94*, 92–95.

Mathews, W. J., & Mosher, D. L. (1988). Direct and indirect hypnotic suggestion in a laboratory setting. *British Journal of Experimental and Clinical Hypnosis, 5*, 63–71.

McConkey, K. M. (1986). Opinions about hypnosis and self-hypnosis before and after hypnotic testing. *International Journal of Clinical and Experimental Hypnosis, 34*, 311–319.

Nadon, R., Hoyt, I. P., Register, P. A., & Kihlstrom, J. F. (1991). Absorption and hypnotizability: Context effects re-examined. *Journal of Personality and Social Psychology, 60*, 144–153.

Orne, M. T. (1959). The nature of hypnosis: Artifact and Essence. *Journal of Abnormal Psychology, 58*, 277–299.

Orne, M. T. (1979). On the simulating subject as a quasi-control group in hypnosis research: What, why, and how. In E. Fromm & R. E. Shor (Eds.), *Hypnosis: Developments in research and new perspectives* (2nd ed., pp. 519–601). Chicago: Aldine.

Rotter, J. B. (1954). *Social learning and clinical psychology.* Englewood Cliffs, NJ: Prentice-Hall.

Saavedra, R. L, & Miller, R. J. (1983). The influence of experimentally induced expectations on responses to the Harvard Group Scale of Hypnotic Susceptibility, Form A. *International Journal of Clinical and Experimental Hypnosis, 31*, 37–46.

Sarbin, T. R. (1989). The construction and reconstruction of hypnosis. In N. P. Spanos & J. F. Chaves (Eds.), *Hypnosis: The cognitive-behavioral perspective* (pp. 18–31). Buffalo, NY: Prometheus Books.

Shor, R. E. (1971). Expectations of being influenced and hypnotic performance. *International Journal of Clinical and Experimental Hypnosis, 19*, 154–166.

Silva, C. E. (1990). *Response expectancy versus interpretational set as mediators of hypnotic response.* Unpublished doctoral dissertation, University of Connecticut.

Silva, C. E., & Kirsch, I. (1987). Breaching amnesia by manipulating expectancy. *Journal of Abnormal Psychology, 96*, 325–329.

Spanos, N. P. (1971). Goal-directed fantasy and the performance of hypnotic test suggestions. *Psychiatry, 34*, 86–96.

Spanos, N. P. (1986). Hypnotic behavior: A social-psychological interpretation of amnesia, analgesia, and "trance logic." *Behavioral and Brain Sciences, 9*, 499–502.

Spanos, N. P., & Barber, T. X. (1972). Cognitive activity during hypnotic suggestion: Goal-directed fantasy and the experience of non-volition. *Journal of Personality, 40*, 510–524.

Spanos, N. P., Cobb, P. C., & Gorassini, D. (1985). Failing to resist hypnotic test suggestions: A strategy for self-presenting as deeply hypnotized. *Psychiatry, 48*, 282–292.

Spanos, N. P., Weekes, J. R., & de Groh, M. (1984). The "involuntarily" countering of suggested requests: A test of the ideomotor hypothesis of hypnotic responsiveness. *British Journal of Experimental and Clinical Hypnosis, 1*, 3–11.

Spinhoven, P., Baak, D., Van Dyck, R., & Vermeulen, P. (1988). The effectiveness of an authoritative versus permissive style of hypnotic communication. *International Journal of Clinical and Experimental Hypnosis, 36*, 182–191.

Tellegen, A., & Atkinson, G. (1974). Openness to absorbing and self-altering experiences ("absorption"), a trait related to hypnotic susceptibility. *Journal of Abnormal Psychology, 83*, 268–277.

Van Der Does, A. J. W., Van Dyck, R., Spinhoven, P., & Kloosman, A. (1989). The effectiveness of standardized versus individualized hypnotic suggestions. *International Journal of Clinical and Experimental Hypnosis, 37*, 1–5.

Vickery, A. R., & Kirsch, I. (in press). The effects of brief expectency manipulations on hypnotic responsiveness. *Contemporary Hypnosis.*

Wickless, C., & Kirsch, I. (1989). The effects of verbal and experiential expectancy manipulations on hypnotic susceptibility. *Journal of Personality and Social Psychology, 57*, 762–768.

Wilson, D. L. (1967). The role of confirmation of expectancies in hypnotic induction. *Dissertation Abstracts, 28*, 4787B. (University Microfilms No. 66-6781)

Wilson, S. C., & Barber, T. X. (1981). Vivid fantasy and hallucinatory abilities in the life histories of excellent hypnotic subjects ("somnambules"): Preliminary report with female subjects. In E. Klinger (Ed.), *Imagery: Concepts, results and applications* (Vol., 2, pp. 340–390). New York: Wiley.

Young, J., & Cooper, L. M. (1972). Hypnotic recall amnesia as a function of manipulated expectancy. *Proceedings of the 80th Annual Convention of the American Psychological Association, 7*, 857–858.

Zamansky, H. S. (1977). Suggestion and countersuggestion in hypnotic behavior. *Journal of Abnormal Psychology, 86*, 346–351.

C H A P T E R   1 5

The Ecosystemic Approach to Hypnosis

DAVID P. FOURIE
University of South Africa

INTRODUCTION

The most successful and influential way of thinking ever introduced into the field of science is often named after Isaac Newton. It rests on the following three notions:

1. *Reductionism or atomism.* According to Newtonian thinking, if an object or phenomenon is to be understood, it needs to be reduced into its most basic elements or building blocks, which are simpler, more easily understandable, and often measurable (Schwartzman, 1984). Once these elements and their properties are known, an understanding of the whole can be achieved by recombining the elements.

2. *Linear causality.* In this mode of thinking, the elements are viewed as connected to one another through cause and effect. For example, the apple is caused to fall from the tree by the action of gravity, which is a property of the earth. Complex phenomena are seen as made up of long causal trains (Hoffman, 1981).

3. *Neutral objectivity.* The fall of the apple is seen as independent of the observer unless the observer actively interferes with the process, such as by shaking the tree. The search for the truth about phenomena should therefore be such that the search itself does not affect this truth. Objectivity of observation is therefore not only possible, but necessary in order to arrive at the truth (Colapinto, 1979).

466

When dealing with relatively simple phenomena, such as those of classical physics, this Newtonian way of thinking is appropriate and very useful. Early in this century, though, it became clear that application of this mode of thinking to more complicated phenomena obscured rather than enhanced understanding. For instance, the observation that light consisted of either particles or waves, depending on the way it was observed, ran counter to the Newtonian notion of objectivity of observation. Physicists such as Einstein and Heisenberg showed that the complexities of quantum physics required a different way of thinking about the world (Capra, 1983).

Despite these observations, the natural sciences continued their adherence to the Newtonian mode of thinking. The social sciences, eager to establish themselves as scientific disciplines, followed suit. In true Newtonian fashion, human behavior, contextually bound as it is, was studied by being reduced into elements that were seen as interconnected via cause and effect and that were regarded as uninfluenced by the process and context of study. The elements to which human behavior was reduced often were hypothetical constructs (MacCorquodale & Meehl, 1948), which were thought to have particular properties and which were then treated as if they were semiconcrete entities. This process of reification, criticized by such eminent theorists as Bateson (1979) and Sarbin and Coe (1972), resulted in the wide acceptance of the existence of such entities as the "ego," the "unconscious," "defense mechanisms," and "hypnotic susceptibility."

As more and more fields of scientific inquiry encountered problems of increasing complexity, the inadequacies of a Newtonian way of thinking became increasingly clear. As gestaltists have long ago realized, one often cannot understand the whole by means of a synthesis of the parts. Criticism of the Newtonian epistemology of science has thus come from the natural sciences (e.g., Capra, 1983; Prigogine & Stengers, 1984), especially biology (e.g., Maturana, 1975, 1983; Varela, 1979); from anthropology (e.g., Bateson, 1972, 1979); and from various branches of psychology, such as counseling (e.g., Cottone, 1988; Ford, 1984) and family therapy (e.g., Keeney, 1979, 1982).

Until recently, hypnosis was conspicuous by its absence from this list. In the last few years, though, various theorists have begun to take cognizance of the limitations of Newtonian thought in the field of hypnosis, and of the possibility of thinking differently about hypnosis. These theorists include Sheehan (1988), Matthews (1985, 1989), Kruse and Gheorghiu (1990), Schmidt (1985), Deissler and Gester (1986), and my colleagues and myself (Fourie, 1983, 1988; Fourie & De Beer, 1986; Fourie & Lifschitz, 1985, 1987, 1988, 1989; Lifschitz & Fourie, 1985). It seems, therefore, that the shift away from reductionism, linear causality, and objectivity that has been going on for some time in other areas of science has now also reached the field of hypnosis. The ecosystemic approach, to be discussed here, is one way in which this shift can be operationalized.

THEORETICAL CONCEPTS AND PRINCIPLES

As the name indicates, the "ecosystemic" approach to hypnosis is based on systems theory. A "system" can by seen as a set of objects and their attributions in interrelationship with one another (Hall & Fagan, 1956). The original general systems theory, as formulated by Von Bertalanffy (1974), was a mechanistic one, applicable to machines that operate within limits set by an outside ("objective") controller. Later developments to the theory led to what is sometimes called "second cybernetics," in which the controller is seen as part of the system and therefore no longer outside of it (Hoffman, 1985). In this development, Bateson's (1972) conception of a system as an "ecology of ideas" became of central importance, particularly in family therapy. The metaphor of "ecology" was used to indicate how ideas in human systems are complexly interwoven and how these ideas continually influence one another in mutual and reciprocal ways (Bogdan, 1984). For this reason, Auerswald (1987) talks of an ecosystemic approach as one that defines a family as a coevolutionary ecosystem. Similarly, Keeney (1983, p. 16) defines an ecosystemic approach as "the epistemological framework representing cybernetics, ecology, and system theory."

So far, this ecosystemic approach has been applied mostly to the study of families and family therapy. However, many other situations lend themselves to be viewed from an ecosystemic perspective; one of these is the hypnotic circumstance. It must be emphasized that this approach to hypnosis is not merely another theory of hypnosis. It embodies a way of thinking (i.e., epistemology) that is radically different from, and in many ways irreconcilable with, the Newtonian epistemology of science. This does not mean that it is better or more "true" than a Newtonian way of thinking. (The search for truth is in itself Newtonian.) Newtonian approaches to hypnosis have been of inestimable value in bringing us to our current level of knowledge of hypnosis. But they suffer from the limitations inherent in this reductionistic and linear way of thinking— limitations that an ecosystemic approach endeavors to circumvent. In doing so, some of the very basic assumptions about hypnosis are questioned, many of which we have become so accustomed to that we seldom realize that they are assumptions and not facts.

The first way in which the ecosystemic approach to hypnosis differs from a Newtonian perspective is that it does not reduce the hypnotic circumstance into elements or parts. Neither does it reify such elements. Accordingly, it does not view hypnosis as an entity, such as a state of consciousness, existing inside the subject. Instead, it perceives of hypnosis as a *concept* denoting a situation in which certain classes of behavior come to be seen as of a type called "hypnotic" or "involuntary." Which classes of behavior these are depend on the ideas of all the people involved in the situation. All participants have opinions and expectations about the situation, and these form the basis on which everybody attributes meaning to whatever occurs in the situation. The definition of the situation is important in this respect. The lifting of an arm in a classroom or on a busy sidewalk would probably be assigned a different meaning than would the same behavior in a situation understood to be one of hypnosis (Schmidt, 1985).

The second difference between an ecosystemic and a Newtonian approach to hypnosis relates to cause. Ecosystemically seen, hypnotic behavior is not caused by anything. When behavior occurs that the participants regard as "hypnotic,"they mutually qualify it as "hypnotic" in many different and subtle ways. The person designated as subject, for instance, lifts a hand in a different way than it would be lifted in some other situation, thereby qualifying it as of a different type. The hypnotist probably acts in such a manner as to indicate acceptance of the hand lifting as "hypnotic"—possibly by suggesting some other "involuntary" behavior, talking mainly to the subject, and otherwise acting as if the subject were an observer of his or her own behavior. Onlookers (if any) probably, by focusing on the subject and by maintaining an intrigued silence, help to qualify the particular behavior as "hypnotic." Their action of refraining from speaking to the subject can be seen as potently qualifying the situation as "hypnotic."

Hypnotic behaviors, therefore, are not caused by anything. They are ordinary behaviors designated as "hypnotic" by means of *ongoing mutual qualification*, which is based on the definition of the situation as one of hypnosis, and on the expectations and ideas of all the participants regarding such a situation. The induction procedure does not cause the hypnosis. Induction has two functions: It serves as a vehicle for the process of mutual qualification, and it punctuates the flow of events in such a way as to indicate that behaviors during and subsequent to induction can be seen and qualified as "hypnotic."

Any behavior can be mutually qualified as "hypnotic," provided that it can fit with the expectations of the people present. Most experienced hypnotists know that if a certain behavior does not occur, then its opposite occurs, and this opposite can often be qualified as "hypnotic." For instance, if eye closure cannot be achieved, then the participants may be amenable to being convinced that the subject shows the rare ability to enter hypnosis with open eyes. Open eyes can then be mutually qualified as a "hypnotic" behavior.

When the first behavior is qualified as "hypnotic," it constitutes an evolutionary step in the developing of the interdependent network of ideas, or ecology of ideas, existing in the system at that time. The participants see that hypnosis is possible with the particular subject in the particular situation. Everybody may then be more amenable to viewing and qualifying the next behavior as "hypnotic." One could say that the ecology of ideas cooperatively strengthens around the view that what is happening is hypnosis. And as every subsequent behavior is seen to belong to the class of behaviors regarded as "hypnotic," the ecology of ideas continues to coevolve so that hypnosis becomes increasingly "real" in the particular system at the particular time. In other words, all participants, including the subject, become increasingly convinced of the "reality" of hypnosis in the particular circumstance. So potent is the process of mutual qualification that even subjectively the subject can have the experiences of so-called "deep" hypnosis, such as amnesia, hallucinations, and analgesia, which again become part of the ecology of ideas in that system.

This ecology of ideas—or "domain of consensus," to use Maturana's (1975) term, is a metaphor for a complicated, ever-evolving network of opinions, expectations, and attributions. Although the so-called "demand characteristics" (Wagstaff, 1981) of the situation can be considered to play a role in its evolution, it cannot be said that these cause hypnosis. In the same vein, although the likes and dislikes, needs and abilities of the subject, like those of everybody else, are part of the ecology of ideas, one cannot say that the subject's hypothesized hypnotizability causes the hypnosis. Similarly, it is reductionistic to say that the intrapsychic strategies that may be used by the subject, such as goal-directed fantasy (Spanos & Gorassini, 1984), bring hypnosis about. Once the hypnotic situation is considered as a whole system, it becomes impossible to think of causal influence of one part on another, especially if it is remembered that many of these "parts" are concepts rather than entities.

Considered in this manner, the third way in which an ecosystemic approach differs from a Newtonian perspective is linked with the well-documented (Bateson, 1972; Dell, 1985; Maturana, 1983) untenability of a notion of objectivity. The hypnotic situation cannot involve an objective observer. All participants are observers of the situation (Maturana, 1975), but none of them can be objective, because all are part of the system. The ecology of ideas that develops and continually evolves in the hypnotic situation is a co-constructed one, meaning that everybody partakes in its construction. And it is constructed by the interplay of the participants' idiosyncratic ideas and attributions; there is nothing "real" or "objective"about it. An ecosystemic approach to hypnosis, therefore, is a "constructivist" (Efran, Lukens, & Lukens, 1988; Von Glasersfeld, 1984) one.

Because this approach so clearly rejects the Newtonian notions of reductionism, linear causality, and objectivity, it has profound implications for hypnosis research and for hypnotherapy.

RESEARCH AND APPRAISAL

Research Implications

The first implication for research has to do with the issue of hypnotic susceptibility or hypnotizability. Behaviors are "hypnotic" only when they are mutually qualified as "hypnotic" within a particular ecology of ideas. Therefore, their occurrence cannot be dependent on any ability of the subject—except, of course, for the fairly universal ability to lift an arm, to close the eyes, to forget, and so forth.

The ecosystemic approach thus does not give credence to the reified concept of susceptibility. In fact, as indicated elsewhere (Fourie & Lifschitz, 1988), it takes issue with the routine employment of susceptibility testing. One reason for this stance is that such testing embodies an attempt to measure something that does not exist, except as an idea. Another reason is that susceptibility testing is not neutral or "objective," as is assumed in a Newtonian perspective. The testing procedure potently defines the situation in a particular way, mostly as structured, limited, and authoritarian. Also, it defines hypnotic behavior for the subject in a certain, limited manner (e.g., closed eyes are "hypnotic" and open eyes are not). These definitions are then part of the ecology of ideas at the particular time. That this must play a role in whatever activity (e.g., research, treatment) takes place subsequently in the system is clear. But adherence to a Newtonian epistemology requires the experimenter(s) or clinician(s) to regard the testing procedure as if it did not have these influences, and as if the susceptibility scores were "objective" and uninfluenced by the testing context. Moreover, the continued use of susceptibility testing reinforces the belief in the existence of susceptibility as a measurable entity.

A good example of the way in which adherence to the Newtonian notion of objectivity of observation has led to questionable research conclusions is to be found in efforts to modify hypnotic susceptibility (e.g., Spanos & Bertrand, 1985). Most such attempts involve pre- and post-training susceptibility testing. But employing standard susceptibility tests before and after some intervening procedure means that both testing situations are defined similarly, precisely because the testing procedure, contrary to the Newtonian assumption, is not neutral or "objective." It is to be expected that susceptibility scores would tend to be of the same order in two such similarly defined situations, regardless of what has happened between the testings. However, by following the assumption of objectivity, researchers have often concluded from the scores that the intervening procedure has not succeeded in modifying susceptibility. Over the years, this has led to the almost universal acceptance of the relative immodifiability of susceptibility. By assuming objectivity of observation in this way, researchers have failed to realize that the relative consistency they have found refers to consistency in the definition of the testing situations, rather than to the immodifiability of hypnotic performance.

In contrast, an ecosystemic conceptualization is that hypnosis occurs in a situation, not in a person. Hypnosis has no absolute reality, but is co-constructed by the people involved in a particular situation. Therefore, it can and does differ from situation to situation. The question of modifiability thus refers to the situation, rather than to the person designated as subject. It can perhaps be stated as follows: How responsive is this system (which includes the observer/questioner) to the qualification of various different behaviors as "hypnotic"? And in which way(s) can this qualification take place? Which behaviors can be so qualified?

Another implication has to do with the functions of the different people in the hypnotic situation. Traditionally, the hypnotist was thought to be the person who induces hypnosis "in" the subject, who in turn was seen as a passive receiver of suggestions. Other people in the context were thought to play no role in the process; they were viewed as "objective" observers. More recently, the emphasis has been reversed. The major factor in hypnosis is considered to be in the subject, rather than in the hypnotist. One school has emphasized the subject's hypnotic talent (see, e.g., E. R. Hilgard, 1982); in the other the hypnotist is thought merely to provide the right "demand characteristics," and it is the subject who is actively engaged in utilizing intrapsychic strategies (e.g., goal-directed fantasy) in order to comply with the demands (e.g., Wagstaff, 1981). Again, the onlookers are considered to play no significant role.

In contrast to both of these views, an ecosystemic perspective considers the hypnotic system to operate as a whole, with every participant functioning according to what is expected of him or her in the particular system. The hypnotist does not induce hypnosis, but he or she plays the role of an executive, organizing the system in such a way that the person designated as the subject is in focus. The onlookers subtly but actively partake in qualifying certain behaviors as "hypnotic." The subject qualifies his or her own behavior in the way it is executed. In our own work, my colleagues and I often find it helpful for the hypnotist actively to engage the onlookers in the qualification process by talking to them rather than to the subject, and by inviting them to comment verbally on the behavior of the subject.

From this perspective, there are no neutral people in the hypnotic context. Researchers and technicians are not "faceless." Even if they operate from behind a one-way screen, they have an input into the evolving ecology of ideas. If they wear white coats and serious expressions, and if they operate scientific-looking apparatus, they communicate a particular definition of the situation—possibly that it is of an authoritarian nature, especially if the subjects are junior students. In such a situation permissive types of suggestions, especially if they are presented by means of a tape recording, may be less appropriate than more authoritarian suggestions may be. Attempting in such a way to compare the effects of different types of suggestions (see, e.g., Van Gorp, Meyer, & Dunbar, 1985) would not make much sense, because the ecology of ideas would be likely to be biased in favor of authoritarian suggestions. This is apart from the fact that such an experiment would be based on the reductionistic idea that suggestions exist independently of the context and that they have a linear causal influence. In the light of this reasoning, ecosystemic research focuses on the context and on all people's ideas in the context, rather than on techniques as if these were independent of the context.

One of the procedures often used in hypnosis research is that of simulation (e.g., Bryant & McConkey, 1989). Often subjects who obtain high scores on a test of hypnotic susceptibility are assigned to one or more experimental groups, while those who obtain low scores are asked to simulate hypnosis and are seen as a control group. They are considered to be unlikely to slip into hypnosis inadvertently, because they are relatively unhypnotizable. The Newtonian assumptions underlying this practice are clear:

1. Hypnotic susceptibility is a relatively unchangeable, but measurable, entity.
2. Susceptibility is independent of the context; no matter how the experimental context differs from the context of testing, a simulator would be unlikely to enter hypnosis in that or any other context.
3. Hypnosis is brought about in some ways (e.g., by means of induction), and not in others (e.g., instructions to simulate).

From an ecosystemic perspective, the practice of simulation involves a situation technically closely akin to the classic one in which a husband is asked whether he has stopped beating his wife. No matter what the answer, the poor man is defined as a wife beater. The simulator is in a similar unenviable situation: The better he or she performs, the more it is defined as simulation (i.e., as not "real").

Ecosystemically seen, people who obtain high scores on a susceptibility test are those who fit well with the structured, authoritarian situation of testing. People who are not comfortable with this situation score low. This latter group might do much better if they were simply asked to perform certain actions in certain ways; for them, this procedure might readily be qualified as hypnosis. But it is not. On the contrary, because they know that they have not done too well on the susceptibility test, it is easy to convince them that although they may perform as well as the experimental group(s), they are not hypnotized. The difference between simulators and "real" subjects thus lies in the way their actions are qualified, and not in any real difference in the actions themselves. Simulation is one of the best ways to show that a person is not judged to be hypnotized on the basis of his or her actions, but on the basis of how the actions are mutually qualified (Fourie, 1990).

If one moves away from the Newtonian assumptions on which simulation is usually based, interesting questions can be raised. For instance, would it be possible to qualify simulation as hypnotic or involuntary? And if so, would the subject then report that he or she could not help acting as if he or she were hypnotized? Would the subject then feel "really" hypnotized, or would the faking feel real? How would simulation of this kind be for people who think that they are highly hypnotizable, in comparison with subjects who think that they are not hypnotizable? And how would it be for other people present? How would knowledge of the subject's hypnotizability level influence the way in which they would qualify the simulation? From all this, it is clear that ecosystemic research must focus on the interplay between the ideas and attributions of all the members of the hypnotic system, and not on the intrapsychic activities of the designated subject.

Treatment Implications

Ecosystemic theorists such as Anderson and Goolishian (1988), Bogdan (1984), Hoffman (1985), and Keeney and Ross (1985) consider problems to exist as ideas in language. According to Maturana (quoted in Efran & Lukens, 1985), a problem does not exist until it is "languaged." From this perspective, depression or alcoholism or schizophrenia is not an entity or a "thing"; it is an idea with accompanying qualifying actions by everybody who is involved with the person designated as the problem carrier, including this person himself or herself. The problem system is thus analogous to the hypnotic system.

Hypnosis can often be used very fruitfully to perturb the ecology of ideas around the problem—not because hypnosis has any intrinsic power, but because clients and families *believe* that hypnosis is powerful. They attribute to hypnosis the power to eliminate problems, and to hypnotic age regression the power to reveal the truth about past traumatic events. In contrast to many other approaches, which advocate the removal of clients' so-called "misconceptions" about hypnosis (e.g., De Betz & Sunnen, 1985), an ecosystemic approach utilizes these conceptions in the process of coevolving, with the client or family, different ideas about the problem. For instance, if through skillful questioning in a situation defined as hypnotic age regression, a family can come to "realize" that the problem carrier's depression is actually frustration with his or her position in the family, then they may begin to be able to do something about the frustration, which they probably could not do if they were to go on thinking about the problem as an intrapsychic entity called depression. Believing that age regression necessarily brings forth the truth may help to convince them that the problem is really one of frustration.

Therefore, in treatment there is no attempt to use hypnosis as a force to rectify some hypothetical malfunctioning in the psyche of the problem carrier. Neither is there, in Ericksonian fashion (e.g., Lankton & Lankton, 1983), an effort to mobilize resources supposedly lying dormant in the unconscious mind of the client. Instead, hypnosis is used as one possible vehicle to perturb the ecology of ideas in which the particular problem is seen to exist.

Because an ecosystemic approach focuses on people's interlinked ideas, beliefs, and attributions, it prefers to deal in treatment with as many as possible of the people involved with a particular problem. Although it therefore often involves whole families, it is also amenable to being used with individuals, couples, or larger groups, depending on the circumstances.

A further implication of an ecosystemic approach to hypnosis, and one following from the idea that it is possible to capitalize on peoples' conceptions of hypnosis, is that the language of operation often differs from the language of conception. In conceptualizing hypnosis or problems, for instance, no credence is given to such reified concepts as the "unconscious," "depth of hypnosis," or "hypnotic susceptibility." However, these and similar terms may all be used in operation because they may be linked with the conceptions of subjects or clients. Therefore, if a client or family believes that hypnotic age regression will bring to the fore traumatic material that has been repressed to the unconscious, then an ecosystemic hypnotherapist will probably go along with this explanation. However, knowing that the responses given in conditions defined as age regression are usually related to the questions asked, and are therefore co-constructions, the therapist will probably ask questions whose answers will be likely to cover a theme subtly different from the one presented as a problem. In this way, as mentioned above, a problem can be redefined (Andolfi, Angelo, Menghi, & Nicoló-Corigliano, 1983), leading to alternative possible solutions. This can, however, only be done if the original conception of hypnotic age regression as a vehicle into the "unconscious" is not questioned.

In ecosystemic hypnotherapy, there is thus no effort to persuade clients or families to view hypnosis or treatment in ecosystemic terms. Whatever the conceptions or attributions of the particular client or family may be, these can potentially be utilized in treatment. Even an exaggerated fear of hypnosis can be employed subtly to imply that hypnosis may have to be used if some other procedure, defined as not hypnosis, fails (Fourie, 1991).

Appraisal: Differences between an Ecosystemic Approach and Other Approaches

Having shown how an ecosystemic approach to hypnosis involves an epistemological shift away from Newtonian thinking, and having indicated some of the implications of such an approach, I can now distinguish more specifically between ecosystemic hypnosis and the three other main perspectives on hypnosis—namely, state theory, social-psychological or nonstate theory, and the Ericksonian position. Although these three perspectives each cover numerous theories that all differ in some respects from one another, for the sake of comparison it is handy to group the various theories into the three broad perspectives.

Probably because many hypnotic behaviors can be quite dramatic, there has through the years been a sustained temptation to focus on the hypnotized person as if he or she were the site of hypnosis. Both in state theory (e.g., J. R. Hilgard, 1970) and in Ericksonian hypnosis (e.g., Lankton & Lankton, 1983), there has been the postulation that hypnosis comprises an altered state of consciousness in the subject. This is often thought to be a situation in which one hypothesized part of the subject (the unconscious) is dissociated from another part (the conscious) (Lankton & Lankton, 1983).

The nonstate theories came to the fore as a reaction against this state conception (T. X. Barber, 1979). Following the early writings of Sarbin (1950), these theories have conceptualized hypnotic behavior as an attempt by the subject to act according to situational demands, as perceived by him or her, as if he or she were hypnotized. It is thought that only certain ("fantasy-prone") subjects can do this (Wilson & Barber, 1982), and that they use cognitive strategies, such as attention diversion and goal-directed fantasy, to do so (e.g., Spanos & Gorassini, 1984; Spanos, Kennedy, & Gwynn, 1984). Although nonstate theory gives more credence than other theories to the environment and the situation, the implication is that environmental and situational factors have a causal influence on the subject's intrapsychic functioning, which is the really important aspect. The subject is still considered to be the site of hypnosis. Other people in the situation are hardly brought into consideration. Because of this continued focus on the subject and his or her intrapsychic functioning, the reified concept of hypnotic susceptibility is retained in nonstate theory.

All of the three broad perspectives on hypnosis thus can be seen to adhere to the Newtonian notion of reductionism. In all of them, albeit in different ways, the richness and interconnectedness of the hypnotic circumstance are reduced to its supposed elements. Although there is nothing wrong with this, it leads to an oversimplified understanding of a complicated situation. The elements assume such importance that the whole gets obscured.

Furthermore, in all three perspectives the elements are seen as connected to each other through cause and effect. In both state and nonstate theory, there is the implication that hypnotic performance is partially caused by the subject's level of hypnotic susceptibility. State theory perceives the induction process as causing dissociation, which in turn causes hypnotic behavior. Nonstate theory seems to conceptualize the intrapsychic strategies used by the subject as causally connected to hypnotic behavior. With its strong emphasis on technique, the Ericksonian position similarly implies that technique causes the activation of unconscious processes, which are seen as a hallmark of hypnosis (Ritterman, 1983).

Matthews (1985) has criticized the linear focus in Ericksonian hypnosis, as well as the concurrent implication that the hypnotist and the technique stand in an objective position with regard to the hypnotic system, being able to influence this system in a linear way from outside of the system. Such an adherence to the Newtonian notion of objectivity of observation is discernible not only in Ericksonian hypnosis, but also in both state and nonstate theory. Both of these schools, for instance, employ the concept of hypnotic susceptibility, and scales for its measurement have been devised by both.

All three of these broad aproaches to hypnosis therefore can be seen to follow Newtonian logic, which is precisely the mode of thinking from which an ecosystemic approach attempts to move away.

CONCLUSION

From this discussion, one could conclude that an ecosystemic approach constitutes no more than a further step in the development of thinking about hypnosis—a process that started a long time ago. State theory developed in an effort to bring order into the chaos of mystical thinking that characterized hypnosis in previous centuries. Contextualist or nonstate theory took the development further, away from a preoccupation with the individual, and toward a consideration of the whole of the hypnotic circumstance. Ecosystemic thinking continues this process, but with the type of change of order that Elkaïm (1981) has called a "bifurcation," or what is more commonly known as an "epistemological jump."

Perhaps the main value of an ecosystemic approach, which is a way of thinking and therefore neither true nor false, lies in its holism. It sensitizes us as hypnosis practitioners to the idea that as observers we influence what we observe, because we cannot help being part of the situation defined mutually by us and others as "hypnotic." In this process our implicit and explicit assumptions play a major role. If we do not continually question and examine these assumptions, we run the risk that our research results may serve to reciprocally validate out pet assumptions rather than to expand our knowledge of hypnosis, or that our treatment may be dictated by these assumptions rather than by the needs of our clients.

Acknowledgments. This chapter is based on an invited paper presented at the Fifth European Congress of Hypnosis in Psychotherapy and Psychosomatic Medicine, Konstanz, Germany, August 18–24, 1990.

REFERENCES

Anderson, H. & Goolishian, H. A. (1988). Human systems as linguistic systems: Preliminary and evolving ideas about the implications for clinical theory. *Family Process, 27*, 371–393.

Andolfi, M., Angelo, C., Menghi, P., & Nicoló-Corigliano, A. M. (1983). *Behind the family mask: Therapeutic change in rigid family systems.* New York: Brunner/ Mazel.

Auerswald, E. H. (1987). Epistemological confusion in family therapy and research. *Family Process, 26*, 317–330.

Barber, T. X. (1979). Suggested ("hypnotic') behavior: The trance paradigm versus an alternative paradigm. In E. Fromm & R. E. Shor (Eds.), *Hypnosis: Developments in research and new perspectives* (2nd ed., pp. 217–271). Chicago: Aldine.

Bateson, G. (1972). *Steps to an ecology of mind.* New York: Ballantine.

Bateson, G. (1979). *Mind and nature.* New York: Dutton.

Bogdan, J. L. (1984). Family organization as an ecology of ideas: An alternative to the reification of family systems. *Family Process, 23*, 375–388.

Bryant, R. A., & McConkey, K. M. (1989). Hypnotic emotions and physical sensations: A real–simulating analysis. *International Journal of Clinical and Experimental Hypnosis, 37*, 305–319.

Capra, F. (1983). *The turning point: Science, society and the rising culture.* London: Flamingo.

Colapinto, J. (1979). The relative value of empirical evidence. *Family Process, 18*, 427–442.

Cottone, R. R. (1988). Epistemological and ontological issues in counseling: Implications of social systems theory. *Counseling Psychology Quarterly, 1*, 357–365.

De Betz, B., & Sunnen, G. (1985). *A primer of clinical hypnosis.* Littleton, MA: PSG.

Deissler, K. G., & Gester, P. W. (1986). Autosystemische transformation: Trancephänomene, systemische Utilisierung oder selbstveränderung. *Familiendynamik, 11*(1), 29–56.

Dell, P. F. (1985). Understanding Bateson and Maturana: Toward a biological foundation for the social sciences. *Journal of Marital and Family Therapy, 11,* 1–20.

Efran, J. S., & Lukens, M. D. (1985). The world according to Humberto Maturana. *The Family Therapy Networker, 9*(3), 23–29, 72–75.

Elkaïm, M. (1981). Non-equilibrium, chance and change in family therapy. *Journal of Marital and Family Therapy, 7,* 291–297.

Ford, D. H. (1984). Reexamining guiding assumptions: Theoretical and methodological implications. *Journal of Counseling Psychology, 31,* 461–466.

Fourie, D. P. (1983). Width of the hypnotic relationship: An interactional view of hypnotic susceptibility and hypnotic depth. *Australian Journal of Clinical and Experimental Hypnosis, 11,* 1–14.

Fourie, D. P. (1988). Hypnosis in dental practice: From awkward add-on to smooth integration. *Journal of the Dental Association of South Africa, 43,* 141–146.

Fourie, D. P. (1990). Simulation in hypnosis research: The "hidden" role of attribution of meaning. *Perceptual and Motor Skills, 71,* 560–562.

Fourie, D. P. (1991). The withholding of hypnosis in family therapy. *Journal of Family Psychotherapy, 2,* 41–53.

Fourie, D. P., & De Beer, M. (1986). Hypnotic analgesia: Some implications of an ecosystemic approach. *British Journal of Experimental and Clinical Hypnosis, 3,* 151–154.

Fourie, D. P., & Lifschitz, S. (1985). Hypnotic behavior: Mutual qualification. *South African Journal of Psychology, 15,* 77–80.

Fourie, D. P., & Lifschitz, S. (1987). Ein Ökosystemischer Ansatz der Hypnose: Rationale Kerngedanken und einige Folgerungen. *Experimentelle und klinische Hypnose: Zeitschrift der Deutschen Gesellschaft für Hypnose, 3*(1), 1–12.

Fourie, D. P., & Lifschitz, S. (1988). Not seeing the wood for the trees: Implications of susceptibility testing. *American Journal of Clinical Hypnosis, 30,* 166–177.

Fourie, D. P., & Lifschitz, S. (1989). Ecosystemic hypnosis: Ideas and therapeutic application. *British Journal of Experimental and Clinical Hypnosis, 6,* 99–107.

Hall, A. D., & Fagan, R. E. (1956). Definition of a system. *General Systems Yearbook, 1,* 18–28.

Hilgard, E. R. (1970). *Personality and hypnosis: A study of imaginitive involvement.* Chicago: University of Chicago Press.

Hilgard, E. R. (1982). Hypnotic susceptibility and implications for measurement. *International Journal of Clinical and Experimental Hypnosis, 30,* 394–403.

Hoffman, L. (1981). *Foundations of family therapy: A conceptual framework for systems change.* New York: Basic Books.

Hoffman, L. (1985). Beyond power and control: Toward a "second order" family systems therapy. *Family Systems Medicine, 3,* 381–396.

Keeney, B. P. (1979). Ecosystemic epistemology: An alternative paradigm for diagnosis. *Family Process, 18,* 117–129.

Keeney, B. P. (1982). What is an epistemology of family therapy? *Family Process, 21,* 153–168.

Keeney, B. P. (1983). *Aesthetics of Change*. New York: Guilford Press.

Keeney, B. P., & Ross, M. (1985). *Mind in therapy: Constructing systemic family therapies*. New York: Basic Books.

Kruse, P., & Gheorghiu, V. A. (1990, August 18–24). *Self-organization theory and radical constructivism: A new concept for understanding hypnosis, suggestion and suggestibility*. Paper presented at the Fifth European Congress of Hypnosis in Psychotherapy and Psychosomatic Medicine, Konstanz, Germany.

Lankton, S. R., & Lankton, C. H. (1983). *The answer within: A clinical framework of Ericksonian hypnotherapy*. New York: Brunner/Mazel.

Lifschitz, S., & Fourie, D. P. (1985). *The hypnotic situation—a systems approach* (Reports from the Psychology Department, No. 13). Pretoria: University of South Africa.

MacCorquodale, K., & Meehl, P. E. (1948). On a distinction between hypothetical constructs and intervening variables. *Psychological Review, 55*, 95–107.

Matthews, W. J. (1985). A cybernetic model of Ericksonian hypnotherapy: One hand draws the other. In S. R. Lankton (Ed.), *Elements and dimensions of an Ericksonian approach* (Ericksonian Monographs No. 1). New York: Brunner/Mazel.

Matthews, W. J. (1989, September 20–24). *Possibility therapy*. Workshop presented at the First European Congress of Ericksonian Hypnosis and Psychotherapy, Heidelberg, Germany.

Maturana, H. R. (1975). The organization of the living: A theory of the living organization. *International Journal of Man–Machine Studies, 7*, 313–332.

Maturana, H. R. (1983). What is it to see? *Archivos Biologia Medicina Experimentales, 16*, 255–269.

Prigogine, I., & Stengers, I. (1984). *Order out of chaos*. New York: Bantam Books.

Ritterman, M. (1983). *Using hypnosis in family therapy*. San Francisco: Jossey-Bass.

Sarbin, T. R. (1950). Contributions to role-taking theory: I. Hypnotic behavior. *Psychological Review, 57*, 25–270.

Sarbin, T. R., & Coe, W. C. (1972). *Hypnosis: A social psychological analysis of influence communication*. New York: Holt, Rinehart & Winston.

Schmidt, G. (1985). Gedanken zum Ericksonschen Ansatz aus einer systemorientierten Perspektive. In B. Peter (Ed.), *Hypnose und Hypnotherapie nach Milton H. Erickson*. München: Pfeiffer-Verlag.

Schwartzman, J. (1984). Family theory and the scientific method. *Family Process, 23*, 223–236.

Sheehan, P. W. (1988, August 31). *Psychology in context—from a cultural perspective*. Presidential address presented at the 24th International Congress of Psychology, Sydney, Australia.

Spanos, N. P., & Bertrand, L. D. (1985). EMG biofeedback, attained relaxation and hypnotic susceptibility: Is there a relationship? *American Journal of Clinical Hypnosis, 27*, 219–225.

Spanos, N. P., & Gorassini, D. R. (1984). Structure of hypnotic test suggestions and attributions of responding involuntarily. *Journal of Personality and Social Psychology, 46*, 688–696.

Spanos, N. P., Kennedy, S. K., & Gwynn, M. I. (1984). Moderating effects of contextual variables on the relationship between hypnotic susceptibility and suggested analgesia. *Journal of Abnormal Psychology, 93*, 285–294.

Van Gorp, W. G., Meyer, R. G., & Dunbar, K. D. (1985). The efficacy of direct versus indirect hypnotic induction techniques on reduction of experimental pain. *International Journal of Clinical and Experimental Hypnosis, 33*, 319–328.

Varela, F. (1979). *Principles of biological autonomy.* New York: Elsevier/North-Holland.

Von Bertalanffy, L. (1974). General system theory and psychiatry. In G. Caplan (Ed.), *American handbook of psychiatry* (Vol. 2, pp. 1095–1117). New York: Basic Books.

Von Glasersfeld, E. (1984). An introduction to radical constructivism. In P. Watzlawick (Ed.), *The invented reality* (pp. 17–40). New York: Norton.

Wagstaff, G. F. (1981). *Hypnosis, compliance and belief.* Brighton, England: Harvester Press.

Wilson, S. C., & Barber, T. X. (1982). The fantasy-prone personality: Implications for understanding imagery, hypnosis, and parapsychological phenomena. In A. A. Sheikh (Ed.), *Imagery: Current theory, research and application* (pp. 340–387). New York: Wiley.

PART FIVE

INTERACTIVE–PHENOMENOLOGICAL MODELS

The Two Disciplines of Scientific Hypnosis: A Synergistic Model

ROBERT NADON
Brock University

JEAN-ROCH LAURENCE and CAMPBELL PERRY
Concordia University

INTRODUCTION

Despite a multitude of experimental and clinical research findings since Hull's classic 1933 treatise on the scientific study of hypnosis, many major theoretical issues remain unresolved. Spanos has represented the theoretical controversy as a clash between "cognitive–behavioral" (Spanos & Chaves, 1989) or "social-psychological" (Spanos, 1986a) versus "special-process" accounts. Because we know of no psychological researcher who argues that hypnotic responses are best understood by concepts drawn from outside mainstream psychology, the special-process label in particular appears to be a convenient fiction around which debate can be polarized. This type of polarization obscures important issues at least as much as it illuminates others, although it is of note that the present schism within the hypnosis community is reminiscent of debates that occurred during the 19th century (Laurence & Perry, 1988).

It is customary, however, to trace the origins of hypnosis to the earlier (though overlapping) period of "animal magnetism," as presented in the theory and practice of Franz Anton Mesmer. As Laurence and Perry (1988) have documented, many of the behaviors and experiences of today's hypnotized individuals were observed also in the magnetized individuals of the late 18th century. Of particular relevance for our approach are 18th-

and 19th-century observations of stable individual differences in response to magnetization and hypnosis. Most of the suggested behaviors contained in current hypnotic scales were borrowed directly from suggestions contained in the 19th-century scales that were developed by Bernheim and his colleagues at Nancy, who in turn had borrowed them from Mesmer and other early practitioners (Bernheim, 1884; Liébeault, 1866).[1]

Indeed, Mesmer was the first to recognize that individuals varied extensively in their response to the influence of the "magnetic fluid" that he believed was actuated by his magnetic passes. As a summary of his system, Mesmer (1779) listed 27 propositions in which he defined animal magnetism as the "property of the animal body that renders it susceptible to the influence of celestial bodies and the reciprocal action of those who surround it" (in Amadou, 1971, p. 77). Mesmer qualified this description of what he considered to be a general law, however, by his next statement: "The action and virtue of animal magnetism, thus defined, can be communicated to other animate and inanimate bodies. *However, both can be found to be more or less susceptible*" (1779; in Amadou, 1971, p. 77, italics added).

Although most authors were aware of these individual differences at the time, few were inclined to theorize about them. In an age rooted in Romanticism, a generalized theory of humankind rather than an explanation of individual variability was sought. Nonetheless, Mesmer's followers continued to document these individual differences. Puységur (1784), for example, noted that no more than 10–15% of his patients could experience artificial somnambulism, a phenomenon thought to be characterized by various responses (e.g., increased intellectual and physical skills, spontaneous amnesia). He was followed by many others who did not share his underlying assumptions about the phenomenon, but who observed the same stable variations in its manifestation: the French Royal Commission of Inquiry into Animal Magnetism (Franklin et al., 1784), Faria (1819/1906), Braid (1843), Liébeault (1866), Bernheim (1884), and Janet (1889), to name a few.

Perhaps the first attempt to explain these observations belongs to the 1784 Royal Commission of Inquiry into Animal Magnetism under the phantom-like leadership of Benjamin Franklin (see Laurence & Perry, 1988, for a detailed account of the inquiry, and McConkey & Perry, 1985, for an analysis of Franklin's private views). The conclusions reached by the commissioners were highlighted by their conviction that three core components (imagination, imitation, and the touch of the magnetist) led to the occurrence of a diversity of behaviors and experiences in magnetized individuals. Subsequently, Faria (1819/1906) argued that response to "lucid sleep" (his term for hypnosis) depended upon the degree of a person's ability to experience the phenomenon in combination with the contextual demands of the situation, as well as the individual's beliefs, expectancies, and motivations (Laurence & Perry, 1988; Nadon, Breton, Perry, & Laurence, 1991). Faria argued further that all lucid sleep phenomena originated with implicit or explicit suggestions, which in turn were acted upon according to the degree of responsiveness of the person. As a clinician, Faria recognized that in order to be most effective, the hypnotic ritual needed to match the hypnotized person's expectations, although he was the first major investigator to recognize that responses in hypnosis were derived mainly from the abilities of the subject, rather than of the *concentrateur* (hypnotist). Indeed, it was on the basis of the stable and differential responsiveness of his subjects that Faria argued in favor of tailoring treatment according to the patient and not according to an all-encompassing theory of disease (either physiological or religious). Faria's approach was radical for an epoch that explained what we now call hypnosis primarily in terms of external influence; the views presented in this chapter owe a particular debt to Faria's (1819/1906) theorizing of interactional mechanisms implicated in hypnotic response (for a more detailed description of this history, see Laurence & Perry, 1988; Perry, 1978).

THEORETICAL CONCEPTS AND PRINCIPLES

In science the competition is not so much between facts and theories as it is between problems and the techniques for solving them.
—M. T. Ghiselin, *Intellectual Compromise: The Bottom Line* (1989, p. 169)

We are advancing a model of hypnosis and hypnotic ability, but more generally we are proposing a spirit of inquiry. In our view, three broad themes need to be addressed.

1. Because over two centuries of (admittedly discontinuous) research has not resolved the single major theoretical *structural* question of what hypnosis is, we are advocating a partial return to a more *functional* approach. The functional questions "Of what use are hypnotic procedures and hypnotic ability?" offer the means to confront many issues for which structural considerations are only of tangential importance. The traditions of William James and John Dewey are sufficiently broad to encompass both laboratory and clinical research, and can highlight concerns (e.g., early development of hypnotic ability, its adaptive and maladaptive consequences, and cognitive processes during hypnosis) that have not usually been of central interest within structural frameworks (see

Kihlstrom & McConkey, 1990, for a discussion of James's views on hypnosis and his digressions into structural considerations).

2. For the debate on structure to be productive, methodological and statistical approaches need to be rethought before some consensus of what constitutes evidence for one position or another can evolve; views within a psychometric framework presented by Tellegen (1978–1979) and by Balthazard and Woody (1985) offer promise in this regard. These potentially fruitful directions notwithstanding, the lack of unanimity concerning criteria for evaluating quality of evidence has significantly obstructed informative theoretical debate, despite early signs of theoretical convergence (e.g., E. R. Hilgard, 1973; Spanos & Barber, 1974). Even a casual observer of hypnosis research over the last two decades is apt to notice that most of the data have been open to numerous interpretations and that no single body of work has been definitive. Clearly, many findings have been "consistent with" a number of alternative views.

3. Finally, as has been expressed by Gould (1989, pp. 50–51) in another context, we reject the notion that the optimal solution to a dichotomous scientific debate lies within a diluted version of the two extreme views. Rather, we propose a model in which contingency plays a central role. That is, whether "dissociative" or "situational" mechanisms, or both (to cite two of the most prominent theories currently offered), best explain what determines a person's hypnotic response depends upon various factors. Which factors are operating in any given circumstance, in what manner, to what extent, and how they interact with other factors are the pivotal questions.

We recognize that this approach may dissatisfy those who favor generalized rules. Indeed, models that emphasize contingencies are often disparaged, incorrectly, for not being lawful (Anderson, 1991; Gould, 1989). Nevertheless, examination of the interrelationships among numerous potentially operating factors can serve as a beginning for sorting out the contingencies that we suspect are integral to hypnotic performance. Examination of personality, cognitive, affective, and social-psychological factors is essential for resolving the present debate and for providing a more extensive empirical underpinning for our central thesis that combined or "synergistic" effects of these four factors will mitigate any dichotomous theoretical interpretation favoring one or the other of the primary views. Indeed, Hollingworth's (1928, p. 83) assertion that *"stimulating details from the same or different contexts may work together,* thus reinforcing each other (synergy)," remains a valid methodological argument for the study of any psychological phenomenon. For optimal pursuit of this multidimensional and synergistic approach, however, correlational and experimental methodologies, which have been identified by Cronbach (1957, 1975) as the two disciplines of scientific psychology, need to be combined within single designs.

The Two Disciplines of Scientific Psychology

[M]ost revolutionary transitions in science have usually
occurred through methodological innovation rather than
grand and bookish theories. A new direction and power is
usually given by devices—as by the microscope, the
telescope, or more subtly by stereochemistry or the
differential calculus. . . . It is this instrumentation—this
capacity to approach old problems in new operational
terms, and to open doors before which bivariate methods
have monotonously marked time— that multivariate
experiment now brings.

—R. B. CATTELL,
Preface to *Handbook of Multivariate
Experimental Psychology* (1966, p. viii)

A cross-disciplinary multidimensional approach of the type envisioned in
part by Cattell is being pursued vigorously within personality research,
which is showing distinct signs of convergence after the spirited
person–situation debate that began in the 1960s. How this consensus is
being achieved, which is occurring almost unnoticed in other psychological disciplines, is noteworthy. Of particular importance, the ongoing
"quiet revolution" within the field of personality (to borrow a telling
phrase from Québec politics of the 1960s) is being fueled primarily by
methodological and statistical advancements, which in turn are generating
empirically driven theoretical refinements (Buss & Cantor, 1989; Cantor,
1990). Cross-fertilization between correlational and experimental methodologies, the respective traditional approaches of personality and social
psychology, has led to the view that neither person nor situation is
primary. Although the inevitable demise of unidimensional person and
situation views has been predicted for some time, notably by K. S. Bowers
(1973), it has taken almost two decades to set aside what has been called
a "pseudo-issue" (Carlson, 1975) and the "fruitless person–situation
debate" (Kihlstrom, 1987, p. 989), prompting Kihlstrom (1986) to call
for an end to the battle of correlation coefficients between Cronbach's two
disciplines. One consequence of the truce (perhaps even a lasting peace) on
this issue is that personality and social psychologists are spending less time
defending or attacking the genuineness of dispositional constructs, and
instead are clarifying their structure and function (Wright & Mischel,
1987).

The present status of the personality debate is contrasted by the
polemic within the hypnosis community, where a search by theorists for an
optimal theoretical framework in which either person or situation is
emphasized has been conspicuous. Because of the significance it attaches to

individual differences in hypnotic ability and mentalistic structures in accounting for hypnotic phenomena, neodissociation theory (E. R. Hilgard, 1977) can be viewed as placing primary explanatory power on the person; caveats notwithstanding (Spanos, 1986b), the social-psychological approach most closely identified with Spanos (1986a) places primary emphasis on situational causes of hypnotic response (see Perry & Laurence, 1986). It is likely that the debate will go the way of the person–situation debate in personality, and that ultimately neither view will be held to be fundamental. The remainder of the present chapter is an attempt to outline the importance of interactions between person and situation for under-standing hypnotic phenomena (Nadon, Laurence, Perry, 1989). Because combined effects of person and situation variables can take forms other than linear interactions, however, we extend our earlier arguments to form a more encompassing synergistic model.

The "Person" in Hypnosis Research

> An unlearned carpenter of my acquaintance once said in
> my hearing: "There is very little difference between one
> man and another; but what little there is, is very
> important." This distinction seems to me to go to the
> root of the matter. It is not only the size of the difference
> which concerns the philosopher, but also its place and its
> kind. An inch is a small thing, but we know the proverb
> about an inch on a man's nose.
> —WILLIAM JAMES, "The Importance of Individuals"
> (1896/1956, pp. 256–257).

Two broad approaches concerning "person" in personality can be de-scribed. According to one view, rooted in Allport's (1937, 1961) notion of trait, the optimal unit of analysis is one of *"personal dispositions*, which are idiosyncratic bases for rendering sets of situations and actions functionally equivalent" (Maddi, 1984, p. 10), and which derive "their significance from the role they play in advancing adaptation within, and mastery of, the personal environment" (Allport, 1937, p. 342). By contrast, and more within Murray's (1938) tradition of motivational influences on behavior and Kelly's (1955) cognitive approach (see also Adams-Webber, 1979), it has been argued that "person" is best understood in terms of ongoing cog-nition brought about in part by exigencies of the situation (e.g., Cantor & Kihlstrom, 1987; Mischel, 1984). This debate within a debate—whether it is advantageous to understand person from an individual-difference per-spective or from a mental-process point of view—has not been a particu-larly quarrelsome issue in hypnosis research. In fact, this is a major area in which hypnosis researchers have anticipated the current trend in the field of personality by examining both aspects of the person in combination.

Unfortunately, from a structural perspective (and as has been the case historically), it has been difficult to differentiate among proposed "person" effects. Spanning three centuries, these effects have been argued to reflect the extent of individuals' investment in the hypnotizable role (e.g., Barber, Spanos, & Chaves, 1974; Sarbin & Coe, 1972) or, similarly, the "imitative tendencies" of the magnetized person (Franklin et al., 1784, cited in Morand, 1889; see Laurence & Perry, 1988, p. 89). Dissociative mechanisms have also been invoked to explain hypnotic response among highly hypnotizable persons (e.g., E. R. Hilgard, 1977; Janet, 1889; Laurence & Perry, 1981). Finally, the effects have been regarded as evidence for the importance of the skill (trait or personal disposition) of hypnotic ability (e.g., K. S. Bowers, 1976; Faria, 1819/1906; J. R. Hilgard, 1970; Liébeault, 1866; Nadon, Laurence, & Perry, 1987). All these approaches can be criticized for their relative theoretical neglect of the vast majority of individuals who are not highly hypnotizable, a practice that Mesmer also criticized in 1799 when he reflected upon the popular enthusiasm surrounding somnambulist patients.

We have generally been identified with the dissociation and the hypnotic ability positions. At the same time, we agree with Sarbin and Coe's (1972; Coe & Sarbin, 1971) emphasis on the total context of hypnotic responding. Nevertheless, we do not accept their argument that individual differences in hypnotic ability can be accounted for by a unitary dimension (for detailed arguments on this point, see E. R. Hilgard, 1965; Sheehan & McConkey, 1982; Tellegen & Atkinson, 1976). In point of fact, our position is quite the opposite: We believe that individual differences in hypnotic ability across the entire range are multidetermined (Nadon et al., 1987).

We view individual differences of various sorts that function outside of the hypnotic context as *a priori* predispositions to act and experience in certain ways, given certain circumstances; that is, we consider pre-existing individual differences to represent the "front end" of an adequate theory of hypnosis, although from a dispositional rather than a causal perspective. The ubiquitous nature of individual differences in global hypnotic ability alone, whether in 19th-century France or in 20th-century North America and Europe (Laurence & Perry, 1988), is sufficient from a functional perspective to recommend this view. Ongoing cognitions and situational cues are therefore seen to act upon various personal dispositions (e.g., absorption, imaginative abilities) in eliciting hypnotic responses.

Another aspect of individual differences that we consider important is the observation of differences among highly hypnotizable persons (Nadon, D'Eon, McConkey, Laurence, & Perry, 1988; Roche & McConkey, 1990). Data gathered on the Revised Stanford Profile Scales (Brenneman, Hilgard, & Kihlstrom, 1991; Weitzenhoffer & Hilgard,

1967), for example, indicate differential response patterns to empirically difficult hypnotic suggestions among virtuoso hypnotic subjects. Although it is not new to assert that these individuals show considerable variability of response to hypnotic suggestions (see E. R. Hilgard, 1965; Perry, 1977), this is particularly promising for the examination of the interaction between and among personal dispositions, beliefs, and subjective experiences.

A systematic pattern of univariate relations between responses to difficult hypnotic suggestions continues to be found in our own work. Examination of various responses, such as the duality experience in age regression (Perry & Walsh, 1978), memory creation (Labelle, Laurence, Nadon, & Perry, 1990; Laurence, Nadon, Nogrady, & Perry, 1986; Laurence & Perry, 1983), the hidden observer (Laurence & Perry, 1981; Nogrady, McConkey, Laurence, & Perry, 1983), and posthypnotic amnesia (Nadon et al., 1988), suggests a predictable and approximate 60–40 split among highly hypnotizable subjects in their responses to these suggestions. Unfortunately, because of the extensive screening and individual testing required, a more thorough multivariate examination of these interesting patterns is beyond the means of most laboratories and the perseverance of most researchers. Recent efforts at modifying the Stanford Hypnotic Susceptibility Scale, Form C (SHSS:C) for group administration by K. S. Bowers, Crawford, and their respective colleagues may provide the methodological tools to pursue these questions with sample sizes more adequately suited to these intrinsically multivariate questions.

Moreover, although the main body of our work until now has been concerned primarily with how various predispositions across all subjects and among highly responsive persons manifest themselves within a quite narrow range of hypnotic situations, our theoretical perspective explicitly recognizes contextualist influences on hypnotic behavior and experience. As Laurence and Perry (1988) concluded:

> Individuals who undergo a hypnotic induction are not monolithic sculptures carved by the context. They bring to the situation many idiosyncratic aspects that will interact with the context in eliciting a behavioral response and a subjective experience that may or may not confirm the experimenter's *and* the individual's perception of the phenomena under study. (p. 392)

One of the critiques of individual-difference approaches, however, is that differences between people typically account for small proportions of variability in actual behavior—the "personality coefficient" of $.20 \leq r \leq .30$ (Mischel, 1968, p. 78). For example, absorption (Tellegen, 1981; Tellegen & Atkinson, 1974), which has been defined recently as "a disposition, penchant, or readiness to enter states characterized by marked cognitive restructuring" (Tellegen, 1987), has been found to correlate positively ($r = .50$ and greater) with interview and self-report measures of imaginative involvement (J. R. Hilgard, 1970), fantasy proneness (Lynn & Rhue, 1988), and openness to experience (McCrae & Costa, 1985). Its correlation with hypnotic behavior, however, has been considerably smaller (Kihlstrom, 1985; Roche & McConkey, 1990), although there is some evidence that the correlation may reach the .40–.50 range when the more empirically difficult SHSS:C (Weitzenhoffer & Hilgard, 1962) is the criterion measure (Nadon, Hoyt, Register, & Kihlstrom, 1991).

In any case, the limitations of effect size estimates have been eloquently described by Rosenthal and Rubin (1982), who have argued that theoretical interpretation of effect magnitude depends upon the context of the question, as James (1896/1956) realized almost 100 years ago (see also Rosenthal, 1990). Thus, although effect size is clearly useful for planning and evaluating experiments for statistical power purposes, its theoretical utility depends upon both the substantive issues at hand and measurement reliability. For this reason, we do not believe that contrasting the magnitudes of situational and person effects is usually a theoretically informative exercise.[2]

The "Situation" in Hypnosis

It is true (Spanos, 1986b) that situational effects on hypnotic response have at times been dismissed; nevertheless, we dispute the argument that they necessarily "run counter to the specific predictions of competing theories" (Spanos, 1986b, p. 496). Because situational effects have not been the focus of our research, we leave it to others to describe recent advances in understanding how situational factors can influence hypnotic response. For example, the reader is referred to an extensive review of reports of subjective involuntariness in hypnosis from a sociocognitive perspective by Lynn, Rhue, and Weekes (1990), which, although differing in emphasis, dovetails quite well with our views; in a transposition of our presentation, they emphasize situational influences on subjective reports while explicitly recognizing the necessity of incorporating individual-difference variables in a comprehensive model. Nonetheless, despite some movement within traditionally situationist theoretical frameworks toward recognizing individual differences as critical sources of response variability, there remains a tendency at times to diminish their role. We discuss below one instance of a strong interpretation of a situational effect that we do not believe was warranted by the data.

In a study of hypnotic depth, Radtke and Spanos (1982; see also Radtke, 1989) found that providing hypnotic subjects with additional nonhypnotic descriptors of their experience dramatically reduced the number of subjects who reported being hypnotized. Scales 1 and 2 in their study provided subjects with a choice of three, of a total of four, responses indicating that they were hypnotized in some fashion; Scale 3 also

provided subjects with three responses indicating that they were hypnotized, but with an additional four responses to indicate that they were not
hypnotized. The proportions of subjects who reported being hypnotized
(regardless of hypnotizability level) were 81%, 80%, and 25% on Scales 1
through 3, respectively. Thus, when subjects were given more opportunity
to indicate that they were not hypnotized, most of them chose this
alternative. Similarly, although not discussed by Radtke and Spanos, there
was a main effect for hypnotizability: Collapsed across scales, 87%, 67%,
and 42% of subjects high, medium, and low in hypnotizability, respectively, reported being hypnotized. (The hypnotizability groups are referred
to hereafter as "highs," "mediums," and "lows," for the sake of brevity.)

From traditional perspectives, a situationist rejoices at the scale
effect, whereas a personologist finds comfort in the effect of hypnotic
ability. There was also an interaction present in the data, although it was
not analyzed formally. The subjects most affected by the additional
descriptors provided in Scale 3 were the mediums; 92% of these subjects
described themselves as hypnotized on Scales 1 and 2 combined, a
proportion that dropped to 18% on Scale 3. The proportion of lows
reporting themselves as hypnotized dropped from 58% to 11%, and for
highs, who were the subjects least affected by the manipulation, the
proportion dropped from 98% to 64%.

Numerous statistical techniques now permit fine dissection of these
data. Cohen (1982, 1989; Cohen & Cohen, 1983, pp. 487–518) has
described a multivariate generalization of multiple regression that he calls
"set correlation" (Cohen & Cohen, 1983, p. 487), which, among other
uses, permits detailed analysis of contingency data. Reanalysis of the
Radtke and Spanos (1982) data along these lines has confirmed the various
ostensible effects in their data. Scale (1, 2, or 3) accounted for 29% of the
variance of the dichotomous dependent variable (hypnotized vs. not
hypnotized), $F (2, 324) = 84.25, p < .001$; hypnotizability level accounted
for 12.5% of the variance, $F (2, 324) = 36.43, p < .001$; and the scale x
hypnotizability level interaction accounted for 2.7% of the variance, $F (4,
324) = 3.87, p < .005$.[3]

Radtke and Spanos (1982) chose to qualify the interaction by noting
that "even among high hypnotizables, less than two thirds defined themselves as 'hypnotized'" (p. 242) when provided with alternative descriptors
on Scale 3, an assessment emphasizing that the scale manipulation exerted
an effect even among these subjects. The "binomial effect size display"
(BESD) technique presented by Rosenthal and Rubin (1982), however,
suggests that effects of this type may be best understood by comparing
effects between groups—for example, by noting that more than twice the
proportion of mediums as highs were affected by the manipulation, despite
having similar proportions of "hypnotized" ratings on Scales 1 and 2.

In the main, Radtke and Spanos (1982) succeeded in drawing attention to an important methodological concern—namely, the powerful impact of question phrasing on subsequent answers, particularly when ambiguous subjective experiences are being assessed. That is, they drew attention to the main effect of scale. As has been argued by Laurence and Nadon (1986), however, Radtke and Spanos's theoretical explanation of the interaction was less than satisfactory. They argued that highly hypnotizable subjects were least affected by the scale manipulation because "these subjects tend to be strongly invested in fulfilling the requirements of the hypnotic role" (p. 243).

This tautological argument, however, is less informative than it might appear at first glance. In part, Radtke and Spanos (1982) recognized this, because they offered a plausible "special 'state' formulation" (p. 242) view and acknowledged that their results could also be interpreted in that light. Other positions could have been presented also: One could account for the results in terms of phenomenological experience that does not assume a special state of any kind, but rather assumes that some subjects experience subjective anomalies following a relatively prescribed ritual— anomalies that nonetheless are not unique to that ritual. Described in this manner, the hypnosis label is merely a point of reference for subjects to indicate that they have undergone unusual (but not unique or "special") subjective experiences. The effect of Radtke and Spanos's (1982) discussion was to minimize the subjective reality of subjects' phenomenological experiences.

All three explanations that have thus far been presented, however, share a tautology that stems from different structural conceptualizations of what hypnosis is. For this reason, they continue to polarize debate. We contend that a more enlightening strategy is to explain the differential effect among subjects while distinguishing between "peripheral nuisance" interactions (which are primarily of methodological concern) and "systematic" interactions that illuminate substantive contingencies (Tellegen, 1981, p. 218). We agree with Radtke and Spanos (1982) that their results point to more than methodological artifacts, but differ with them on their theoretical significance.

We are led to question why the high subjects were less susceptible to this type of situational manipulation in their study than were the lows. Part of the reason is probably a floor effect: lows were less likely to describe their experiences as hypnotic, regardless of scale. This does not explain, however, the greater effect on the medium subjects relative to the highs; both groups described themselves as hypnotized in similar proportions on Scales 1 and 2, but showed vastly different responses to Scale 3.

Radtke and Spanos's (1982) depiction of the interaction, although tautological within the confines of their experiment, is nonetheless testable. If they are correct in maintaining that many of the high subjects continued to define themselves as hypnotized on Scale 3 despite extensive opportunity to do otherwise, because they were invested in the role requirements of the hypnotic context, then all that is required is an independent measurement of this tendency. Lynn, Snodgrass, Rhue, Nash, and Frauman (1987), for example, have shown that subjects who attribute greater skill to the hypnotist tend to report greater involuntariness accompanying their hypnotic responses, even when the potentially confounding factor of individual differences in hypnotic behavior is statistically removed. Lynn et al. (1987) have thus provided direct, if not independent, evidence for their argument that "subjects' ratings of involuntariness are associated with the belief that their hypnotic behavior is a function of the hypnotist's ability" (Lynn et al., 1990, p. 172).[4]

One would prefer, however, to find a relation between response to the hypnotic depth scales and an indicator of role investment, as hypothesized by Radtke and Spanos (1982), that is assessed independently of the hypnotic context. If Radtke and Spanos are correct, the way in which subjects respond to a measure of role investment would be subject to the same contextual influences hypothesized to be operating on the depth scales. For this reason, it would be necessary to administer another measure (outside of the hypnotic context) that might moderate responses to the depth scales in the hypnotic context. For example, if subjects' attributions of being hypnotized represent attempts to maintain a self-image or public image of being hypnotizable, measures of private and public self-consciousness (Fenigstein, Scheirer, & Buss, 1975), respectively, might tap role fulfillment mechanisms. Alternatively, although measures of social desirability have not fared well in explaining hypnotic response (K. S. Bowers, 1976), they might interact with other factors (such as wording of scales) in predicting self-reports. That is, the high subjects in the Radtke and Spanos (1982) study who continued to define themselves as hypnotized on Scale 3, which provided alternatives to the "hypnotized" description, may have scored higher on a measure of social desirability than highs who reported not being hypnotized.

The strategy of independently assessing measures of psychological mechanisms thought to moderate experimental effects has general applicability. For example, similar patterns of immunity to situational demands among some, but not all, high subjects have been observed in studies of breaching posthypnotic amnesia (K. S. Bowers, 1966; Kihlstrom, Evans, Orne, & Orne, 1980; Schuyler & Coe, 1981). As Kihlstrom et al. (1980) noted, the various findings are at odds with unidimensional theories of hypnosis and "appear to place boundaries on both the traditional and alternative views of posthypnotic amnesia" (p. 614).

Here again, the battle between the two predominant views of hypnosis has resulted in a theoretically unsatisfying stalemate. The nature of the boundaries referred to by Kihlstrom et al. (1980), we suggest, can be clarified by examination of various person variables. As already described, one facet of the person that may explain these types of differences among high subjects may be some aspect of social desirability, or similarly, some aspect of what Tellegen (1978–1979) has defined broadly as a "compliance dimension" (p. 228) in hypnotic response.

A second potentially important factor in hypnotic response, which is theoretically distinct but related to behavioral response, is the subjective experiences that accompany hypnotic behavior, particularly the empirically difficult suggestions (P. G. Bowers, Laurence, & Hart, 1988; Kirsch, Council, & Wickless, 1990). Tellegen (1978–1979) has labeled this aspect of hypnotic response "the tendency to experience hypnotic suggestions as real" (p. 228). Similarly, P. G. Bowers et al. (1988) have argued that subjective experiences vary according to the cognitive demands of the hypnotic suggestions. These experiential aspects of hypnosis have been the foundation of hypnosis research and therapeutic intervention since Mesmer's time, and have been described as the "classic suggestion" effect (K. S. Bowers, 1981; P. G. Bowers, 1982; E. R. Hilgard, 1981; Kihlstrom, 1985; Laurence & Perry, 1988; Lynn et al., 1990; Weitzenhoffer, 1980). To the extent that hypnotic experience is seen as partially orthogonal to hypnotic behavior, multivariate procedures can offer an informative solution. By providing the means to statistically remove individual variability common to both hypnotic behavior and experience, prior to analysis of independent variables' effects, these procedures offer promise for tapping hypnotic behavior and experience (as criterion variables) independently.

As we discuss in the next section, absorption (Tellegen, 1981; Tellegen & Atkinson, 1974) is a promising candidate to index the experiential aspects of hypnosis in an independent fashion. The relation between absorption and global hypnotic response, like that between attitudinal variables and global response, has been disappointingly small (K. S. Bowers, 1976; Nadon, Hoyt, et al., 1991). As we demonstrate in the next section, however, its explanatory power can probably best be tapped in combination with other variables. This description is consistent with Tellegen's (1981) conceptualization of absorption as a personal disposition that influences behavior and experience given particular circumstances. For example, if the thesis that the highly hypnotizable subjects who continued to define themselves as hypnotized on Scale 3 in the Radtke and Spanos (1982) study did so because of more potent subjective experiences within the hypnotic context (but experiences that can also occur outside of hypnosis), then these subjects may score higher on absorption; that is, subjects for whom the subjective experiences are more potent may need to rely less on external cues, such as scale wording, for labeling those experiences (Laurence & Nadon, 1986). Alternatively, high-absorption subjects who are predisposed to have unusual subjective experiences in other contexts may not attribute their unusual hypnotic experiences to hypnosis, and they thus may report that they were not hypnotized if given adequate opportunity to do so. In either case, the synergistic effect of hypnotizability and absorption would be evidenced by their interaction.

A Synergistic Model

In the tradition within personality research that began with Allport (1937), Tellegen (1981) has argued that "the manifestation of a trait . . . jointly depends on personal characteristics and current conditions" (p. 219). We use the term "synergy" to describe the application of this principle to our own thinking, although like Tulving (1983), we use the term advisedly and despite its present trendy status within psychology. By "synergy," we mean the effects of various influences on hypnotic response *in combination*.

Statistically, the synergistic model subsumes cumulative models in which predictors have both zero-order and unique correlations (i.e., with all other predictors partialed out) with the criterion or criteria of interest; it allows also for empirically rare but theoretically interesting suppressor effects, in which predictors can account for response variability not by their zero-order relations with the criterion, but rather by virtue of their relations to other predictors (see Wiggins, 1973, for a discussion of the advantages and failings of these models in personality research). One advantage of this approach is that a broad range of correlational and experimental variables can be examined with maximum power, while at the same time design structure is simplified. Indeed, one can bypass the difficulty of trying to obtain subjects to complete relatively rare combinations of independent variables, such as high absorption and low imagery ability, by retaining the full range of information provided by quantitative scales. In this manner, various combined effects of continuous and discrete variables, which are examined inefficiently within traditional analysis of variance (ANOVA) designs, can be evidenced with utmost simplicity within correlational–experimental designs.

Clearly, designs that capture the multidimensionality of response to hypnotic procedures require equally multidimensional data-analytic strategies. Although this point of view is perhaps anachronistic (Faria expressed it in nonstatistical terms over 150 years ago!), we are restating it because it occurs infrequently in practice and because it implicitly rejects strict adherence to a reductionistic psychology of hypnosis derived primarily from experimentally manipulated variables. Exercising experimental control of various aspects of hypnotic performance deemed to reflect sources of statistical error is all to the good, provided that researchers can agree on what is error and what is substance—that is, the "artifact" and "essence" discussed by Orne (1959). The intervening three decades since 1959 suggest, however, that agreement on this issue is not forthcoming within the present climate of research (see Jones & Flynn, 1989). Moreover, it can be argued that experimental control is often not uniform across subjects who differ on important (for the question at hand) individual-difference factors, a situation akin to the violation of the homogeneity-of-regression-slopes assumption in analysis of covariance. For the moment, it will probably be informative to sort out how individual differences interact with sources of error from one perspective and substance from another. To be most informative, however, such designs will need to tap the full range of statistical power of all variables, to the extent that their measurement permits. The multivariate general linear model seems particularly well suited to this task, because it allows univariate and multivariate ANOVA approaches (which are special cases of the model) to be integrated with more general and widely applicable multiple-regression approaches; psychological research will increasingly tap the flexibility and power of this statistical paradigm, well into the next century (Cohen, 1989; Cohen & Cohen, 1983; Edwards, 1976; Keppel & Zedeck, 1989; Morrison, 1990; Pedhazer, 1982).

Our emphasis on statistical issues, however, should not be regarded as a neglect of methodological or substantive concerns; rather, it is because hypnosis researchers such as T. X. Barber, E. R. and J. R. Hilgard, and M. T. and E. C. Orne, among others, have made major contributions to the methodology of psychological research that we are able to focus on statistical questions within a synergistic framework. Theoretical refinement of absorption, for example, has been obtained within a synergistic correlational–experimental framework in a series of recent studies (Nadon, Dywan, Ogilvie, & Simons, 1991; Qualls & Sheehan, 1979, 1981a, 1981b).

In their studies, Qualls and Sheehan speculated that absorption might moderate performance on a muscle tension reduction task. Two conditions from Qualls and Sheehan (1981a, Experiment 2) are representative. In one condition, subjects were asked to generate their own internal strategies for relaxing (*internal* attentional demand); in a second condition, subjects were asked to attend to the experimenter's relaxation instructions (*external* attentional demand). Qualls and Sheehan found that high-absorption subjects performed well in the internal demand condition but poorly in the external condition; low-absorption subjects showed the reverse pattern. The authors argued that the relation between absorption and muscle tension was mediated by situation-induced attentional demand.

Tellegen (1981) offered a different theoretical perspective on these findings. Although agreeing that the relation between absorption and tension was contingent upon other factors in the Qualls and Sheehan studies, he argued that the operational mechanism was not attentional demand, but rather the presence or absence of an experiential set. According to this view, asking subjects to generate their own internal strategies for relaxing encouraged them to focus on the *experience* of the activity rather than on the outcome—a strategy that benefited high-absorption subjects, but that was difficult for low-absorption subjects, who did not have the prerequisite imaginative skills to focus as extensively on an experiential activity. By contrast, asking subjects to attend to the experimenter's instructions encouraged them to focus on the requirements of the task, or in other words to adopt an *instrumental* set—a strategy that benefited low-absorption subjects, but that served to detract from the enjoyable aspects of the experience for the high-absorption subjects (see also Harackiewicz, 1989, for a similar distinction between intrinsic enjoyment and goal accomplishment concerning a wide range of tasks).

To examine the question, Nadon, Dywan, et al. (1991) designed a three-way factorial experiment in which the synergistic effect of a personal disposition (absorption), ongoing cognition (instructions encouraging subjects to adopt either an experiential or an instrumental set), and a situational manipulation that contrasted external with internal attentional demand conditions (music vs. no music) was examined. Nadon, Dywan, et al. reasoned that a strong version of Qualls and Sheehan's hypothesis would predict a two-way interaction between absorption and attentional demand, to the exclusion of main effects or other interactions. A similarly strong interpretation of Tellegen's hypothesis would predict a different two-way interaction—that is, between absorption and instructional set.[5] Nadon et al. hypothesized, however, that the contingencies for the relation between absorption and muscle tension were themselves contingent upon each other. Specifically, they agreed with Tellegen that an experiential set would benefit high-absorption subjects, whether attentional demands were internal or external; they also argued, however, that whereas an instrumental set would benefit low-absorption subjects, it would only do so when a specific rather than a diffuse attentional focus was presented to them (e.g., in the form of musical passages). That is, they predicted the three-way interaction illustrated in Figure 16.1, $F (1, 24) = 5.15, p < .05; sr^2 = .15$.

The direction of the relationship between absorption and muscle tension depended on attentional demand, as Qualls and Sheehan predicted, but only within the instrumental factor: the negative slope in the instrumental/no-music cell, $r = -.45$, differed from its positive counterpart in the instrumental/music cell, $r = .40; t (24) = 1.97; p < .10$. Contrary to what was predicted based on a strong version of Qualls and Sheehan's model, however, the slope between absorption and tension was negative in both the no music ($r = -.24$) and the music ($r = -.72$) cells within the experiential factor: Further contrary to their model, the negative slope in the latter cell, in which an external attentional focus was presented to subjects, was different from zero, $t (6) = 2.51, p < .05$.

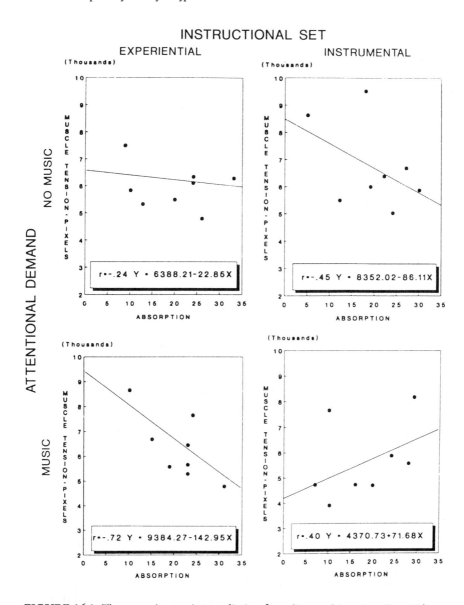

FIGURE 16.1. Three-way interaction predicting frontalis muscle tension. From *Absorption and Muscle Tension: Moderating Effects of Instructional Set and Attentional Demand* by R. Nadon, C. Dywan, R. Ogilvie, and I. Simons, 1991, unpublished manuscript, Brock University, St. Catharines, Ontario, Canada.

Similar conclusions can be drawn with respect to the predictions derived from a strong Tellegen model. As predicted by Tellegen, an experiential set determined the sign of the regression coefficient predicting tension from absorption, but only within the music factor: the negative slope in the experiential/music cell, $r = -.72$, differed from the positive slope, $r = .40$, in the instrumental/music cell; $t(24) = 2.32$, $p < .05$. The differences between the slopes of the experiential/no music and the instrumental/no music cells, however, were in the direction opposite to that predicted by Tellegen, although they did not differ significantly from each other, $r = -.24$ vs. $-.45$, $t(24) < 1$.

It is customary to extol the virtues of replicating new findings, and we do not oppose this tradition. The various comparisons we have reported between the cells of the design were based on small sample sizes and were nonorthogonal. Although this was necessary for purposes of comparing different models, the nonindependence of the comparisons complicates interpretation, particularly concerning the magnitude of the effect sizes within the cells (the correlation of $-.72$ in one cell is suspiciously high). The overall pattern was statistically reliable, however, despite the relatively small sample size, illustrating the advantages of combining correlational and experimental methodologies within a multiple-regression framework.

Moreover, the results lend substantial support to Tellegen's (1981, 1987) theorizing that absorption is an inherently interactive construct. This evidence suggests that attentional demand may moderate tension reduction for low-absorption subjects, but that the most important factor for high-absorption subjects is the extent to which the task encourages experiential activity. Thus, the findings lend support to Tellegen's (1981) view that a high capacity for absorption reflects an ability and preference to adopt an experiential set as dictated by circumstances—a conclusion that has also been reached independently in a recent doctoral dissertation (Donovan, 1989; P. W. Sheehan, personal communication to R. Nadon, September 10, 1990) that used a substantially different methodology. They also begin to hint at why absorption correlates at best moderately with hypnotic response. Although research to date has focused primarily on how absorption correlates with measures of global hypnotic response, how absorption relates to hypnosis probably depends on a host of cognitive, affective, and situational factors that have yet to be delineated. This idea has guided some of our research, which we present in the following section.

RESEARCH AND APPRAISAL

Our central thesis is that hypnosis can most profitably be understood from a multivariate and functional perspective that combines correlational and experimental methodologies. Although we have not yet fully realized this view in our own research, four recent studies have provided early insights concerning the conceptual clarity afforded by this approach.

There has been much discussion recently about contextual effects in hypnosis research, especially concerning the relation between absorption (Tellegen, 1981; Tellegen & Atkinson, 1974) and hypnotic behavior, but more generally the relation between any self-report measure and any aspect of hypnotic behavior or experience. This line of research has in part drawn upon methodological issues within personality research concerning the impact of responses to early items within self-report instruments on responses to later items (e.g., Knowles, 1988). In a more theoretical vein, the research stems from Kirsch's (1985) analysis of how response expectancies may affect behavior.

The initial study that elicited the attention of researchers was that of Council, Kirsch, and Hafner (1986). The most theoretically interesting finding of that study (and the one discussed most extensively by the authors) was an interaction ($p < .10$) between absorption and testing context in the prediction of a 10-item, modified, group-administered SHSS:C. When the interaction was examined, Council et al. found that the relation between absorption and hypnotizability was statistically significant when absorption was assessed within the hypnotic context just prior to hypnosis testing, but not when absorption was measured earlier in a context that was divorced of hypnosis. This finding prompted the authors to conclude:

> [T]he relation of the Absorption Scale . . . and similar measures to hypnotic responsivity is *highly reactive* to contextual factors and is probably mediated by subjects' expectancies. Administering the Absorption Scale to hypnotic subjects may implicitly suggest that imaginative processes are important in hypnosis, which in turn could influence levels of expectancy for successful hypnotic responding. The likelihood that past research has been confounded in this way must be considered when one evaluates theories and research that have stressed imaginative involvement and related constructs in explanations of hypnotic behavior. (Council et al., p. 188; italics added).

There were at least three consequences of these findings if they proved to be reliable. First, the generalizability of the evidence supporting the relation among absorption, other individual-difference variables, and hypnosis was in doubt, because most of the evidence from the various studies had been gathered within distinctly hypnotic contexts, either just before hypnosis or under conditions that were clearly related to hypnosis testing. Second, because much of the evidence supporting the construct validity of absorption has come from hypnosis research, the Council et al. (1986) findings placed the validity of the absorption construct in doubt. Third, additional studies on correlates of hypnotic response would be hampered by the necessity of keeping both testing contexts entirely separate, a difficult task within laboratories known for their hypnosis work.

For these reasons, the Council et al. (1986) study generated considerable interest. A subsequent study from the Carleton University laboratory by de Groot, Gwynn, and Spanos (1988) claimed a replication of Council et al.'s findings for women but not for men. With large-n, mixed-model designs, Nadon, Dywan, et al. (1991), however, failed to find evidence supportive of either Council et al. or de Groot et al., and argued that the conclusions drawn by the latter authors were derived from inadequate statistical analyses—a view buttressed by a recent failure to replicate either the de Groot et al. or the Council et al. findings within the Carleton laboratory (Perlini, Lee, & Spanos, 1990).[6] Debate is ongoing, but the upshot of the pattern of results since the original findings is that contextual effects, if genuine, are most likely to be small and to pose little (if any) threat to the validity of past research that has found relations between hypnotic ability and various experiences and processes outside of the hypnotic context. Indeed, Kirsch has proposed that "some preliminary data from a current study in our lab seems to be showing a significant correlation between absorption and the Harvard Scale, with context kept separate. Maybe there *is* a real relation between the two constructs" (I. Kirsch, personal communication to R. Nadon, May 4, 1990; but see also Kirsch, Chapter 14, this volume).

Additional evidence for the relation between hypnotic and nonhypnotic experiences and behavior comes from a series of recent studies on perceptual processing. Dixon, Brunet, and Laurence (1990; see also Dixon, 1990) found a reliable relation between hypnotizability and the manner in which language is processed. The derivation of their hypothesis stemmed primarily from the fundamental importance of language to hypnosis. That is, although hypnosis can be administered either in a dyad involving the hypnotist and the person being hypnotized or in groups (by either a hypnotist who is present or by a tape-recorded voice), responses to suggestions are elicited through the use of language (K. S. Bowers & Kelly, 1979). Given that hypnotic suggestions are almost always conveyed verbally, Dixon et al. argued that what may differentiate subjects who are highly hypnotizable (highs) from their relatively unhypnotizable counterparts (lows) is the manner in which they process verbal information. Specifically, they postulated that highs process language with greater automaticity.

Based on the work of Macleod and Dunbar (1988; Dunbar & MacLeod, 1984), Dixon et al. (1990) quantified automaticity in terms of performance on the Stroop color-naming task, in which reaction time is assessed for naming the physical color of words (e.g., BLUE, RED), or nonwords (e.g., XXXXX) presented in different colors (blue, red). For congruent trials (e.g., the word RED colored in red), the automatic processing of the color word facilitates faster reaction times relative to control trials (XXXXX colored in red). For incongruent trials (e.g., RED colored in blue), the automatic processing of the word creates interference in naming the color, which leads to increases in reaction time relative to control trials. Thus, the more automatically the words are processed, the greater the discrepancies between congruent and incongruent color-naming reaction times.

In one of a series of experiments, Dixon (1990) supported the automaticity hypothesis by showing that although no differences existed between highs and lows for congruent and control trials, highs had significantly longer incongruent reaction times than lows. In two other experiments, Dixon et al. (in press) replicated this hypnotizability–automaticity relation and showed that automaticity effects were not a by-product of differential use of strategies by highs and lows. In these studies, automaticity was assessed by the magnitude of the differences between congruent and incongruent trials, whereas strategy was assessed by varying the probability of congruent trials. Although these studies failed to reveal differences in the propensity to adopt performance optimization strategies in the Stroop task, highly hypnotizable subjects were shown to have greater discrepancies between congruent and incongruent trials in both strategy-aided and strategy-free conditions.

These Stroop findings are difficult to reconcile with a strictly social-psychological or response expectancy view of hypnosis and hypnotizability. In a recent review, Jones and Flynn (1989) argued that performance differences on perceptual tasks between highs and lows are attributable to the propensity of subjects to "strategically adjust their behavior to meet the demands of an experimenter for perceptual enhancement or degradation" (p. 174). Several factors suggest, however, that such a "strategic adjustment" hypothesis cannot adequately explain the data from the current series of studies. In all three experiments, performance differences were obtained in a setting that was removed from the hypnotic testing context. Subjects were tested under the auspices of a cognition laboratory, and no mention was made of possible links to hypnosis until after the experiment was completed. Furthermore, the experimenter conducting the Stroop experiments was blind to the susceptibility level of the subjects being tested. Finally, despite explicit instructions to name the colors as quickly as possible, "better" hypnotic subjects were shown to have poorer reaction time performance for incongruent trials.

These Stroop findings, combined with other findings on perceptual processes and hypnotizability in and out of hypnosis (Blatt, 1990; Jones & Flynn, 1989), suggest that a primarily social-psychological account of hypnosis is untenable; they provide additional support for the idea that hypnotic susceptibility is multidetermined. Viewed within a synergistic framework, the relatively greater automaticity with which highly hypnotizable subjects process verbal input may, in conjunction with social psychological mechanisms, allow other cognitive resources to be devoted to other skills such as absorption and imagery, which seem to aid in the production of a hypnotic response (see, e.g., Miller & Bowers, 1986). As such, verbal automaticity can be seen as a triggering mechanism that can actuate a series of cognitive processes, which in turn allows highly hypnotizable subjects to experience hypnotic suggestions.

In a different study, we (Button et al., 1990) adopted a more explicitly synergistic framework by examining eyewitness recall in and out of hypnosis within a multivariate framework. In Experiment 2, 39 subjects were shown a short videotape of a mock armed robbery (Yuille, 1985). Subjects were asked to recall specific aspects of the film (such as the suspect's description) in a free-recall format on six occasions. They recalled details of the film twice immediately after its presentation. A week later, they recalled the details again twice before hypnosis was introduced. They were then hypnotized and were asked to recall the details in hypnosis. A final recall was administered after hypnosis. Individual-difference data had already been gathered on hypnotizability (SHSS:C), imagery preference (Preference for an Imagic Cognitive Style, or PICS; Isaacs, 1982; Nadon et al., 1987), and absorption. Recall data were coded as correct, incorrect, or attributional (e. g., "The robber was ugly").

Net and cumulative recall were assessed at each recall trial. "Cumulative recall" was defined as new items recalled during a particular recall, plus any other items that had been recalled previously (see Payne, 1987, for a discussion of the merits of assessing both net and cumulative recall). Results were examined through a series of hierarchical mixed-model regression analyses. Because subjects had been sampled primarily on the basis of their hypnotizability scores, SHSS:C classification (high vs. low) was entered first into the hierarchy, followed by imagery preference (high vs. low) and absorption (high vs. low); thus, absorption effects reported below refer to effects of absorption scores with hypnotizability and imagery preference statistically removed (partialed), whereas effects of hypnotizability are unpartialed.[7]

Of particular interest for the present discussion were the hypnotizability × trial and the absorption × trial interactions. High- but not low-hypnotizability subjects recalled more cumulative correct items in hypnosis (Recall 5) than they did just before hypnosis. Both high- and low-absorption subjects recalled more correct items in hypnosis, although the effect was significantly more pronounced for the high-absorption subjects. Somewhat differently, both high- and low-hypnotizability subjects made more cumulative errors during hypnosis than just prior to hypnosis; the effect, however, was significantly larger for the highs. There was no absorption × trial interaction for errors.

How are these results to be explained? Klatzky and Erdelyi (1985) and others have argued that hypnotized individuals, particularly those who are highly responsive, adopt a looser report criterion in hypnotic than in nonhypnotic recall. That is, hypnotized subjects simply produce more information and thus show an increase in both errors and correct information. The Button et al. (1990) findings that highly hypnotizable subjects produced both more correct and incorrect information in hypnosis is consistent with this model. The criterion shift hypothesis is supported further by the finding that new correct information and new errors produced in hypnosis were related, r (37) = .72, p < .01. This pattern supports the possibility that the hypnotizability × trial interaction may have been due to high-hypnotizability subjects' adoption of a lower report criterion in hypnosis relative to their low-hypnotizability counterparts.

Additional multivariate regression analyses (Cohen, 1989; Cohen & Cohen, 1983, pp. 487–518), however, suggested that more than a criterion shift occurred. For correct recall during hypnosis, a significant effect of hypnotizability was observed even when productivity was held constant. When the cumulative correct information from Recall 4, and the cumulative errors and attributional information from Recall 5, were partialed from correct recall in hypnosis, high-hypnotizability subjects recalled 3.4 more new correct items of information than subjects low in hypnotizability (standard error = 1.2). (When Recall 4 cumulative correct information only was held constant, the groups differed by 4.8 correct items; standard error = 1.4). Similarly, a significant hypnotizability effect for cumulative errors was found. When productivity was held constant, the highs made 2.9 more errors (standard error = 1.4) in hypnosis than the lows. (When Recall 4 cumulative errors only were held constant, the groups differed by 4.5 errors; standard error = 1.4.)

These results suggest that contextual and phenomenological mechanisms may both be implicated in hypnotic recall. The press and popular media, dating to the 18th century (Laurence & Perry, 1988), have encouraged the popular belief that normal capabilities can be transcended in hypnosis (Nadon & Kihlstrom, 1987). The introduction of any new procedure after numerous recall attempts encourages the belief, at least implicitly, that performance will improve. When combined with popular notions about hypnosis, the introduction of hypnosis in the Button et al. (1990) study probably motivated subjects to try harder and possibly encouraged them to adopt a looser report criterion. Moreover, to the extent that individual differences in imagination and perceptual alteration are tapped in hypnosis, the blend of contextual pressures and phenomenological experiences may have created a powerful elixir for eliciting correct and incorrect recall. The Button et al. results suggest that for some individuals the primary effect is to increase correct recall (although new errors are also introduced), and that for others the major effect is to increase errors (although new correct information is obtained also).

Similar to the observation that one cannot tell without independent corroboration which information produced in hypnosis is correct, it is not presently possible to identify subjects for whom hypnosis is likely to increase correct recall relative to errors. Within a synergistic framework, however, individual differences in risky behavior can be seen as potential moderators of responses to contextual pressures and phenomenological experiences in hypnotic recall. The Control subscale of the Multidimensional Personality Questionnaire (MPQ; Tellegen, 1982) is a candidate for tapping this process. Tellegen (1982, p. 8) has described a low scorer on the subscale (which has the highest loading on the higher-order Constraint dimension) as "impulsive and spontaneous; can be reckless and careless; prefers to 'play things by ear.' " Because these individuals might be expected to adopt lower report criterions, examination of the potentially moderating effect of the Control subscale on hypnotic recall would probably inform the criterion-shift-versus-phenomenology debate, and might also begin to differentiate subjects likely to provide greater relative increases in errors from those likely to increase their correct recall.

Finally, a recent study by our group (Labelle et al., 1990) illustrates how examining the combined effects of individual-difference variables can improve prediction and theoretical understanding of memory phenomena in hypnosis. The Labelle et al. study replicated earlier findings (Laurence & Perry, 1983; see also Laurence et al., 1986) of an approximate 45% incidence among highly hypnotizable subjects of accepting a hypnotically suggested memory as veridical. Forty-six percent of moderately highly hypnotizable subjects in the Labelle et al. study also reported pseudomemories, whereas none of the low-hypnotizability subjects did so. Their finding that very high hypnotizability was not necessary for eliciting false memories suggested the possibility of other mechanisms. Drawing from Johnson and Raye's (1981) reality-monitoring model, we (Labelle et al., 1990) hypothesized that imagery might play a moderating role. Hierarchical regression analyses supported this hypothesis. Hypnotizability (SHSS:C) and imagery preference (PICS), both measured on a continuous scale, predicted significant variance in the dichotomous criterion measure of pass–fail on the pseudomemory item at their respective steps in the analysis. In addition, a hypnotizability × imagery preference interaction indicated that subjects who scored high on both measures were most likely to report a pseudomemory; by contrast, low-hypnotizability subjects, even if they reported a preference for imagic thought, did not appear to believe their imaginings and consequently did not report pseudomemories.

CONCLUSIONS

[P]ersonality is complex and multifaceted, and . . .
personality theories must come to terms with individuals
both as they *construe* their worlds and as they *function* in
those worlds.
—D. M. Buss and N. Cantor,
Introduction to *Personality Psychology:
Recent Trends and Emerging Directions* (1989, p. 6)

Perhaps because of the hypnosis community's traditional interest in
individual differences, Buss and Cantor's (1989) description of the task
confronting personality researchers and theorists is also an apt description
of the challenge that faces the field of hypnosis. How individuals construe
the hypnotic context, either as a function of their life experiences and
abilities or as a function of situational manipulations, has been of interest
historically and is also a presently active line of inquiry. Despite the
observation that subjects' expectations of hypnosis are not always validated
(McCord, 1961), they clearly play a role in hypnotic behavior (Kirsch,
Chapter 14, this volume). How these expectations are formulated,
however, and whether they represent epiphenomena or substantive
contingencies, are matters of debate.

Individual differences of various kinds will continue to play a central
role in theoretical frameworks of hypnosis, despite experimental psychology's attempts to minimize between-subjects variability by either ignoring individual differences in personality traits or treating them as
statistical error. Experimental psychology's undisputed success notwithstanding, we believe that this strategy is fundamentally misguided. The
Fisherian ANOVA techniques in which experimentalists have been
typically trained are usually inefficient for assessing individual-difference
effects (but see footnote 7). Paradoxically, there is evidence that R. E.
Fisher, the "father of modern statistics" (Cohen, 1990, p. 1308), first
conceptualized a data-analytic system much like modern regression, which
would have facilitated the examination of individual differences within
experimental designs; however, he opted for the more limited ANOVA
techniques because the hand calculations for the regression models were
too onerous.

Today's computers make the artificial boundaries between regression
techniques and the special case of the various ANOVA techniques
unnecessary and should allow for the development of a more general
psychology of hypnosis, which includes effects that are measured on both
continuous and categorical scales. For example, there are clear advantages
for assessing how subjects construe the hypnotic situation and how they
function within it by examining personality traits and by manipulating

the situation and subjects' cognitions within single designs; optimally, the effects should be examined within one analysis (or a series of hierarchical analyses). This type of more broadly based methodological foundation will inevitably lead to a more general theoretical understanding of hypnosis, as the increasingly fuzzy boundaries between social psychology and personality would indicate. Because of the myriad of possibilities for moderator effects and nonlinear relations, however, future work will need to be theoretically driven, but with sufficient theoretical comprehensiveness and flexibility to permit exploration of contingencies that are incompatible (or at least inconsistent) with one's theoretical orientation. Moreover, despite the methodological and theoretical advantages of this general approach, there will probably be resistance to adopting them among some researchers because of the extensive investment of "retooling" required to become proficient in their use (Ghiselin, 1989, p. 20). For this reason, the conceptual elegance of the model, rather than its technical aspects, will need to be highlighted in theoretical discussions of substantive issues.

The model for hypnosis research that we have outlined has emphasized a unidirectional approach. That is, we have stressed how aspects of the testing context can act upon pre-existing individual differences to elicit hypnotic experiences and behaviors, although we have purposely avoided questions of environmental influences on early development of this ability. As such, our model is more readily applicable to adults and to constrained laboratory situations, in which the influence of the subject upon the experimenter is minimal. The reciprocal-deterministic model (Bandura, 1978) that has been outlined by Sheehan and McConkey (1982) is needed for adequate conceptualization of clinical applications, particularly those that are unstandardized. This is not to say, however, that our synergistic model cannot generate generalizable results. Because it advances models that capitalize on the advantages of both correlational and experimental methodologies, it is especially suited for initiating findings that have wide applicability.

Finally, to paraphrase Gould (1989), complex, contingent, interactive, and hierarchical do not mean "special" (Spanos, 1986a). Rather, singling out particulars of human experience (whether social-psychological, cognitive, or personality) to explain hypnotic phenomena is to assign them an unwarranted special status that is divorced from mainstream psychology. Because of its comprehensiveness, the multivariate general linear model can provide the means for developing a truly general theory of hypnosis that is informed by the respective insights afforded by the two scientific disciplines of psychology. Because of its deceptively simple elegance at the conceptual level, however, the model presents risks of overdetermination when the techniques are used inappropriately; these risks must be understood and minimized. Nonetheless, in order to arrive at the consensus envisioned by Spanos and Barber (1974) and E. R.

Hilgard (1973), hypnosis will of necessity be conceptualized in multivariate terms.

Acknowledgments. The writing of this chapter and the research reported here were supported in part by Social Sciences and Humanities Research Council of Canada Research Fellowship Grant No. 455-90-0072 and by SSHRC Grant No. 410-91-0737 to Robert Nadon. In addition, Jean-Roch Laurence and Campbell Perry were supported by Natural Sciences and Engineering Council of Canada Grant No. U0440 (to J.-R. L.) and Grant No. A6361 (to C. P.), and by the Fonds pour la Formation de Checheurs et l'Aide à la Recherche of Québec (Principal Investigator, Jean-Roch Laurence).

NOTES

1. For example, one can find the first gustatory and olfactory hallucinations described in Mesmer (1781). Mesmer did not refer to these behaviors as suggested, however. He viewed the alteration of taste and smell as the end result of a change of direction in the magnetic fluid elicited by the magnetist (see Mesmer, 1781, pp. 33–34).
2. There is much to recommend in the increased reporting of how large an effect is (Cohen, 1988, 1990). Effect magnitude estimates provide the means for more precise discussion than mere, and ultimately arbitrary, statistical significance dichotomies. It also encourages development of sufficiently powerful replication studies (Hunt, 1990; Tukey, 1986). Along the lines proposed by Rosenthal and Rubin (1982), Cohen (1988) has argued that "the size of an effect can only be appraised in the context of the substantive issues involved" (p. 534). Concerning a subject dear to the hearts of many North Americans, Cohen cites an intriguing finding by Abelson (1985) to illustrate the point. Astonishingly, Abelson found that among major league baseball players, the percentage of variance in obtaining a hit in any single appearance at bat that was accounted for by batting average was less than 0.33%!
3. Because the criterion measure in Radtke and Spanos (1982) was dichotomous, the analysis can proceed with univariate regression procedures, which are special cases of set correlation. Other procedures, such as logistic regression, are also available (see Tabachnick & Fidell, 1989, for a nontechnical discussion).
4. Interestingly, Faria (1819/1906) made a similar argument.
5. The term "strong model" is used here to refer to the emphasis placed by Tellegen (1981) on the experiential–instrumental dimension and by Qualls and Sheehan (1981a) on the internal–external dimension. Tellegen's argument that subjects in an instrumental condition could "be asked to perform a specific task . . . [such as] to count silently . . . and at each count of 5 they could rate for themselves their state of relaxation" (Tellegen, 1981, p. 224), however, suggests that Tellegen's model does not neglect attentional mechanisms, inasmuch as subjects in this

instrumental condition are asked to attend to a specific, rather than a diffuse, task. Similarly, Qualls and Sheehan's reply that "low-absorption subjects may be instructed in such a way as to generate internal stimuli that could serve as an attentional focus" (1981b, p. 229) indicates that attentional demand per se, rather than external or internal focus, is central to their model.

6. de Groot et al. (1988) analyzed women and men separately, despite the fact that they did not provide evidence that women and men differed in demonstrating the context effect. That is, they relied on a significant (for women) versus not significant (for men) dichotomy to essentially argue for differences between men and women (see Nadon, Hoyt et al., 1991, for a more complete discussion). Cohen (1990) presents an interesting summary of an apparently caustic debate between R. A. Fisher and K. Pearson on this same issue.

7. Whether it is theoretically more informative to consider hypnotizability in terms of discrete levels or in terms of continuous measurement is uncertain. Clearly, creating discrete categories of a variable that is continuous at the conceptual level is inefficient and can introduce distribution distortions into the data set (Cohen, 1988; Tukey, 1986). Nevertheless, the debate concerning the viability of hypnotizability types is ongoing (Balthazard & Woody, 1985).

REFERENCES

Abelson, R. P. (1985). A variance explanation paradox: When a little is a lot. *Psychological Bulletin, 97*, 129–133.

Adams-Webber, J. (1979). *Personal construct theory: Concepts and applications.* New York: Wiley.

Allport, G. W. (1937). *Personality: A psychological interpretation.* New York: Holt, Rinehart & Winston.

Allport, G. W. (1961). *Pattern and growth in personality.* New York: Holt, Rinehart & Winston.

Amadou, R. (Ed.). (1971). *F. A. Mesmer: Le magnétisme animal.* Paris: Payot.

Anderson, J. L. (1991). Rushton's racial comparisons: An ecological critique of theory and method. *Canadian Journal of Psychology, 32*, 51–60.

Balthazard, C. G., & Woody, E. Z. (1985). The "stuff" of hypnotic performance: A review of psychometric approaches. *Psychological Bulletin, 98*, 283–296.

Bandura, A. (1978). The self system in reciprocal determinism. *American Psychologist, 33*, 344–358.

Barber, T. X., Spanos, N. P., & Chaves, J. F. (1974). *Hypnosis, imagination, and human potentialities.* Elmsford, NY: Pergamon Press.

Bernheim, H. (1884). *De la suggestion dans l'état de veille.* Paris: Octave Doin.

Blatt, T. (1990). *Hypnotic susceptibility differences in the acquisition of automatic behavior.* Unpublished master's Thesis, Concordia University, Montréal, Québec, Canada.

Bowers, K. S. (1966). Hypnotic behavior: The differentiation of trance and demand characteristic variables. *Journal of Abnormal Psychology, 71*, 42–51.

Bowers, K. S. (1973). Situationism in psychology: An analysis and critique. *Psychological Review, 80,* 307–336.

Bowers, K. S. (1976). *Hypnosis for the seriously curious.* Monterey, CA: Brooks/Cole.

Bowers, K. S. (1981). Do the Stanford scales tap the "classic suggestion effect"? *International Journal of Clinical and Experimental Hypnosis, 26,* 184–202.

Bowers, K. S., & Kelly, P. (1979). Stress, disease, psychotherapy and hypnosis. *Journal of Abnormal Psychology, 88,* 490–505.

Bowers, P. G. (1982). The classic suggestion effect: Relationship with scales of hypnotizability, effortless experiencing, and imagery vividness. *International Journal of Clinical and Experimental Hypnosis, 30,* 270–279.

Bowers, P. G., Laurence, J. -R., & Hart, D. (1988). The experience of hypnotic suggestions. *International Journal of Clinical and Experimental Hypnosis, 36,* 336–349.

Braid, J. (1843). *Neurypnology: or The rationale of nervous sleep, considered in relation with animal magnetism.* London: John Churchill.

Brenneman, H. A., Hilgard, E. R., & Kihlstrom, J. F. . (1991). *Patterns of hypnotic abilities.* Unpublished manuscript, University of Saskatchewan, Saskatchewan, Canada.

Buss, D. M., & Cantor, N. (1989). Introduction. In D. M. Buss & N. Cantor (Eds.), *Personality psychology: Recent trends and emerging directions* (pp. 1–12). New York: Springer-Verlag.

Button, J., Blatt, T., Lamarche, M.-C., Laurence, J.-R., Nadon, R., & Perry, C. (1990). *The effects of imagery preference, absorption, and hypnotizability in memory.* Unpublished manuscript, Concordia University, Montréal, Québec, Canada.

Cantor, N. (1990). From thought to behavior: "Having" and "doing" in the study of personality and cognition. *American Psychologist, 45,* 735–750.

Cantor, N., & Kihlstrom, J. F. (1987). *Personality and social intelligence.* Englewood Cliffs, NJ: Prentice-Hall.

Carlson, R. (1975). Personality. *Annual Review of Psychology, 26,* 393–414.

Cattell, R. B. (1966). Preface. In R. B. Cattell (Ed.), *Handbook of multivariate experimental psychology* (pp. vii–x). Chicago: Rand McNally.

Coe, W. C., & Sarbin, T. R. (1971). An alternative interpretation to the multiple composition of hypnotic scales: A single role relevant skill. *Journal of Personality and Social Psychology, 18,* 1–8.

Cohen, J. (1982). Set correlation as a general multivariate data-analytic method. *Multivariate Behavioral Research, 17,* 301–341.

Cohen, J. (1988). *Statistical power analysis for the behavioral sciences* (2nd ed.). Hillsdale, NJ: Erlbaum.

Cohen, J. (1989). *SETCOR: A supplementary module for SYSTAT and SYGRAPH.* Evanston, IL: SYSTAT.

Cohen, J. (1990). Things I have learned (so far). *American Psychologist, 45,* 1304–1312.

Cohen, J., & Cohen, P. (1983). *Applied multiple regression/correlation analysis for the behavioral sciences* (2nd ed.). Hillsdale, NJ: Erlbaum.

Council, J. R., Kirsch, I., & Hafner, L. P. (1986). Expectancy versus absorption in the prediction of hypnotic responding. *Journal of Personality and Social Psychology, 50,* 182–189.

Cronbach, L. J. (1957). The two disciplines of scientific psychology. *American Psychologist, 12,* 671–684.

Cronbach, L. J. (1975). Beyond the two disciplines of scientific psychology. *American Psychologist, 30,* 116–127.

de Groot, H. P., Gwynn, M. I., & Spanos, N. P. (1988). The effects of contextual information and gender on the prediction of hypnotic susceptibility. *Journal of Personality and Social Psychology, 54,* 1049–1053.

Dixon, M. (1990). *Hypnotic susceptibility differences in the automaticity of verbal information processing.* Unpublished doctoral dissertation, Concordia University, Montréal, Québec, Canada.

Dixon, M., Brunet, A., & Laurence, J. R. (1990). Hypnotizability and automaticity: Towards a PDP model of hypnotic responding. *Journal of Abnormal Psychology, 99,* 336–343.

Donovan, P. B. (1989). *Task explication of trait (absorption) differences in performance using Stroop interference.* Unpublished doctoral dissertation, University of Queensland, St. Lucia, Queensland, Australia.

Dunbar, K., & MacLeod, C. M. (1984). A horse race of a different color: Stroop interference patterns with transformed words. *Journal of Experimental Psychology: Human Perception and Performance, 10,* 622–639.

Edwards, A. L. (1976). *An introduction to linear regression and correlation* (2nd ed.). San Francisco: W. H. Freeman.

Faria, J. C. de Abbé. (1906). *De la cause du sommeil lucide: ou Étude de la nature de l'homme* [*On the cause of lucid sleep: Or the study of human nature*]. Paris: Henri Jouvre. (Original work published 1819)

Fenigstein, A., Scheier, M. F., & Buss, A. H. (1975). Public and private self-consciousness: Assessment and theory. *Journal of Consulting and Clinical Psychology, 43,* 522–527.

Franklin, B., de Bory, G., Lavoisier, A. L., Bailly, J. S., Majault, Sallin, D'Arcet, J., Guillotin, J. I., & LeRoy, J. B. (1784). *Rapport des commissaires chargés par le Roy de l'examen du magnétisme animal.* Paris: Bibliothèque Royale. (Reprinted *in extenso* in C. Burdin & F. Dubois [Eds.], *Histoire académique du magnétisme animal.* Paris: Baillière, 1841.)

Ghiselin, M. T. (1989). *Intellectual compromise: The bottom line.* New York: Paragon House.

Gould, S. J. (1989). *Wonderful life: The Burgess Shale and the nature of history.* New York: Norton.

Harackiewicz, J. M. (1989). Performance evaluation and intrinsic motivation processes: The effects of achievement orientation and rewards. In D. M. Buss & N. Cantor (Eds.), *Personality psychology: Recent trends and emerging directions* (pp. 128–137). New York: Springer-Verlag.

Hilgard, E. R. (1965). *Hypnotic susceptibility.* New York: Harcourt, Brace & World.

Hilgard, E. R. (1973). The domain of hypnosis: With some comments on alternative paradigms. *American Psychologist, 23,* 972–982.

Hilgard, E. R. (1977). *Divided consciousness: Multiple controls in human thought and action.* New York: Wiley.

Hilgard, E. R. (1981). Hypnotic susceptibility scales under attack: An examination of Weitzenhoffer's criticisms. *International Journal of Clinical and Experimental Hypnosis, 29,* 24–41.

Hilgard, J. R. (1970). *Personality and hypnosis: A study of imaginative involvement.* Chicago: University of Chicago Press.

Hollingworth, H. L. (1928). General laws of redintegration. *Journal of General Psychology, 1,* 79–90.

Hull, C. L. (1933). *Hypnosis and suggestibility: An experimental approach.* New York: Appleton-Century-Crofts.

Hunt, E. B. (1990). The traditional editorial statement. *Journal of Experimental Psychology: General, 119,* 3–4.

Isaacs, P. (1982). *Hypnotic responsiveness and the dimensions of thinking style and imagery.* Unpublished doctoral dissertation, University of Waterloo, Waterloo, Ontario, Canada.

James, W. (1956). The importance of individuals. In W. James, *The will to believe and other essays in popular philosophy and human immortality* (pp. 255–262). New York: Dover. (Original work published 1896)

Janet, P. (1889). *L'automatisme psychologique.* Paris: Alcan.

Johnson, M. K., & Raye, C. L. (1981). Reality monitoring. *Psychological Review, 88,* 67–85.

Jones, W. J., & Flynn, D. M. (1989). Methodological and theoretical considerations in the study of "hypnotic" effects in perception. In N. P. Spanos & J. F. Chaves (Eds.), *Hypnosis: The cognitive–behavioral perspective* (pp. 149–174). Buffalo, NY: Prometheus Books.

Kelly, G. (1955). *The psychology of personal constructs.* New York: Norton.

Keppel, G., & Zedeck, S. (1989). *Data analysis for research designs: Analysis of variance and multiple regression/correlation approaches.* San Francisco: W. H. Freeman.

Kihlstrom, J. F. (1985). Hypnosis. *Annual Review of Psychology, 36,* 385–418.

Kihlstrom, J. F. (1986). More on determinants of delay of gratification. *American Psychologist, 41,* 477–479.

Kihlstrom, J. F. (1987). Introduction to the special issue: Integrating personality and social psychology. *Journal of Personality and Social Psychology, 53,* 989–992.

Kihlstrom, J. F., Evans, F. J., Orne, E. C., & Orne, M. T. (1980). Attempting to breach posthypnotic amnesia. *Journal of Abnormal Psychology, 89,* 603–616.

Kihlstrom, J. F., & McConkey, K. M. (1990). William James and hypnosis: A centennial reflection. *Psychological Science, 1,* 174–178.

Kirsch, I. (1985). Response expectancy as a determininant of experience and behavior. *American Psychologist, 40,* 1189–1202.

Kirsch, I., Council, J., & Wickless, C. (1990). Subjective scoring for the Harvard Group Scale of Hypnotic Susceptibility, Form A. *International Journal of Clinical and Experimental Hypnosis, 38,* 112–124.

Klatzky, R. L., & Erdelyi, M. H. (1985). The response criterion problem in tests of hypnosis and memory. *International Journal of Clinical and Experimental Hypnosis, 33,* 246–257.

Knowles, E. S. (1988). Item context effects on personality scales: Measuring changes the measure. *Journal of Personality and Social Psychology, 55,* 312–320.

Labelle, L., Laurence, J.-R., Nadon, R., & Perry, C. (1990). Hypnotizability, preference for an imagic cognitive style, and memory creation in hypnosis. *Journal of Abnormal Psychology, 99,* 222–228.

Laurence, J.-R., & Nadon, R. (1986). Reports of hypnotic depth: Are they more than mere words? *International Journal of Clinical and Experimental Hypnosis, 34*, 215–233.

Laurence, J.-R., Nadon, R., Nogrady, H., & Perry, C. (1986). Duality, dissociation, and memory creation in highly hypnotizable subjects. *International Journal of Clinical and Experimental Hypnosis, 34*, 295–310.

Laurence, J.-R., & Perry, C. (1981). The "hidden observer" phenomenon in hypnosis: Some additional findings. *Journal of Abnormal Psychology, 90*, 334–344.

Laurence, J.-R. & Perry, C. (1983). Hypnotically created memory among highly hypnotizable subjects. *Science, 222*, 523–524.

Laurence, J.-R., & Perry, C. (1988). *Hypnosis, will, and memory: A psycholegal history.* New York: Guilford Press.

Liébeault, A. A. (1866). *Du sommeil et des états analogues surtout au point de vue de l'action du moral sur le physique.* Paris: Masson.

Lynn, S. J., & Rhue, J. W. (1988). Fantasy proneness: Hypnosis, developmental antecedents, and psychopathology. *American Psychologist, 43*, 35–44.

Lynn, S. J., Rhue, J. W., & Weekes, J. R. (1990). Hypnotic involuntariness: A social cognitive analysis. *Journal of Personality and Social Psychology, 97*, 169–184.

Lynn, S. J., Snodgrass, M., Rhue, J. W., Nash, M. R., & Frauman, D. C. (1987). Attributions, involuntariness, and hypnotic rapport. *American Journal of Clinical Hypnosis, 30*, 36–43.

MacLeod, C. M., & Dunbar, K. (1988). Training and Stroop-like interference: Evidence for a continuum of automaticity. *Journal of Experimental Psychology: Learning, Memory, and Cognition, 14*, 126–135.

Maddi, S. R. (1984). Personology for the 1980s. In R. A. Zucker, J. Aronoff, & A. I. Rabin (Eds.), *Personality and the prediction of behavior* (pp. 7–41). New York: Academic Press.

McConkey, K. M., & Perry, C. (1985). Benjamin Franklin and mesmerism. *International Journal of Clinical and Experimental Hypnosis, 33*, 122–130.

McCord, H. (1961). The "image" of the trance. *International Journal of Clinical and Experimental Hypnosis, 9*, 305–307.

McCrae, R. R., & Costa, P. T. (1985). Openness to experience. In R. Hogan & W. H. Jones (Eds.), *Perspectives in personality* (Vol. 1, pp. 145–172). Greenwich, CT: JAI Press.

Mesmer, F. A. (1781). *Précis historique des faits relatifs au magnétisme animal jusques en avril 1781.* London: No publisher available.

Mesmer, F. A. (1799). *Mémoire de F. A. Mesmer, docteur en médecine, sur ses découvertes.* Paris: Didiot le Jeune.

Miller, M. E., & Bowers, K. S. (1986). Hypnotic analgesia and stress inoculation in the reduction of pain. *Journal of Abnormal Psychology, 95*, 6–14.

Mischel, W. (1968). *Personality and assessment.* New York: Wiley.

Mischel, W. (1984). Convergences and challenges in the search for consistency. *American Psychologist, 39*, 351–364.

Morand, J. S. (1889). *Le magnétisme animal: Étude historique et critique.* Paris: Garnier.

Morrison, D. F. (1990). *Multivariate statistical methods* (3rd ed.). New York: McGraw-Hill.

Murray, H. A. (1938). *Explorations in personality: A clinical and experimental study of fifty men of college age.* New York: Oxford University Press.

Nadon, R., Breton, G., Perry, C., & Laurence, J.-R. (1991). *Faria's contributions to psychotherapy and hypnosis: Placebo and beyond.* Unpublished manuscript, Brock University, St. Catharines, Ontario, Canada.

Nadon, R., D'Eon, J., McConkey, K. M., Laurence, J.-R., & Perry, C. (1988). Posthypnotic amnesia, the hidden observer effect, and duality during hypnotic age regression. *International Journal of Clinical and Experimental Hypnosis, 36,* 19–37.

Nadon, R., Dywan, C., Ogilvie, R., & Simons, I. (1991). *Absorption and muscle tension: Moderating effects of instructional set and attentional demand.* Unpublished manuscript, Brock University, St. Catharines, Ontario, Canada.

Nadon, R., Hoyt, I. P., Register, P. A., & Kihlstrom, J. F. (1991). Absorption and hypnotizability: Context effects re-examined. *Journal of Personality and Social Psychology, 60,* 144–153.

Nadon, R., & Kihlstrom, J. F. (1987). Hypnosis, psi, and the psychology of anomalous experience. *Behavioral and Brain Sciences, 10,* 597–599.

Nadon, R., Laurence, J.-R., & Perry, C. (1987). Multiple predictors of hypnotic susceptibility. *Journal of Personality and Social Psychology, 53,* 948–960.

Nadon, R., Laurence, J.-R., & Perry, C. (1989). Interactionism: Cognition and context in hypnosis. *British Journal of Experimental and Clinical Hypnosis, 6,* 141–150.

Nogrady, H., McConkey, K. M., Laurence, J.-R., & Perry, C. (1983). Dissociation, duality, and demand characteristics in hypnosis. *Journal of Abnormal Psychology, 86,* 543–552.

Orne, M. T. (1959). The nature of hypnosis: Artifact and essence. *Journal of Abnormal and Social Psychology, 58,* 277–299.

Payne, D. G. (1987). Hypermnesia and reminiscence in recall: A historical and empirical review. *Psychological Bulletin, 101,* 5–28.

Pedhazur, E. J. (1982). *Multiple regression in behavioral research* (2nd ed.). New York: Holt, Rinehart & Winston.

Perlini, A. H., Lee, S. K. A., & Spanos, N. P. (1990, August). *The relationship between imaginal ability and hypnotic susceptibility: Contextual artifact or essence.* Paper presented at the 98th Annual Convention of the American Psychological Association, Boston.

Perry, C. (1977). Variables influencing the posthypnotic persistence of an uncancelled hypnotic suggestion. *Annals of the New York Academy of Sciences, 296,* 264–273.

Perry, C. (1978). The Abbé Faria: A neglected figure in the history of hypnosis. In F. H. Frankel & H. S. Zamansky (Eds.), *Hypnosis at its bicentennial* (pp. 37–45). New York: Plenum.

Perry, C., & Laurence, J.-R. (1986). Social and psychological influences on hypnotic behavior. *Behavioral and Brain Sciences, 9,* 478–479.

Perry, C., & Walsh, B. (1978). Inconsistencies and anomalies of response as a defining characteristic of hypnosis. *Journal of Abnormal Psychology, 87,* 574–577.

Puységur, A. M. J. Chastenet, Marquis de. (1784). *Détails des cures opérées à Buzancy, par le magnétisme animal.* Paris: Soissons.

Qualls, P. J., & Sheehan, P. W. (1979). Capacity for absorption and relaxation during electromyograph biofeedback and no-feedback conditions. *Journal of Abnormal Psychology, 88,* 652–662.

Qualls, P. J., & Sheehan, P. W. (1981a). Role of the feedback signal in electromyograph biofeedback: The relevance of attention. *Journal of Experimental Psychology: General, 110,* 204–216.

Qualls, P. J., & Sheehan, P. W. (1981b). Trait–treatment interactions: Reply to Tellegen. *Journal of Experimental Psychology: General, 110,* 227–231.

Radtke, H. L. (1989). Hypnotic depth as social artifact. In N. P. Spanos & J. F. Chaves (Eds.), *Hypnosis: The cognitive–behavioral perspective* (pp. 64–75). Buffalo: Prometheus Books.

Radtke, H. L., & Spanos, N. P. (1982). The effect of rating scale descriptors on hypnotic depth reports. *Journal of Psychology, 3,* 235–245.

Roche, S., & McConkey, K. M. (1990). Absorption: Nature, assessment, and correlates. *Journal of Personality and Social Psychology, 59,* 91–101.

Rosenthal, R. (1990). How are we doing in soft psychology? *American Psychologist, 45,* 775–778.

Rosenthal, R., & Rubin, D. A. (1982). A simple, general purpose display of magnitude of experimental effect. *Journal of Educational Psychology, 74,* 166–169.

Sarbin, T. R., & Coe, W. C. (1972). *Hypnosis: A social psychological analysis of influence communication.* New York: Holt, Rinehart & Winston.

Schuyler, B. A., & Coe, W. C. (1981). A physiological investigation of volitional and nonvolitional experience during posthypnotic amnesia. *Journal of Personality and Social Psychology, 40,* 1160–1169.

Sheehan, P. W., & McConkey, K. M. (1982). *Hypnosis and experience: The exploration of phenomena and process.* Hillsdale, NJ: Erlbaum.

Spanos, N. P. (1986a). Hypnotic behavior: A social-psychological interpretation of amnesia, analgesia and trance logic. *Behavioral and Brain Sciences, 9,* 449–467.

Spanos, N. P. (1986b). More on the social psychology of hypnotic behavior. *Behavioral and Brain Sciences, 9,* 489–497.

Spanos, N. P., & Barber, T. X. (1974). Toward a convergence in hypnosis research. *American Psychologist, 29,* 500–511.

Spanos, N. P., & Chaves, J. (1989). Hypnotic analgesia and surgery: In defence of the social-psychological position. *British Journal of Experimental and Clinical Hypnosis, 6,* 131–139.

Tabachnick, B. G., & Fidell, L. S. (1989). *Using multivariate statistics* (2nd ed.). New York: Harper & Row.

Tellegen, A. (1978–1979). On measures and conceptions of hypnosis. *American Journal of Clinical Hypnosis, 21,* 219–237.

Tellegen, A. (1981). Practicing the two disciplines for relaxation and enlightenment: Comment on "Role of the feedback signal in electromyograph biofeedback: The relevance of attention" by Qualls and Sheehan. *Journal of Experimental Psychology: General, 110,* 217–226.

Tellegen, A. (1982). *Brief manual for the Multidimensional Personality Questionnaire.* Unpublished manuscript, University of Minnesota.

Tellegen, A. (1987). *Discussion of symposium: Hypnosis and absorption.* Paper presented at the 38th Annual Meeting of the Society for Clinical and Experimental Hypnosis, Los Angeles.

Tellegen, A., & Atkinson, G. (1974). Openness to absorbing and self-altering experiences ("absorption"), a trait related to hypnotic susceptibility. *Journal of Abnormal Psychology, 83,* 268–277.

Tellegen, A., & Atkinson, G. (1976). Complexity and measurement of hypnotic susceptibility: A comment on Coe and Sarbin's alternative interpretation. *Journal of Personality and Social Psychology, 33*, 142–148.

Tukey, J. W. (1986). Data analysis and behavioral science or learning to bear the quantitative man's burden by shunning badmandments. In L. V. Jones (Ed.), *The collected works of John W. Tukey* (pp. 187–389). Monterey, CA: Brooks/Cole.

Tulving, E. (1983). *Elements of episodic memory*. Oxford: Clarendon Press.

Weitzenhoffer, A. M. (1980). Hypnotic susceptibility revisited. *American Journal of Clinical Hypnosis, 22*, 130–144.

Weitzenhoffer, A. M., & Hilgard, E. R. (1962). *Stanford Hypnotic Susceptibility Scale, Form C*. Palo Alto, CA: Consulting Psychologists Press.

Weitzenhoffer, A. M., & Hilgard, E. R. (1967). *Revised Stanford Profile Scales of Hypnotic Susceptibility, Forms I and II*. Palo Alto, CA: Consulting Psychologists Press.

Wiggins, J. S. (1973). *Personality and prediction: Principles of personality assessment*. Reading, MA: Addison-Wesley.

Wright, J. C., & Mischel, W. (1987). A conditional approach to dispositional constructs: The local predictability of social behavior. *Journal of Personality and Social Psychology, 53*, 1159–1177.

Yuille, J. (1985). *Video as a medium for eyewitness research*. Unpublished manuscript. University of British Columbia, Vancouver, British Colombia, Canada.

C H A P T E R   1 7

Hypnosis, Context, and Commitment

PETER W. SHEEHAN
University of Queensland

INTRODUCTION

The field of hypnosis has a powerful attraction to those who do research in it. The phenomena of hypnosis are intriguing, because seemingly simple communications are associated with quite radical shifts in behavior and reports of experience. It is not just the phenomena that are intriguing, however; there is the lure of the pursuit of theoretical agreement. The field has not yet arrived at a reasonable consensus about how to explain the phenomena of hypnosis, and sharp disagreement exists in the area about the validity of the different viewpoints. For example, some perspectives emphasize normal psychological processes of functioning, and others which focus upon processes that are said to reliably distinguish the hypnotic and waking states. My view of hypnosis falls somewhere between these two broad alternatives. It would be naive to deny that normal social-psychological processes of influence shape and determine hypnotic behavior and experience. Yet there seems to be value in exploring those processes that are relatively distinctive in the way that they operate in the hypnotic context.

At the outset, and before establishing some historical precedents for my view, it seems useful to summarize my position. According to this view, a deeply susceptible subject given hypnotic instruction will evidence a positive motivation to cooperate with the hypnotist—not simply to conform, but to work cognitively upon suggestion in an active way toward solving the problem or tasks posed by the hypnotist in the suggestion communication. Aptitude factors are important, but they must be seen to interact with contextual influences so as to shape and determine the final outcome of hypnotic suggestion. Such a theory depends rather more heavily than others on the meaning of the variability of response that exists in hypnosis, and on individual differences among (as opposed to between) hypnotic groups differing in level of susceptibility. The diversity and complexity of hypnotic behavior, and especially the experience that accompanies it, are theoretically most rewarding; and the study of style rather than competency will help most usefully to integrate the data. The interactions between and among task, setting (of which task is a component), and susceptibility to hypnosis are not additive ones, but reflect complex relationships. These are considered to be appropriately captured by a model that acknowledges the existence of reciprocal relationships among situation, behavior, and trait. The interactions that occur are not static in character, but fluid and dynamic, and frequently result in variable and complex response.

Some Historical Antecedents

The model that has just been summarized is influenced substantially by the theorizing in the field of personality—in particular, by the thinking of Mischel (1979) and Bandura (1978), and by the work on cognitive style of Witkin (1978). Bandura's concept of "reciprocal determinism," for example, emphasizes the give-and-take between the cognitively appraising organism and the environment in which that organism is placed. Comparably, the hypnotic subject is conceived (Sheehan and McConkey, 1982) as essentially engaged in an active, problem solving task. Consistent with defining response in terms of an interactionist perspective of psychological functioning, the hypnotic subject processes suggestions that are given by the hypnotist so as to respond in a socially appropriate way, but the meaning of "appropriate" needs to be understood in terms of the subject's cognitive appraisal of the situation in which he or she is placed. The term "appropriate" can only really be understood by gaining access to the subject's private comprehension of the hypnotist's suggestion communications. I would argue that the major goal of hypnosis, from the subject's point of view, is to be consistent with his or her personal and motivated involvement in the hypnotic situation. It takes skill to become involved intensely in hypnotic events, but the impact of that skill can only be assessed fully by considering the influence of aptitude within the framework of the subjects' private and subjective conception of the events surrounding him or her.

Historically speaking, such a view relates to a number of other theories, although it can be distinguished from them. Consider the social psychological theorizing of Sarbin and Coe (1972), for example. According to their view, theorizing in hypnosis should focus on the interactions and communications that take place between subject and hypnotist. The character of hypnotic behavior depends for these theorists on the constraints of the hypnotic environment and special contextual influences that are relevant to it, including cognitive and motoric skills, role perception, and prior knowledge of the hypnotic role. The reasons for behavior are not located internally, but externally in peripheral events. The ultimate test of credibility of a proposition to Sarbin (1982) is behavior, not mental structures (Sheehan, 1986a).

Sarbin's early focus on the social-psychological character of hypnotic behavior was carried forward in its most extreme form by Barber in his 1969 treatise, *Hypnosis: A scientific approach*. The thinking of both Sarbin and Barber influenced in turn the more current models of hypnosis proposed by Spanos and Wagstaff (see Spanos, 1986; Wagstaff, 1981), which focus heavily on the concept of compliant behavior and the processes of conformity and obedience. The theorizing of Spanos and Wagstaff, however, does not emphasize at all the phenomenal meaning of suggestion events.

Experience is emphasized heavily by other theorists in terms of the assumptions of the models of explanation that they adopt. Consider, for instance, the work of Fourie (1983). Fourie and his associates adopt an ecosystemic, epistemological point of view that explicitly rejects the analysis of hypnotic behavior and experience in terms of discrete, analytical events. Fourie's ecosystemic theory places primary emphasis on the complexity of the web of interrelated influences, and conceptualizes hypnotic responsiveness in terms of "interfacing" among the hypnotist, the subject, and observers. According to this view, the phenomena of hypnosis are extremely complex, and efforts to analyze discrete parts of them lead to what Keeney (1982) might call "fractionation of complexity and destruction of patterns that connect" (p. 156). This perspective recognizes the complexity of interrelating factors of influence in the hypnotic setting in a way that other social-psychological theories do not, but it argues for them in the absence of a methodology that is distinctively attuned to studying the consequences of the array of interactive events.

Within Australia, where my view of hypnosis clearly has its origins—and in its development over time with colleagues (Sheehan & McConkey, 1982)—the early historical influences have been those models of explanation that have pursued essential (vs. artifactual) features of hypnosis (e.g., Sutcliffe, 1958; Hammer, 1961). Sutcliffe, for example, argued for delusion as the central concept of his theoretical model, whereas Hammer appealed primarily to the special relevance of the process of dissociation. My theory, however, though influenced by these theorists in their analytical accounts of hypnosis and the focus placed jointly by them on individual differences in level of susceptibility, came to take on a separate identity that was determined more by the interactionist debate occurring in the general personality literature. It was this debate that posed the important question of the relative strength of contribution of trait (vs. situation). Finally, with the development of the "Experiential Analysis Technique" (EAT; Sheehan & McConkey, 1982), a method sympathetically attuned to investigating the phenomenal meaning of subjects' cognitions about the suggestions they received was constructed, and a theoretical point of view acquired procedures to match it. At this point, the model moved pointedly away from the prevailing Zeitgeist of behavioristic investigation and explanation.

Essentially, then, the model being proposed is a contextual one, and the relevance of context can perhaps be best understood by relating it to fields of study outside hypnosis. Contextualism, for example, emerged as a major organizational philosophy within the field of developmental psychology during the 1970s (Lerner, Hultsch, & Dixon, 1983). Changes in development, for example, were argued to occur as a result of reciprocal relations between an active organism and an active context. As context influences and affects on the individual, the individual alters it; as such, "by being a product and a producer of their context, individuals affect their own development" (p. 103). It is important to recognize, however, the special relevance of a major principle advocated by contextualism in the wider debate. This is what Lerner et al. (1983) and Rosnow (1981) have called "methodological pluralism." This principle states that there is no single mode of critical examination, or method, that is valid for the assessment of the multiple levels of analysis associated with processes occurring at different moments of historical time.

Related Perspectives

Having canvassed the general properties and features of this model, which should perhaps be placed within the general category of contextual models of explanation, I want to look briefly at two specific theoretical perspectives that relate to it: the framework of Diamond (1987), which places its emphasis on relational dimensions, and Shor's (1962, 1979) theory, which focuses on archaic involvement. There are other relevant theoretical frameworks outside the field of hypnosis that have not been directly pursued as yet in hypnotic research, and some of these are examined briefly.

Diamond's Perspective

Diamond (1987) argues for "a discernible and vital quality to an individual's hypnotic experiencing that differs from, and is seemingly unrelated to, either the hypnotisability score or depth of trance per se. Moreover, this qualitative, experiential involvement does not necessarily co-vary with objective or subjectively reported susceptibility" (p. 96). Like our (Sheehan & McConkey, 1982) model, Diamond's model stresses the complex nature of this elusive quality, and emphasizes the idiosyncratic and complicated nature of hypnosis.

Diamond's perspective focuses primarily on relational dimensions. Two of these include the enacting of former object relations, and the notion of a symbiotic or fusional alliance (whereby the hypnotist is experienced as a purely internal figure). The first of these (the forming of object relations) is very similar to Shor's (1962) postulation of "archaic involvement." The second, concerning a symbiotic alliance, probes further into uncharted realms of consciousness. The description my colleagues and I (see Dolby & Sheehan, 1977; Sheehan & Dolby, 1979; Sheehan & McConkey, 1982) give to the motivated commitment of the hypnotic subject seems particularly relevant to the second of these relational dimensions: Commitment is defined in terms of subjects' imbuing the hypnotist and what is communicated by the hypnotist with special significance and importance, leading subjects to make a special motivational effort to respond according to the hypnotist's intent.

Shor's Perspective

Shor's notion of archaic involvement bears a close relation to this concept of motivated cognitive commitment. Both ideas depend in their origins on the concept of transference, which emphasizes the importance of the relationship between hypnotist and subject and the maintenance of rapport. According to Shor, archaic involvement processes include the displacement or transference of basic personality emotive attitudes evolving from early life onto the hypnotist. Thus, archaic and primitive ways of relating to the hypnotist derive from the very early relationships of life. Hence, the hypnotist may assume a form for the subject as if he or she were an object of emotional attachment. Accordingly, the subject overevaluates the hypnotist as a person to a degree that is disproportionate with the objective situation. Essentially, the subject experiences a strong desire to please the hypnotist and infuses the hypnotist with a special significance that has personal meaning. In a similar fashion, and offering data in support of the argument, I have contended (Sheehan, 1971, 1980) that hypnotic subjects perceive the implicit demands of the hypnotist in a way that necessitates an appeal to subjective involvement by them in the hypnotic context, and that the process is characterized by the hypnotist's being infused with particular significance. Finally, it must be emphasized that concepts such as archaic involvement and motivated cognitive commitment are distinct from accounts by theorists (e.g., Wagstaff, 1981) who talk of conforming, compliant subjects' wishing to obey the hypnotist by responding in a correct manner. This alternative view recognizes contextual influences, but fails to acknowledge the deeper, more profound dynamics of the hypnotic situation to which transference or relational theorizing alerts us.

Other Perspectives

There are a number of theories lying outside the field of hypnosis that have potential relevance to the explanation of hypnotic events, but have not been generally discussed or researched by investigators concerned with hypnosis. One such theory contends that each person in an interaction (in this instance, the subject and the hypnotist) constitutes the other's major environmental cue. "Social exchange theory," as this model is labeled, maintains that social exchange is based upon trust and often creates feelings of personal obligation; it is also entered into voluntarily (see Blau, 1964). Social exchange theory appears to describe a situation not unlike that encountered in the hypnotic setting.

It seems probable, however, that the interpersonal dynamics of hypnosis need to be explained in a deeper, more intense fashion and in a way that is more compatible with the concepts underlying the notion of commitment. It can be argued, for example, that the subject is generally more responsive than the hypnotist in the dyadic interactions that occur in hypnosis (Sheehan & Statham, 1988; Shor, 1962), there being an inequality in the extent of responsiveness shown in the hypnotic context by the two participants (hypnotist and subject). In contrast, the concept of "motivated cognitive commitment" seems better suited than the concept of "social exchange" to explain the particular dynamics of the hypnotist–subject interaction, and can be viewed as a more refined elaboration of the concepts of transference and archaic involvement. The concept of motivated cognitive commitment, for example, appropriately emphasizes the nature of the hypnotized subject's cognitive involvement in the suggestions that are communicated by the hypnotist, while nevertheless focusing also on the relational dimensions that characterize the exchange.

THEORETICAL CONCEPTS AND PRINCIPLES

Clearly, expectations about hypnotic response, attitudes toward hypnosis, and inference making about what the hypnotist requires can all be documented as powerful determinants of what a subject does in the hypnotic setting. It is the character of the subject's motivations and cognitions as aroused in the hypnotic setting, however, that sets the study of hypnosis apart from that of normal waking behavior. Behavior in hypnosis is motivated by the desire of the subject to repond in a socially appropriate way, but the effort is an active one: The task of responding to hypnotic suggestion can be viewed as akin to planful problem solving in a context that is defined and regulated by rules set by the hypnotist, and that engages the hypnotist and hypnotic subject in an active interaction. The process is not to be identified with conformity, or passive obedience to what the hypnotist demands. Rather, it is the reflection of a motivated cognitive effort by the subject to respond to suggestions as they are understood, within a context defined by the hypnotist. The most appropriate focus for helping us understand the nature of the subject's commitment to this task is the style of a subject's response, rather than his or her competence.

In the task of isolating those processes responsible for hypnotic behavior and experience, it is helpful to distinguish those influences that are nonhypnotic in kind from those that are hypnotic. To some, this may appear to prejudge that "hypnosis" is a meaningful concept; on the other hand, looking for distinctive determinants of the quality of hypnotic response by acknowledging the concept of hypnosis as a useful exploratory tool, provides us with a means for possibly isolating what Orne (1959) calls "essence" from "artifact." In determining essence, it seems to me that the most rewarding theoretical strategy, is to examine the fine-grained variation in responsiveness to suggestion that exists among subjects who are very deeply susceptible to hypnosis. Particular methods are required to do this, however, and this is a point to which I return later.

No matter which view one may adopt on the issues implicated by the discussion above, it is relevant to stress that strong individual differences in the degree of responsiveness to hypnotic test suggestions characterize performance in the hypnotic setting. We know that different hypnotic tasks tap particular skills and capacities (such as ideomotor involvement and cognitive/delusory thinking), yet marked differences exist in the responsiveness of highly susceptible subjects themselves. Among deeply susceptible subjects, for example, not all subjects will pass trance logic tests, and only about 50% will illustrate hidden-observer effects when standard methods are used to study them. It seems, then, that any theory purporting to explain phenomena in hypnosis must address the primary question of what explains individual differences among hypnotic subjects themselves. This is a separate (though related) issue, of course, from the description and explanation of individual differences existing among subjects in the total population.

Motivated Cognitive Commitment

The key concept in the theory being outlined here is that of "motivated cognitive commitment." This process reflects the positive motivations of the deeply susceptible subject to respond cooperatively with the hypnotist—not simply to conform, but rather to process the hypnotist's communications in a cognitively active way in order to solve the problem of responding appropriately to suggestion. Hypnotic suggestion poses a problem that the susceptible subject is motivated positively to solve. With the development of the EAT (Sheehan & McConkey, 1982), the main support for the theory comes from work done on the analysis of the meaning of experiences communicated by hypnotized subjects, and on the relevance of rapport to producing relatively distinctive hypnotic effects that tap into the essential quality of hypnotic responsiveness.

Characteristic of other models of hypnosis that pursue essential (vs. artifactual) features of hypnotic performance, the model appeals ultimately to processes that are internal rather than peripheral, and places special emphasis on the reported subjective experience of the hypnotized subject. It affords, for example, a degree of significance to experience that many other contextual models do not. The concept of "motivated cognitive commitment" indicates the special utility of acknowledging the variability in commitment to respond that exists among highly susceptible subjects themselves. This variability is not attributable to hypnotic skill or to aptitude differences in skills related to hypnotizability (such as imaginative capacity). Rather, it highlights particular processes of motivation at work that characterize the differences in level of involvement that hypnotic subjects are willing to display. These individual-difference variables and their cognitive correlates need to be studied in interaction with process and situational variables, as they operate conjointly to influence overall performance in the hypnotic setting.

Awareness of Reality

Another key theoretical feature recognized implicitly by the model, and important in its formulation, is the extent to which the hypnotized subject is capable of experiencing the world as perceived and the world as it exists at one and the same time. This is not simply a restatement of the discussion in the general literature of dualistic thinking as a cognitive style that is associated with the performance of some hypnotic subjects (see Laurence & Perry, 1981). Rather, the model highlights the relationship between suggestion and the activity of the mentation on the subject's part that is created by suggestion. It emphasizes, for instance, the cognitively active problem solver who works upon suggestions to respond in a positive and motivated way; it thus recognizes the capacity of the hypnotized subject to reformulate his or her comprehension of a suggestion, especially if it conflicts with reality or needs to be redefined as "inappropriate" in the context of hypnotic testing.

The Interactionist Properties of the Model

Essentially, the model is an interactionist one and argues strongly for features that are relevant to the current debate about the influence of trait versus situation in personality functioning. Consistent with Emmons, Diener, and Larsen (1986), for example, it argues for a move away from the additive or mechanistic account of how much variance in responsiveness can be accounted for by trait, situation, and/or interaction, and recognizes that the relationship between trait and situation is reciprocal (see also Lerner & Lerner, 1986; Vondracek, 1987). It also explicitly argues for the hypnotized individual as actively involved in constructing his or her own environment, in a goal-directed, problem-solving manner (Pervin, 1987). The hypnotic situation should be viewed as one that is created by the persons involved in it (Schneider, 1987), and the interpersonal relationships between hypnotist and subject can be seen as those of two systems both seeking to satisfy different needs in the created situation (for extensions of this argument outside the field of hypnosis, see Aronoff & Wilson, 1985; and Spokane, 1987).

Information Processing and Hypnosis

Finally, it seems appropriate to discuss the relevance of information-processing theories to this model of hypnosis. A review of cognitive psychologists' efforts to realize their goal of understanding the strategies used by individuals to process information may add valuable insights to our comprehension of the idiographic responses observed in the hypnotic setting.

It is relevant in information processing terms to distinguish among the various stages of the processing of information: acquisition, processing, and goal setting (Aronoff & Wilson, 1985). During the acquisition stage, a person scans and attends to limited sets of information that may or may not be encoded in guiding a response to a situation; strategies of search flexibility may relate to these scanning procedures. After selecting the information for attention, the person engages in solving the task for which the selection is made. Two important characteristics of processing per se are flexibility and persistence; the former is the degree to which the person is prepared to explore the problem using divergent or convergent thinking, and the latter is the degree to which the person continues in his or her attempts to encode, transform, and assimilate the information. According to such an information-processing account, the ability to use certain mechanisms efficiently in selective attention may vary, depending on the particular task involved and the ability of the person (see Tipper & Baylis, 1987). Such a view highlights the potential relevance of individual-difference factors, such as the ability to focus attention, which are so important in the hypnotic setting.

In the 1960s and 1970s, theorists perceived human information processing primarily in terms of serial processing. McClelland and Rumelhart (1986) propose that although thought and problem solving have a sequential character when viewed over a given time frame, each step in the sequence is the result of what they term "parallel distributed processing." They argue that each step in the sequence of problem solving is the result of the simultaneous activity of a large number of simple computational elements in interaction, each influencing others and being influenced by them. In this way, they oppose the type of processing suggested by E. R. Hilgard's (1977) neodissociation concept of a number of control systems arranged in a hierarchical order with a dominant or master control system, although Hilgard does suggest parallel processing (see Stava & Jaffa, 1988).

Such notions appear to tie in meaningfully with the concept of the hypnotic subject as an active participant in the hypnotic context. They are compatible, for example, with the concept of the hypnotic subject as a problem solver striving to accomplish what the hypnotist suggests, and relaxing as a solution is found and the task accomplished. Within this broad perspective, it is the interaction between the systems that holds most promise of yielding fruitful insights. At the core of the "parallel distributed processing" model of human information processing lies a dynamic, interactive, and self-organizing system. The person does not sit idly by and let the world change and then passively monitor it. Rather, the individual acts on the world. This in turn changes the environment, which then feeds back into the system and leads to another interpretation and another action. The observer has the ability to create mental models of the world, to simulate "what would happen if . . ." and then to decide to act according to the output of these models. Such concepts seem relevant to responsiveness both within and outside the hypnotic setting.

RESEARCH AND APPRAISAL

This section examines some of the relevant research that has been conducted in relation to the concepts and principles that have been outlined above. The review is not exhaustive, and evidence is sampled insofar as it seems appropriate to the model that has been outlined.

Relevance of Rapport

Lying behind the model that has been discussed is the assumption that the rapport existing between hypnotist and subject is an especially important mediating process. For the most part, the literature on hypnosis acknowledges rapport as one of many social-psychological factors that may influence hypnotic response. Barber (1969), for example, defines it as a relevant antecedent factor that has potential links with hypnotic outcomes. Orne (1959), in his original article on essence versus artifact, strongly hints at motivationally toned variables other than demand characteristics as essential determinants of hypnotic responsiveness, but does not pursue the point. There are relatively few studies, in fact, that have addressed rapport as a primary mediating variable.

I addressed the significance of rapport directly in two extensive programs of research involving numerous studies, which were reported in 1971 and 1980 respectively. The first of these programs (Sheehan, 1971) applied the real–simulating model to test the basic hypothesis that hypnotic subjects would stop responding when they perceived that the hypnotist was about to remove a suggestion, whereas simulators would not, even though both groups of subjects were led outside the hypnotic context to believe that a good hypnotic subject will continue to respond compulsively right up until the moment suggestions are finally removed. The phenomenon isolated in the work was labeled "countering," and it was proposed as an objective index of hypnotized subjects' motivated involvement with the hypnotist. It was hypothesised that deeply susceptible subjects, committed to respond in accord with the hypnotist's intent, would lay aside a preconception about hypnosis that was counter to the hypnotist's intent if the actual intent of the hypnotist and the preconception were subsequently placed in direct conflict. Results showed that subjects who were susceptible to hypnosis countered their preconception in favor of the hypnotist and stopped responding by reason of their subjective involvement with trance events, while simulators (see Orne, 1979) exposed to the same influences did not. The phenomenon of countering was shown to be durable and particular interpersonal orientations characterized the susceptible group. Collectively, the data from the five studies reported in the 1971 program of work indexed susceptible subjects' distinctive involvement in hypnotic events and highlighted the special importance to susceptible subjects of their relationship with the hypnotist.

Later work (Sheehan, 1980) further investigated the phenomenon of countering by exploring the parameters of the index. This research investigated the special relevance of rapport processes to the hypnotic setting, and manipulated rapport across a range of studies that varied either the warmth or genuineness of the hypnotist. It was predicted from theorizing about transference and motivated cognitive commitment that countering would decrease in the negative context, but would increase in the positive one. Results confirmed predictions for deeply susceptible subjects tested in the former context, but not the latter. In the negative setting, subjects were inhibited in their rate of countering, but maintained their previous level of response to the hypnotist when rapport was facilitated. The data highlighted, as before, the relevance of interpersonal processes to theorizing about hypnosis. A particularly interesting aspect of the data reported, however, was that, on the average, counterers passed fewer Stanford Hypnotic Susceptibility Scale, Form C (SHSS:C) items than did noncountering subjects in 90% of the comparisons that were made. Only in one comparison was there a trend for this particular pattern of data to be reversed. The quite remarkable stability of the data in this respect suggested that it is inaccurate to associate the pattern of responsiveness of hypnotized subjects with greater behavioral compliance with suggestion, or overall conformity to respond. The same persons who detected and responded to the hypnotist's intent were *not* those subjects who responded best to the hypnotist's overt, direct communications on standard test tasks. The argument here, in favor of the model that has been outlined, is that hypnotic skill is not unimportant to the occurrence of hypnotic phenomena; however, there are interindividual differences in behavior among deeply susceptible subjects that defy explanation in terms of simple compliance or of ability to perform routinely in the hypnotic context.

The data from both programs of work are consistent with the theory that hypnotized subjects will work in a committed fashion to cognitively process the communications that they receive, so as to respond appropriately to what the hypnotist wants. They point to the relevance of isolating the "cohesive cognitive organizations" (Rapaport, 1951) that appear to differentiate hypnotic from waking consciousness.

Among the few investigators who have extensively researched the variable of rapport are Lynn and his associates. Essentially arguing for the relevance of studying the interactions between and among contextual influences, attitudes and beliefs about hypnosis, trait levels of hypnotizability and degree of rapport existing between subject and hypnotist, Lynn believes that these and other phenomena interact actively to produce the final behavioral and subjective responses that are observed in the hypnotic context.

Frauman, Lynn, Hardaway, and Molteni (1984) subtly manipulated affective interpersonal factors by subliminally exposing subjects to the message "Mommy and I are one." Another group were presented with a neutral subliminal stimulus ("People are walking"). The message that the experimental group was shown was congruent with Shor's (1962) concept of archaic involvement. Results showed that the "Mommy" group, given a choice, was willing to discuss topics with the hypnotist that were significantly more positive in nature than the topics the neutral group was willing to discuss. Frauman et al. (1984) inferred from this that the "Mommy" subjects felt more positive rapport toward the hypnotist than did the control group. Although there was no concrete behavioral effect, data were supportive of the notion of affective factors as important in hypnosis.

In a later study involving three groups of subjects, Gfeller, Lynn, and Pribble (1987) tested subjects under conditions designed to create a high level of rapport between subject and hypnotist. A second group was manipulated so as to facilitate a lower level of rapport, while a third group had no rapport enhancement at all. Subjects rated their feelings of rapport on a 5-pt. scale. Analysis indicated that the subjects in the two rapport enhancing conditions rated levels of rapport as higher than subjects in the control condition. However, rapport ratings did not differ significantly between the two treatment groups. These results are congruent with my own data (Sheehan, 1980), which showed that once rapport is facilitated (even in small amounts), it is difficult to produce large objective changes in hypnotic performance by further increasing (or attempting to increase) rapport. This points to rapport's existing as an "either–or" phenomenon, rather than on a continuum where it occurs in strongly varying degrees.

In a more recent study, Lynn, Weekes, Matyi, and Neufeld (1988) tested 274 subjects to investigate the effects of direct versus indirect suggestions of archaic involvement with the hypnotist. A newly developed test for measuring archaic involvement based on nineteen 7-point Likert-type scales, was used (see Nash & Spinler, 1989). Indirect suggestions created more archaic involvement among subjects than direct suggestions on two of the three factors that characterized the new test ("positive emotional bond to the hypnotist" and "fear of negative appraisal"). Thus, the wording of hypnotic communications affects subjects' experience of the hypnotist and the hypnotic relationship. This sits comfortably with our interactionist account of hypnosis (Sheehan & McConkey, 1982), which gives considerable weight to situational factors as well as the influence of trait.

Results across the programs of research conducted by Lynn and his associates and myself are not entirely comparable (e.g., Lynn, Nash, Rhue, Frauman, & Sweeney, 1984); however, sufficient congruity exists to point to the importance of further pursuing rapport as a variable of considerable influence. There is a need, however, to develop appropriately subtle measures of rapport to detect the effects that can be observed. Across existing studies reported in the literature, for example, there has been frequent support for effects' being stronger for subjective than for objective measures. It may well be that we must wait for the construction of subtle measures to illustrate the objective accompaniments of the subjective effects that have been demonstrated.

"Rapport" also may only be a partially suitable term to describe the complexity of the involvement that exists between hypnotist and subject. Certainly, measures have been designed to assess it that do not seem appropriate to the process that is at issue. Young (1927), for example, concluded that rapport was not important to our understanding of hypnosis, on the basis of his finding that subjects' decisions prior to hypnosis (i.e., that they would not be responsive to a particular hypnotic suggestion during hypnosis) proved more powerful than the hypnotist's later contrary instructions. The comparison that was made, however, confounded auto- and heterosuggestion. If a heterosuggestion is ignored during hypnosis, it may simply mean that the initial autosuggestion and accompanying rapport have remained potent throughout the hypnotic session.

As previously discussed, Diamond has importantly emphasized the significance of the relational dimension to the explanation of hypnotic behavior, yet relatively few studies have borne directly upon his model. As noted earlier, Frauman et al. (1984) showed that the unconscious activation of symbiotic fantasies before trance induction increased rapport with the hypnotist ($p < .044$, based on those subjects choosing more positive topics for disclosure) this provides some support for the importance of symbiotic alliances in hypnosis. Another study with 18 male schizophrenics (Silverman, Spiro, Weissberg, & Candell, 1969) also appears to offer support for the relevance of symbiotic alliances. In this study, subjects rated themselves as being relatively differentiated from a presented mother figure. When subliminally exposed to the message "Mommy and I are one" and an accompanying picture of a man and woman fused at the shoulders, subjects exhibited a decrease in pathology. Silverman and Weinberger (1985) claim that at least 12 experiments have since replicated these results (e.g., Bronstein & Rodin, 1983). At a clinical level, Chertok (1983) argues also that the hypnotised person may fuse with the hypnotist, and details five case histories that illustrate the successful use of hypnosis incorporating this element, in the treatment of various ailments. Symbiotic alliance, then, appears to be a reliable and clinically sensitive phenomenon, and data suggest the value of pursuing it further in hypnotic research.

Cognitive Discriminability

One of the common theoretical processes that appears to characterize contextual models of hypnosis is the emphasis these models place, in various ways, on the capacity of the hypnotic subject to process suggestion communications in an active fashion. In essence, this issue refers to the definition of the relationship between suggestion and mode of processing the information that is communicated. Spanos (1986), for example, talks of strategic enactment in hypnosis, which highlights the role cognitive strategies play in hypnotic subjects' execution of their hypnotic response. The same emphasis is also implied strongly in Wagstaff's (1981) account of the compliant, conforming subject's wanting to obey the hypnotist and respond in an appropriate way. Kruse (1989) talks in a related fashion about the process of discrimination—a conception on his part that focuses on subjects' constructing cognitions in response to suggestions.

Kruse's faculty of discrimination is not unlike our own (Sheehan & McConkey, 1982) concept of problem solving and Spanos's notions about the strategies that subjects employ to enact suggestions. All share the same active, cognitive character in the influences that are argued. Data are needed, however, to test for the complexity that my model argues is essential. The complexity of possible contextual responses is recognized through Bandura's (1978) concept of reciprocal determinism, but even this concept seems poorly equipped to handle the degree of complexity implied by the constantly changing flux of influences that can occur in the hypnotic context, from one participant of the hypnotic interaction to the other (for further discussion, see Sheehan, 1989).

Some data do exist that address this possible complexity, and results again are not compatible with a strictly compliance-based account of hypnosis. They do not, for example, lend themselves readily to the view that socio-cognitive factors operate routinely in the hypnotic setting to shape subjects' reactions in a purely conforming way. My colleagues and I (Sheehan, Donovan, & McLeod, 1988), for example, investigated Stroop interference in subjects who were either high or low in susceptibility to hypnosis, and found that highly susceptible subjects freely selected appropriate strategies when hypnotized. When not instructed to use strategies on the Stroop task, they did not use strategies. However, later when provided with an attention-focusing instruction under hypnosis, high-susceptibility subjects sharply reduced the Stroop effect by using strategies, while low-susceptibility subjects decreased it only slightly. The total absence of reported strategies for highly susceptible subjects in the one condition, and the increased interference that these same individuals displayed later, suggest that it is not simply a matter of subjects in hypnosis doing what is appropriate. If strategic enactment is routine, then strategies ought to have been used by hypnotic subjects in hypnosis even when not instructed to use them.

In some respects, the effects obtained in this study are akin to seemingly earlier paradoxical findings elsewhere (e.g., Sheehan, 1979) that subjects who are clearly motivated to resolve conflict to favor the hypnotist's intent, and who counter preconceptions about hypnosis, nevertheless perform reliably less well on standard suggestion tasks than do nonhypnotic, low-susceptibility subjects. The nature of the subjective involvement of susceptible subjects is clearly paramount. Deeply suscepti-ble subjects solve the problem of responding to suggestion in ways that are appropriate to them and that are congruent with their personal commit-ment to perform. This raises, of course, the issue of cognitive styles of responding and individual differences in them.

Styles of Responding

There are meaningful consistencies in the data with respect to the various styles and modes of responding that hypnotic subjects demonstrate (for a detailed discussion of these, see Sheehan & McConkey, 1982). The cognitive styles that we isolated initially (Sheehan & McConkey, 1982) were labeled "concentrative," "independent," and "constructive," and particular styles have been linked with specific levels of aptitude in interaction with suggestion tasks of specific difficulty. These three styles, however, are far from exhaustive of the different modes of processing that exist. There is now substantial evidence, for example, of individual differences in "cognitive flexibility." Data collected by Laurence and Perry (1981), for example, have demonstrated flexible acceptance of multiple cognitive perspectives among some hypnotic subjects. These same subjects were those who could experience the hidden-observer effect. The evidence suggests also that cognitive flexibility is a style that is relatively pervasive. It has been isolated, for instance, in work by Crawford and Allen (1983) where holistic versus detailed modes of processing were relevant to explaining individual differences in memory for picture material. Finally, integral to the concept of style are assumptions about the variability, individuality, and complexity of hypnotic reaction; all of these reflect key features of the general model that has been outlined.

An Illustration of Contextual Influences at Work

At this point, it seems appropriate to illustrate the investigation of hypnosis and context in a study that represents the model under discussion. The example serves to highlight the potential of the model for useful research, as well as the difficulties that may remain in attempting to measure the processes at issue.

The major focus of the study (Keegan, 1987), which was conducted in the hypnosis laboratory at the University of Queensland, was on the phenomenon of duality in age regression. This phenomenon is especially relevant to the model, in that it addresses the capacity to experience fantasy and reality simultaneously; the notion of active problem solving incorporated within the model implies at least some evidence of contact with reality, as well as with suggestion. In Keegan's study, the communications of the hypnotist were examined in detail for the impact of the linguistic references made to the fantasy aspects of regression and to objective reality. Typically, references both to fantasy and to reality vary frequently through standard hypnotic communications on this (and other) items. In accord with the methodology underlying the model under discussion, a fine-grained analysis of moment-by-moment variations in subjects' experiences was conducted using the EAT procedures (Sheehan and McConkey, 1982). The contextual variable that was the focus of the research was classified as "pragmatic ambiguity," (PA) defined as the relative strength of reality messages over suggestion messages. When PA is low, for example, references to the testing (real) context are kept as indirect as possible, and suggestion messages are strong (e.g., "You are at home with your mother, enjoying a game"); when pragmatic ambiguity is high, all references to the testing context are direct and strong, and suggestion messages are weak (e.g., "And you write that sentence for me now"). It was expected that PA would relate meaningfully to the capacity of subjects to recognize suggested and real frames of reference simultaneously (illustrating duality).

The PA of the hypnotist's communications was manipulated across eight segments of the age regression item. The item was administered by one experimenter (the hypnotist), and an EAT session was conducted by an independent experimenter to explore the phenomenological impact of the regression item on the subjects who were tested. Ratings of EAT interviews were conducted for 29 highly susceptible hypnotic subjects. These ratings indicated that approximately 50% of the subject sample (as one would expect) reported duality. As PA became extreme, however, reality awareness predominated for most but not all subjects. Evidence overall showed a strong relationship between levels of PA and duality: Increasing PA across the course of the age regression item generally produced increased reality awareness, as measured by the duality rating scale. Results also supported the notion that duality response is a stable individual difference response style; duality ratings were relatively consistent, for example, across similar (e.g., moderate) levels of PA.

Keegan's (1987) study can be viewed as an analysis of the effect of metacontext (experimental context) intrusion into the context established by age regression communications. The fine-grained analysis of subjects' reactions over short time segments highlighted meaningful effects, as predicted from a contextualist frame of reference. However, the research only went some distance toward achieving the methodological ideals of a contextual model. The relationship under test, for example, was essentially conceptualized in analytical terms (e.g., it was hypothesized that the wording of the hypnotist's communications would lead to [cause?] changes in experience). Furthermore, the wording and the hypnotist's behavior were controlled, thereby placing inevitable constraints on the hypnotist–subject dyad. Although the EAT probed appropriately for the influence of expectancies, impressions, and subjective involvement, the hypnotist offered no indication that she felt any freedom to adapt her performance to subjects' reactions.

Having evaluated the work from within the framework of the contextual model, however, I must add that if the hypnotist and subject had both been free to interact as they wished, then the independent variable under scrutiny (the level of ambiguity of the hypnotist's verbal communications) would have been far less controlled than it in fact was. Although the research highlighted a new contextual variable in operation, and allowed fresh insights to be developed about duality as a cognitive style, the dynamic give-and-take between subject and hypnotist could not have been fully studied by the relatively analytical procedures that were adopted without interfering with the predictive strength of the experimental design. To depart radically from controlled procedures, however, would have been to forgo adherence to what we know as good experimental design. Clearly, more work is required to research the theoretical possibilities raised by the contextualist perspective (while continuing to maintain methodological strength).

CONCLUSION

There are several different ways to classify the model that is expounded in this chapter. One may view it, as I have argued elsewhere (Sheehan, 1986b), as an individual-differences model of hypnosis, because it emphasizes the significance of intragroup differences in the pattern of hypnotic performance. Alternatively, one may view it as a phenomenologically based model, in the way that is conveyed by another work (Sheehan and McConkey, 1982). Invariably, however, single categories fail to do justice to the nature of theories, and hence it is perhaps wisest to view this theory as a means of exploring particular hypotheses about hypnotic phenomena that focus primarily on the meaning of suggestion as perceived by susceptible subjects. This model focuses, in a way that most other theories do not, on the motivational implications of the cognitive involvement of the susceptible subject in the events of the hypnotic setting. It offers a variant of contextual theories of psychological functioning, but is experiential in its emphasis rather than simply behavioral.

The motivated cognitive commitment of hypnotic subjects is the central concept of the theory, and it expresses more than the simple cooperation of subjects, their response to demand characteristics, or their response to the pressure to conform. Essentially, it is an expression of the internal process that defines the hypnotic subject's problem solving attempts to respond appropriately to hypnotic suggestion.

It has not been my intention in this chapter to attempt to define conditions that would critically differentiate the model proposed here from others. There are points of similarity and contrast in my theory with models that are described elsewhere in this book. Pointed differentiation of theories from one another is an elusive goal and serves more to polarize differences among theorists than to demonstrate the ways in which different perspectives may usefully converge on the meaning of phenomena. Theories should be seen not as ways of claiming exclusive rights to truth, but as devices to forge a path through the data we collect. In that sense, I hope that the model I have outlined is useful. Only continued research, of course, will establish the limits of that utility.

Acknowledgments. The research for this chapter was supported by a grant from the Australian Research Council made to the author. I wish to thank Scott Ferguson and Patricia Truesdale for their help in the preparation of the chapter.

REFERENCES

Aronoff, J., & Wilson, J. P. (1985). *Personality in the social process.* Hillsdale, NJ: Erlbaum.

Barber, T. X. (1969). *Hypnosis: A scientific approach.* New York: Van Nostrand Reinhold.

Bandura, A. (1978). The self system in reciprocal determinism. *American Psychologist, 33,* 344–358.

Blau, P. (1964). *Exchange and power in social life.* New York: Wiley.

Bronstein, A., & Rodin, G. (1983). An experimental study of internalization fantasies in schizophrenic men. *Psychotherapy: Theory, Research and Practice, 20,* 408–416.

Chertok, L. (1983). Psychoanalysis and hypnosis theory: Comments on five case histories. *American Journal of Clinical Hypnosis, 25,* 209–224.

Crawford, H. J., & Allen, S. N. (1983). Enhanced visual memory during hypnosis as mediated by hypnotic responsiveness and cognitive strategies. *Journal of Experimental Psychology: General, 112,* 662–685.

Diamond, M. J. (1987). The interactional basis of hypnotic experience: On the relational dimensions of hypnosis. *International Journal of Clinical and Experimental Hypnosis, 35,* 95–115.

Dolby, R., & Sheehan, P. W. (1977). Cognitive processing and expectancy behavior in hypnosis. *Journal of Abnormal Psychology, 86,* 334–345.

Emmons, R. A., Diener, E., & Larsen, R. J. (1986). Choice and avoidance of everday situations and affect congruence: Two models of reciprocal interaction. *Journal of Personality and Social Psychology, 51,* 815–826.

Fourie, D. P. (1983). Width of the hypnotic relationship: An interactional view of hypnotic susceptibility and hypnotic depth. *Australian Journal of Clinical and Experimental Hypnosis, 11,* 1–14.

Frauman, D. C., Lynn, S. J., Hardaway, R. A., & Molteni, A. L. (1984). Effect of subliminal symbiotic activation on hypnotic rapport and susceptibility. *Journal of Abnormal Psychology, 93,* 481–483.

Gfeller, J. D., Lynn, S. J., & Pribble, W. E. (1987). Enhancing hypnotic susceptibility: Interpersonal and rapport factors. *Journal of Personality and Social Psychology, 52,* 586–595.

Hammer, A. G. (1961). Reflections on the study of hypnosis. *Australian Journal of Psychology, 13,* 3–22.

Hilgard, E. R. (1977). *Divided consciousness: Multiple controls in human thought and action.* New York: Wiley.

Keegan, F. J. (1987). *Duality and context: A fine grained experiental analysis of the effects of hypnotist communications.* Unpublished honours dissertation, University of Queensland, St. Lucia, Queensland, Australia.

Keeney, B. P. (1982). What is an epistemology of family therapy? *Family Processes, 21*, 153–168.

Kruse, P. (1989). Some suggestions about suggestion and hypnosis: A radical constructivist view. In V. A. Gheorghiu, P. Netter, H. J. Eysenck, & R. Rosenthal (Eds.), *Suggestion and suggestibility: Theory and research.* Berlin: Springer-Verlag.

Laurence, J. R., & Perry, C. W. (1981). The "hidden observer" phenomenon in hypnosis: Some additional findings. *Journal of Abnormal Psychology, 90*, 334–344.

Lerner, R. M., Hultsch, D. F., & Dixon, R. A. (1983). Contextualism and the character of developmental psychology in the 1970s. In J. W. Dauben & V. S. Sexton (Eds.), *Essays in the Philosophy of Science* (pp. 101–128). New York: New York Academy of Sciences.

Lerner, R. M., & Lerner, J. V. (1986). Contextualism and the study of child effects in development. In R. L. Rosnow & M. Georgoudi (Eds.), *Contextualism and understanding in behavioral science: Implications for theory and research* (pp. 89–104). New York: Praeger.

Lynn, S. J., Nash, M. R., Rhue, J. W., Frauman, D. C., & Sweeney, C. A. (1984). Nonvolition, expectancies, and hypnotic rapport. *Journal of Abnormal Psychology, 93*, 295–303.

Lynn, S. J., Weekes, J. R., Matyi, C. L., & Neufeld, V. (1988). Direct versus indirect suggestions, archaic involvement, and hypnotic experience. *Journal of Abnormal Psychology, 97*, 296–301.

McClelland, J. L., & Rumelhart, D. E. (1986). *Parallel distributed processing: Explorations in the microstructure of cognition.* Cambridge, MA: MIT Press.

Mischel, W. (1979). On the interface of congition and personality: Beyond the person-situation debate. *American Psychologist, 34*, 740–754.

Nash, M. R., & Spinler, D. (1989). Hypnosis and transference: A measure of archaic involvement with the hypnotist. *International Journal of Clinical and Experimental Hypnosis, 37*, 129–144.

Orne, M. T. (1959). The nature of hypnosis: Artifact and essence. *Journal of Abnormal and Social Psychology, 58*, 277–299.

Orne, M. T. (1979). On the simulating subject as a quasicontrol group in hypnosis research: What, why, and how. In E. Fromm & R. E. Shor (Eds.), *Hypnosis: Developments in research and new perspectives* (2nd ed., pp. 519–565). Hawthorne, NY: Aldine.

Pervin, L. A. (1987). Person-environment congruence in the light of the person-situation controversy. *Journal of Vocational Behavior, 31*, 222–230.

Rapaport, D. (1951). *Organization and pathology of thought.* New York: Columbia University Press.

Rosnow, R. L. (1981). *Paradigms in transition: The methodology of social inquiry.* New York: Oxford University Press.

Sarbin, T. R. (1982). Contextualism: A world view for modern psychology. In W. L.

Allen & K. E. Scheibe (Eds.), *The social context of conduct: Psychological writings of Theodore Sarbin* (pp. 15–34). New York: Praeger.

Sarbin, T. R., & Coe, W. C. (1972). *Hypnosis: A social psychological analysis of influence communication.* New York: Holt, Rinehart & Winston.

Schneider, B. (1987). E = f(P,B): The road to a radical approach to person–environment fit. *Journal of Vocational Behavior, 31*, 353–361.

Sheehan, P. W. (1971). Countering preconceptions about hypnosis: An objective index of involvement with the hypnotist. *Journal of Abnormal Psychology Monograph, 78*, 299–322.

Sheehan, P. W. (1979). Expectancy reactions in hypnosis. In G. D. Burrows, & D. R. Collison (Eds.), *Hypnosis 1979* (pp. 25–32). Amsterdam: Elsevier.

Sheehan, P. W. (1980). Factors influencing rapport in hypnosis. *Journal of Abnormal Psychology, 89*, 263–281.

Sheehan, P. W. (1986a). [Review of *The social context of conduct: Psychological writings of Theodore Sarbin*]. *International Journal of Clinical and Experimental Hypnosis, 34*, 55–59.

Sheehan, P. W. (1986b). An individual differences account of hypnosis. In P. L. N. Naish (Ed.), *What is hypnosis? Current theories and research* (pp. 145–161). Milton Keynes, England: Open University Press.

Sheehan, P. W. (1989). The nature of Australian psychology— From cross cultural analysis of theorising about the role of context in hypnosis. *International Journal of Psychology, 24*, 315–331.

Sheehan, P. W., & Dolby, R. (1979). Motivated involvement in hypnosis: The illustration of clinical rapport through hypnotic dreams. *Journal of Abnormal Psychology, 88*, 573– 583.

Sheehan, P. W., Donovan, P., & McLeod, C. (1988). Strategy manipulation and the stroop effect in hypnosis. *Journal of Abnormal Psychology, 4*, 455–460.

Sheehan, P. W., & McConkey, K. M. (1982). *Hypnosis and experience: The exploration of phenomena and process.* Hillsdale, NJ: Erlbaum.

Sheehan, P. W., & Statham, D. (1988). Associations between lying and hypnosis: An empirical analysis. *British Journal of Experimental and Clinical Hypnosis, 5*, 87–94.

Shor, R. E. (1962)., Three dimensions of hypnotic depth. *International Journal of Clinical and Experimental Hypnosis, 10*, 23–28.

Shor, R. E. (1979). A phenomenological method for the measurement of variables important to an understanding of the nature of hypnosis. In E. Fromm, & R. E. Shor (Eds.), *Hypnosis: Developments in research and new perspectives* (pp. 105–135). Hawthorne, N.Y.: Aldine.

Silverman, L. H., Spiro, R. H., Weissberg, J. S., & Candell, P. (1969). The effects of aggressive activation and the need to merge on pathological thinking in schizophrenia. *Journal of Nervous and Mental Diseases, 148*, 39–51.

Silverman, L. H., & Weinberger, J. (1985). Mommy and I are one: Implications for psychotherapy. *American Psychologist, 40*, 1296–1308.

Spanos, N. P. (1986). Hypnotic behavior: A social psychological interpretation of amnesia, analgesia and "trance logic." *Behavioral and Brain Sciences, 9*, 449–467.

Spokane, A. R. (1987). Conceptual and methodological issues in person– environment fit research. *Journal of Vocational Behavior, 31*, 217–221.

Stava, L. J., & Jaffa, M. (1988). Some operationalizations of the neodissociation concept and their relationship to hypnotic susceptibility. *Journal of Personality and Social Psychology, 54,* 989–996.

Sutcliffe, J. P. (1958). *Hypnotic behavior: Fantasy or simulation?* Unpublished doctoral dissertation, University of Sydney, Sydney, New South Wales, Australia.

Tipper, S. P., & Baylis, G. C. (1987). Individual differences in selective attention: The relation of priming and interference to cognitive failure. *Personality and Individual Differences, 8,* 667–675.

Vondracek, F. W. (1987). Comments with a focus on Pervin's paper. *Journal of Vocational Behavior, 31,* 341–346.

Wagstaff, G. F. (1981). *Hypnosis, compliance and belief.* Brighton, England: Harvester.

Witkin, H. A. (1978). *Cognitive styles in personal and cultural adaptation.* Worcester, MA: Clark University Press.

Young, P. C. (1927). Is rapport an essential characteristic of hypnosis? *Journal of Abnormal Psychology, 22,* 130–139.

The Construction and Resolution of Experience and Behavior in Hypnosis

KEVIN M. McCONKEY
Macquarie University

INTRODUCTION

Hypnotized subjects shape their subjective experiences in a way that is consistent with their interpretation of the communications of the hypnotist. The experience and behavior of hypnotized subjects reflect an interplay of the cognitive skills of the subjects and the social cues of the hypnotic setting. In this chapter, I present a perspective on hypnosis that emphasizes that the experience and behavior of hypnotized subjects should be understood in terms of particular cognitive and social processes. Moreover, I consider that the complexity of the interaction between those processes should not be underestimated. From this perspective, I attempt to assist understanding of hypnosis, and to provide a particular framework for the further investigation of hypnotic phenomena.

Some Influential Views

Much of the current theorizing about hypnosis can be traced to the work of White (1937, 1941), who pointed to the various types of responses that could occur in hypnotized subjects. In his examination of the responses of active and passive subjects during hypnosis, in particular, White (1937) made a number of points that are relevant to the perspective I present in this chapter. For example, he highlighted that the hypnotic setting contains a number of paradoxes if the communications of the hypnotist are taken literally. When the hypnotist says, for instance, that the subjects are getting sleepier and sleepier and falling into a deep sleep, the hypnotist obviously does not mean this in a literal sense. Similarly, when the hypnotist says that the subjects are now 5 years of age, or now can see nothing, or now can remember nothing, it is clear that the hypnotist does not mean this literally. Rather, the hypnotist is asking the subjects to experience at a phenomenal level the state of affairs that would occur if the communications of the hypnotist were correct in a literal sense. As White (1937) argued, the hypnotist is conveying his or her wishes about a particular state of affairs. The communication of these wishes by the hypnotist is inherently paradoxical, however, and must be interpreted by the subjects in a way that makes sense to them. Thus, the subjects' interpretations of the communications of the hypnotist, rather than the communications themselves, shape the responses that occur in the hypnotic setting.

White (1937) also pointed to the importance of understanding how a subject's own expectations and wishes influence and ultimately determine the hypnotic responses that occur. Thus, the relationship between the hypnotized subject and the hypnotist was an important element in his theorizing. He spoke, for instance, of the "pleasure of obedience" in which, at least for the period of their dyadic interaction, carrying out the wishes of the hypnotist becomes the wishes of the subject. Moreover, White (1937) argued that hypnotized subjects bring "natures predisposed" to interpret and respond to the communications of the hypnotist in a way that is consistent with their role as hypnotic subjects. That is, hypnotized subjects process information on the basis of a preparedness to respond in a particular way, and this allows them to make sense of the communications of the hypnotist. Hypnotized subjects, in this sense, should be seen as working to resolve the demands that impinge upon them from a number of different sources of influence.

In an extension of these views that placed a greater emphasis on the social psychology of the interaction between hypnotized subjects and the hypnotist, White (1941) argued that "hypnotic behavior is meaningful, goal-directed striving, its most general goal being to behave like a hypnotized person as this is continuously defined by the operator and understood by the subject" (p. 483). White's notion that goal-directed striving is central to the responses of hypnotized subjects importantly underscored that both the subjects and the hypnotist are in the hypnotic setting for a reason. This reason is for the subjects to experience phenomenal events and display behavior that they may not experience and display in a nonhypnotic setting. As White (1941) noted, however, even if the behavior that occurs in the hypnotic setting also occurs in nonhypnotic settings, this does not exempt theorists and researchers from explaining why the behavior occurs in the hypnotic setting.

For White (1941), the fact that "mere words" from the hypnotist could initiate a variety of profound changes in the experience and behavior of subjects was an intriguing state of affairs. The diversity of views presented in this volume indicates that this state of affairs maintains its intrigue 50 years later. White (1941) argued that the goal-directed striving of a subject in the hypnotic setting "takes place in an altered state of the person" (p. 489). Thus, he saw hypnosis as involving a change in the phenomenal experience of subjects. That change was defined in part by the social characteristics of the setting and in part by the cognitive skills that the subjects used to respond in accord with the communications of the hypnotist. At this level, the views of White (1937, 1941) provide an important preface to my own views.

Shor (1959, 1962) extended the theorizing of White (1937, 1941) and presented a series of propositions that attempted to explain the alterations of experience characteristic of hypnosis and related phenomena. An essential concept in these propositions was that of the "generalized reality orientation," which he defined as the "structured frame of reference in the background of attention which supports, interprets, and gives meaning to all experiences" (Shor, 1959, p. 585). Shor (1959) argued that specific task orientations also occur within the generalized reality orientation, and highlighted that the occurrence of these two cognitive processes is central to the experience of hypnosis. Specifically, he argued that hypnosis involves both the relative fading of the generalized reality orientation, and the construction of a specific orientation to the tasks defined by the communications of the hypnotist and understood by the subjects. Consistent with the perspective that I am presenting, Shor (1959, 1962) argued also that the phenomenon of hypnosis is characterized by a special relationship between the subjects and the hypnotist, and by a particular preparedness of the subjects to experience events consistent with their personal commitment to behave as hypnotic subjects.

Attentional processes and awareness were central aspects of the views of Shor (1959). He used the notion of the generalized reality orientation, or the subject's overall frame of reference, to argue that information can both exist and be influential either inside or outside the awareness of the subject. Whether the information is processed inside or outside the awareness of the subject depends on the subject's generalized reality orientation and on the specific task orientation that is occurring. Importantly, he argued also that a specific task orientation can itself be outside the awareness of the subjects, and can influence their experience and behavior even though they may not be aware of that influence. The emphasis that Shor (1959, 1962) placed on attentional processes and awareness anticipated, in an essential sense, much of the current theoretical and empirical work in hypnosis specifically and cognitive psychology generally on the construct of awareness (e.g., see Kihlstrom, 1987).

Although he drew upon White (1937, 1941), Shor (1959, 1962) emphasized much more the importance of understanding the experience of the hypnotized subject. He offered insights into that experience by focusing on the cognitive processes at work in the hypnotized subject. For instance, Shor (1962) argued that much of the experience of the hypnotized subject is a consequence of the subject's own "structured strivings," and that these strivings, or goal-directed personal activities, are based on both cognitive and motivational aspects within the subject. Moreover, he clarified that the subject who is striving to play the role of the hypnotized subject is not necessarily doing this with awareness. Rather, the experience and behavior of the hypnotized subject can occur "without the experience of conscious intention" (Shor, 1962, p. 29). Consistent with this notion, my perspective underscores that hypnotized subjects intend to respond, at least at some level, to the communications of the hypnotist. I consider, however, that this intention does not necessarily occur within the awareness of the subjects. Rather, the intention to experience the suggested effects, as well as the strategies that are used to enact those effects, may occur outside the awareness of subjects.

At about the period of Shor's (1959, 1962) writings, there was intense activity on both theoretical and methodological fronts in the area of hypnosis. The work of Orne (1959) and Sutcliffe (1960, 1961), for instance, was highly influential. In his classic paper on differentiating the "valid and significant aspects" of hypnosis from the artifactual elements that surround the behavior of subjects in the hypnotic setting, Orne (1959) pointed to the importance of understanding the subjective experience of the hypnotized subject. As he emphasized, "an important attribute of hypnosis is a potentiality for the [subject] to experience as subjectively real suggested alterations in his environment that do not conform with reality" (Orne, 1959, p. 297). In this respect, Orne (1959) argued that the hypnotized subject develops a transient belief that the state of affairs is as conveyed by the communications of the hypnotist rather than by the information that comes from objective reality. Thus, the subject's interpretation and experience of events, rather than the objective features of the situation, play the major role in the occurrence of hypnotic phenomena. The notion that the subjective experience of the hypnotized subject is the critical feature in need of explanation has been long argued by Orne (1959, 1977). That notion is central to my perspective as well.

Sutcliffe (1960, 1961) focused on the observation that hypnotized subjects develop a belief in the genuineness of the subjective effects that they experience. In his analysis of hypnotic phenomena and their explanation by various investigators, Sutcliffe (1960, 1961) highlighted the dichotomy between "credulous" and "skeptical" views about hypnosis, which saw hypnotic phenomena as being like actual phenomena or as being based on imagination, respectively. He illustrated how these different views made different assumptions, involved different methodologies, and accepted different data as admissible evidence. That dichotomy, albeit in more modern guise, can be seen in many of the chapters in this volume. Moreover, Sutcliffe's (1960, 1961) analysis of the dichotomy remains valid today, in the sense that neither extremely credulous nor extremely skeptical views can provide a full explanation of the phenomena associated with hypnosis. To avoid the major problems associated with these extreme views, Sutcliffe (1961) argued that "the main feature of [hypnosis] is the hypnotized subject's emotional conviction that the world is as suggested by the hypnotist" (p. 200). Moreover, he argued that attempts to explain hypnosis should focus on this feature. Consistent with this, I also consider that systematic research is needed on the precise relevance of transient delusion (I use the term "delusion" in a nonpejorative sense) to the occurrence of hypnotic phenomena. In a basic sense, the development of a false belief on the part of the hypnotized subject can be said to be a central feature of hypnosis.

Sutcliffe (1960, 1961) believed that this development of a false belief or "delusory conviction" occurs because of both the cognitive and the social events associated with hypnosis. Specifically, Sutcliffe (1960, 1961) considered that the emotional conviction of hypnotized subjects occurs because of their use of cognitive strategies that selectively focus attention on some but not other information, and because of the social or interpersonal features of their dyadic interaction with the hypnotist. The interaction of these cognitive and social processes encourages the establishment of a context of credibility, in which the subjects accept the genuineness of the events suggested by the hypnotist and experienced by themselves.

The views of investigators such as White (1937, 1941), Shor (1959, 1962), Orne (1959, 1977), and Sutcliffe (1960, 1961) not only converged to some extent, but also provided distinct emphases that have shaped much contemporary research in the area of hypnosis. Moreover, the approach of Barber (1969), the theorizing of Sarbin and Coe (1972), and the perspective of Hilgard (1977) each provided distinct emphases and contrasts whose influence can be seen in virtually all contemporary research and theory in the area. Because these positions are represented elsewhere in this volume, I turn now to summarize some recent work that underlies the specific perspective I am presenting here.

Understanding Subjective Experience

Understanding more about the subjective experience of the hypnotized subject was a major focus of my work with Sheehan (Sheehan & McConkey, 1982), and stimulated the development of the "experiential analysis technique" (EAT). In that work, we viewed hypnotized subjects as cognitively active participants who process the information that they receive, both from the communications of the hypnotist and from objective reality, in a way that allows them to enact their desired role in the hypnotic setting. Moreover, we highlighted that researchers should not lose sight of the fact that the hypnotized subject is a functioning subject who thinks, feels, and strives to respond in a social setting of considerable complexity. Our emphasis (Sheehan & McConkey, 1982) on both cognitive and social processes underscored the basic notion that behavior is ultimately the outcome of a bidirectional interaction between internal personal factors and external environmental influences.

The EAT was designed to be a procedure of subjective inquiry. It involves subjects' watching videotapes of their hypnotic testing and commenting about their experience and behavior during that testing. We used the EAT to explore the processes involved in a range of hypnotic phenomena, and the details of these investigations are presented elsewhere (Sheehan & McConkey, 1982). In commenting on the findings from these applications of the EAT, however, we (Sheehan & McConkey, 1982) adopted a cognitive and subject-oriented framework that emphasized the degree to which hypnotized subjects work toward hypnotic responding by processing information that they receive in a way that allows them to construct their responses and resolve any problems of responding in accord with the role of the hypnotic subject. Moreover, we noted that the construction of hypnotic responses involves a shift in the way in which subjects process information, and that this shift occurs because of both the facilitative social features of the hypnotic setting and the essential cognitive skills of the subjects.

From this perspective, we (Sheehan & McConkey, 1982) emphasized that more attention needs to be given to the different cognitive strategies or styles that hypnotized subjects use to experience the events suggested by the hypnotist. We argued also that there is much more variability in the experience of hypnotized subjects than has been recognized previously. Our emphasis on the subjective experience of hypnotized subjects, the cognitively active way in which subjects respond to hypnotic suggestions, and the essential variability and individual differences in hypnotic responding underscored the need to understand the experience and behavior of the experiencing subject in the hypnotic setting in a way that does not emphasize one type of process to the exclusion of the other.

THEORETICAL CONCEPTS AND PRINCIPLES

In this section, I would like to discuss in more detail how hypnotized subjects construct their suggested experiences and resolve the problems associated with being a responsive subject in a hypnotic setting. At the outset, it is important to underscore that the subjects bring a particular set of expectations, skills, and traits to a setting that reflects an unusual amalgam of social demands, interpersonal dynamics, and behavioral constraints. The subjects who come to the hypnotic setting are being guided by an anticipatory schema that will determine, at least in part, their experience and behavior in the setting. Moreover, both the cognitive and the social events that occur in the hypnotic setting will influence and be influenced by the schema of the subjects in a way that eventually shapes the phenomena that occur.

Example of the Problem

Before I turn to an overview of a model, it may be useful to consider in a concrete fashion the complexity and variability of the responses that can be seen in subjects who demonstrate hypnotic phenomena. In a basic sense, this complexity and variability constitute a major part of the theoretical dilemma that occurs in the area of hypnosis. In an individual comparison study, my colleagues and I (McConkey, Glisky, & Kihlstrom, 1989) tested two highly hypnotizable subjects on a range of hypnotic items, and observed a number of illustrations of this theoretical dilemma. For instance, what these subjects reported to be the most interesting aspect of their hypnotic testing was not what we thought would be the most interesting to them, or the most theoretically meaningful to researchers at large. Specifically, the subjects reported that they found a hand levitation item to be the most interesting part of the hypnosis session, even though many researchers would see this ideomotor item as a relatively simple instance of responding. This divergence between the meaning that the subjects assigned to a particular experience and the importance that researchers typically attach to this type of item suggests that researchers should look more closely at hypnosis from the point of view of the subjects. After all, it is the meaning that subjects assign to the communications of the hypnotist, rather than the communications themselves, that determines subjects' behavior and also allows them to interpret their responses in a meaningful fashion.

The comments of the two subjects indicated that they cognitively processed the suggestions offered by the hypnotist in quite different ways. Specifically, whereas one subject was relatively passive in her processing of the suggestions, the other was very active and reported using a range of personal strategies in order to respond positively. That is, although the suggested effects "just happened" for the first subject, those effects were created by the second subject through her use of particular cognitive strategies. This difference between apparent "happenings" (for the first subject) and "doings" (for the second subject) lies at the heart of much of the theoretical debate in the area of hypnosis research (see Sarbin & Coe, 1972). Faced with this variability, different theoretical views seem to fit the different experiences of these subjects. For instance, an emphasis on processing outside awareness and nonvolitional responding appears to describe the first subject well, whereas an emphasis on goal-directed fantasy and responsiveness to social demands appears to describe the second subject well. What needs to be kept in mind, however, is that these differential emphases should be relative. That is, both cognitive and social processes should be seen as interactively determining the way in which both of the subjects approached, displayed, and interpreted the hypnotic phenomena.

The behavior of the two subjects was similar on the majority of hypnotic items, but there were subtle differences that need to be explained in a theoretical sense. For instance, on an item that involved the visual hallucination of an assistant, both of the subjects reported that the assistant was sitting in a chair, even though the quality of their hallucinations differed markedly. Whereas one subject's hallucination was relatively incomplete, the other's was reportedly clear and vivid. Nevertheless, the comments of the subject with the incomplete hallucination seemed to indicate that she held a greater belief in the genuineness of the hallucinated assistant than did the comments of the other subject; of course, this may reflect their use of different criteria to personally define their belief in the hallucinated image, as it were. Nevertheless, in a counterintuitive way one subject reported that she knew the assistant was not there even though she could see her clearly, whereas the other subject acted as if the assistant was there even though she could not see her very well. The relationship between the completeness of a suggested experience and the belief that the hypnotized subject develops in the genuineness of that experience is an issue that needs to be addressed more specifically and examined in greater detail. The virtual reality that can be said to be constructed by the hypnotized subject may be compelling in a subjective sense, even if it is incomplete.

From my perspective, further investigations of hypnotized subjects' belief in the genuineness of their suggested experiences are critical to the development of a full theoretical appreciation of hypnosis. Although substantial data indicate that hypnotized subjects can process both reality and suggested features of the hypnotic setting (Sheehan & McConkey, 1982), it is striking that this mixing of percept and imagination does not necessarily challenge the belief of subjects in the primacy of their suggested experiences. This theoretical problem is thrown into bold relief when we consider the responses of hypnotized subjects who are faced with apparently paradoxical situations. For instance, we (McConkey et al., 1989) asked the two subjects to indicate the feelings that they experienced when they were looking at pages for which they had reported hypnotic blindness. For both of the subjects, there was a perfect correspondence between the happy, neutral, and sad faces on the pages and the happy, neutral, and sad feelings that they reported experiencing. That is, the two subjects both believed that they did not see the faces and responded as if they were processing the visual information.

The comments of the subjects about their experiences of this negative visual hallucination item are instructive. During the inquiry, one subject reported that she still did not know what was on the pages, and she seemed at a loss to explain the feelings that she had. In contrast, the other subject reported that she thought that faces were on the pages, and she attributed her feelings to these faces. Whether the responses of these subjects were based on the processing outside of awareness of the visual information (for the first subject) or on the active denial of the visual information that was nevertheless in awareness (for the second subject) is an important theoretical issue (e.g., see Kihlstrom, 1987; Spanos, 1986). Whatever the case, it is clear that both of the subjects held a firm belief, at least for a time, that they could not see the visual information that was before them.

Another example of the variability that occurs in hypnosis was seen in the responses of the subjects on a suggested anesthesia item. This item involved the apparent paradox of asking the subjects to say "No" when they did not feel a touch. One of the subjects responded in strict accord with these instructions and displayed apparently incongruous behavior. That is, this subject reported that she could feel nothing, and also answered "No" every time that the hypnotist touched her in the area of tactile insensitivity, thus indicating that she was processing the information conveyed by the touches of the hypnotist. During the inquiry, this subject did not appear to be concerned about the illogicality of the instructions and did not appear to recognize the apparent paradox in her behavior. By contrast, the other subject typically made no response when the hypnotist touched her in either the anesthetized or the normal area. This subject reported that she recognized the illogical nature of the instructions given by the hypnotist, and commented during the inquiry that she felt confused by these instructions. Thus, this particular subject's lack of verbal responses when she was touched could perhaps be explained in terms of the confusion causing her simply to give no particular response. This explanation is not consistent, however, with her behavior on the item that involved hypnotic blindness for faces. On that item, she accurately reported the feelings conveyed by the pages, while at the same time she reported blindness for the material on the pages. In this sense, the behavior of this particular subject highlights the intraindividual differences that can occur in hypnotic responding.

In summary, this consideration of the subjects we tested (McConkey et al., 1989) points to a number of issues that are central to a theoretical appreciation of hypnosis. The subjects assigned personal meaning and special importance to an event during the hypnotic testing (viz., the ideomotor item) that researchers would typically consider to be of little importance. Moreover, the subjects displayed quite different ways of approaching and thinking about the suggestions offered by the hypnotist. Whereas one subject reported passive concentration on the words of the hypnotist, the other subject reported that she used personally relevant strategies in an active manner in order to experience the suggested effects. When they were experiencing the suggested effects (e.g., hallucination of the assistant), the subjects varied in the reality status that they ascribed to their experience. Counterintuitively, however, the reality value that they placed on their experience did not seem to be tied directly to the completeness of the experience. Finally, the subjects differed in their responses to items that involved paradoxical features or conflicting communications from the hypnotist. This was perceived as a situation of conflict and concern by one subject, but not by the other. Of course, the inferences that can be drawn from such an analysis of individual subjects are limited (see McConkey et al., 1989), but the findings nevertheless point to the issues that need to be addressed by researchers on both theoretical and empirical levels.

Overview of a Model

At this stage, it is appropriate to note that I am concerned mostly with understanding the experience and behavior of subjects who do, rather than those who do not, display hypnotic phenomena. That is, my perspective relates more to the reactions of subject who are high, rather than medium or low, in hypnotizability. By definition, however, hypnotizability plays a major role in the reactions of subjects in the hypnotic setting, and I assume that high hypnotizability reflects a particular constellation of cognitive skills (e.g., attention) and personal traits (e.g., absorption) that is relevant to the experience of hypnotic phenomena. The subjects bring these skills and traits to the hypnotic setting, and their activation is potentiated by the social influences that exist in that setting.

The subjects are motivated by the social influences of the hypnotic setting and by their own expectations concerning hypnosis to adopt a role that involves a willingness and commitment to respond positively to the suggestions of the hypnotist. The communications of the hypnotist provide subjects with relatively clear information about the reactions that are consistent with the role of the hypnotic subject. In addition, those communications motivate the subjects and potentiate cognitive events that ultimately shape the experience of hypnotized subjects. Thus, through social influences that define the role responsibility of the hypnotic subject, hypnotized subjects are motivated to respond in a way that is appropriate.

The impact of social influences in the hypnotic setting is mediated by the meaning that the subjects assign to them, and this meaning is determined in large part by the cognitions of the subjects. Hypnotized subjects may differ in terms of the specific cognitive styles or strategies that they employ to respond to the communications of the hypnotist, but it is clear that the positive responding involves the allocation of attention. Thus, the allocation of attention by hypnotized subjects is a critical determinant of the degree to which the subjects succeed in responding to the communications of the hypnotist. If highly hypnotizable subjects employ appropriate cognitions and allocate attentional resources in a way that is consistent with their motivation to respond to the suggestion given by the hypnotist, then they will experience the suggested effect in a compelling manner.

A characteristic of this experience is the subjects' interpretation of information, both internal and external, in a way that leads them to experience the suggested effect and to develop a belief in the genuineness of their internal, subjective experience. In essence, hypnotized subjects' processing of information that is both consistent and inconsistent with the suggested effect allows them to develop and maintain a belief that the event suggested by the hypnotist and experienced by them approaches virtual reality. Even when hypnotized subjects process information that is inconsistent with the suggested effect, they tend to do so in a way that serves to reinforce, rather than to challenge, their belief in the genuineness of the experience suggested by the hypnotist.

Because the phenomenal experience of hypnotized subjects is shaped by the cognitive and social processes that occur, changes in these processes or in their interaction may change the nature of the experience at any time. In that sense, the phenomenal experience of hypnotized subjects should be seen as a fluid rather than a static event, and as being influenced by changes in both the personal and the situational influences that impinge upon the subjects. Moreover, it seems plausible that the belief of hypnotized subjects in the genuineness of their subjective experiences will be shaped by the events that occur before, during, and after those experiences. That is, the events that occur before, during, and after a particular hypnotic experience may influence not only how subjects interpret and make attributions about that experience, but also how they approach and respond to subsequent experiences during hypnosis.

From this perspective, further research is needed on the attributions that hypnotized subjects make about their experiences, and on the ways in which those attributions may shape their future experiences and behavior during hypnosis. Before, during, and after their experience of suggested effects, it appears that hypnotized subjects work to give meaning to their experience, and the nature of their cognitive activity in this respect needs to be determined more specifically. Overall, though, it is clear that hypnotized subjects try to make sense of their experiences, at least within the constraints of their role as participants in a particular interaction in the hypnotic setting.

In summary, particular cognitive and social processes are operating in the hypnotic setting, and these processes shape the experience of hypnotized subjects. A number of questions remain to be addressed by the model in both theoretical and empirical terms, but it is nevertheless important to point to those components that appear to be relatively influential. Of course, there is a risk of highlighting the relevance of some components rather than others before sufficient data are in hand. Accordingly, I emphasize the need for research about the precise relevance of particular cognitive and social processes.

RESEARCH AND APPRAISAL

I turn now to consider representative research that relates to the major issues raised by the perspective presented here. The research considered is not reviewed comprehensively, but rather is presented in a way that illustrates the conceptual issues of central concern. Where appropriate, the specific work that needs to be undertaken in the future is also presented.

Expectations and Skills

Subjects bring particular expectations to the hypnotic setting about the events that will occur, and they also bring particular skills that will be instrumental in determining whether or not those events actually do take place. The expectations that hypnotized subjects typically bring to the setting have been assessed in a number of analyses of attitudes and opinions about hypnosis. For instance, in one study (McConkey, 1986), I surveyed subjects just before they participated in group hypnosis sessions; at that point, subjects believed that hypnosis is quite different from normal waking consciousness, and that hypnotized people experience suggested effects without having to consciously try to make those effects happen. Moreover, the subjects felt that the experience of hypnosis depends more on the ability of the person than on the ability of the hypnotist, and that hypnotized people experience a sort of double awareness in which they experience what is suggested but also know things that contradict the suggestions.

About a week after these subjects had participated in group hypnosis sessions, they were surveyed again. At this point in time, more of the subjects believed that hypnosis is a normal state of consciousness that essentially involves focusing attention and thinking along with and imagining the suggestions. In addition, an even greater number of subjects felt that the experience of hypnosis depends on the ability of the person rather than the ability of the hypnotist. Moreover, on the basis of their own hypnotic testing, the subjects believed that their own experience had been largely determined by what they wanted to do, and only partly influenced by the hypnotist. Notably, however, their own experience of hypnosis was generally not what these subjects thought it would be. Although information about the expectations of hypnotized subjects is inevitably limited by the procedures that are used to gather that information, my findings indicated that subjects had particular opinions about hypnosis and hypnotic suggestions that influenced and were influenced by their own experience of hypnosis. In this sense, the expectations that subjects bring and how those expectations are either reinforced or challenged by the hypnotic setting will play an essential role in determining the responses of hypnotized subjects (McConkey, 1986).

More important determinants of the positive responses of hypnotized subjects, perhaps, are the cognitive skills and personal traits that the subjects bring with them to the hypnotic setting. A major aspect in this respect is the degree to which subjects can become absorbed in ongoing experience. Since the work of Tellegen and Atkinson (1974), research has pointed to the construct of "absorption" as a relatively consistent correlate of hypnotizability, even though the exact nature of that relationship is controversial. A colleague and I (Roche & McConkey, 1990), for instance, reviewed work on the construct of absorption and argued that although the trait of absorption appears to be an aspect of hypnotizability, much more research is needed to determine the precise role that absorption plays in the subject's experience of hypnotic phenomena. The construct of absorption is important, however, not only because of its relevance to understanding hypnotizability, but also because it provides a strong and important connection between hypnosis research and research in personality psychology generally. For instance, the construct of absorption is linked closely to the dimension of "openness to experience" that is part of the model of personality developed by McCrae and Costa (1983). In this respect, it should be noted that theorizing in the area of hypnosis needs to be linked much more obviously to theorizing about phenomena and process outside the area than has often been the case. Additional work on absorption, openness to experience, and hypnotizability would seem to allow that link to occur in an essential way.

Communications of the Hypnotist

When the subjects are in the hypnotic setting, they are exposed to a wide variety of information from the hypnotist, the procedures employed, the physical situation itself, and their own thoughts and feelings. Collectively, though, the evidence indicates that the messages received from the hypnotist exert a substantial influence on the responses of hypnotized subjects. Moreover, this is the case even when those messages are challenged by directly conflicting instructions and influences (see McConkey, 1983a, 1983b). In such a situation of conflict, where subjects are exposed to statements that are inconsistent with the suggestions given by the hypnotist, hypnotized subjects appear to work to interpret the communications of the hypnotist in a way that involves a considerable preparedness to respond in accord with the hypnotic suggestions as subjects understand them. That is, it seems that hypnotized subjects are cognitively predisposed to process information in a way that leads to a positive response.

It is important to underscore that this preparedness should not be viewed in terms of simple acquiescence or compliance, but rather as a position of cognitive readiness by the subjects to construct incoming information in a way that allows them to experience the suggested effect and enact the role of hypnotic subjects. In an earlier paper (McConkey, 1983a), I reviewed a number of instances in hypnosis research where hypnotized subjects had been exposed either intentionally or unintentionally to conflicting influences, and concluded that even in the face of direct challenges to their positive responding many subjects worked to maintain their experience and their commitment to the role of hypnotic subjects. At a theoretical level, the way in which hypnotized subjects resolve the conflict between the communications of the hypnotist and the state of affairs conveyed by objective reality is an essential issue in understanding hypnosis. The critical theoretical issue here, perhaps, is whether this resolution occurs within or without the awareness of hypnotized subjects. The resolution of problems outside the hypnotic setting does not necessarily involve the processing of all information within awareness, and the resolution of problems inside the hypnotic setting would not seem to be any different in this respect.

In another paper (McConkey, 1983b), I reported that subjects often expended considerable effort to respond within a framework of suggestion that prevented objective reality information from interfering with their experience. For these subjects, the interpretation of reality information was determined in large part by their desire to meet the suggestions given by the hypnotist. The subjects cognitively managed diverse information in a way that allowed them to initiate and to maintain their experience as it was suggested by the hypnotist and interpreted by themselves. When faced with reality constraints, some hypnotized subjects attempted to incorporate that information within a framework of experience that was consistent with their preparedness to respond positively. In other words, hypnotized subjects cognitively processed reality information in a way that matched the suggestions they were given and met the strivings consonant with their role as hypnotic subjects.

As noted earlier, substantial variability occurs in the responses of hypnotized subjects to suggestions from the hypnotist. A process variable that helps to explain some of the individual differences in hypnotized subjects' ways of approaching, initiating, and understanding the experiences suggested by the hypnotist is that of "cognitive style." In essence, cognitive style reflects the ways in which hypnotized subjects move toward experiencing and displaying hypnotic phenomena, and the relevance of this variable in a theoretical sense has been highlighted elsewhere (Sheehan & McConkey, 1982). Recent empirical work has supported that relevance also. For instance, a colleague and I (Bryant & McConkey, 1990a) contrasted the responses of hypnotized subjects who employed a constructive style, which involved using active strategies to experience the suggested effect, with the responses of subjects who employed a concentrative style, which involved simply focusing on the words of the hypnotist. The subjects who employed a constructive style were more likely to experience hypnotic blindness following an appropriate suggestion from the hypnotist than those who employed a concentrative style. That is, the subjects who approached the suggestion in a cognitively strategic way were more likely to experience the suggested effect than those who adopted a relatively passive style. In this sense, the notion of cognitive style appears to be a useful one for understanding some aspects of hypnotic responding, although additional theoretical and empirical work is needed (Sheehan & McConkey, 1982). Nevertheless, the variable emphasizes that hypnotized subjects differ in the way in which they approach and structure their experiences, and theoretical views on hypnosis need to specify the relevance of that difference more precisely.

Cognition and Awareness

The role of particular cognitions in, and the relevance of awareness to, hypnotic phenomena are controversial issues in the area of hypnosis. Denying that information can be processed and can exert an influence from outside the awareness of subjects would seem to reject much of the work in contemporary cognitive psychology (e.g., Kihlstrom, 1987). By the same token, however, arguing that virtually all events in hypnosis occur outside the awareness of subjects would seem to reflect a lack of appreciation of the active way in which hypnotized subjects strive to meet their role responsibilities. Although a great deal more work is needed to delineate the role of cognition and awareness in hypnosis, some recent research on hypnotic blindness has pointed to the relevance of these constructs.

Hypnotic blindness is an interesting and challenging phenomenon, and we (Bryant & McConkey, 1989a) investigated both the behavioral and experiential aspects of the phenomenon. In that research, the real–simulating model of hypnosis was used, and real/hypnotizable and simulating/unhypnotizable subjects were tested. Also, the EAT was used to inquire into the phenomenal experience of hypnotically blind subjects. The subjects were asked to perform a decision task while they were also reporting hypnotic blindness. This task involved choosing one of three switches to stop a tone that was being emitted by a machine in front of the subjects. There was a visual display of triangles above the switches, and the triangle above the switch that stopped the tone was oriented differently from those above the other switches. The subjects were asked to perform the task when these triangles were illuminated and when they were not—that is, when visual information was available to influence their decision and when it was not.

The hypnotically blind real subjects made more correct responses on the decision task when the visual information was available; moreover, they made more correct responses than simulating subjects when the visual information was available. In terms of the phenomenal experience of subjects, the majority of hypnotically blind real subjects reported that they used a constructive cognitive strategy, which enabled them to construe reality features of the setting in a way that allowed them to experience blindness for the visual information. This was consistent with other findings that hypnotized subjects often use active strategies to meet the demands placed on them by the communications of the hypnotist (e.g., Sheehan & McConkey, 1982). Consistent with my perspective, many of the real subjects who experienced hypnotic blindness seemed to approach the overall situation as one that involved a problem-solving task. That is, they perceived themselves as needing to use whatever strategies were appropriate to experience the effect suggested by the hypnotist, as well as to perform appropriately on the decision task with which the hypnotist confronted them. From the point of view of the subjects, the multiple, conflicting demands of the setting had to be resolved, and they worked to resolve those demands within the particular nexus of cognitive and social influences.

The emphasis on the active way in which some hypnotized subjects approach and respond to hypnotic suggestions should not be seen, however, as questioning the phenomenal genuineness of their experience. Rather, it should be seen as reflecting the commitment of hypnotized subjects to experiencing the events suggested by the hypnotist. By contrast, we (Bryant & McConkey, 1989a) reported that simulating subjects, who were responding in a nongenuine way, reported passive cognitive processing. That is, simulating subjects apparently believed that real subjects would experience blindness easily and that the presentation of visual information would not interfere with that experience. The data from real subjects, however, indicated that this was not the case. Rather, they worked actively to experience and to maintain their experience of blindness, as well as to meet the other demands that the hypnotist placed on them when he presented them with the decision task.

This research suggested that hypnotized subjects were processing visual information in a way that was outside their reported awareness. This is consistent with other work on hypnotic blindness that also employed the decision task. Specifically, we (Bryant & McConkey, 1990b) reported that hypnotically blind subjects took longer to respond on the decision task when the visual information was present than when it was not. That is, the presence of visual information slowed the responding of subjects on the decision task. This suggests that subjects were allocating attentional resources to maintain their experience of blindness to this information. Moreover, when hypnotized subjects were experiencing blindness and the visual information was present, they took longer to respond on a secondary task than when they were not experiencing blindness. This suggests that the allocation of attentional resources by subjects to manage the visual information left relatively fewer attentional resources available to be allocated to a task that was unrelated to their experience of blindness.

Overall, these findings indicated that hypnotized subjects allocated attentional resources to initiate and maintain their experience of blindness when they were faced with conflicting reality information in their visual field. For hypnotized subjects, however, this did not involve the simple denial of visual information that they were aware of in an explicit way. Rather, it involved the attention-demanding management of the reality information that conflicted with the suggested experience. That information was obviously processed by the subjects, but it was not necessarily processed in a way that allowed them to know it consciously when they were experiencing hypnotic blindness.

Belief and Attribution

A striking feature of the experience of many hypnotized subjects is the degree of subjective conviction that they exhibit regarding the genuineness of their experience. This feature, together with the degree to which subjects work to protect the integrity of their hypnotic experience, was seen in another investigation of hypnotic blindness (Bryant & McConkey, 1989b). In this study, we focused on the attributions that subjects made about their experience of blindness and their performance on a task that was presented to the subjects while they were experiencing hypnotic blindness. In this research, highly hypnotizable subjects who were experiencing hypnotic blindness were visually presented with the uncommon spellings of a number of homophones. Later in the session, when they were no longer experiencing blindness, the subjects were asked to spell a number of words (including the previously presented homophones). Following hypnosis, the EAT was used to explore the subjects' experience of blindness and their attributions about their performance on the spelling task. The findings indicated that subjects' spelling was influenced by the words that were presented during hypnotic blindness. This is consistent with the effects that we observed on the decision task (Bryant & McConkey, 1989a, 1990b). That is, hypnotized subjects both reported blindness and were influenced by the presence of visual information. Notably, however, the hypnotized subjects who were tested on the spelling task by Bryant and McConkey (1989b) typically made attributions about their performance that did not involve awareness of the words that were presented during hypnotic blindness. Rather, the subjects typically explained their spelling in terms of idiosyncratic, personal reasons, rather than in terms of any awareness of seeing the words during hypnotic blindness. In essence, the subjects made attributions that can be said to have confirmed for them the genuineness of their experience of blindness. This suggests that hypnotized subjects support the emotional conviction that they develop in the reality of their suggested experiences through the attributions that they subsequently make about those experiences.

This research highlights the relevance of further understanding the development of subjective conviction in the genuineness of suggested experiences during hypnosis. Although additional research is needed on this issue, I consider that just as hypnotized subjects work to actively construct the experiences that are suggested by the hypnotist, they also work to develop and maintain their emotional conviction in the genuineness of those experiences. In other words, the development of delusion during hypnosis may be a result, at least in part, of an active cognitive construction by subjects within a social context that fosters a belief in the reality of genuineness of suggested experiences. The limits of this notion, however, obviously need to be determined more fully in further empirical work.

One way to investigate the limits of suggested experiences and the belief that hypnotized subjects hold in their genuineness is to attempt to challenge or break down those experiences. In research on posthypnotic amnesia, for instance, we (McConkey & Sheehan, 1981; see also McConkey, Sheehan, & Cross, 1980) played the videotape of their hypnosis session to real and simulating subjects who reported that they could not remember the events of the session following a suggestion for posthypnotic amnesia. Relevant to the belief that subjects hold in the genuineness of their suggested experiences, we (McConkey & Sheehan, 1981) found that when they were confronted with the videotape, the real, but not the simulating, subjects made a distinction between remembering their behavior during hypnosis and not remembering the experiences that were associated with their behavior. Of course, the reports of the real amnesic subjects concerning behavioral versus experiential recall may relate either to features of posthypnotic amnesia itself or to aspects of being confronted with a videotape of material for which they were experiencing amnesia. The relevant point, however, is that even though some hypnotized subjects acknowledged the occurrence of their behavior as they observed it on the videotape, they nevertheless reported that they were amnesic for the experiences associated with that behavior. In this sense, the subjects adopted a position of cognitive resolution that allowed them to maintain a belief in the genuineness of their experience of amnesia, while at the same time meeting the conflicting demands of the setting to acknowledge the occurrence of the events of hypnosis.

CONCLUDING COMMENT

I have presented a perspective on hypnosis and hypnotic phenomena that emphasizes the role of particular cognitive and social processes. The influence of investigators such as White (1937, 1941), Shor (1959, 1962), Orne (1959, 1977), and Sutcliffe (1960, 1961) can be seen in the perspective that I have presented here. Moreover, the emphasis on the active participant who employs appropriate cognitive strategies to resolve the multiple problems posed by the hypnotic setting can obviously be seen as well (Sheehan & McConkey, 1982). I have given further emphasis here, however, to the belief that subjects develop in the virtual reality of their subjective experience during hypnosis. I have also emphasized the relevance of the attributions that subjects make about their experiences during hypnosis, and especially the way in which these attributions appear to be used to protect the integrity of hypnotic responses. It is plausible that both cognitive and social processes in the hypnotic setting contribute to the beliefs and attributions of hypnotized subjects, and systematic research is needed to explore those processes in detail.

A major conceptual issue that I have raised here is the relevance of cognition and awareness to the experience of hypnotized subjects. Indeed, this is a major conceptual issue in psychology generally, and the body of evidence seems to indicate that information can be processed and can exert an influence when it is outside the awareness of subjects, whether they are hypnotized or not. However, a major stumbling block to the resolution of this issue is that no fully articulated models of awareness exist in psychology; because of this, it is difficult to predict what information will be inside and what information will be outside the awareness of subjects, whether they are hypnotized or not. In this respect, however, advances are being made on both theoretical and empirical fronts, and researchers in hypnosis have an opportunity to contribute to a more complete understanding of the nature and function of awareness generally.

The issues that I have discussed do not exhaust those that are relevant to the experience and behavior of hypnotized subjects, and the specific importance of other variables is highlighted in other chapters in this volume. For example, the importance of the interpersonal relationship between the subject and hypnotist, and the affective qualities of their dyadic interaction, may be central to the responses of hypnotized subjects to the communications of the hypnotist. The relevance of emotional processes clearly needs to be explored in future research and incorporated into the perspective that I have presented. Nevertheless, I have emphasized a number of variables that influence the management of reality information by hypnotized subjects in a way that allows them both to experience the effects suggested by the hypnotist and to develop a belief in the genuineness of those experiences. This emphasis recognizes the importance of the phenomenal experience of the hypnotized subject.

Finally, some 50 years ago White (1941) noted that "the atmosphere of magic" tended to linger around hypnosis, and called for the "light of reason" to bear upon the phenomenon. As the chapters in this volume indicate, although the atmosphere of magic rarely lingers around contemporary hypnosis, we are faced with the light of reason shining from multiple sources and illuminating various features of the phenomenon to different degrees. This situation illustrates not only the complexity of the phenomenon of hypnosis, but also the vitality of the area of research as a whole. Only by the systematic examination of the core features of the phenomenon and the major processes identified in this chapter will we fully appreciate the construction and resolution of experience and behavior in hypnosis.

Acknowledgments. The perspective presented here is based in part on research supported by a grant from the Australian Research Council. I prepared the chapter while visiting the University of Arizona, and I am grateful to John Kihlstrom and Jacquelyn Cranney for their intellectual companionship during that visit.

REFERENCES

Barber, T.X. (1969). *Hypnosis: A scientific approach.* New York: Van Nostrand Reinhold.

Bryant, R.A., & McConkey, K.M. (1989a). Hypnotic blindness: A behavioral and experiential analysis. *Journal of Abnormal Psychology, 98,* 71–77.

Bryant, R.A., & McConkey, K.M. (1989b). Hypnotic blindness, awareness, and attribution. *Journal of Abnormal Psychology, 98,* 443–447.

Bryant, R.A., & McConkey, K.M. (1990a). Hypnotic blindness and the relevance of cognitive style. *Journal of Personality and Social Psychology, 59,* 756–761.

Bryant, R.A., & McConkey, K.M. (1990b). Hypnotic blindness and the relevance of attention. *Australian Journal of Psychology, 42,* 287–296.

Hilgard, E.R. (1977). *Divided consciousness: Multiple controls in human thought and action.* New York: Wiley.

Kihlstrom, J.F. (1987). The cognitive unconscious. *Science, 237,* 1445–1452.

McConkey, K.M. (1983a). Challenging hypnotic effects: The impact of conflicting influences on response to hypnotic suggestion. *British Journal of Experimental and Clinical Hypnosis, 1,* 3–10.

McConkey, K.M. (1983b). The impact of conflicting communications on response to hypnotic suggestion. *Journal of Abnormal Psychology, 92,* 351–358.

McConkey, K.M. (1986). Opinions about hypnosis and self-hypnosis before and after hypnotic testing. *International Journal of Clinical and Experimental Hypnosis, 34,* 311–319.

McConkey, K.M., Glisky, M.L., & Kihlstrom, J.F. (1989). Individual differences among hypnotic virtuosos: A case comparison. *Australian Journal of Clinical and Experimental Hypnosis, 17,* 131–140.

McConkey, K.M., & Sheehan, P.W. (1981). The impact of videotape playback of hypnotic events on posthypnotic amnesia. *Journal of Abnormal Psychology, 90,* 46–54.

McConkey, K.M., Sheehan, P.W., & Cross, D.G. (1980). Posthypnotic amnesia: Seeing is not remembering. *British Journal of Social and Clinical Psychology, 19,* 99–107.

McCrae, R.R., & Costa, P.T., Jr. (1983). Joint factors in self-reports and ratings: Neuroticism, extraversion and openness to experience. *Personality and Individual Differences, 4,* 245–255.

Orne, M.T. (1959). The nature of hypnosis: Artifact and essence. *Journal of Abnormal and Social Psychology, 58,* 277–299.

Orne, M.T. (1977). The construct of hypnosis: Implications of the definition for research and practice. *Annals of the New York Academy of Sciences, 296,* 14–33.

Roche, S.M., & McConkey, K.M. (1990). Absorption: Nature, assessment, and correlates. *Journal of Personality and Social Psychology, 59,* 91–101.

Sarbin, T.R., & Coe, W.C. (1972). *Hypnosis: A social psychological analysis of influence communication.* New York: Holt, Rinehart & Winston.

Sheehan, P.W., & McConkey, K.M. (1982). *Hypnosis and experience: The exploration of phenomena and process.* Hillsdale, NJ: Erlbaum.

Shor, R.E. (1959). Hypnosis and the concept of the generalized reality orientation. *American Journal of Psychotherapy, 13,* 582–602.

Shor, R.E. (1962). Three dimensions of hypnotic depth. *International Journal of Clinical and Experimental Hypnosis, 10,* 23–38.

Spanos, N.P. (1986). Hypnotic behavior: A social-psychological interpretation of amnesia, analgesia, and "trance logic." *Behavioral and Brain Sciences, 9,* 449–502.

Sutcliffe, J.P. (1960). "Credulous" and "skeptical" views of hypnotic phenomena: A review of certain evidence and methodology. *International Journal of Clinical and Experimental Hypnosis, 8,* 73–101.

Sutcliffe, J.P. (1961). "Credulous" and "skeptical" views of hypnotic phenomena: Experiments on esthesia, hallucination, and delusion. *Journal of Abnormal and Social Psychology, 62,* 189–200.

Tellegen, A., & Atkinson, G. (1974). Openness to absorbing and self-altering experiences ("absorption"), a trait related to hypnotic susceptibility. *Journal of Abnormal Psychology, 83,* 268–277.

White, R.W. (1937). Two types of hypnotic trance and their personality correlates. *Journal of Psychology, 3,* 279–289.

White, R.W. (1941). A preface to the theory of hypnotism. *Journal of Abnormal and Social Psychology, 36,* 477–505.

CHAPTER 19

Toward a Social-Psychobiological Model of Hypnosis

ÉVA I. BÁNYAI
Eötvös Loránd University

INTRODUCTION

I grew up in a country where the discipline of psychology and the "mystic" phenomena of hypnosis were regarded with suspicion. It is no wonder that the study of hypnosis, as a "forbidden fruit of the tree of knowledge," was so personally alluring. Yet today—after 20 years of actively studying hypnosis, at a time when hypnosis has achieved broad-based academic and clinical acceptance in Hungary—hypnosis still fascinates me, albeit for somewhat different reasons. In the course of pursuing hypnosis research, I have come to realize that hypnosis poses some of the most tantalizing intellectual challenges for the student of human nature.

Hypnosis is challenging for a number of reasons. As a psychotherapeutic procedure effective in alleviating if not removing physical symptoms, it exemplifies the "mystic leap" from mind to body, which has always been a central problem in psychology. It is also challenging because no explanation or definition of hypnosis has been widely accepted, despite a history of suggestive techniques dating back to the ancient Egyptians, and a modern history of more than 200 years. Furthermore, reconciling or placing in perspective the seemingly contradictory explanations of hypnosis constitutes an even greater intellectual challenge.

The debates of the past three decades over state versus trait views, cognitive versus social approaches, and subject-centered versus hypnotist-centered explanations has spurred me to search for a different way of understanding the mechanisms central to hypnosis. Instead of conceptualizing the various issues in an "either–or" manner, I have attempted to integrate interpersonal and intrapersonal aspects of hypnosis into a multidimensional interactional framework; in so doing, I have formulated what I term a "social-psychobiological" model of hypnosis.[1]

The Social-Psychobiological Model: A Brief Overview

The social-psychobiological model that I advance in this chapter represents an attempt to respond to the challenges that have captured my interest. The model conceptualizes hypnosis as an altered state of consciousness that may have an adaptive value. This state arises in a special social context as a result of reciprocal interactions between the subject and the hypnotist. According to this model, hypnosis is influenced by personal characteristics and physiological predispositions of both the hypnotist and the subject, including their attitudes, expectations, characteristic cognitive styles, and relationship to each other. The unfolding of hypnosis is also influenced by the physiological, behavioral, and subjective experiential modifications accompanying the process of inducing and testing hypnosis. The social-psychobiological model views hypnosis as an ever-changing process, and seeks to delineate the interdependence of diverse elements of the hypnotist–subject interaction; in so doing, it rejects the search for linear causal relationships as simplistic and ultimately fruitless. Before I sketch the lineage of this approach, and briefly discuss its relationship with other theories, I present key concepts that are the rudiments of the model.

When I use the term "altered state of consciousness," I do not regard this state as an "all-or-nothing" change from the usual normal waking state. Rather, I use the term to represent a fuzzy set that, according to the prototypical model of concept formation, is helpful in delineating the family resemblance of disparate hypnotic phenomena, which converge in their being accompanied by perceived alterations in experience. As opposed to social-psychological theorists (e.g., Barber, 1979; Sarbin & Coe, 1972; Spanos, 1982a, 1982b; Wagstaff, 1981), I find it useful to adopt the term "altered state" because it serves the function of organizing our knowledge about hypnosis in a manner similar to the way natural concepts are organized in everyday life. The term "hypnotic state" is thus no more ill defined than many psychological concepts.

Beyond that, the subjective experience of alteration in consciousness is an essential feature of hypnosis. In order to characterize an altered state of consciousness, it is not enough to test whether the subject performs suggestions. On the one hand, the term "altered state" necessarily implies subjectively detectable alterations in consciousness; on the other hand, despite generally high correlations between behavioral response to suggestion and subjective alterations, responsiveness to suggestion and subjective alterations in experience often diverge. The model therefore focuses not only on traditional manifestations of hypnosis, as measured by the widely used scales of susceptibility, but also on the subjective experiences of the subject.

The model also emphasizes the role of the special social context. No other altered state of consciousness exists that is so closely related to an interaction between two persons. This altered state, nested within a special social context, is the very essence of hypnosis. The social-psychobiological model (see also Diamond, 1984, 1987; Nash, Chapter 6, this volume; Sheehan, Chapter 17, this volume) thus stresses the importance of the relationship between hypnotist and subject. This relational dimension is considered not only at the level of current personal attraction, but also at deeper, more archaic layers of the personality. This two-tiered approach is necessary because I believe that the hypnotic situation is especially effective in mobilizing archaic patterns of relating to another person.

I use the term "reciprocal interactions" to highlight the subject's active role in the interaction and the fact that the subject and hypnotist affect each other. As opposed to the traditional view of the subject as being a passive "wax" molded by the "magic hands" of the hypnotist, the subject plays an active role in the transactions that occur during hypnosis. The subject is active not only in the sense that he or she uses active cognitive strategies and expresses emotions when experiencing hypnosis (as emphasized by the accounts of Sheehan & McConkey, 1982; Lynn, Nash, Rhue, Franman, & Sweeney, 1984), but also in the sense that this activity in turn influences the hypnotist's behavior and affect in relation to the subject in a recursive fashion.

Physiological mechanisms may bring about somatic as well as behavioral and experiential changes during hypnosis. For this reason, the physiological concomitants of hypnosis in subjects who vary in hypnotizability level are subjects of interest. In addition to recognizing alterations in the subjects' state of consciousness, the model also highlights the role of personal characteristics and physiological predispositions (i.e., the "traits" of the interactants). I use the term "trait" in a manner consistent with its use in contemporary psychology—as referring to a characteristic that differs from person to person in a relatively permanent and consistent way within the bounds of relatively stable situational parameters. Although the hypnosis literature takes scant notice of the personal characteristics of the hypnotist, our research (Bányai, Gosi-Greguss, Vágó, Varga, & Horváth, in press) suggests that the role of the hypnotist's personal style is as important as the characteristics of the subject.

Finally, the model emphasizes the adaptive value of hypnosis. From a social-psychobiological perspective, the very fact that hypnotic-like techniques have existed for thousands of years suggests that hypnosis serves to modulate psychic tension and facilitates the acquisition of new experiences and insights. It accomplishes this by engaging the participants in an intensive interpersonal relationship without undue risk to themselves or other persons. Hypnosis thus helps the participants to function more adequately, constructively, and creatively in the social-biological milieu.

Intellectual, Theoretical, and Research Background of the Model

The roots of my thinking about hypnosis originated outside the realm of hypnosis research. In the 1970s, when I first became acquainted with hypnosis research, psychology in Hungary was in a very special position. On the surface, at least, the only kind of psychology that was acceptable had some connection with "higher nervous system activity"—that is, with Pavlovian physiological conceptions of psychological phenomena. Under the surface, however, a mainly gestalt-oriented experimental tradition, along with the very influential psychoanalytic tradition of the Budapest school, still survived. It might be said that the "manifest" psychology had a strong associative and physiological orientation, whereas the "latent" psychology maintained a holistic and dynamic emphasis. Although in the early 1970s this situation was beginning to change, my orientation to hypnosis research was fundamentally influenced by these three seemingly mutually exclusive traditions.

As a student, I received training at the laboratory of Dr. Endre Grastyán, a well-known neurophysiologist. As a young researcher, I began my work in the area of hypnosis at the Department of Comparative Physiology of Eötvös Loránd University (Budapest), chaired by Dr. György Adám, whose work on interoception began at the Pavlov Laboratory in Koltushi in the USSR. Given these formative influences, it seemed quite natural to initiate my study of hypnosis by testing a physiological theory of hypnosis—namely, the "partial sleep" theory of Pavlov (1923).

The development and study of an activity-increasing "active/alert" hypnotic induction procedure, to be discussed in more detail later in the chapter (Bányai & Hilgard, 1976; Bányai, 1987), appeared to indicate that the sleep-like quality of hypnosis was not an essential feature of the hypnotic state. Despite this finding, I still believe that inhibitory central nervous system processes, stressed by Pavlov, play a central role in the psychophysiological mechanisms of hypnosis. My understanding of the effects of active/alert hypnosis, and my present views regarding the nature of the inhibitory processes associated with hypnosis, were strongly influenced by Grastyán and his colleagues' research on the dynamics of subcortical (hypothalamic and hippocampal) excitatory and inhibitory processes in animals (Grástyan, 1981; Grastyán, Lissák, Madarász, & Donhoffer, 1959), as well as by Grastyán's views on the adaptive role of play and regressive states in devoplopment (Grastyán, 1985). The idea that not only central, but also peripheral, alterations may accompany hypnosis is in accordance with the spirit of the research on interoception at Adám's department, demonstrating that interoceptive processes regulated by the so-called "autonomic" nervous system can be conditioned both by classical and instrumental methods (Adám, 1967).

It follows from this approach's tradition that my initial research on hypnosis, conducted in collaboration with Dr. Istvan Mészáros, was on the effect of hypnosis on verbal learning (Mészáros, Osman, & Bányai, 1972). Although learning is a classical field of study of behaviorism, the analysis of the findings pertinent to the effects of hypnosis on learning convinced me of the necessity of exploring the data in a wider context, based on a more cognitive approach (Bányai, 1973). The findings of Hilgard and his colleagues on the cognitive changes that result in dissociations in hypnosis (e.g., E. R. Hilgard, 1965), Shor's (1959) notion of the alteration of generalized reality orientation during hypnosis, and Orne's (1959) emphasis on the importance of subjective experiences as the essence of hypnosis encouraged me to search beyond purely behavioristic or physiological conceptualizations of hypnosis for a more complete explanation of hypnotic phenomena.

Hilgard's research had a particularly important influence on the development of my thinking about hypnosis. In 1973, I had the opportunity to spend a postdoctoral year at his Laboratory of Hypnosis Research at Stanford University. His rigorous but flexible scientific approach toward a traditionally mystical field like hypnosis; his critical but tolerant attitude, rooted in American functionalism; his somewhat eclectic position regarding explanatory principles; and his searching for relationships among quite distant fields of psychology exerted a determining influence on my own research. The sprit of investigation in his laboratory, which incorporated the clinical interest of his wife, Josephine Hilgard, encouraged me to conduct research that controlled input–output variables (which was a natural consequence of my "manifest" Hungarian heritage) and examined subjective reports, interview data, the cognitive style of the subject, and the diverse effects of social influence processes. At the theoretical level, I found the Hilgards' developmental–interactive theory (E. R. Hilgard, 1965; J. R. Hilgard, 1970; J. R. Hilgard & Hilgard, 1962) very appealing.

The year spent in the United States acquainted me with the promising applications of hypnosis in therapy. As a direct consequence, I pursued clinical training in the psychoanalytic tradition of the Budapest school. As a result of this experience, psychoanalytic theories stressing the importance of the relational dimension (Ferenczi, 1909/1965; Freud, 1921; Gill & Brenman, 1959) gained more primary ground in my thinking. Yet it was not until I began practicing hypnotherapy myself that I realized the strong, at times even organismic, involvement of the *hypnotist* in the development and curative effect of hypnosis, particularly with respect to psychosomatic diseases. To illustrate, let me briefly describe the final, eye-opening experience I had with a colitis patient. It was this experience that led me to develop the interactional experimental paradigm, which constitutes the experimental basis of my social-psychobiological model of hypnosis.

With this patient, I applied the "affect bridge" technique of Watkins (1971) to explore the roots of her disease. As part of this technique, I administered an age regression suggestion for her to regress to the age when she had experienced something connected to her present symptoms. As I counted to help her regress, she suddenly turned white, her breathing became irregular, and beads of perspiration appeared on her forehead. Simultaneously with the appearance of her symptoms, *I myself* had a strange sensation. For a moment, *I* felt a sharp pain at exactly the same place in my body where she experienced pain as a result of her colitis (although I myself have never in my life had any indigestion problems). Although, as she reported later, she had never thought she had problems at that early age, strongly repressed material emerged when we explored that age together. This single experience with hypnosis, and the following 3 months of psychotherapy working through this experience, were sufficient for her colitis symptoms to disappear completely, with no remission for the 10 years following.

Social-psychological research directed my attention to the possibility of analyzing hypnosis in terms of social influence. Sarbin and Coe's role enactment theory (Sarbin & Coe, 1972, 1979; Coe & Sarbin, 1977; Coe, 1978), and Barber and his associates' studies of the relevance of situational factors (e.g., Barber, 1979; Barber, Spanos, Chaves, 1974; Spanos, 1982a, 1982b), pointed to the importance of including the social context among the fundamental factors influencing hypnosis.

Related Approaches and Theories

The interactive aspects of hypnosis stressed by my social-psychobiological model have never been alien to the experimental investigators to whom hypnosis owed its revival in the 1950s. The Hilgards' developmental–interactive theory has been mentioned above, and Orne (1962) emphasized the importance of the hypnotist's entering into the hypnotic relation-ship— or, as he expressed it, participating in a *folie à deux*. Shor (1962), in his very influential theoretical paper, recognized three separate dimensions of hypnotic depth: "hypnotic role-taking involvement," "trance," and "archaic involvement," each of which was thought to be capable of varying independently of the other two dimensions. I agree with these distinctions, although I prefer to use different names for the three dimensions: "behavioral," "experiential," and "relational" dimensions, respectively. My model, however, includes a physiological dimension, attempts to explain how these dimensions are interrelated, and explicitly recognizes contextual factors as response determinants.

I therefore believe that my model resembles the "newer generation" of hypnosis theories (Kihlstrom, 1985) more than it does the classical theories. The "newer" theories that emerged in the 1980s incorporate concepts derived from general systems theory (Cavallo, 1979; von Berta-lanffy, 1974) in their study of objects and events in the contexts in which they occur. Whereas psychological explanations of behavior were previously conceptualized in terms of a limited set of determinants, which were viewed as independent entities that combine to produce behavior, contemporary theorizing has shown a steady progression to more compli-cated accounts that emphasize reciprocal interactions. According to this emerging approach, behavior, internal personal and cognitive factors, and environmental influences operate mutually as interlocking determinants of one another (Bandura, 1978).

Hypnosis researchers who theorize about hypnosis within this interactive framework stress different dimensions of complex reciprocal processes. Diamond (1984) calls attention to the "neglected importance of the hypnotist in an interactive hypnotherapeutic relationship" (p. 3). On the basis of recent psychoanalytic work, he differentiates four relational dimensions: "transference," "working (therapeutic) alliance," "narcissistic or fusional alliance," and the "real relationship" (Diamond, 1987). My research group's findings, which I discuss below, provide empirical justification for Diamond's plea to devote attention to relational factors in hypnosis. The sociocognitive theoretical positions adopted by Baker, Levitt, Lynn, Nash, and Sheehan are related to the social-psychobiological model. Because my model relies on their findings, their work pertinent to my theory is discussed later in this chapter, together with research from my laboratory.

To my knowledge, none of the approaches mentioned above integrates physiological explanations into an interactional framework. Because a distinctive feature of the social-psychobiological model is the inclusion of a physiological explantion within an interactional framework, the model relies to a great extent on our research concerning physiological concomitants of hypnosis.

Before I conclude this section, it is useful to specify in what respects the model is interactional: (1) On the basis of a multidimensional approach in which behavioral, experiential, relational and physiological dimensions are considered to be equally important, it emphasizes the interaction among these dimensions; (2) instead of limiting its focus to either the subject or the hypnotist, it considers the interaction between these two persons. Despite this interactional emphasis, the most distinctive feature of my model is its social-psychobiological perspective.

THEORETICAL CONCEPTS AND PRINCIPLES

An adequate hypnosis theory should be able to explain the intriguing fact that in a hypnotic situation two unique persons, who meet as strangers, can soon engage in a meaningful interaction in which dramatic changes occur in at least one of the interactants (usually the hypnotized subject). These changes radically modify not only their relationship, behavior, and conscious experience, but also their somatic functioning.

Intrapersonal and Interpersonal Motivation

To understand the relatively effortless appearance of these changes, it is helpful to assume that the participants in the hypnotic interaction actively seek to enter the situation. Personality research and the psychoanalytic literature emphasize motivations such as sensation seeking, dependency needs, and so forth. Recent social-psychological theories note that in interpersonal relationships, the interactants seek to satisfy diverse needs in the situations they create (Aronoff & Wilson, 1985). For example, they may be motivated to maximize their own rewards, as Thibaut and Kelley (1959) originally assumed; or, according to Kelley and Thibaut's more recent theorizing (Kelley, 1979; Kelley & Thibaut, 1978), they may feel personally rewarded when another's needs are met. In either case, they are both motivated to enter an interdependent situation.

Unfortunately, until recently, systematic research on what motivates the participants in the hypnosis interaction has been lacking. An ongoing research program, conducted in our Hypnosis Laboratory at the Department of Experimental Psychology of Eötvös Loránd University, has attempted to address this question. Data secured in an interactional experimental situation (Bányai, Mészáros, Csókay, 1982, 1985) has consistently shown that both intrapersonal and interpersonal needs affect the hypnotist and the subject. Subjects expect to have a mind-altering experience, which they typically think will be sleep-like, and expect to be taken care of by the hypnotist. In a complementary fashion, hypnotists often express a desire to help another person have new experiences. Undoubtedly, this desire to help may in part reflect the need to control others, as psychoanalytic authors (e.g., Gill & Brenman, 1959; Pardell, 1950) have stressed.

Expectation: An Insufficient Explanation

When the subject and the hypnotist agree to participate in a hypnosis session, it seems self-evident that their knowledge, beliefs, attitudes, and expectations will have an impact on their behavior and experience. It has been argued (Kirsch, 1985) that expectation alone may be sufficient to account for the effects of hypnosis—that is, that hypnosis can be reduced to the effects of expectation.

In my opinion, this cannot be a sufficient account of the most characteristic hypnotic effects. Although expectations play an important role, fundamental changes occur in hypnosis that do not conform to the prior expectations of the participants. It is commonplace for hypnotists to encounter subjects who exhibit surprise at experiencing something completely unexpected during hypnosis. In experimental research, Shor, Pistole, Easton, and Kihlstrom (1984) found that persons' expectations about their hypnotic responsiveness accounted for relatively little variance in their performance on standardized hypnotic susceptibility scales.

Our results further confirm the finding that there may be a discrepancy between what is expected and what is experienced during hypnosis. In fact, at times, subjects' experiences are contrary to their previous expectations. After an active/alert hypnotic induction (Bányai & Hilgard, 1976), in which subjects were asked to pedal a stationary bicycle while listening to the hypnotist's suggestions, subjects reported experiencing a hypnotic, genuinely altered state of consciousness that did not bear the slightest resemblance to sleep or relaxation. Instead, they experienced a highly aroused, vigorous state. What is interesting is that this state was very different from their preconceptions about hypnosis-related alterations in consciousness. It is thus not surprising that after subjects are hypnotized for the first time, their attitudes toward hypnosis change significantly (McConkey, 1986).

The Hypnotic Context

An important contextual factor is the definition of the situation as hypnosis. Evidence is accumulating that when procedures are defined as "hypnosis," they have a radically different effect—mainly phenomenologically—than when similar or identical procedures are *not* labeled "hypnosis" (e.g., Pekala & Forbes, 1988; Spanos, Kennedy, & Gwynn, 1984; Spanos, Voorneveld, & Gwynn, 1987). Apart from labeling, other contextual factors (e.g., the prestige and location of the research laboratory; its atmosphere; and the style, age, and clothing of the staff), have been shown to influence the outcome of hypnosis. Furthermore, whether the context is labeled or perceived as hypnotic or not has an effect on the correlations between hypnotic susceptibility and various personality measures (for reviews see Spanos, Gabora, Jarrett, & Gwynn, 1989). This so-called "context effect" is taken up later.

Hypnotic Susceptibility: Stable and Modifiable

There has been intense debate about whether hypnotic susceptibility is a reasonably stable personality trait (e.g., E. R. Hilgard, 1965) or whether it is a set of sociocognitive skills and attitudes (e.g., Diamond, 1977; Gorassini & Spanos, 1986). By now, compelling evidence suggests that it remains stable over a long period of time, despite substantial changes in the personal life and social and economic circumstances of the individual (Morgan, Johnson, & Hilgard, 1974; Piccione, Hilgard, & Zimbardo, 1989). The high correlations among susceptibility scores assessed by different methods also suggests that susceptibility is stable (E. R. Hilgard, 1979).

Although there is an impressive degree of consistency over time and across methods, opinion is nevertheless divided about the factors that account for this response stability. Some explanations emphasize an aptitude dimension of hypnotic responsiveness (e.g., E. R. Hilgard, 1965, 1977; J. R. Hilgard, 1979; Tellegen, 1979), whereas other accounts attribute the high cross-time, cross-test correlations to the "situational commonalities inherent in the structure of even different hypnotizability tests" (Spanos et al., 1989, p. 271). Despite these opposing views, there may be a way to resolve the apparent contradictions.

The fact that some investigators report significant changes in hypnotic responsiveness as a result of specially designed modification procedures has been interpreted as evidence against the hypothesis that hypnotizability is a trait (see Spanos, 1986). Early efforts to modify hypnotizability (see reviews by Diamond, 1974, 1977) were criticized on methodological grounds. More recent studies (Gfeller, Lynn, & Pribble, 1987; Gorassini & Spanos, 1986; Spanos et al., 1987, 1989) are also flawed by methodological problems: They use somewhat misleading instructions; they place strong demands on subjects to conform to the instructions; they use only a single pretest, failing to control for anxiety reduction attendant on retesting; and generalization of training effects is not tested across the complete spectrum of cognitive and affective measures. However, even if methodological problems were eliminated, it would not change the fact that a certain proportion of subjects remain resistant to even the most concerted efforts to modify susceptibility. I therefore agree with Gfeller et al.'s (1987) opinion that "there is no intrinsic conflict between the contention that hypnotizability can be modified and enhanced and the notion that certain personal attributes and abilities exist that are stable, enduring, and perhaps resistant to modification" (p. 594).

Flexibility as the Common Factor

The discussion above suggests that it is worthwhile to address this question: What stable and enduring abilities are associated with hypnotic susceptibility? Investigators have attempted to address this question by conceptualizing the ability central to hypnosis as "tranceability" (Shor, 1979), a capacity for "imaginative involvement" (J. R. Hilgard, 1979), "absorption" (Tellegen & Atkinson, 1974), a physiological predisposition for preference for right-hemispheric use (Bakan, 1969; Gur & Gur, 1974; Sackheim, Paulus, & Weiman, 1979), "hemispheric specificity" (MacLeod-Morgan, 1985), and "attentional capacity" (Graham & Evans, 1977).

In my view, a common factor among these various abilities is *flexibility in changing the ways of functioning*. In an important paper entitled, "Cognitive and Physiological Flexibility: Multiple Pathways to Hypnotic Responsiveness, " Crawford (1989) expresses a similar viewpoint, stating that highly susceptible subjects are more flexible cognitively and possibly physiologically than their less susceptible counterparts. (These two groups are referred to hereafter as "highs" and "lows," for the sake of brevity.) Evans takes a similar position and summarizes research relevant to the issue of cognitive flexibility in Chapter 5 of this volume.

This flexibility is reflected in the fact that highs *generally* seem to be more flexible in altering their consciousness: They fall asleep more rapidly and take more daytime naps than lows (Evans, 1977), and they have more unusual experiences in everyday life than lows (see Kihlstrom et al., 1989, for a review). Pekala and his associates found that alterations in consciousness, as measured by the Phenomenology of Consciousness Inventory (Pekala, 1982), were able to predict hypnotizability scores of subjects with a validity coefficient of .63–.65 (Pekala & Kumar, 1984, 1987).

In a series of experiments (reviewed by Crawford, 1989), Crawford and her colleagues found that highs demonstrated a greater ease in shifting cognitive strategies from analytic to nonanalytic, and from a detail-oriented to a holistic manner of information processing, than lows. A study conducted in our laboratory (Greguss, Bányai, Mészáros, Csókay, 1980) revealed that highs, as compared to lows more easily ignored the temporal sequence of stimulus presentation in free recall. This difference in cognitive styles appeared not only after hypnosis or posthypnotic suggestions (as was reported by Evans & Kihlstrom, 1973), but also in the waking state. This finding indicates that highs and lows may differ in the flexibility of attending to temporal and sequential cues necessary for information processing. Combined, the data suggest that highs are able to regress to an earlier, more archaic way of processing information (for a review, see Nash, 1988).

Mounting evidence suggests that high susceptible subjects are more flexible than low subjects in the alternate use of the two cerebral hemispheres when tasks are administered that demand such an alteration. Data from our laboratory (e.g., Bányai, 1985a, 1985b; Mészáros, Bányai, & Greguss, 1985) and from other laboratories (e.g., MacLeod-Morgan, 1979, 1985; MacLeod-Morgan & Lack, 1982) have demonstrated that highs, relative to lows, exhibit greater task-specific shifts in differential electroencephalographic (EEG) activation of the hemispheres as measured by power spectra.

Both behavioral and central electrophysiological data (40-Hz EEG) indicate that hypnotizability is also related to flexibility in shifting the focus of selective attention. In general, highs have a greater ability to focus on a task and to ignore stimuli unrelated to the task (e.g., DePascalis & Penna, 1990; Graham & Evans, 1977; Karlin, 1979; Wallace, Knight, & Garrett, 1976). A difference in physiological flexibility was also evident in a study of regional cerebral blood flow, with highs again being more flexible than lows (Crawford, Skolnick, Benson, Gur, & Gur, 1985). Furthermore, heart rate, the most sensitive peripheral physiological index of vegetative arousal, showed greater variation in highs than in lows when subjects were performing test suggestions (Sturgis & Coe, 1990), and when subjects had to imagine frightening scenes in the waking state (Hughes & Bowers, 1987).

It should be emphasized that *all* the above-cited data showing greater flexibility in various physiological functions were secured *within a hypnotic context*. Even if a hypnotic induction was not administered, the experiements were conducted in a hypnosis laboratory by hypnosis researchers; thus, the "atmosphere" of hypnosis was usually unavoidably present.

Interaction between Hypnotic Responsiveness and Context

As noted above, research has demonstrated that if subjects are tested outside the context of hypnosis, the typical correlations between different personality measures and hypnotizability are no longer evident (see Kirsch, Chapter 14, this volume). Beyond absorption (Council, Kirsch, & Hafner, 1986), de Groot and his associates (de Groot, Gwynn, & Spanos, 1988) found this effect in questionnaire measures of mystical experience, daydreaming frequency, and paranormal beliefs. Spanos and his colleagues (Spanos et al., 1989) reported that the correlation between the scores on the Creative Imagination Scale (CIS) and the Carleton University Responsiveness to Suggestion Scale (CURSS) was as high as the correlation that is typically secured among hypnotizability scales if the CIS was defined as a test of hypnotizability. However, if the CIS was introduced as a test of imagination, there was no significant correlation with the CURSS.

Sociocognitive theorists interpret this context effect as evidence against the hypothesis that hypnotic susceptibility is a stable personality trait. In my view, however, it may also be a relatively stable characteristic of a person, whether or not he or she is flexible enough to manifest his or her flexibility *within a social context.* Although low subjects may have a capacity for absorption or imagination outside the hypnotic context, it is possible that they do not express it in hypnotic contexts where they fear relinquishing control to the hypnotist. A number of studies provide indirect support for this possibility. Virtually every hypnotist has encountered lows who move their arms *up*ward when they receive a hand-lowering suggestion. Jones and Spanos (1982) and Lynn et al. (1986) reported that in a hypnotic context, certain lows do more than simply fail to cooperate; they actively oppose the suggestions.

Thus, when I use the term "flexibility" as it pertains to hypnosis, I use it in a broader sense than do Crawford (1989) and Evans (see Chapter 5): In addition to cognitive and physiological flexibility, I include *flexibility in the social context* within the purview of this construct. This type of flexibility can be thought of as the ease with which one enters into a social relationship in which strong mutual regulatory processes will be set in motion. Because this is a developmental characteristic of functioning in intimate relationships, the model and archetype of which is the early parent–child relationship, this social flexibility can be thought of as a capacity to enter into a regressed relationship.

In summary, changes caused by contextual factors do not pose a serious challenge to the idea that hypnotic susceptibility is a stable personality trait. Hypnotizability develops in the process of socialization, and, as J. R. Hilgard (1979) observed, it is therefore "natural" that early modes of social relating influence it. However, the fact that Morgan (1973) found a significantly higher correlation of hypnotic susceptibility between monozygotic twins than between dizygotic twins or siblings suggests that there may also be a genetic component contributing to the stability of hypnotic responsiveness. This fact provides indirect support for the social-psychobiological hypothesis that hypnosis and hypnotic susceptibility have a socially and biologically adaptive value.

The Hypnotist's Personal Style

The concept of the hypnotist's "personal style" or "personal working style" is new in the hypnosis literature. By this term I mean the characteristic way in which the hypnotist enters the interaction defined as hypnosis. We (Bányai et al., in press) found it necessary to introduce this term because comparative analysis of hypnotic sessions of different hypnotists revealed that even under standard experimental circumstances, hypnotists utilized different cues in perceiving subtle changes in the subjects' behavior and alterations of consciousness.

As I describe in more detail later in the chapter, we have so far identified two characteristic hypnotist styles: a "physical/organic" style, relying more on bodily cues, and an "analytic/cognitive" style, relying more on thoughts. The two styles are characterized by complex, distinctive patterns of behavioral, phenomenological, and relational features (Bányai et al., in press). The hypnotist's style is important insofar as it contributes to the outcome of hypnosis interactions, although in a manner distinct from what is measured by a standard susceptibility score. That is, whereas a behavioral score on a standardized scale of hypnotic susceptibility is primarily a function of the subject's hypnotic responsiveness, subjective experiences and the intensity of the relationship appear to be related to the hypnotist's personal style.

The Hypnotic State: Altered but Not Necessarily Sleep-Like

The traditional view of hypnosis emphasizes its sleep-like nature. Even the name "hypnosis" comes from the Greek word for sleep, *hypnos*. Since one of the most important physiological theories of hypnosis, that of Pavlov (1923), conceptualizes hypnosis as partial sleep, it is not surprising that the first physiological investigations of hypnosis (e.g., Loomis, Harvey, & Hobart, 1936) sought to identify sleep-like EEG indices. As we concluded elsewhere (Mészáros & Bányai, 1978), the research does not confirm these expectations: none of the studies in which the hypnotic state has been sufficiently controlled has demonstrated sleep-like changes in the background EEG (for a similar review, see Evans, 1979). Nor does hypnosis increase triggered alpha afterdischarge (a finer index of synchronization tendency), which is considered to be a sign of active cortical inhibition (Bányai, Mészáros, Greguss, Andrejva, & Neumann, 1979; Mészáros, Bányai, & Greguss, 1980).

The occurrence of spontaneous ecstatic trance states during certain tribal ceremonies (e.g., the trance dances in Bali and the dances of the whirling dervishes), together with the highly aroused states that appear in special therapeutic settings, led me to question whether the sleep-like quality of the state is an essential aspect of hypnosis or a by-product of the type of induction employed. To address this question, I, together with E. R. Hilgard (Bányai & Hilgard, 1976), devised an activity-increasing *active/alert* hypnotic induction procedure. This method requires that the subject ride a bicycle ergometer under load with the eyes open, while verbal suggestions are given to enhance alertness, attentiveness, and a feeling of freshness. No mention is ever made of sleepiness, relaxation, or eye closure. In a series of studies, we showed (Bányai, 1976, 1980, 1987; Bányai & Hilgard, 1976; Bányai, Mészáros, & Greguss, 1981) that subjects achieved a genuinely altered state of consciousness after the active/alert induction.

From the beginning of my theorizing about hypnosis, I have believed that hypnosis, just like any other state of consciousness, should be regarded as a complex state "which can be differentiated and characterized only by taking into consideration three factors simultaneously: the subjective experience of the hypnotized person, his/her observable behavior, and his/her physiological changes" (Bányai, 1973, p. 38; a similar view is expressed by Tellegen, 1979). Thus, in order to explore the essence of the hypnotic state, all three dimensions were studied. The comparative analysis of the traditional and active/alert hypnosis showed that although there were differences in subjective experiences, in behavior, and in physiological characteristics reflecting the decrease and increase in induced arousal, the direction of change in activity/arousal level was a by-product of the induction procedures used (Bányai et al., 1981). It can therefore be concluded that hypnosis is not a sleep-like state. It is also important to point out that our research indicated that hypnosis can be induced in a context completely different from the traditional relaxation-based context in which suggestions are typically administered.

The Hypnotic State: A Socially Altered State of Consciousness?

One of our most interesting findings was that, regardless of whether a traditional relaxation-based or an active/alert induction was administered, more than three-quarters of the subjects (78%) spontaneously reported a narrowing of attention after the induction. Because the modification of selective attention was a common feature of response to both inductions, we studied it in its own right. We reached the conclusion that "independently of the changes of the general level of activation evoked by different types of hypnotic induction—relaxational and active–alert—it is the modification of selective attention that lies behind the characteristic behavioral and subjective changes in hypnosis" (Mészáros, Bányai, & Greguss, 1981, p. 474).

In our research on selective attention, we found that subjects reacted to subtle (sometimes even nonverbal) cues in the hypnotist's communication, in accordance with the demands of the task. For example, when subjects had to focus their attention on the interval between a warning tone signal and a visual stimulus, the latencies of the late components of the visual evoked potentials (VEPs) decreased; in avoidance conditioning, when they had to delay their motor responses, the latencies of the VEPs increased (Bányai et al., 1981; Mészáros et al., 1981).

Later research (e.g., Bányai et al., 1985; Cikurel & Gruzelier, 1989; Mészáros et al., 1985) revealed that attention to the hypnotist's communications was accompanied by a relative preponderance of right-hemispheric activity in both traditional and active/alert hypnosis. In fact, numerous studies originating from different laboratories have confirmed these findings (for a review, see DeBenedittis & Carli, 1990). Although the hopes raised by laterality research of finding clear-cut, well-separated functional differences between the two hemispheres seem to be vanishing (see Gosi-Greguss, Bányai, Vágó, Varga, & Horváth, 1988), the right hemisphere still seems to be superior in the distribution of attention across space and in the production and perception of emotion (for a review, see Hellige, 1990). It is also generally agreed that this superiority indicates that the right hemisphere is superior in processing interpersonal communication.

Our research on the effects of active/alert hypnosis, especially the findings regarding its effects on attentional processes, appears to yield direct support for a social-psychobiological conceptualization of hypnosis. The findings indicate that the essential feature of the hypnotic state, which differentiates it from other altered states of consciousness, may lie in its social character. The alteration of consciousness appears in an interpersonal situation in which attention is focused on the partner's communication so that the direction of attention is controlled by this communication.

With this view of the hypnotic state in mind, the flexibility in the social context that I have described earlier as the common factor underlying hypnotic susceptibility means that in a hypnotic context, high susceptible subjects are apt to direct their attention toward or away from internal or external stimuli in accordance with the communications of the hypnotist. In contrast, subjects low in susceptibility are not flexible enough to attune themselves to the hypnotist's suggestions in a manner comparable to that of highs. This difference between highs and lows is not reflected in the same way with regard to physiological, behavioral, and experiential dimensions of hypnosis. That is, recent research (Bányai et al., in press) shows that although behavioral and physiological differences are conspicuous, highs and lows are equally likely to report alterations of consciousness when subjective reports are secured by appropriate nonsuggestive methods.

The Induction of Hypnosis: Cognitive and Interpersonal Attunement

Research on interactional processes, which extends beyond the field of hypnosis, has highlighted the mutual regulatory functions of participants in close relationships. In their studies of parent–infant interactions, Brazelton and his colleagues (Brazelton, Koslowski, & Main, 1974) found that reciprocity was evident even in early mother–infant interactions. Furthermore, in both animals and humans, social emotions and interactions are accompanied by marked neurophysiological and hormonal changes (Reite & Field, 1985). As Field (1985) states, "Attachment might . . . be viewed as a relationship that develops between two or more organisms as their behavioral and physiological systems become attuned to each other. Each partner provides meaningful stimulation for the other and has a modulating influence on the other's arousal level" (p. 415). According to Field, the individual has differential stimulation and arousal modulation needs, and they may be met by diverse individuals in different life stages.

When the hypnotist and the subject agree to enter into a situation defined as hypnosis, one of their (perhaps unconscious) motives may be to engage in an interaction in which mutual regulatory functions become more intensive than in their everyday interactions. Although more systematic research is needed to clarify this issue, our research (Bányai et al., 1982, 1985) concerning the complementary motives of the hypnotist and subject, alluded to above, seems to support this hypothesis.

The hypnotic situation is generally constructed so as to isolate the participants from their usual, everyday environment. It has long been established that the deprivation of everyday environmental and social cues increases susceptibility to alterations of consciousness (e.g., Heron, Doane, & Scott, 1956). As a result of prolonged isolation, (rare) social cues become more influential. As Sargant (1957) pointed out, the ancient technique of brainwashing is based on this principle. Barabasz (1980) reported that after nine persons' wintering-over isolation in Antarctica, they showed a significant increase in waking suggestibility as measured by the Barber Suggestibility Scale (Barber & Glass, 1962).

In my view, the hypnotic induction plays an important role in helping a subject to direct attention to cues selected by the hypnotist and to develop a special regressed relationship with the hypnotist. In the course of the hypnotic induction the hypnotist gives verbal feedback to the subject about perceivable sensations in the subject's body that are usually out of awareness, but can be brought into the focus of awareness (e.g., breathing, muscle tone). As a result, a high susceptible subject usually begins to narrow attention to these sensations in accordance with the hypnotist's instructions. As the proceedings continue, the subject is likely to attribute these changes to the effects of hypnosis or the hypnotist. Sooner or later, the subject starts to respond to the hypnotist's suggestions, as if the hypnotist has become the "structured frame of reference in the background of attention which supports, interprets, and gives meaning to all experiences" (Shor, 1959, p. 586).

The verbal feedback given in the course of the induction procedure typically has a twofold effect on high susceptible subjects: (1) because of the marked changes in selective attention, cognitive, behavioral, and even physiological changes appear; (2) because these changes are attributed to the hypnotist (which is similar to the way a child attributes omnipotence to its parents), they begin to develop a special regressed relationship with the hypnotist. Low subjects, for the most part, even when they are able to direct their attention to what the hypnotist communicates, are unwilling and unable to relinquish their mundane reality orientation. They maintain analytical and sometimes critical attitudes, and typically avoid experiencing a regressed relationship with the hypnotist.

Regrettably, the regulatory role of the subject has been neglected in the hypnosis literature. Although clinicians have sporadically referred to the effect of subjects in modifying their own (i.e., the hypnotists') state of consciousness, sometimes resulting in "spontaneous trance" experiences (for reviews, see Diamond, 1980, 1984, 1987), I believe that ours is the only laboratory to systematically investigate this aspect of the hypnotic interaction. As I discuss below, the systematic analysis of behavioral, physiological, experiential, and relational data pertinent to hypnotists reveals that subtle cues emanating from subjects direct hypnotists' attention and, in turn, influence the hypnotists' communications to their subjects (Vágó, et al., 1988). Furthermore, the hypnotists' characteristic style moderates this effect.

In summary, the social-psychobiological model conceptualizes the hypnotic induction as a process of mutual attunement in which the hypnotist and the subject become sensitive and responsive to each other's stimulation. This process may have an adaptive function, because evidence suggests that attunement or "being on the same wavelength" (Field, 1985, p. 415) generally characterizes close relationships that have a crucial role in maintaining the comfort and the optimal level of arousal of the organism.

In a social-psychobiological model of hypnosis, it is not enough to study one participant of an interaction *and then* the other participant. To study the process of attunement beyond sequential analysis, a more holistic approach is required. It is therefore important to introduce the concept of "interaction synchrony"—a central concept of modern interaction research—into the field of hypnosis. "Interaction synchrony" is a term applied to the matching of rhythms present in individuals. Interaction researchers have reported interaction synchrony with respect to diverse physical activities and physiological processes. For example, Condon and Ogston (1967) have noted movement synchrony between therapist and client; Stern (1982) has discussed the functions of rhythm changes between mothers and infants; and Chapple (1982) has recognized the importance of the "musical language of body rhythms" in interactions.

I conceive of interaction synchrony in a broader sense: In human interactions synchrony may come about not only in physical and physiological activites, but in terms of subjective experiences as well. The study of interaction synchrony in overt and covert processes within the hypnotic interaction may yield valuable information about the nature of rapport between the subject and hypnotist. As I elaborate below, our findings (Bányai, 1988; Bányai et al., in press) concerning interaction synchrony in hypnosis indicate that the relation between interactional synchrony and rapport varies as a function of the hypnotist's style.

RESEARCH AND APPRAISAL

The review of the research supporting the social-psychobiological model outlined above is not exhaustive. Although data in the classical hypnosis literature point in the direction of the social-psychobiological model, I cite only those results that have direct relevance to the model. These data were obtained within an interactive framework. Few laboratories have extended the scope of their investigation to interactive processes. Thus, the main body of research I review is based on studies conducted in our laboratory since 1982, when we first adopted an explicitly interactive framework of analysis.

I preface this discussion with a description of the interactional experimental paradigm of hypnosis. According to this research model, interactions are studied in a complex way. First, prehypnotic attitudes and expectations are recorded. Then the behavioral manifestations of hypnosis, physiological indices, subjective experiences, and data pertinent to the relational dimension of hypnosis are recorded simultaneously with respect to the hypnotist and the subject. The experimental sessions, including interviews to obtain information about subjective experiences, are video-taped so that both participants in the interaction can be observed. Data are analyzed separately for the different dimensions of interest with respect to both participants, and are then intercorrelated. Measures of interaction synchrony are also analyzed. Raw data are assessed by independent judges and raters who are naive with respect to the aim, procedures, and other findings of the experiements. Raters who content-analyze subjective experiences therefore know nothing about subjects' hypnotic susceptibility or that of the experimental groups.

Interactional Experiential Analysis Technique

In order to obtain reliable information about the subjective experiences of both the subject and the hypnotist, we developed the "interactional experiential analysis technique" (IEAT; Varga, 1986; Varga, Bányai, Gosi-Greguss, Vágó, & Horváth, 1988). In addition to Sheehan and

McConkey's (1982) "experiential analysis technique," in which the subject's reports on his or her subjective feelings and thoughts are stimulated by the video playback of the original hypnosis session, the hypnotist is asked to relate his or her experiences in a similar way, but completely separated from the subject. In this situation, independent inquirers, who have not been involved in any way in the hypnosis interaction, listen to the subject's and hypnotist's reports.

Data secured with the IEAT have demonstrated that the hypnotist and subject are experientially attuned. I (Bányai, 1986) reported that during certain periods of the hypnotic process, subjective experiences of the hypnotist and the subject converged, at least symbolically and in terms of mood: At the beginning of the video playback of the hypnotic interaction, the hypnotist and the subject reported completely different experiences; however, as the session progressed, they began to relate similar feelings. They often used identical metaphors to describe their experiences; they had common associations to events; the colors appearing in their fantasies had the same tones; and they reported sadness and happiness, for example, at the same point during the hypnotic interaction. Similar interaction synchrony in subjective experiences has been observed in the therapeutic context (Smith, 1990).

A systematic analysis of the intercorrelations of the verbal reports of hypnotists interacting with different subjects revealed (Bányai et al., in press; Varga et al., 1988) that interaction synchrony in subjective experiences was unrelated to the "success" of hypnosis, measured in terms of behavioral response to test suggestions and judgments of hypnotic depth. The synchrony in the interactants' verbal reports was, however, related to measures of the relational dimension of hypnosis.

Subjective Experiences versus Behavioral Scores

Perhaps the most conspicuous finding secured in our laboratory is that subjects high, medium, and low in susceptibility are comparable with respect to the number of experiences they report that indicate an alteration of their usual awareness (Varga, 1986, 1991; Varga, Bányai, Gosi-Greguss, Vágó, & Horváth, 1987; Varga et al., 1988). For example, lows experience spontaneous amnesia, disturbed time sense, body image change, and trance logic—indices of altered conconsciousness—as often as do highs.

Yet perhaps even more striking is the finding that the frequency of experiences indicating alterations of consciousness are not correlated with measures of the subjective depth of hypnosis. One possible interpretation of these surprising results is that subjective depth reports reflect a difference in attributional processes across hypnotizability levels. That is, although low and high subjects experience alterations of consciousness with equal frequency, lows may not attribute these alterations to the hypnotist or to the effect of hypnosis. This interpretation is consonant with Bowers's (1973) attributional analysis of hypnosis, and with Lynn and his colleagues' report (Lynn, Snodgrass, Rhue, Nash, & Frauman, 1987) that "high and low susceptible subjects differ in their judgments about the degree to which their responses are a function of their own versus the hypnotist's abilities and efforts even before they are hypnotized" (p. 42).

Interaction Synchrony

In order to study the relation between subjective deepening of hypnosis and other phenomena of the hypnotic interaction, we (Bányai, Mészáros, & Csókay, 1984; Bányai, 1985b, 1986) collected depth reports in different phases of the hypnosis session. It was noticed that sudden deepenings of hypnosis occurred after a number of phenomena comprehensively termed "interaction synchrony."

Interaction synchrony appeared either in overt movements (e.g., joint movements of the limbs when the subject performed motor suggestions) and postures (e.g., posture mirroring), or in some covert processes (e.g., breathing and electromyographic activity). These movements were involuntary and out of awareness. An interaction rhythm was reported at the end of the hypnotic induction: If hypnosis was sufficiently deep, a swaying motion of the hypnotist's body was observed in synchronization with the subject's breathing. Linton, Travis, Kuechenmeister, and White (1977) reported a similar finding: In their experiments, heart rate concordance between hypnotist and subject increased in the course of the hypnotic induction in some subjects. These experimental findings lend empirical support to anecdotal observations that point to the importance of the hypnotist's "being on the same wavelength" as the subject.

The Style of the Hypnotist

We have systematically studied the the relation between interaction synchrony and different dimensions of hypnosis. We (Vágó et al., 1988; Bányai et al., in press) discovered that hypnotists differed in the occurrence of interaction synchrony. For example, for one hypnotist, the percentage of time of common breathing rhythm during hypnosis was three times greater than that of another hypnotist ($p < .01$). The percentage of time of joint rhythmic movements (i.e., the hypnotist's unwittingly moving back and forth or from left to right in the breathing rhythm of the subject) was also significantly higher for that hypnotist. These differences were interpreted as signs of being physically more "tuned in" to the subject.

Analysis of the subjective experiences of the hypnotists (Bányai et al., in press; Varga et al., 1988) revealed that observable differences in interaction synchrony paralleled verbal reports. The hypnotist with more signs of physical attunement made many comments on her bodily involvement in the process. She described various sensations in her body and the ways in which these sensations affected her during the hypnosis session. She stated that in many instances she relied on her own bodily sensations in order to assess the state of the subject, as if acquiring information about the subject through this channel. In contrast, the reports of the other hypnotist, who showed less observable signs of physical attunement, reflected a more cognitive/rational involvement. He reported his impressions of the subject's personality, and "analyzed" the process of hypnosis as well as his own style and attitude.

On the basis of the intercorrelations of physical attunement and verbal reports of different hypnotists, we have described two distinct hypnotist styles: a physical/organic style, which is characterized by the frequent occurrence of interaction synchrony and by the use of bodily cues during the hypnotic proceedings; and an analytic/cognitive style, characterized by maintaining greater distance from the subject and relying on thoughts rather than bodily cues (Bányai et al., in press). Although there was no correlation between hypnotists' personal style and subjects' behavioral responsiveness to standardized test suggestions, we found that hypnotists' personal style had an effect on the subjective experiences and the relationship of the interactants.

"Maternal" and "Paternal" Hypnosis

The difference in the hypnotists' characteristic working styles described above closely resembles Ferenczi's (1909/1965) hypothesized distinction between "maternal" and "paternal" hypnosis. According to Ferenczi, these two types of hypnosis are based on the "same feelings of love or fear, the same conviction of infallibility, as those with which his [the subjects'] parents inspired him as a child" (p. 178). The physical/organic style we have identified resembles Ferenczi's maternal hypnosis, whereas the analytic/cognitive style resembles paternal hypnosis.

Research on verbal communication supports this distinction. We (Vágó et al., 1988) noted that the hypnotist with the physical/organic style called subjects by their first names in order to establish better rapport with highly susceptible males (as if being more "maternal" with them), whereas the hypnotist with the analytic/cognitive style inhibited the frequency of subjects' speech (similar to a "restricting father"). Thus, the terms "maternal" and "paternal" appear to be useful metaphors for describing the styles of the hypnotists.

We regard these data as preliminary. The present interpretation of the findings requires further testing with additional hypnotist–subject dyads. To elaborate the construct validity of hypnotist style, it will be important to determine whether the initial description of hypnotist styles is valid, and whether additional styles can be identified in an interactional framework in which subjects' responses to varying styles can be studied as well. From a social-psychobiological perspective, however, we can postulate that hypnosis styles will resemble the styles of the most important relationships in life that have regulatory functions. That is, beyond maternal and paternal hypnosis, there may exist "sibling" and other types of hypnosis.

The Relational Dimension

Interest in the relational dimension of hypnosis has come to the fore as the result of renewed interest on the part of clinicians (for reviews, see Diamond, 1984, 1987). Although Shor (1962) argued that "archaic involvement"—as he termed the transference-like phenomena appearing in hypnosis—is unlikely to develop under experimental conditions, several lines of experimental research have addressed the relational dimension of hypnosis. Sheehan and his colleagues (Sheehan, 1971; Sheehan & Dolby, 1975; Dolby & Sheehan, 1977) developed a special experimental paradigm based on "countering," by which they were able to obtain an objective index of involvement with the hypnotist. They reported that some high susceptible subjects showed such a strong involvement with the hypnotist that they were able to counter their preconceptions about hypnosis in favor of responding in accordance with the hypnotist's intent.

Studies on the ability to resist hypnotic suggestions (e.g., Baker & Levitt, 1989; Levitt, Baker, & Fish, 1990; Spanos et al., 1984) are also relevant to this topic. These studies show that even high susceptible subjects are able to resist hypnotic suggestions if an appropriate relationship develops between the resistance instructor and the subject; as a result, the subjects perceptions about appropriate behavior will include resistance. Lynn et al. (1984) found that hypnotic rapport, in addition to normative expectancies about appropriate hypnotic behavior, affected hypnotizable subjects' ability to resist suggestions.

Findings pertinent to the relational dimension of hypnosis, taken together with our findings regarding the involvement of the hypnotist, cast doubt on theoretical formulations (e.g., Barber, 1979; Sarbin & Coe, 1972; Spanos, 1982a, 1982b; Wagstaff, 1981) that emphasize situational factors at the expense of relational factors. The phenomena of countering and the hypnotist's involvement suggest that deeper, more "archaic" bonds exist in hypnotic situations.

In the course of pursuing our research program, we repeatedly became aware of the development of a special regressed relationship between the hypnotist and the subject. The development of this relationship either facilitated the induction of deep hypnosis (e.g., when a male subject reported that the hypnotist reminded him of his father) or interfered with it (e.g., when a female hypnotist miscalled the subject by the name of her divorced husband) (Bányai et al., 1984).

The relation between archaic involvement and other hypnosis dimensions was studied in our laboratory by using the Archaic Involvement Measure (Nash & Spinler, 1989). We extended the scale to the negative side of involvement, and also to the archaic involvement of the hypnotist with the subject (Horváth, Bányai, Varga, Gosi-Greguss, & Vágó, 1988; Bányai et al., in press). We found that archaic involvement and behavioral and subjective measures of hypnotic depth were related only if subjects had had at least one prior experience with hypnosis. This finding indicates that having experienced hypnosis once shapes not only expectations and attitudes (as is usually emphasized), but also the deeper layers of the hypnotic experience.

Interaction synchrony data, subjective experiences, and data derived from diverse paper-and-pencil tests of the relational dimension may be useful in better understanding the four dimensions of hypnotic relationships hypothesized by Diamond (1987). For example, the occurrence of interaction synchrony in overt and covert processes found with certain hypnotists in some phases of the hypnotic interaction may be an objective index of the narcissistic or fusional alliance described by Diamond (1987). Data on the archaic involvement of hypnotists and subjects may contribute to our understanding of the transference dimension, whereas verbal reports may be used to secure data pertinent to the real relationship and the working alliance. I suspect that from these data an ever-changing, dynamic, complex pattern of relational processes will emerge, the further study of which will be necessary in order to capture the essence of hypnosis.

Possible Mediating Mechanisms

The intercorrelation of physiological, behavioral, phenomenological, and relational data secured within an interactional paradigm, along with related findings, suggests tentative hypotheses concerning the processes that mediate the development of a hypnotically altered state of consciousness. The subject's hypnotic susceptibility and the hypnotist's style interact to affect the development of hypnosis. Hypnotists characterized by different working styles react differently to subjects' cues as a function of their own hypnotic susceptibility (Bányai et al., in press).

When hypnotists with low susceptibility encounter signs of high susceptibility, they tend to react with "maneuvers" that foster attunement with the subject. It can be hypothesized, in the case of the maternal style, that interaction synchrony provides a bridge between subjects' and hypnotists' feelings. Interaction rhythm, then, can be used as a "tool" to help hypnotists "get on the same wavelength" as subjects. Perhaps this explains why, in the case of the maternal hypnotist, the number of interactionally synchronous phenomena correlated positively with the subjects' positive comments about their relationship, and also with the subjects' positive archaic involvement with the hypnotist: If a hypnotist uses this "tool" effectively, then a subject will feel taken care of and a feeling of comfort will ensue.

When more hypnotically susceptible hypnotists, on the other hand, encounter signs of high susceptibility, they tend to increase the "distance" between themselves and subjects by employing "cooler" cognitive maneuvers. In this case, the analytic/cognitive style of a paternal hypnotist could serve to maintain control or regulate the situation. This could explain why, after hypnosis sessions with the paternal hypnotist, the subjects' verbal reports were more positive if the hypnotist acted in ways consistent with a cognitive/analytic working style. It appeared that under these circumstances subjects felt more secure in the interaction.

From the data secured so far, we have the impression that if hypnotists use their characteristic working style, then the atmosphere of hypnosis sessions becomes more positive than otherwise: The interactants report more positive mutual feelings, and the subjects report greater hypnotic depth. It is noteworthy that under strictly controlled laboratory conditions, we found that with maternal hypnotists, occasional slight physical discomfort (e.g., headache) often disappeared when the hypnotist acted in a manner consistent with her maternal style. This finding may contribute to our understanding of the somatic curative effects of hypnosis. It suggests that attunement itself may have a healing effect.

In order to formulate even preliminary working hypotheses regarding the physical mechanisms mediating the experience of hypnosis, it is necessary to search for relationships among quite distant fields of inquiry. One relationship that is worthy of study is the possible link between regulatory brain mechanisms and the effects of a hypnotic induction on hemispheric preponderance. Tucker and Williamson (1984) proposed that there are two major cortical regulatory systems: Arousal is externally oriented, located primarily in the right hemisphere and parietal regions, and controlled by noradrenergic neurotransmission, whereas activation is internally oriented, associated with the left hemisphere and frontal regions, and controlled by dopaminergic transmission. A recent study (Mészáros, Crawford, Szabó, Nagykovács, & Révész, 1989) documenting differential activation of parieto-occipital and fronto-central regions in high susceptible subjects as a result of hypnosis may indicate that the frontal region of the left hemisphere and the parietal region of the right hemisphere may be involved in the central physiological processes mediating the effects of a hypnotic induction. Researchers (e.g., Pribram & McGuinnes, 1975) have suggested that the system that coordinates externally oriented arousal and internally oriented activation is located in the hippocampus. Thus it seems reasonable to hypothesize that the differential activation of the hemispheres is based on a mechanism involving the hippocampus. Kissin (1986), on the basis of studies of the behavioral consequences of certain psychoactive drugs, and of physiological studies during various hypnagogic states other than hypnosis, proposed that "physiologically hypnagogic states are activated through the inhibitory effect of the septal–hippocampal circuit upon amygdaloid control" (p. 323).

An important series of studies by DeBenedittis and Sironi (for a review, see DeBenedittis & Sironi, 1988) on the electrical recording and stimulation of deep brain structures in humans reported controlled experimental evidence of the role of the limbic system in mediating the experience of hypnosis. Electrical stimulation of the amygdala aroused patients from hypnosis, but electrical stimulation of the hippocampus did not have a comparable effect. The authors concluded that hypnotic behavior is mediated at least in part by a dynamic balance of antagonizing effects of discrete limbic structures, the amygdala and the hippocampus.

Additional control in this type of research (e.g., hypnotic vs. nonhypnotic conditions) is needed, along with studies that describe how the hypothesized fronto-limbic mechanisms are involved in mediating the effects of the hypnotic induction. However, the results described above, together with recent studies using brain-mapping techniques (DeBenedittis & Carli, 1990), hold promise for studying the physiological mechanisms of hypnosis.

The hypothesized crucial role of the hippocampus and of right cerebral activation as physiological mechanisms in hypnosis is in accordance with the role of the hippocampus in sensory reorganization of adaptive behavior proposed by Grastyán (1981). He suggested that hippocampal function may correspond to a motivational separation and leveling of environmental stimulus configurations and their fixation in a flexible manner in memory. This role seems to be crucial in changing strategies, so necessary for the adaptive exploration of the environment. The hippocampus may have a role in initiating what Grastyán has termed "hypothesis behavior, " which includes play, creative acts, sensation seeking, and so forth. These activities may help to extend the scope of the organism; thus, they may have a biologically adaptive value.

CONCLUSION

According to the social-psychobiological model of hypnosis I have proposed, a hypnotically altered state of consciousness may have a socially and biologically adaptive value. By helping two individuals engage in a close relationship in which mutual attunement and meaningful cognitive and emotional experiences emerge, hypnosis may broaden the horizons of both participants in the interaction.

From this perspective, hypnosis can be regarded as a manifestation of a common and archaic realm of humanity, manifesting itself in intensive intimate interpersonal relationships (e.g., parent–child or love relationships), Jungian archetypes, religious states, peak experiences, creative acts, and so forth. Because hypnosis is a situation that can be studied under rigorously controlled laboratory conditions, it can be useful as a model for studying those human functions mentioned above, which are evolutionarily archaic but may constitute the driving force of development.

Acknowledgments. The research for this chapter was supported in part by a grant from the Hungarian Research Support Fund (OTKA 1667/86). I wish to express my gratitude to Anna Csilla Gosi-Greguss for her valuable help in the preparation of this chapter. I also thank Katalin Varga and Róbert Horváth for their critical comments on earlier versions of the chapter.

NOTE

1. The social-psycho*biological* model is based on the social-psycho*physiological* approach my colleagues and I have been applying since 1982.

REFERENCES

Adám, G. (1967). *Interoception and behavior.* Budapest: Akadémiai Kiadó.

Aronoff, J., & Wilson, J. P. (1985). *Personality in the social process.* Hillsdale, NJ: Erlbaum.

Bakan, P. (1969). Hypnotizability, laterality of eye movements and functional brain asymmetry. *Perceptual and Motor Skills, 28,* 927–932.

Baker, E. L., & Levitt, E. E. (1989). The hypnotic relationship: An investigation of compliance and resistance. *International Journal of Clinical and Experimental Hypnosis, 37,* 145–153.

Bandura, A. (1978). The self system in reciprocal determinism. *American Psychologist, 33,* 344–358.

Bányai, É. I. (1973). *A hipnózis hatása a tanulásra* [*The effect of hypnosis on learning*]. Unpublished doctoral dissertation, Eötvös Loránd University, Budapest.

Bányai, É. I. (1976). A new way to increase suggestibility: Active–alert hypnotic induction. *International Journal of Clinical and Experimental Hypnosis, 24,* 358.

Bányai, É. I. (1980). A new way to induce a hypnotic-like altered state of consciousness: Active–alert induction. In L. Kardos & C. Pléh (Eds.), *Problems of the regulation of activity* (pp. 261–273). Budapest: Akadémiai Kiadó.

Bányai, É. I. (1985a). A social psychophysiological approach to the understanding of hypnosis: The interaction between hypnotist and subject. *Hypnos: Swedish Journal of Hypnosis in Psychotherapy and Psychosomatic Medicine, 12,* 186–210.

Bányai, É. I. (1985b, August). *On the interactional nature of hypnosis: A social psychophysiological approach.* Paper presented at the 10th International Congress of Hypnosis and Psychosomatic Medicine, Toronto.

Bányai, É. I. (1986, November). *Psychophysiological correlates of the interaction between hypnotist and subject.* Paper preseted at the I. Convegno Interregionale sulle Applicazioni Cliniche dell 'Ipnossi, Trieste.

Bányai, É. I. (1987). *Aktivitás-fokozással létrehozható módosult tudatállapot: Aktív-éber hipnózis* [*Activity increasin altered state of consciousness: Active–alert hypnosis*]. Unpublished dissertation for the title of Candidate of Science, Eötvös Loránd University, Budapest.

Bányai, É. I. (1988, August). *Can an interactional approach bridge the gap between clinical and experimental hypnosis?* Keynote address presented at the 11th International Congress of Hypnosis and Psychosomatic Medicine, Leiden, The Netherlands.

Bányai, É. I., Gosi-Greguss, A. C., Vágó, P., Varga, K., & Horváth, R. (in press). Interactional approach to the understanding of hypnosis: Theoretical background and main findings. In R. Van Dyck, P. Spinhoven, A. J. W. Van der Does, & W. De Moor (Eds.), *Hypnosis: Current theory, research and practice.* Amsterdam: Free University Press.

Bányai, É. I., & E. R. Hilgard (1976). A comparison of active–alert hypnotic induction with traditional relaxation induction. *Journal of Abnormal Psychology, 85,* 218–224.

Bányai, É. I., Mészáros, I., & Csókay, L. (1982). Interaction between hypnotist and subject: A psychophysiological approach. *International Journal of Clinical and Experimental Hypnosis, 30,* 193.

Bányai, É. I., Mészáros, I., & Csókay, L. (1984, May). *Further data on the psychophysiological factors of the interaction between hypnotist and subject.* Paper presented at the 2nd European Congress of Hypnosis, Abano Terme-Padova, Italy.

Bányai, É. I., Mészáros, I., & Csókay, L. (1985). Interaction between hypnotist and subject: A social psychophysiological approach. (Preliminary report.) In D. Waxman, P. C. Misra, M. Gibson, & M. A. Basker (Eds.), *Modern trends in hypnosis* (pp. 97–108). New York: Plenum Press.

Bányai, É. I., Mészáros, I., Greguss, A. C., Andrejeva, N. G., & Neumann, L. (1979). Modification of evoked alpha afterdischarge in hypnosis. *Acta Physiologica Academiae Scientiarum Hungaricae, 53,* 233.

Bányai, É. I., Mészáros, I., & Greguss, A. C. (1981). Alteration of activity level: The essence of hypnosis or a byproduct of the type of induction? In G. Adám, I. Mészáros, & É. I. Bányai (Eds.), *Advances in physiological sciences: Vol. 17. Brain and behavior* (pp. 457–465). Budapest: Pergamon Press/Akadémiai Kiadó.

Barabasz, A. F. (1980). EEG alpha, skin conductance and hypnotizability in Antarctica. *International Journal of Clinical and Experimental Hypnosis, 28,* 63–74.

Barber, T. X. (1979). Suggested ("hypnotic") behavior: The trance papadigm versus an alternative paradigm. In E. Fromm, & R. E. Shor (Eds.), *Hypnosis: Developments in research and new perspectives* (2nd ed., pp. 217–274). Chicago: Aldine.

Barber, T. X., & Glass, L. B. (1962). Significant factors in hypnotic behavior. *Journal of Abnormal and Social Psychology, 64,* 222–228.

Barber, T. X., Spanos, N. P., & Chaves, J. F. (1974). *Hypnosis, imagination, and human potentialities.* Elmsford, NY: Pergamon Press.

Bowers, K. S. (1973). Hypnosis, attribution, and demand characteristics. *International Journal of Clinical and Experimental Hypnosis, 21,* 226–238.

Brazelton, T. B., Koslowski, B., & Main, M. (1974). The origins of recirpocity: The early mother–infant interaction. In M. Lewis, & L. Rosenblum (Eds.), *The effect of the infant on its caregiver.* New York: Wiley.

Cavallo, R. E. (Ed.). (1979). Systems research movement: Characteristics, accomplishments, and current developments. A report sponsored by the Society for General Systems Research [Special issue]. *General Systems Bulletin, 9,* 1–131.

Chapple, E. D. (1982). Movement and sound: The musical language of body rhythms in interaction. In M. Davis (Ed.), *Interaction rhythms. Periodicity in communicative behavior* (pp. 31–51). New York: Human Sciences Press.

Cikurel, K., & Gruzelier, J. (1989). *The affect of an active–alert hypnotic induction on lateral asymmetry in haptic processing.* Manuscript submitted for publication.

Coe, W. C. (1978). The credibility of posthypnotic amnesia: A contextualist's view. *International Journal of Clinical and Experimental Hypnosis, 26,* 218–245.

Coe, W. C., & Sarbin, T. R. (1977). Hypnosis from the standpoint of a contextualist. *Annals of the New York Academy of Sciences, 296,* 2–13.

Condon, W. S., & Ogston, W. D. (1967). A segmentation of behavior. *Journal of Psychiatric Research, 5,* 221–235.

Council, J. R., Kirsch, I., & Hafner, C. P. (1986). Expectancy versus absorption in the prediction of hypnotic responding. *Journal of Personality and Social Psychology, 50,* 182–189.

Crawford, H. J. (1989). Cognitive and physiological flexibility: Multiple pathways to hypnotic responsiveness. In V. A. Gheorghiu, P. Netter, H. J. Eysenck, & R. Rosenthal (Eds.), *Suggestion and suggestibility: Theory and research.* Berlin: Springer-Verlag.

Crawford, H. J., Skolnick, B. E., Benson, D. M., Gur, R. E., & Gur, R. C. (1985, August). *Regional cerebral blood flow in hypnosis and hypnotic analgesia.* Paper presented at the 10th International Congress of Hypnosis and Psychosomatic Medicine, Toronto.

DeBenedittis, G., & Carli, G. (1990). Psiconeurobiologia dell 'ipnosi. *Seminari sul Dolore, 3,* 59–116.

DeBenedittis, G., & Sironi, V. A. (1988). Arousal effects of electrical deep brain stimulation in hypnosis. *International Journal of Clinical and Experimental Hypnosis, 36,* 96–106.

De Groot, H. P., Gwynn, M. I., & Spanos, N. P. (1988). The effects of contextual information and gender on the prediction of hypnotic susceptibility. *Journal of Personality and Social Psychology, 54,* 1049–1053.

DePascalis, V., & Penna, P. M. (1990). 40-Hz EEG activity during hypnoitc induction and hypnotic testing. *International Journal of Clinical and Experimental Hypnosis, 38,* 125–138.

Diamond, M. J. (1974). Modification of hypnotizability: A review. *Psychological Bulletin, 81,* 180–198.

Diamond, M. J. (1977). Hypnotizability is modifiable: An alternative approach. *International Journal of Clinical and Experimental Hypnosis, 25,* 147–166.

Diamond, M. J. (1980). The client-as-hypnotist: Furthering hypnotherapeutic change. *International Journal of Clinical and Experimental Hypnosis, 28*, 197–207.

Diamond, M. J. (1984). It takes two to tango: Some thoughts on the neglected importance of the hypnotist in an interactive hypnotherapeutic relationship. *American Journal of Clinical Hypnosis, 27*, 3–13.

Diamond, M. J. (1987). The interactional basis of hypnotic experience: On the relational dimensions of hypnosis. *International Journal of Clinical and Experimental Hypnosis, 35*, 95–115.

Dolby, R. M, & Sheehan, P. W. (1977). Cognitive processing and expectancy behavior in hypnosis. *Journal of Abnormal Psychology, 86*, 334–345.

Evans, F. J. (1977). Hypnosis and sleep: The control of altered states of awareness. *Annals of the New York Academy of Sciences, 296*, 162-174.

Evans, F. J. (1979). Hypnosis and sleep: Techniques for exploring cognitive activity during sleep. In E. Fromm, & R. E. Shor (Eds.), *Hypnosis: Developments in research* (2nd ed., pp. 139–183). Chichago: Aldine.

Evans, F. J., & Kihlstrom, J. F. (1973). Posthypnotic amnesia as disrupted retrieval. *Journal of Abnormal Psychology, 82*, 317–323.

Ferenczi, S. (1965). Comments on hypnosis (E. Jones, Trans.). In R. E. Shor, & M. T. Orne (Eds.), *The nature of hypnosis: Selected basic readings*. New York: Holt, Rinehart & Winston. (Original work published in 1909)

Field, T. (1985). Attachment as psychobiological attunement: Being on the same wavelength. In M. Reite, & T. Field (Eds.), *Behavioral biology: The psychobiology of attachment and separation* (pp. 415–454). Orlando: Academic Press.

Freud, S. (1921). *Massenpsychologie und Ich-analyse*. Leipzig: Internationaler Psychoanalysticher Verlag.

Gfeller, J. D., Lynn, S. J., & Pribble, W. E. (1987). Enhancing hypnotic susceptibility: Interpersonal and rapport factors. *Journal of Personality and Social Psychology, 52*, 586–595.

Gill, M. N., & Brenman, M. (1959). *Hypnosis and related states*. New York: International Universities Press.

Gorassini, D. R., & Spanos, N. P. (1986). A sociocognitive skills approach to the successful modification of hypnotic susceptibility. *Journal of Personality and Social Psychology, 50*, 1004–1012.

Gosi-Greguss, A. C., Bányai, É. I., Vágó, P., Varga, K., & Horváth, R. J. (1988, August). *Interactional approach to the understanding of hypnosis: Electrophysiological indices*. Paper presented at the 11th International Congress of Hypnosis and Psychosomatic Medicine, Leiden, The Netherlands.

Graham, C., & Evans, F. J. (1977). Hypnotizability and the development of waking attention. *Journal of Abnormal Psychology, 86*, 631–638.

Grastyán, E. (1981). Sensory reorganization of adaptive behavior by the hippocampus. In E. Grastyán, & P. Molnár (Eds.), *Advances in physiological sciences: Vol. 16. Sensory functions* (pp. 275–289). Budapest: Pergamon Press/ Akadémiai Kiadó.

Grastyán, E. (1985). *A játék neurobiológiája. Akadémiai székfoglaló (1983. ápr. 19)* [*Neurobiology of play*]. Budapest: Akadémiai Kiadó.

Grastyán, E., Lissák, K., Madarász, Il, & Donhoffer, H. (1959). Hippocampal electrical activity during the development of conditioned reflexes. *Electroencephalography and Clinical Neurophysiology, 11*, 409–430.

Greguss, A. C., Bányai, É. I., Mészáros, I., & Csákay, L. (1980). Hypnotic susceptibility and memory organization. In M. Pajntar, E. Roskar, & M. Lavric

(Eds.), *Hypnosis in psychotherapy and psychosomatic medicine* (pp. 8–12). Ljubljana, Yugoslavia: University Press.

Gur, R. C., & Gur, R. E. (1974). Handedness, sex and eyedness as moderating variables in the relation between hypnotic susceptibility and functional brain asymmetry. *Journal of Abnormal Psychology, 83*, 635–643.

Hellige, J. B. (1990). Hemispheric asymmetry. *Annual Review of Psychology, 41*, 55–80.

Heron, W., Doane, B.K., & Scott, T. H. (1956). Visual distrubances after prolonged perceptual isolation. *Canadian Journal of Psychology, 10*, 13–16.

Hilgard, E. R. (1965). *The experience of hypnosis* (a shorter version of *Hypnotic susceptibility*). New York: Harcourt, Brace & World.

Hilgard, E. R. (1977). *Divided consciousness: Multiple controls in human thought and action.* New York: Wiley-Interscience.

Hilgard, E. R. (1979). The Stanford Hypnotic Susceptibility Scales as related to other measures of hypnotic responsiveness. *American Journal of Clinical Hypnosis, 21*, 68–82.

Hilgard, J. R. (1970). *Personality and hypnosis: A study of imaginative involvement.* Chicago: University of Chicago Press.

Hilgard, J. R. (1979). *Personality and hypnosis: A study of imaginative involvement* (2nd ed.). Chicago: University of Chicago Press.

Hilgard, J. R., & Hilgard, E. R. (1962). Developmental–interactive aspects of hypnosis: Some illustrative cases. *Genetic Psychology Monographs, 66*, 143–178.

Horváth, R. J., Bányai, É. I., Varga, K., Gosi-Greguss, A. C., & Vágó, P. (1988, August). *Interactional approach to the understanding of hypnosis: Relational Dimensions.* Paper presented at the 11th International Congress of Hypnosis and Psychosomatic Medicine, Leiden, The Netherlands.

Hughes, D. E., & Bowers, K. S. (1987). *Hypnotic ability as a mediator of heart rate responsiveness to imagery.* Paper presented at the 38th Annual Meeting of the Society for Clinical and Experiemental Hypnosis, Los Angeles.

Jones, B., & Spanos, N. P. (1982). Suggestions for altered auditory sensitivity, the negative subject effect and hypnotic susceptibility: A signal detection analysis. *Journal of Personality and Social Psychology, 43*, 637–647.

Karlin, R. A. (1979). Hypnotizability and attention. *Journal of Abnormal Psychology, 88*, 92–95.

Kelley, H. H. (1979). *Personal relationships: Their structures and processes.* Hillsdale, NJ: Erlbaum.

Kelley, H. H., & Thibaut, J. W. (1978). *Interpersonal relations: A theory of interdependence.* New York: Wiley-Interscience.

Kihlstrom, J. F. (1985). Hypnosis. *Annual Review of Psychology, 36*, 385–418.

Kihlstrom, J. F., Register, P. A., Hoyt, I. P., Albright, J. S., Grigorian, E. M., Heindel, W. C., & Morrison, C. R. (1989). Dispositional correlates of hypnosis: A phenomenological approach. *International Journal of Clinical and Experimental Hypnosis, 37*, 249–263.

Kirsch, I. (1985). Response expectancy as a determinant of experience and behavior. *American Psychologist, 40*, 1189–1202.

Kissin, B. (1986). *Psychobiology of human behavior: Vol. 1. Conscious and unconscious programs in the brain.* New York: Plenum.

Levitt, E. E., Baker, E. L., & Fish, R. C. (1990). Some conditions of compliance and resistance among hypnotic subjects. *American Journal of Clinical Hypnosis, 32*, 225–236.

Linton, P. H., Travis, R. P., Kuechenmeister, C. A., & White, H. (1977). Correlation between heart rate covariation, personality and hypnotic state. *American Journal of Clinical Hypnosis, 19*, 148–154.

Loomis, A. L., Harvey, A. N., & Hobart, G. A. (1936). Brain potentials during hypnosis. *Science, 83*, 239–241.

Lynn, S. J., Nash, M. R., Rhue, J. W., Frauman, D. C., & Sweeney, C. (1984). Nonvolition, expectancies, and hypnotic rapport. *Journal of Abnormal Psychology, 93*, 295–303.

Lynn, S. J., Snodgrass, M., Rhue, J. W., Nash, M. R., & Fraumann, D. C. (1987). Attributions, involuntariness, and hypnotic rapport. *American Journal of Clinical Hypnosis, 30*, 36–43.

Lynn, S. J., Weekes, J., Snodgrass, M., Abrams, L., Weiss, F., & Rhue, J. (1986). *Control and countercontrol in hypnosis.* Paper presented at the meeting of the American Psychological Association, Los Angeles, California.

MacLeod-Morgan, C. (1979). Hypnotic susceptibility, EEG theta and alpha waves, and hemispheric specificity. In G. D. Burrows, D. R. Collison, & L. Dennerstein (Eds.), *Hypnosis 1979.* Amsterdam: Elsevier/North-Holland.

MacLeod-Morgan, C., & Lack, L. (1982). Hemispheric specificity: A physiological concomitant of hypnotizability. *Psychophysiology, 19*, 687–690.

McConkey, K. M. (1986). Opinions about hypnosis and self-hypnosis before and after hypnotic testing. *International Journal of Clinical and Experimental Hypnosis, 34*, 311–319.

Mészáros, I., & Bányai, É. I. (1978). Electrophysiological characteristics of hypnosis. In K. Lissák (Ed.), *Neural and neurohumoral organization of motivated behavior* (pp. 173–187). Budapest: Akadémiai Kiadó.

Mészáros, I., & Bányai, É. I., & Greguss, A. C. (1980). Psychophysiological correlates of hypnosis. *Wiessenschaftliche Zeitschrift der Karl-Marx-Universitat Leipzig, Mathematisch-Naturwissenschaftliche Reihe, 29*, 235–240.

Mészáros, I., & Bányai, É. I., & Greguss, A. C. (1981) Evoked potential, reflecting hypnotically altered state of consciousness. In G. Adám, I. Mészáros, & É. I. Bányai (Eds.), *Advances in physiological sciences: Vol. 17. Brain and behavior* (pp. 467–475). Budapest: Pergamon Press/Akadémiai Kiadó.

Mészáros, I., & Bányai, É. I., & Greguss, A. C. (1985). Evoked potential correlates of verbal versus imagery coding in hypnosis. In D. Waxman, P. C. Misra, M. Gibson, & M. A. Basker (Eds.), *Modern trends in hypnosis* (pp. 161–168). New York: Plenum Press.

Mészáros, I., Crawford, H. J., Szabó, C., Nagykovács, A., & Révész, Z. (1989). Hypnotic susceptibility and cerebral hemisphere preponderance: Verbal–imaginal discrimination task. In V. A. Gheorghiu, P. Netter, H. J. Eysenck, & R. Rosenthal (Eds.), *Suggestion and suggestibility: Theory and research* (pp. 191–203). Berlin: Springer-Verlag.

Mészáros, I., Osman, J. S., & Bányai, É. I. (1972). Factors of human learning under hypnotic effect. *Acta Physiologica Academiae Scientiarum Hungaricae, 41*, 298.

Morgan, A. H. (1973). The heritability of hypnotic susceptibility in twins. *Journal of Abnormal Psychology, 82*, 55–61.

Morgan, A. H., Hohnson, D. L., & Hilgard, E. R. (1974). The stability of hypnotic susceptibility: A longitudinal study. *International Journal of Clinical and Experimental Hypnosis, 22,* 249–257.

Nash, M. R. (1988). Hypnosis as a window on regression. *Bulletin of the Menninger Clinic, 52,* 383–403.

Nash, M. R., & Spinler, D. (1989). Hypnosis and transference: A measure of archaic involvement. *International Journal of Clinical and Experimental Hypnosis, 37,* 129–143.

Orne, M. T. (1959). The nature of hypnosis: Artifact and essence. *Journal of Abnormal and Social Psychology, 58,* 277–299.

Orne, M. T. (1962). Implications for psychotherapy derived from current research on the nature of hypnosis. *American Journal of Psychiatry, 118,* 1097–1103.

Pardell, S. S. (1950). Psychology of the hypnotist. *Psychiatric Quarterly, 24,* 483–491.

Pavlov, I. P. (1923). The identity of inhibition with sleep and hypnosis. *Science Monthly, 17,* 603–608.

Pekala, R. J. (1982). *The Phenomenology of Consciousness Inventory (PCI).* Thorndale, PA: Psychophenomenological Concepts.

Pekala, R. J., & Forbes, E. J. (1988). Hypnoidal effects associated with several stress management techniques. *Australian Journal of Clinical and Experimental Hypnosis, 16,* 121–132.

Pekala, R. J., & Kumar, V. K. (1984). Predicting hypnotic susceptibility by a self-report phenomenological state instrument. *American Journal of Clinical Hypnosis, 27,* 114–121.

Pekala, R. J., & Kumar, V. K. (1987). Predicting hypnotic susceptibility via a self-report instrument: A replication. *American Journal of Clinical Hypnosis, 30,* 57–66.

Piccione, C., Hilgard, E. R., & Zimbardo, P. G. (1989). On the stability of measured hypnotizability over a 25-year period. *Journal of Personality and Social Psychology, 56,* 289–295.

Pribram, K. H., & McGuinnes, D. (1975). Arousal, activation, and effort in the control of attention. *Psychological Review, 82,* 116–149.

Reite, M., & Field, T. (Eds.). (1985). *Behavioral biology: The psychobiology of attachment and separation.* Orlando: Academic Press.

Sackeim, H. A., Paulus, D., & Weiman, A. L. (1979). Classroom seating and hypnotic susceptibility. *Journal of Abnormal Psychology, 88,* 81–84.

Sarbin, T. R., & Coe, W. C. (1972). *Hypnosis: A social psychological analysis of influence communication.* New York: Holt, Rinehart & Winston.

Sarbin, T. R., & Coe, W. C. (1979). Hypnosis and psychopathology: Replacing old myths with fresh metaphors. *Journal of Abnormal Psychology, 88,* 506–526.

Sargant, W. (1957). *Battle for the mind.* Garden City, NY: Doubleday.

Sheehan, P. W. (1971). Countering preconceptions about hypnosis: an objective index of involvement with the hypnotist. *Journal of Abnormal Psychology Monograph, 78,* 299–322.

Sheehan, P. W., & Dolby, R. M. (1975). Hypnosis and the influence of most recently perceived events. *Journal of Abnormal Psychology, 84,* 331–345.

Sheehan, P. W., & McConkey, K. M. (1982). *Hypnosis and experience: The exploration of phenomena and process.* Hillsdale, NJ: Erlbaum.

Shor, R. E. (1959). Hypnosis and the concept of the generalized reality-orientation. *American Journal of Psychotherapy, 13,* 582–602.

Shor, R. E. (1962). Three dimensions of hypnotic depth. *International Journal of Clinical and Experimental Hypnosis, 10*, 23–28.

Shor, R. E. (1979). A phenomenologicl method for the measurement of variables important to an understanding of the nature of hypnosis. In E. Fromm, & R. E. Shor (Eds.), *Hypnosis: Developments in research and new perspectives* (2nd ed., pp. 105–135). Chicago: Aldine.

Shor, R. E., Pistole, D. D., Easton, R. D., & Kihlstrom, J. F. (1984). Relation of predicted to actual hypnotic responsiveness, with special reference to posthypnotic amnesia. *International Journal of Clinical and Experimental Hypnosis, 32*, 376–387.

Smith, A. (1990). The hypnotic relationship and the holographic paradigm. *American Journal of Clinical Hypnosis, 32*, 183–193.

Spanos, N. P. (1982a). A social psychological approach to hypnotic behavior. In G. Weary, & H. L. Mirels (Eds.), *Integrations of clinical and social psychology* (pp. 231–271). New York: Oxford University Press.

Spanos, N. P. (1982b). Hypnotic behavior: A cognitive social psychological perspective. *Research Communications in Psychology, Psychiatry and Behavior, 7*, 199–213.

Spanos, N. P. (1986). Hypnotic behavior: A social psychological interpretation of amnesia, analgesia, and trance logic. *Behavioral and Brain Science, 9*, 449–502.

Spanos, N. P., Gabora, N. J., Jarrett, L. E., & Gwynn, M. J. (1989). Contextual determinants of hypnotizability and of relationships between hypnotizability scales. *Journal of Personality and Social Psychology, 57*, 271–278.

Spanos, N. P., Kennedy, S. K., & Gwynn, M. I. (1984). Moderating effects of contextual variables on the relationship between hypnotic susceptibility and suggested analgesia. *Journal of Abnormal Psychology, 93*, 285–294.

Spanos, N. P., Voorneveld, P. W., & Gwynn, M. I. (1987). The mediating effects of experimentation on hypnotic and nonhypnotic pain reduction. *Imagination, Cognition and Personality, 6*, 231–245.

Stern, D. (1982). Some interactive functions of rhythm changes between mother and infant. In M. Davis (Ed.), *Interaction rhythms: Periodicity in communicative behavior* (pp. 101–117). New York: Human Sciences Press.

Sturgis, L. M., & Coe, W. C. (1990). Phsiological responsiveness during hypnosis. *International Journal of Clinical and Experimental Hypnosis, 38*, 196–207.

Tellegen, A. (1979). On measures and conceptions of hypnosis. *American Journal of Clinical Hypnosis, 21*, 219–237.

Tellegen, A., & Atkinson, G. (1974). Openness to absorbing and self-altering experiences ("absorption"), a trait related to hypnotic susceptibility. *Journal of Abnormal Psychology, 83*, 268–277.

Thibaut, J. W., & Kelley, H. H. (1959). *The social psychology of groups*. New York: Wiley.

Tucker, D. M., & Williamson, P. A. (1984). Asymmetric neural control systems in human self-regulation. *Psychological Review, 91*, 185–215.

Vágó, P., Bányai, É. I., Nagy-Gergely, I., Gosi-Greguss, A. C., Varga, K., & Horváth, R. (1988, August). *Interactional approach to the understanding of hypnosis: Behavioral manifestations*. Paper presented at the 11th International Congress of Hypnosis and Psychosomatic Medicine, Leiden, The Netherlands.

Varga, K. (1986). *A hipnózis élménye: Elméleti és módszertani megfontolások [The experience of hypnosis: Theoretical and methodical considerations*]. Unpublished master's thesis, Eötvös Loránd University, Budapest.

Varga, K. (1991). *Comparative analysis of the behavioral and experiential levels of hypnosis.* Doctoral dissertation in preparation (in Hungarian), Eötvös Loránd University, Budapest.

Varga, K., Bányai, É. I., Gosi-Greguss, A. C., Vágó, P., & Horváth, R. (1987). Hypnotic interaction: The method of experimental analysis [Abstract]. In *Abstracts of the Sociophysiology Satellite Symposium of the Second World Congress of Neurosciences (IBRO), Gálosfa, Hungary, August 22–25, 1987.*

Varga, K., Bányai, É. I., Gosi-Greguss, A. C., Vágó, P., & Horváth, R. (1988, August). *Interactional approach to the understanding of hypnosis: Subjective experiences.* Paper presented at the 11th International Congress of Hypnosis and Psychosomatic Medicine, Leiden, The Netherlands.

Von Bertalanffy, L. (1974). General system theory and psychiatry. In G. Caplan (Ed.), *American handbook of psychiatry* (Vol. 2). New York: Basic Books.

Wagstaff, G. F. (1981). *Hypnosis, compliance and belief.* Brighton, England: Harvester.

Wallace, B., Knight, T. A., & Garrett, J. B. (1976). Hypnotic susceptibility and frequency reports to illusory stimuli. *Journal of Abnormal Psychology, 85,* 558–563.

Watkins, J. G. (1971). The affect bridge: A hypnoanalytic technique. *International Journal of Clinical and Experimental Hypnosis, 19,* 21–27.

PART SIX

CONCLUSIONS

CHAPTER 20

Hypnosis Theories: Themes, Variations, and Research Directions

STEVEN JAY LYNN and JUDITH W. RHUE
Ohio University

Kuhn (1962) insists that the real work of science begins once a community of workers has adopted a paradigm. We take issue with this conclusion, at least as it pertains to the field of hypnosis. Workers in the field are still divided about which paradigm provides the most accurate, consistent, and fruitful explanation of the transactions that constitute hypnosis. Nevertheless, the contributors to our book have not been deterred from proposing hypotheses to account for the phenomena that comprise the domain of hypnosis, and from conducting vigorous research to test theory-driven hypotheses. The tensions that exist among theories, and the research stimulated by areas of disagreement, have extended knowledge about hypnosis in many directions. In short, the "work of science"—the meticulous study of hypnosis—is well underway, even though thinking about hypnosis has not coalesced into a unified theoretical paradigm.

In our concluding chapter, we review some of the main themes we have encountered as we examine some of the points of divergence and confluence among hypnosis theories. We do so by considering three broad questions that have captured the attention of theorists who represent quite different schools of thought: (1) Is hypnosis an altered state of consciousness? (2) Is hypnotic behavior involuntary? (3) How stable, trait-like, and modifiable is hypnotizability? At the conclusion of the chapter, we discuss research issues and directions for future research.

IS HYPNOSIS AN ALTERED STATE OF CONSCIOUSNESS?

For more than 40 years, one of the pre-eminent themes in contemporary hypnosis theory has been what Fellows (1990) has dubbed the "state–nonstate" issue. Following Sarbin's (1950) attack on the traditional conception of hypnosis as a state (e.g., "hypnotic trance," "hypnotic state") that arises in subjects after exposure to a hypnotic induction, controversy has swirled around the issue of whether hypnosis evokes an altered state of consciousness that produces or enhances hypnotic responses. As Fellows notes, T. X. Barber (1969) later criticized the state concept on two grounds: first on the basis of logical circularity (i.e., hypnotic responsiveness can both indicate the existence of a hypnotic state and be explained by it), and second because a hypnotic induction is not necessary for the production of a wide variety of phenomena associated with hypnosis.

More recently, Kirsch, Mobayed, Council, and Kenny (1991) have summarized the data that nonstate theorists have used to support their position: (1) Unique physiological markers of the hypnotized state have not been identified; (2) all of the phenomena produced by suggestion following a hypnotic induction can also be produced without a hypnotic induction; and (3) increases in suggestibility that occur after a hypnotic induction are small and can be duplicated or even surpassed by a variety of other procedures (e.g., task motivation instructions, placebo pills, and imagination training). Although nonstate theorists dispute the idea that a unique, specific, or somehow special state of consciousness flows from a hypnotic induction, most do not deny the subjective reality of the hypnotic experience or believe that hypnotic responses are necessarily faked or the product of mere compliance.

The data claimed by nonstate theorists to support their position have not entirely quelled theoretical tensions and disagreements in this area. Hypnosis theorists are still divided about the utility of invoking the concept of a hypnotic state or condition. At least three distinct viewpoints have been adopted by theorists and researchers; a number of exemplars of each viewpoint in the present volume are presented below.

The first view is that hypnosis involves characteristic changes in the person's state or condition. These changes are held to play an important if not dominant role in determining the subject's response to suggested events. This position is epitomized by J. Barber's theory (see Chapter 8), which posits that hypnosis is an altered state of consciousness or a "condition [that] allows the individual to be inordinately responsive to such suggestions, so that he or she is able to alter perception, memory, and physiological processes that under ordinary conditions are not susceptible to conscious control." The altered state involves a shift to an alternate perspective characterized by a reduction of defenses, greater than usual levels of emotional contact, and access to not-conscious processes.

Nash (Chapter 6) is also explicit about the characteristic changes in the hypnotized subject's condition that are attendant on psychological regression, the central process thought to underlie hypnotic responsiveness. These changes include an increase in primary-process material, more spontaneous and intense emotion, unusual body sensations, the experience of nonvolition, and the tendency to displace core attributes of important others onto the hypnotist and to maintain a posture of receptivity to inner and outer experience.

Edmonston (Chapter 7) believes that the notion of an altered state of consciousness is "appropriate, even mandatory" to account for phenomena such as hallucinations and age regression experienced by talented hypnotic subjects. For Edmonston, the question is not whether a change in the hypnotized person's condition occurs, but rather what the fundamental nature of the change is. According to Edmonston, the fundamental change is relaxation (or "anesis," in his parlance). The important role of relaxation-based alterations in condition or state is evident in Edmonston's observation that it "precedes and provides the agar in which the subjective ideas can develop and thus influence the hypnotic phenomena."

According to Bányai (Chapter 19), the hypnotic state can be characterized by a special pattern of physiological concomitants, a characteristic way of processing information, and characteristic ways of organizing behavior and relating to the inner and outer environment. Bányai goes so far as to suggest that the hypnotically altered state of consciousness may have a socially and biologically adaptive value for both the subject *and* the hypnotist.

Even though a number of the theories (e.g., those of Bányai and Nash) we have referred to invoke a variety of factors, including social factors, to explain hypnotic behavior, the altered state or condition of the person is nevertheless seen as an important determinant of hypnotic behavior, not merely a description of how the subject perceives or interprets hypnotic events.

A second view is that hypnosis involves a change in the person's state or condition; however, the altered state or condition is viewed in a descriptive rather than in an explanatory sense. For example, neither E. R. Hilgard nor other neodissociation theorists shy away from discussing alterations in the person's "state" following a hypnotic induction. Hilgard (Chapter 3) argues that from the point of view of the subject, the experimenter, and "any other unbiased observer," hypnosis appears to induce alterations in the "total condition or state, just as drunkenness and sleep are described as altered states, subject to differences in the profundity of the change at any given time." Hilgard, however, prefers to speak of a "hypnotic condition," and notes that because dissociations can be partial, hypnosis does not necessarily involve an all-or-nothing change from the normal waking condition. Although Hilgard embraces the idea of an altered state of the person as a characteristic of hypnosis on the descriptive level, since 1965 (Hilgard, 1965), he has increasingly edged away from using the construct of an altered state in an explanatory sense.

Zeig and Rennick (Chapter 9) contend that the concept of trance is irrelevant, and that it is best to dispense with it so that hypnosis can more easily be viewed as an interpersonal process. This would imply that the authors believe that the concept of trance has little explanatory value. Nevertheless, they repeatedly use descriptive phrases such as "trance," "formal trance," and "trance phenomena," rendering their position regarding the altered state issue somewhat ambiguous. Furthermore, they state that, at least from the patient's point of view, hypnosis can be experienced as a state of focused awareness on whatever is immediately relevant, in which previously unrecognized psychological and physiological potentials are accessed to some avolitional extent.

It is worth noting that whether dissociation, relaxation, or regression is thought to be at the heart of hypnosis, none of these psychological processes is claimed to be unique or specific to hypnosis (see Nadon, Laurence, & Perry, Chapter 16). Rather, hypnosis is viewed as a situation or context that activates or potentiates processes that are operative in certain everyday life circumstances. These processes, in conjunction with a hypnotic induction and suggestions that access or facilitate them, are responsible for the alterations in behavior and consciousness that accompany hypnotic communications.

A third view is that the concept of trance not only lacks utility but is misleading. It is widely believed that hypnotized subjects experience relaxation, along with a variety of other sensations and alterations in perceptions of the environment (see Brentar, 1990). Sociocognitive theorists do not view these alterations in the subjects' phenomenology as an explanation of hypersuggestibility or hypnotic phenomena. Instead, perceived changes in subjective experience are thought to be the by-products of subjects' attitudes, beliefs, expectancies, and actions—that is, their prehypnotic expectancies; their ongoing and retrospective interpretations and attributions of suggestion-related sensations; and their active, goal-directed attempts to have the experiences implicitly and explicitly called for by hypnotic communications. In addition, the standards that subjects adopt to evaluate their behavior and experiences may in turn shape their experience of hypnosis. Given this variegated blend of determinants and interactive processes, there is no single or unique "trance" state that is the *sine qua non* of hypnosis; rather, various somatic and perceptual changes are possible, depending on the particular social and cognitive factors that come into play in the hypnotic context.

According to sociocognitive theorists, the hypnotic induction conveys information and cues about hypnosis that serve to shape the hypnotic experience. The hypnotic induction procedures help subjects to "locate their roles" (Coe & Sarbin, Chapter 10); establish expectancies that an altered state will ensue (Kirsch, Chapter 14; Wagstaff, Chapter 12); and contain words and phrases that are commonly associated with passive or receptive mental states (our view, Chapter 13). Sociocognitive theorists thus underscore the informational, expectancy-inducing function of hypnotic procedures, in contrast with state theorists, who believe that the induction engenders or activates a process or mechanism (dissociation, relaxation, psychological regression, or physiological processes) associated with important modifications in consciousness.

Sociocognitive and interactive-phenomenological theorists converge in the view that subjects' experience is not a static, fixed, and invariant state or condition. Descriptors of hypnotized subjects' phenomenology as an "experiential stream" (ourselves, Chapter 13), "fluid" (McConkey, Chapter 18), an "ever-changing process" (Bányai, Chapter 19), and "unfolding" (Spanos, Chapter 11; Fourie, Chapter 15) capture the ebb and flow of hypnotic experience. This dynamic quality is thought to reflect the complex interaction of multiple factors, including variations in subjects' motivation, attention, expectancies, self-evaluations, rapport with the hypnotist, and interpretations of hypnotic behavior.

Some theorists (e.g., Wagstaff, Spanos, ourselves) have proposed that the concept of trance is misleading because it implies that there is a single explanation for all hypnotic phenomena, when, in actuality, disparate phenomena such as amnesia and age regression require somewhat different explanations. In fact, even subjects' *failure* to generate subjectively compelling experiences may account for certain phenomena, such as transparency of hallucination and incongrous responses during age regression (see Spanos, 1986; Chapter 13, this volume).

Some years ago, Bowers (1966) wrote, "Most investigators interested in hypnosis believe that there is a hypnotic state which fundamentally differs from the waking state." Given the diversity of opinions about the "altered state" issue, it is clear that many contemporary workers in the field have moved away from the view that a particular state of consciousness or trance constitutes a sufficient explanation for the diversity of hypnotic phenomena. In fact, the terms "state" and "nonstate" no longer appear to be particularly fashionable, at least among hypnosis researchers. Nevertheless, as Engstrom (1976) has observed, basic theoretical differences center around " . . . whether hypnosis is best defined as the private, internal responses of the hypnotized subject or by external characteristics implicit in the hypnotic situation." (Engstrom, 1976, p. 174).

Even though consensus regarding this issue is unlikely to be achieved in the near future, discourse on this topic would be abetted if theorists were more specific and precise regarding a number of questions: In what sense are alterations in consciousness variable and related to subjects' active efforts to experience specific suggestions, as opposed to relatively static and unsuggested? What is the relation between so-called state changes and prehypnotic expectancies, imaginative/dissociative abilities, demand characteristics, and situational factors, including the hypnotic relationship? And finally, if the concept of an altered state or condition is invoked, is it used in a descriptive or an explanatory sense?

IS HYPNOTIC BEHAVIOR INVOLUNTARY?

Not only do subjects often report perceptual and somatic alterations during hypnosis, but they frequently report a sense of diminished control of suggestion-related behavior. Descriptions such as "automatic," "compelled," and "effortless" color many subjects' accounts of their hypnotic experience. Many years ago, White (1941) maintained that suggestion-related involuntariness was so central to the experience of hypnosis that it was incumbent upon theorists to address this domain of experience. Many of the theorists in our book have risen to the challenge of attempting to account for what Weitzenhoffer (1974) has termed the "classical suggestion effect": The subject's "transformation of the essential, manifest, ideational content of a communication" (p. 238) into behavior that is considered as involuntary.

Depending on how "involuntariness" is construed, theorists either agree or disagree with one another. The term "involuntary" can be defined in at least three ways (I. Kirsch, personal communication, February 18, 1989; see Lynn, Rhue, & Weekes, 1990). An action can be termed involuntary if it is beyond one's control, so that one cannot act otherwise even if one wishes to. Since the so-called "golden age" of hypnotism (the 1880s and 1890s), the view of the hypnotized subject as a passive automaton under the sway of a powerful hypnotist has faded in popularity. In fact, this rather extreme position is not endorsed by any of the theorists whose ideas are represented in our book. It is perhaps most explicitly rejected by social-psychological theorists, who contend that hypnotized subjects are conscious agents who actively pursue their personal goals and agendas. It is in this pursuit that subjects come to think of their goal-directed actions as involuntary "happenings." Perceptions of involuntariness notwithstanding, hypnotized subjects can resist suggested actions if they so desire.

Adopting a very different perspective, Nash (Chapter 6) agrees that hypnotic subjects retain the ability to refuse to comply with suggestions; in fact, he uses the fact that subjects can resist suggestions to support the idea that the topographic regression only involves a subsystem of the ego. That subjects retain control of their ability to respond to (or resist) suggestions is also implied by theorists (McConkey, Chapter 18; Sheehan, Chapter 17; Kirsch, Chapter 14) who argue that hypnotized subjects *intend* to respond to the hypnotist's suggestions, even though this intention may not be fully consciously articulated. Even neodissociation theorists fall short of arguing that people exercise no control whatsoever over their hypnotic behavior; rather, as Bowers and Davidson (Chapter 4) point out, the theory holds that this control is "dissociated from high-level, executive plans, intentions, and effort."

It is not surprising that authors (J. Barber, Chapter 8; Zeig & Rennick, Chapter 9) whose theoretical approach derives in part from the practice of hypnotherapy focus on the client-centered nature of the hypnotherapeutic relationship, and think of the hypnotic subject as cognitively active and involved. This image of the subject as intimately involved in the hypnotic proceedings, rather than as passive and fully subject to the hypnotist's control, is consistent with contemporary movements within the fields of psychotherapy (and within the broader societal context) to legitimize a more egalitarian, less authoritarian "doctor–patient" relationship (T. X. Barber, 1985).

In Chapter 13, we cite data that provide a solid foundation for concluding that hypnotized subjects can indeed resist suggestions, particularly when resistance is defined as consistent with the role of good hypnotized subjects. Even research conducted by Hilgard (1963), who maintains in Chapter 3 that "effective suggestions from the hypnotist take much of the normal control away from the subject," suggests that hypnotized subjects do not fully relinquish their ability to control their hypnotic responses. That is, even though hypnotizable subjects experience considerable conflict when instructed to resist the hypnotist's suggestions, they are generally able to resist one or more suggestions successfully. In short, there is widespread agreement that subjects retain at least a measure of control during hypnosis, so that, at the very least, they are capable of resisting suggestions under certain circumstances.

A second meaning of the term "involuntary" can be that the suggested response occurs automatically, without effort or activity to make it occur, even if the subject is able to prevent it from occurring if he or she so desires. One area of disagreement among theorists centers around the question of whether hypnotic behavior is strategic, or whether it occurs in the absence of goal-directed strategies and is instead directly activated by suggestions. Cognitive strategies encompass a variety of imaginative (e.g.,

goal-directed fantasies) and attentional (e.g., distraction) activities believed to increase the probability that subjects will experience or respond
to hypnotic suggestions.

Social-psychological theorists view cognitive strategies as particularly
important determinants of the experience of nonvolition. The use of
specific cognitive strategies, in combination with prehypnotic expectancies and contextual features (e.g., suggestion wording) that prime the use
of these strategies, is highlighted by Spanos (Chapter 11) and by ourselves
(Chapter 13). According to Coe and Sarbin (Chapter 10), cognitive
strategies are intimately associated with hypnotized subjects' evolving
self-narrative. Cognitive strategies, which include "spelling out" certain
aspects of experience and not "spelling out" others, can promote the
experience of such hypnotic phenomena as posthypnotic amnesia. For
instance, by attending to feelings of relaxation while not attending to the
material to be forgotten or to retrieval cues, subjects can convince
themselves that they are amnesic for hypnotic events.

Subjects' active cognitive efforts to interpret, understand, and devise
creative ways of responding to suggestions are also integral to Sheehan's
(Chapter 17) and McConkey's (Chapter 18) models. These theorists
conceptualize the hypnotized subject not as a passive or inert recipient of
suggestions, but as a cognitively active problem solver. It is the motivated
cognitive activity of the subject that shapes the hypnotic experience.

McConkey and Sheehan are perhaps less concerned about cataloguing
particular strategies or studying their effects than are the social-psychological theorists. They observe that some subjects appear to use cognitive
strategies to facilitate their responses to suggestions, whereas the use of
cognitive strategies is less obvious or not apparent in other subjects'
reports. There is little doubt that hypnotized subjects who respond
successfully to suggestions focus their attention on the hypnotist's
communications. However, Sheehan's and McConkey's work suggests that
what is even more interesting is the individualistic, constructive, problem-
solving nature of subjects' responses to diverse suggestions, as well as the
cognitive styles they apply to augment their responses. Barber (Chapter 8)
and Zeig and Rennick (Chapter 9) also believe that hypnotized subjects
actively processes suggested information. However, it is unclear whether
they believe that a link exists between cognitive strategies and subjective
reports, including feelings of involuntariness.

A number of theorists are dubious about the central or exclusive role
of cognitive strategies in producing hypnotic experiences, including
reports of nonvolition. Wagstaff (Chapter 12) states that subjects use
cognitive strategies to make hypnotic experiences veridical or believable,
in line with expectations and situational demands. However, he also notes
that if this is not possible, then they will behaviorally comply or sham if
this course of action is deemed appropriate. In short, cognitive strategies

will not necessarily be successful in achieving desired ends; if they are not, other actions will be undertaken (such as compliance) in order to achieve particular goals.

Kirsch (Chapter 14) and Wagstaff agree that hypnotic subjects' strategic behaviors are aimed toward generating compelling hypnotic experiences. They also agree that subjects can engage in strategic actions or cognitions, yet fail to experience a hypnotic response. However, unlike Wagstaff, Kirsch argues that this attempt to have a particular hypnotic experience and the subsequent failure to achieve this objective indicate that hypnotic responses are not fully under voluntary control, and that they should be viewed as outcomes, rather than as actions. Although "outcomes" may depend on cognitive strategies, Kirsch withholds judgment about whether cognitive strategies play a role in nonvolitional experiences that is independent of the direct effects of expectancies on subjective reports.

Fourie (Chapter 15), in turn, maintains that cognitive strategies do not *cause* hypnotic responses, as he feels is implied by the social psychological perspective. Instead, Fourie believes that cognitive strategies are enmeshed in the unfolding ecology of the whole system, which is not appropriately divisible into parts (e.g, goal-directed fantasies) that influence one another (e.g., behaviors). In actuality, contemporary social-psychological theories do not state explicitly that goal-directed fantasies *cause* hypnotic responses independently of other factors, such as role-related expectancies. However, social-psychological theories do maintain that goal-directed fantasies either serve to legitimize suggestion-related responses or contribute to the attribution of actions as "happenings." Clearly, more research and greater theoretical specificity are called for with respect to this issue.

Bowers and Davidson (Chapter 4) are unabashedly skeptical about the ability of active cognitive strategies to produce such hypnotic phenomena as analgesia. In their critique of Spanos's social-psychological postion, Bowers and Davidson argue that research does not support Spanos's assertion that hypnotic analgesia and cognitive strategies constitute similar mechanisms. Executive initiative, allocation of attention, and effort do not appear to be required to produce hypnotic analgesia; rather, suggestion-activated subsystems of pain control are believed to be associated with analgesia. Similarly, they maintain that hypnotic amnesia involves a breakdown of mnemonic mechanisms associated with ordinary access to memories and their representation in conscious experience, rather than strategic and motivated enactments. Not surprisingly, these assertions have been vigorously challenged by Spanos.

In a recent paper, Bowers and colleagues (Woody, Bowers, & Oakman, 1991) make the interesting argument that even though many hypnotized subjects who receive an analgesia suggestion report cognitive strategies along with reduced pain, it does not necessarily follow that the cognitive strategies mediate the pain reduction. Instead, the strategies and analgesia experienced could be independent responses that co-occur because they both are suggested as part of the initial analgesia suggestion.

Our discussion suggests that the debate about the role of cognitive strategies is far from settled. In what sense, if any, cognitive strategies mediate suggested responses and involuntariness reports awaits more definitive research. At the present time it is unclear whether cognitive strategies directly mediate hypnotic behaviors and the experience of involuntariness, whether they merely legitimize them, or whether cognitive strategies represent co-occurring responses to suggestion in responsive subjects.

A third sense in which a response can be classified as "involuntary" is that the subject simply has the *experience* of an action as occurring without direct volitional effort. Kirsch (Chapter 14), for example, states that "responses are defined as nonvolitional if they are experienced as occurring without direct volitional effort." According to some theorists, a response that is devoid of the experience of nonvolition should not be classified as "hypnotic" in nature. For Zeig and Rennick (Chapter 9), the litmus test of an "essential hypnotic response" versus a compliance-based response is that it is experienced nonvolitionally, at least to some degree. According to Edmonston (Chapter 7), the subjective impression of nonvolition is a "defining characteristic change" that accompanies anesis. And Barber (Chapter 8) states that every example of prototypical hypnotic behavior includes either the experience of nonvolition or a lack of awareness of a stimulus.

Whatever their theoretical persuasion, workers in the field are in agreement that the experience of involuntariness frequently accompanies hypnotic responses. Sociocognitive theorists have no quarrel with neodissociation theorists about the fact that hypnotic responses are often perceived as "involuntary" from the subjects' perspective. Neodissociation or state theorists, however, take subjects' responses at face value as reflecting fundamental changes in executive control or alterations in consciousness. In contrast, social-psychological and nonstate theorists view reports of involuntariness as reflecting multiple determinants, including pre-existing expectancies and schemas, goal-directed fantasies, and the wording of hypnotic suggestions.

Bowers and Davidson (Chapter 4) note that Spanos's earlier writings do not capture the distinction between goal-directed behavior and behavior that is enacted volitionally (i.e., on purpose). Moreover, Bowers and Davidson state that Spanos "places all his eggs in the basket of conscious control and purposes." The contributions to our book would suggest a somewhat different conclusion: The view that not all hypnotic behavior or thought is deliberate, in the sense that it is deliberated or consciously articulated, is increasingly shared by a wide variety of theoreticians (including Spanos).

There seems to be a growing recognition that subjects can intend to respond to suggestions and have suggested experiences, yet may not necessarily be conscious of the contextual determinants and cognitive operations that shape their hypnotic experiences (see the chapters by Coe & Sarbin, Spanos, ourselves, Wagstaff, Nash, McConkey, Sheehan, and Zeig & Rennick). Nash (Chapter 6), for example, states that reports of nonvolition during hypnosis do not reflect diminished behavioral control, but instead reveal "an experienced separation between intent (to comply) and awareness of that intent." Spanos's (Chapter 11) concept of tacit understanding implies that subjects may not consciously articulate their expectancies or the situational demands that guide their behavior, unless these are made salient. According to Zeig and Rennick (Chapter 9), responses become increasingly autonomous or "avolitional" as the cues that prompt them become increasingly obscure. Coe and Sarbin (Chapter 10) note that subjects may actually do things that facilitate their experience of a hypnotic phenomenon such as amnesia, yet may not be aware that they are engaged in certain actions to achieve their ends. And as McConkey (Chapter 18) has noted, even the hypnotized subjects' intention to respond to the hypnotist may occur outside the field of awareness. Finally, strategic cognitions and actions are not necessarily effortful or dependent on the allocation of a great deal of attention. In short, several different theories admit the possibility that cognitive processes, contextual demands, and even intentions that guide behavior may not reach the threshold of awareness.

What our discussion suggests is that sharp paradigmatic distinctions are breaking down in terms of the issue of whether hypnotic behavior and thought are purposive, in the sense that they are consciously articulated and deliberated on an ongoing basis. This increased recognition of the unavailability to introspection of contextual determinants and cognitive processes during hypnosis parallels a growing awareness in cognitive psychogy of the unavailability to conscious scrutiny of cognitive events, bodily feelings, and even mental states.

HOW STABLE, TRAIT-LIKE, AND MODIFIABLE IS HYPNOTIZABILITY?

The "Stable Trait" Controversy

Proponents of the idea that hypnotizability is dispositional have generally argued that hypnotic responsiveness is best construed as a relatively stable, aptitudinal capacity of the individual. Bányai (Chapter 19) is one of many theorists who conceptualize hypnotic ability as a relatively stable personality trait. Bányai's use of the term "trait" is compatible not only with its use in modern psychology, but also with its use by other theorists who contend that hypnotic responsiveness is trait-like. Here, "trait" refers to a characteristic that differs from person to person in a relatively permanent and consistent way, within relatively stable situational parameters. Hypnotic ability is thought to predispose or potentiate subjects' responsiveness to suggestion, and can, according to some theorists (e.g., Nadon et al., Chapter 16; McConkey, Chapter 18; Sheehan, Chapter 17), interact with a variety of contextual and interpersonal determinants that potentiate hypnotic abilities.

Of course, hypnotic ability is characterized in very different ways by different theorists represented in this volume. It is variously conceptualized as the capacity for dissociation (Hilgard and Bowers & Davidson); as a cognitive flexibility in accessing multiple cognitive and/or psychodynamic pathways (Evans); as a flexibility in changing ways of functioning, including physiological flexibility (Bányai); as the capacity for psychological regression (Nash) or relaxation (Edmonston); as responsiveness to minimal cues (Zeig & Rennick); and finally, as personal dispositions such as absorption, imaginative and dissociative abilities, and openness to experience (Nadon et al., Sheehan, McConkey, Barber, and Coe & Sarbin).

Regardless of how hypnotic ability is conceptualized, the idea that hypnotic responsiveness is trait-like is supported not only by high test–retest reliability among different hypnosis measures, but also by correlations between disparate scales that are typically in excess of .60 (Bowers, 1976). Even after a retest period of 25 years, one study found that the test–retest correlation was .71, and that mean hypnotic performance was stable over time (Piccione, Hilgard, & Zimbardo, 1989).

As Hilgard (Chapter 3) observes, the issue of whether to consider hypnotizability as a "trait" (of more or less enduring ability or skill) is controversial not only because of the critique of personality traits in general by social psychologists, but also because of the controversy over the extent to which individual differences in measured hypnotizability can be modified. Just how modifiable hypnosis is thought to be varies among theorists. Bowers and Davidson (Chapter 4) observe that the trait of hypnotic ability does not imply that hypnotic responsiveness is immutable. Rather, it implies constraints on the degree to which hypnotic responsiveness will vary as a function of experience.

There is at least the implicit suggestion that hypnotizability is modifiable to some degree in theories that acknowledge the impact of social and contextual variables. Bányai's (Chapter 19) model, for example, accords importance to both trait (aptitude) and situational/relational influences, which interact to create a more encompassing hypnotic process. Bányai in turn maintains that hypnotizability can be stable *and* modifiable, within limits. Despite Barber's (Chapter 8) contention that imaginative and dissociative capacities predict responsiveness to hypnotic suggestions, he argues that hypnotizability is mutable. Tailoring hypnotic procedures to the person's unique personality or counteracting inhibitions against experiencing hypnosis make it possible for the therapist to "unlock" hypnotic capacities, and thereby to facilitate responsiveness, even in low-hypnotizable subjects. Zeig and Rennick (Chapter 9) make a similar argument in noting that hypnotizability can be maximized by capitalizing on patients' responsiveness and learnings, and by respecting their personalities and customizing techniques to fit their needs and situations.

The limits of hypnotizability are not specifically addressed by Barber and by Zeig and Rennick (in their chapters). However, from a clinical perspective, there is much to be gained by developing procedures to enhance hypnotic response. Hypnotizability may have clinical relevance in diminishing patients' response to pain (see Chaves, 1989; Stam, 1989), and in treating disorders and conditions (e.g., asthma, warts) that have an involuntary component (Perry, Gelfand, & Marcovitch, 1979; Wadden & Anderton, 1982).

Social-psychological theories adamently reject the proposition that individual differences in hypnotizability are a function of differences in trait-like abilities. Instead, they construe hypnotizability as a composite of potentially modifiable cognitive skills, attitudes, and expectancies. Spanos (Chapter 11), for example, contends that stability in hypnotic responding does not reflect a stable trait. Instead, it reflects stability in subjects' attitudes, expectations, and interpretations about hypnosis. Although stable cognitive abilities (e.g., imaginal propensities or other cognitive abilities) may play an important role in hypnotizability, their effects are apparent only in interaction with attitudes and interpretations that constitute subjects' understandings of hypnosis and their motivation to respond (see Nadon et al., Chapter 16). According to social-psychological theories, hypnotic responsiveness is so malleable that many low-hypnotizable subjects, with proper training, can learn to respond like "hypnotic virtuosos."

Spanos (Chapter 11; see also Gorassini & Spanos, 1986) has described a highly successful multifaceted cognitive skill training program (The Carleton Skills Training Program, or CSTP) that targets subjects' attitudes, expectancies, and interpretations of suggestions for change. It also emphasizes the importance of enacting responses rather than assuming a passive response set, and teaches subjects imagery strategies to promote the experience of suggestions as involuntary. Like Spanos, Wagstaff (Chapter 12) expresses confidence in the ability of hypnotizability modification procedures to enhance hypnotic responsiveness. He attributes much of the stability in hypnotic performance to the subjects' conscious wish to perform at a certain hypnotizability level as well as to compliant responding, which may remain stable across testings. He maintains that by making expectations and cognitive strategies congruent, hypnotizability modification procedures are actually likely to minimize rather than produce compliance.

Kirsch (Chapter 14) is open to the possibility that an ability factor can account for the stability of hypnotic responsiveness. Nevertheless, Kirsch questions whether this factor operates independently of expectancy. One possibility is that expectancies become stabilized by testing procedures, so that each hypnosis test confirms and reinforces expectancies, rendering them resistant to change. This hardening of expectancies thus accounts for the stability of hypnotic responsiveness across repeated testings. However, engendering powerful expectations that convince subjects they are having suggestion-related experiences makes it possible to produce high levels of responsiveness in even initially low-hypnotizable subjects.

Like Kirsch, Fourie (Chapter 15) argues that performance stability is a function of how subjects come to feel about and define the susceptibility-testing situation, which is typically structured and authoritarian. So persons who feel comfortable in this sort of test situation are likely to score as highly hypnotizable; in contrast, people who are not comfortable are likely to score low on susceptibility tests. Because the susceptibility-testing situation and subjects' definition of it are likely to remain stable, hypnotic performance is likely to remain stable as well. Modifying subjects' expectations about hypnosis or adapting the test situation to the expectations of subjects should make it possible to modify hypnotizability.

Hypnotizability Modification: The Question of Compliance

Theories that tout the modifiability of hypnotic responsiveness are bolstered by the documented success (see Spanos, 1986) of Gorassini and Spanos's (1986) hypnotizability modification program, the CSTP. However, despite the apparent success of the CSTP, it has been criticized on the grounds that posttraining gains do not reflect valid enhancements of hypnotizability. Hilgard (Chapter 3) and Bowers and Davidson (Chapter 4) maintain that external demands and expectancies for compliance with suggestions inherent in the training procedures result in trained subjects' simply acquiescing to suggestions in the absence of suggestion-related experiences. Relatedly, Bányai (Chapter 19) argues that the training procedures place strong demands on subjects to conform with instructions. A crucial issue is thus whether the CSTP actually changes skills and aptitudinal capacities that underlie hypnotic responding, or whether the

CSTP functions more like a "coaching program" that improves performance on specific tests without essentially altering subjects' fundamental skills, abilities, and experiences.

The most complete and focused critique of the CSTP has been provided by Bates and colleagues (Bates, Miller, Cross, & Brigham, 1988; Bates & Brigham, 1990; Bates, in press). Bates (in press) notes that there are at least two reasons to suspect that CSTP gains reflect compliance rather than, or in addition to, enhanced hypnotic ability. First, subjects are informed that the goal of training is to increase hypnotic responsiveness. Second, the procedures themselves indicate that compliance is an essential part of successful hypnotic responding. Consider the following examples of parts of suggestions administered during the instructional training (Bates, in press) that exemplify the latter point:

Arm-raising suggestion: "Of course, your arm will not really go up by itself, you must raise it."
Hand lock suggestion: "Do not move your hands apart. You want it to seem that this is not happening through any effort on your part."

These concerns may be well founded. Two studies (Bates & Brigham, 1990; Spanos, Robertson, Menary, & Brett, 1986) deleted instructional elements of the CSTP (e.g., telling subjects that responses must be enacted and giving them information about how to interpret suggestions) and found that treatment gains were degraded as a result; two studies (Bates et al., 1988; Bates & Brigham, 1990) showed that subjective experiences were not necessarily affected by training procedures; and one study (Bates et al., 1988) indicated that when the training and testing sessions were defined as part of separate experiments, training gains were compromised relative to when subjects were informed that training and testing were part of the same experiment.

Spanos acknowledges that compliance with situational demands may play a role in the hypnotizability gains produced by skill training, but he also maintains that compliance is not a sufficient explanation. Spanos has defended the CSTP on the grounds (Spanos, 1986; Spanos & Flynn, 1989) that treatment gains generalize to novel suggestions (see Spanos, Lush, & Gwynn, 1989); that gains are maintained for 9–30 months, even when retesting is conducted by a different hypnotist (Spanos, Cross, Menary, & Smith, 1988); and that subjects who demonstrate posttreatment hypnotizability gains typically obtain scores on hypnotizability and subjective involvement indices comparable to those of subjects who test as highly hypnotizable without the benefit of training (see Spanos, 1986).

Research with the CSTP has contributed to the debate about whether compliance is an important determinant of suggestion-related responding.

Although it would be naive to argue that compliance is never a factor, most hypnosis theorists downgrade the importance or ignore the role of compliance in hypnosis. It is widely believed that outright faking or simulation is negligible during hypnosis (e.g., Hilgard, Chapter 3); that actions of hypnotic subjects represent serious efforts at adopting and enacting a social role (Coe & Sarbin, Chapter 10); and that hypnotic responses are generally not acts of deliberate deception (Kirsch, Chapter 14; ourselves, Chapter 13). However, a number of theorists, including Wagstaff (Chapter 12) and Spanos (Chapter 11), maintain that there are multiple pathways to a suggestion-related responses (including compliance), and that subjects sometimes exaggerate and purposely misdescribe their experiences in order to fulfill suggested demands.

It would be worthwhile for workers in the field to articulate more precisely what they mean by the term "compliance." That is, theoreticians generally do not distinguish among the effects of social pressure on subjects to respond in a certain manner; subjects' voluntarily enacting responses in the absence of concomitant subjective effects; and subjects' attuning their behavioral and subjective responses to the implicit and explicit demands conveyed by the test suggestions while successfully experiencing suggested effects. If compliance is defined in the latter sense, it can be argued that cooperating with or conforming to test demands is probably a requirement of high hypnotizability (see Spanos, 1986). This type of conformity does not, then, pose a serious challenge to the validity of treatment-related gains, inasmuch as many of the theoreticians represented in our book acknowledge that social-psychological variables (including sensitivity to demand characteristics) constitute important determinants of hypnotic responding and subjective experience.

Crucial experiments are necessary to clarify the role of compliance and demand characteristics in producing CSTP gains, and in hypnosis more generally. Research is needed to provide a comprehensive analysis of the CSTP task demands, to examine the relation between demands to enact suggestions and treatment outcomes, and to examine setting × response interactions in testing the generalization of treatment effects to a variety of measures germane to the cognitive and interpersonal domains of hypnosis. Furthermore, the precise contribution of compliance to hypnotic responding, and the conditions in which subjects are most likely to feel pressed to comply, remain unclear and await concerted research attention. Spanos's attempts to distinguish compliance, the reinterpretation or reclassification of experience, and changes in sensory experiences are promising.

We wish to sound a cautionary note about regarding subjects' responses as "compliant." To be sure, certain subjects willfully enact suggestion-related behaviors. They do so in the absence of any attempt to imagine or experience suggested effects, or they are totally unable to have suggestion-related experiences but respond nevertheless. Perhaps more commonly, subjects are able to generate some suggestion-related experiences. If a disparity exists between subjects' actual experience and their standards about what constitutes a "good enough" experiential response, then they may report that suggestion-related behaviors are accompanied by minimal imagery or sensations, for example. Under these circumstances, an experimenter may mistakenly regard the response as "compliant." A careful assessment of subjects' motivation to respond, performance standards, imagery, and suggestion-related sensations is necessary before we assume that subjects are merely engaging in compliant behavior, rather than actively attempting to "be hypnotized" or experiencing suggested effects to a limited degree.

Before we conclude this section, it is worth noting that, in all likelihood, hypnotizability modification research will eventually show that hypnotic responsiveness is considerably more malleable than was generally recognized. However, it may also shed light on aspects of hypnotic responsiveness that remain intractable to even the most concerted and clever modification efforts. It may perhaps be ironic, if not paradoxical, if learning more about our ability to modify hypnotizability ultimately broadens our understanding of the stable or "trait-like" properties of hypnotic responsiveness.

HYPNOSIS RESEARCH: ISSUES AND FUTURE DIRECTIONS

In our comments about important issues and points of convergence and divergence among theories, we have drawn attention to a number of directions for future research. In this section, we delineate additional conceptual and methodological issues and research questions that can profitably be addressed. In so doing, we feel that the heuristic value of the theories presented herein will become increasingly evident.

Theoretical approaches differ in terms not only of what is studied, but of how it is studied. Theories dictate the range of phenomena that are subject to experimental inquiry. The theories we have considered vary with respect to the number of variables and processes or mechanisms thought to determine hypnotic response and experience. Edmonston (Chapter 7) and Evans (Chapter 5), for example, contend that relaxation and dissociation, respectively, are essential substrates of hypnosis, and largely confine their research to demonstrating the parallels between these mechanisms and their manifestations and hypnosis. Hilgard (Chapter 3) and Bowers and Davidson (Chapter 4), who regard dissociation as central to hypnosis, have targeted phenomena for study that have a particular dissociative quality. Hilgard, for example, has studied the so-called "hidden observer," whereas Bowers and colleagues have studied analgesia and amnesia, in research designed to show that high-level cognitive work is not required to "achieve [a] hypnotically suggested state of affairs." Because hypnotic ability is accorded a prominent role, studies in this tradition often compare the performance of subjects high and low in hypnotzability, in order to highlight the impact of individual differences in ability. Although a great deal of research has been spurred by these theories, they may be said to have a relatively narrow focus or bandwidth.

In contrast, sociocognitive and interactive-phenomonological theories have a wider bandwidth, and have made a broad range of determinants fair game for study. Not only are multiple variables pertinent to situational (e.g., demand characteristics, interpersonal factors, instructional set), cognitive (e.g., cognitive strategies, distraction, attentional focus), dispositional (e.g., absorption, fantasy proneness, hypnotizability), and even physiological dimensions of hypnosis deemed worthy of study, but so too is their interaction. Designs that manipulate expectancies and characteristics of the situation are common in this tradition, as are studies that examine the interaction of contextual features and personal dispositions. Nadon et al. (Chapter 16) suggest that research designs taking into account the multidimensionality of hypnotic responses require equally multidimensional data-analytic strategies, which ideally combine experimental and correlational statistical techniques.

As Hilgard (1986) has observed, in hypnosis, as in any area of psychology, the empirical method does not eliminate controversies over experimental design and over the theoretical interpretations of findings. It is therefore not surprising that the value of certain control groups, so often dictated by theory-driven considerations, has also become the subject of controversy. Studies derived from sociocognitive theories, which emphasize the mundane nature of hypnotic responses, often include nonhypnotic control groups to illustrate that when subjects are properly instructed and motivated to respond, hypnotic and nonhypnotic behaviors and experiences are often indistinguishable. Designs that use task motivated subjects have been criticized by neodissociation theorists (see the chapters by Hilgard and by Bowers & Davidson) for being deceptive in their implication that hypnotic subjects invariably can have particular responses (e.g., hallucinations) if they wish to, and for bringing inordinate pressure to bear on subjects to acquiesce or conform to instructional demands.

At the same time, sociocognitive theorists (see the chapters by Coe & Sarbin, Spanos, Wagstaff, and ourselves) have been skeptical of interpreting differences between hypnotized and simulating subjects as evidence for a special hypnotic state or process. They argue not only that hypnotizable and simulating subjects differ in terms of hypnotizability, but that the task demands of simulating instructions are so distinctive that they could account for any group differences secured. Investigators (Spanos, 1986;

Stanley, Lynn, & Nash, 1986; Wagstaff & Benson, 1987) have called attention to the occasional tendency of simulators to "overplay" their role plays when task demands are clear-cut by responding in an exaggerated fashion, representative of only a minority of "excellent" hypnotic subjects. Conversely, simulators may adopt a conservative, cautious response set, and may not respond when in doubt (see Sheehan, 1970).

Questions about the inferences that can be drawn from the use of different control groups have contributed to the failure of research to resolve important theoretical issues. Some theoretical questions are difficult to resolve because there is no consensus about the kind of data necessary to resolve them. For a better understanding of the strengths and limitations of task motivation and simulation control groups, as well as the extent to which these control groups can help to resolve theoretical questions, research should be undertaken that "dismantles" these procedures so that their disparate components can be isolated and their effects ascertained. Future evaluation of these designs should include a detailed postexperimental inquiry, preferably utilizing evocative procedures such as Sheehan and McConkey's (1982) experiential analysis technique. In conclusion, the study of hypnotic control groups is interesting and valuable in its own right.

Hypnotic Experience

A task of hypnosis theories is to explain not only variations in hypnotic responses but also variations in hypnotic experiences. We must disagree with Wagstaff's (Chapter 12) contention that there is little profit in attempting to introduce elaborate designs to tease out the finer details of the "experience of hypnosis." Unfortunately, programmatic analyses of subjects' cognitive processes and subjective experiences are for the most part lacking, with the notable exceptions of Sheehan and McConkey's (1982), Spano's (see Chapter 11), and Bányai's (see Chapter 19) work. Researchers have neglected to capture the richness and complexity of subjects' cognitive activities in responding to hypnotic communications. Additional information is needed regarding how subjects perceive hypnotic procedures on an ongoing basis, how they arrive at attributions about their responses, how they resolve conflict during hypnosis, and under what conditions particular strategies are preferred. The relation between the choice of cognitive strategies (e.g., imagination vs. distraction in analgesia) and personality dispositions (e.g., fantasy proneness and absorption) would also be a worthwhile focus of research attention.

Exploiting descriptive phenomenological methods, including clinical interviews (see Coe & Sarbin, Chapter 10), could help to unravel the relations between and among contextual factors, cognitive processes, and subjective experiences. It could also contribute to a better understanding of when and under what stimulus conditions subjects consciously produce their hypnotic responses.

Imagination and Hypnosis

Few theorists would contest the statement that imaginative processes and abilities play a role in hypnosis. Nevertheless, a great deal remains to be learned about the relation between imagination and hypnotizability. Studies designed to examine this link have generally failed to assess diverse yet potentially interrelated aspects of imaginative involvement, including degree of involvement, intrusive cognitions, and credibility and vividness of imagining. Their relative independence of one another remains to be ascertained, as does whether certain aspects of imaginative involvement are more influential determinants of hypnotic responding than others.

The issue of whether the testing context mediates the relations between and among measures of imagination, absorption, and hypnotizability is controversial (see Kirsch, Chapter 14, vs. Nadon et al., Chapter 16). To be sure, crucial studies have yet to be performed. Even if a small "context effect" proves to be reliable, it will be important to examine explanations for this effect. One such explanation is that screening and testing subjects in the same context primes them to imagine—that is, to use their nascent imaginative abilities during hypnosis. Studying subjects under these conditions should provide an optimal assessment of the relation between absorption and hypnotizability, and may facilite the emergence of the "true" relation between the two.

To test the "priming hypothesis," groups of primed subjects (e.g., subjects imagining the sorts of things mentioned on the absorption scale) and nonprimed subjects can be tested for hypnotizability when absorption is measured in and apart from the hypnosis context. If priming is a viable explanation, then subjects who have been primed to use their imagination prior to hypnosis should be expected to show some degree of response consistency across absorption and hypnotizability measures, even though these measures are administered in different contexts. Of course, this relation should not obtain when subjects are tested "out of context" but not primed to imagine during hypnosis.

Another possible explanation for the "context effect" is that demand characteristics for correspondent responding across measures are established by the administration of absorption and hypnotizability measures in the same testing context. That is, are correlations between measures of hypnotizability and absorption mediated by the perception that there is a relation between the two measures? This hypothesis can be tested by providing subjects with differing information regarding the connection between absorption and hypnotizability (e.g., "Absorption is an indicator of hypnotizability" vs. "The measures are independent") and testing subjects for hypnotizability when absorption is measured in and apart from the hypnosis context. Other interesting research avenues include examining whether context effects are apparent when the range of measures tested is extended to dissociation, and whether context effects are equally apparent across the entire range of hypnotizability or whether they are particularly pronounced in subjects high, medium, or low in hypnotizability.

Clinical Hypnosis

Despite the recent surge of interest in the application of hypnosis to the treatment of a wide range of psychological and physiological disorders, hypnotic treatments have yet to be adequately evaluated on any dimension of theoretical interest or in terms of effectiveness (Spanos & Chaves, 1989). The study of the effectiveness of hypnotherapy is complicated by the fact that the dynamics of therapy are superimposed on the dynamics of hypnosis, rendering it difficult to determine whether treatment gains are due to hypnosis, psychotherapy, or an interaction between the two. Studies are needed to parcel out the effects of hypnosis and psychotherapy, as well as the role of "common factors" (e.g., positive therapeutic alliance, client motivation and expectancy, modeling of "healthy" behaviors) versus specific hypnotic effects as mediators of treatment success.

Previous research has not clearly or consistently operationalized hypnotic procedures or what constitutes "hypnosis." This has limited the conclusions that can be drawn about hypnotic effects in clinical studies. For example, because Erickson did not operationalize hypnosis in terms of precise criteria, it is unclear what part, if any, hypnosis played in Erickson's treatment. He often stated that clients were hypnotized, even though they did not manifest classical hypnotic responses (e.g., analgesia, posthypnotic amnesia) or report subjective characteristics typically regarded as "hypnotic" (i.e., involuntariness). Failure to quantify the client's responses or to outline the boundary conditions of what constitutes a "hypnotic" response makes it impossible to specify the relation between therapeutic techniques and treatment success to hypnotizability, at least as it is conventionally defined. In short, the term "hypnosis," as used by therapists who do not specify what constitues "hypnosis" or a hypnotic response, is perhaps best thought of as a descriptive metaphor that lends a semblance of coherence to a constellation of therapeutic techniques (Kirmayer, 1988).

The failure to operationalize hypnosis does not preclude field observations and naturalistic methods (see Zeig & Rennick, Chapter 9), which can yield rich anecdotal impressions. However, precise specifications of procedures and of criteria as to what constitutes a hypnotic response are required in order to examine the specific effects of hypnosis in controlled outcome research. Research designs that artfully combine naturalistic methods and controlled scientific studies are therefore a priority.

Studies that bridge the gap between experimental and clinical settings are few in number. This is unfortunate, because many of the processes and variables (e.g., imagination, demand characteristics) that appear to play a role in laboratory studies have potential relevance in clinical contexts. Studies that examine the generalizability of determinants from the laboratory to the clinical setting therefore merit attention.

To make strides in our understanding of the curative effects of hypnosis, the tools of the researcher can be applied to a wide range of problems in clinical and quasi-clinical contexts. For example, we are currently studying the effects of integrating hypnotic and self-hypnotic techniques in a personal development program. This program teaches subjects assertive skills, the control of unwanted habits, and cognitive–behavioral approaches for coping with stress and regulating emotions. We are evaluating the long-term effects of this treatment against the outcomes of no-hypnosis and no-treatment control groups, with self-identified depressed and anxious college students. Outcome is evaluated in terms of measures of college adjustment, psychopathology, and changes in preidentified target behaviors.

Clinicians and researchers share interests in learning more about the factors that maximize hypnotic responding, including the wording and perceptions of hypnotic communications. Researchers (e.g., ourselves and Spanos) have attached significance to suggestion wording, because it has a bearing on perceptions of involuntariness. Clinicians in turn have emphasized tailoring suggestions to clients' needs and problems, and have touted the benefits of admistering so-called "indirect" suggestions to recalcitrant clients. Unlike traditional, authoritative "direct" suggestions, indirect suggestions are generally permissively worded, and are characterized by a greater range of response choices than direct suggestions (see Lynn, Neufeld, & Maré, 1991). Unfortunately, investigators have generally failed to distinguish adequately among three types of suggestions— permissive, individually tailored, and indirect. The tendency to label these different types of suggestions as "indirect" may obscure potential differences in their impact on subjects or clients.

However, another possibility is that similar cognitive, affective, and behavioral processes underlie diverse types of suggestions. Variations in wording may be trivial in comparison with the demand characteristics of hypnotic communications and subjects' unique perceptions of them. Communication style may not be as important as the way communications are perceived by the subject. What the subject hears, rather than what the hypnotist says, may thus be the most critical feature of the hypnotist–subject interaction.

The complexity of the hypnotist's communication transcends the direct–indirect distinction. Studies should address syntactic and grammatical aspects of verbal messages, along with the effects of varying tonal and intonational qualities of the hypnotist's patter and of changes in volume, pitch, rate, and stress, on subjects' responses to direct versus indirect suggestions. Finally, hypnotizability and treatment outcome should be studied as a function of subjects' preference for different types of hypnotic communications.

So many types of inductions are used clinically that it is questionable whether researchers have even begun to study all of them. It would be worthwhile to survey clinicians to determine what inductions are used on an everyday basis in clinical work. Beyond that, it would be of interest to contrast traditional experimental inductions with inductions that are more representative of those used in clinical practice. For example, it would be useful to compare traditional inductions with both inductions that stimulate sensory awareness by focusing subjects on immediate sensory experiences (e.g., breathing, the space between the eyes, and the sound of the hypnotist's voice) and inductions that involve supportive or ego-strengthening suggestions, commonly used in clinical practice (see Barber, 1985).

Clinicians and researchers also share an interest in learning more about the relationship dimension of hypnosis and the physiological mechanisms that mediate hypnotic responding. Despite the fact that many hypnosis theories define hypnosis as a social encounter or emphasize the social aspects of the hypnotic proceedings, little attention has been devoted to the systematic study of motivation and relationship factors in hypnosis, with the exception of Bányai's, Nash's, Sheehan's, and our own research. Comprehensive hypnosis theories have neglected to systematically explicate subjects' motives and goals and their relation to hypnotic responsiveness and perceptions of the hypnotic relationship. For instance, we know very little about how subjects' motives to experience versus resist hypnosis reflect their rapport with the hypnotist.

Other questions pertinent to the affect-laden, relationship dimension of hypnosis are equally important to address: To what degree is positive rapport with the hypnotist an antecedent to successful responding versus a consequence of it? To what extent are more subtle (e.g., indications of rapport with the hypnotist in hypnotic dreams) versus more obvious (e.g., questionnaires with high face validity) measures of rapport differentially sensitive to fluctuations in the nature and quality of the hypnotic relationship? Do subtle and more obvious rapport measures tap a unitary dimension or construct? To what extent is "archaic involvement" truly divorced from contemporary aspects of the relationship, and to what extent (and in what sense) do "archaic" perceptions of the hypnotist represent a distortion of the hypnotist and the hypnotic relationship? Does psychotherapy, relative to the traditional experimental test context, promote feelings of archaic involvement? Does relaxation increase involvement with the hypnotist and sensitivity to role demands, or does the experience of anxiety or negative affect bond the subject and the hypnotist, who is seen as a "protector"?

Bányai's research on hypnotist styles and physiological mechanisms opens up new territory for investigators to explore. Yet before firm conclusions can be drawn about hypnotist styles, it is necessary to conduct controlled research on experimenter/hypnotist working styles in nonhypnotic as well as hypnotic test contexts, and to ascertain whether hypnotist style is consistent across subjects and situations or varies as a function of subject behavior. Of course, the need for rigorously controlled research also applies to the study of physiological mechanisms of hypnosis. Very few well-controlled studies have been conducted, as Bányai is the first to acknowledge. Her work, however, stands alone in its consideration of hypnosis as a truly reciprocal process within an interactive framework that examines multiple dimensions of hypnosis simultaneously.

The research proposed above is but one of many possible agendas for investigators to pursue. No doubt, as many research questions and programs of research could be generated as there are readers of this volume. This, we believe, is a healthy state of affairs; it reflects the richness and heuristic value of the theories presented herein, as well as the quality of the discourse and debate among competing models and perspectives.

A FINAL WORD

Theories and research are driven by curiosity, by the will to understand puzzling phenomena, and by data that do not match our existing blueprints of reality. Theoretical insights can provide schemas for organizing research data. However, we would do well to remember that our theories represent only approximations of "reality"; ideally, they must be open to revision to accommodate new insights and observations. In fact, there is no reason to suppose that there ever will be a final hypnosis theory that represents a single "true reality." The fact that major theoretical issues are still unresolved, and that many research questions remain to be addressed, augurs well for the advancement of scientific methodology and for the refinement and creative evolution of theories of hypnosis.

REFERENCES

Barber, T. X. (1969). *Hypnosis: A scientific approach*. New York: Van Nostrand Reinhold.

Barber, T. X. (1985). Hypnosuggestive procedures as catalysts for psychotherapies. In S. J. Lynn & J. P. Garske (Eds.), *Contemporary psychotherapies: Models and methods* (pp. 333–375). Columbus, OH: Charles E. Merrill.

Bates, B. L. (in press). Compliance and the Carleton Skills Training Program. *British Journal of Experimental and Clinical Hypnosis*.

Bates, B. L., & Brigham, T. A. (1990). Modifying hypnotizability with the Carleton Skills Training Program: A partial replication and analysis of components. *International Journal of Clinical and Experimental Hypnosis, 38*, 183–195.

Bates, B. L., Miller, R. J., Cross, J. J., & Brigham, T. A. (1988). Modifying hypnotic suggestibility with the Carleton Skills Training Program. *Journal of Personality and Social Psychology, 55*, 120–127.

Bowers, K. S. (1966). Hypnotic behavior: The differentiation of trance and demand characteristic variables. *Journal of Abnormal Psychology, 71*, 42–51.

Bowers, K. S. (1976). *Hypnosis for the seriously curious*. Monterey, CA: Brooks/Cole.

Brentar, J. P. (1990). *The Posthypnotic Experience Scale: A construct validation study*. Unpublished doctoral dissertation, Ohio University.

Chaves, J. F. (1989). Hypnotic control of clinical pain. In N. P. Spanos & J. F. Chaves (Eds.), *Hypnosis: The cognitive–behavioral perspective*. Buffalo, NY: Prometheus.

Fellows, B. J. (1990). Current theories of hypnosis: A critical overview. *British Journal of Experimental and Clinical Hypnosis, 7*, 81–92.

Gorassini, D. P., & Spanos, N. P. (1986). A sociocognitive skills approach to the successful modification of hypnotic susceptibility. *Journal of Personality and Social Psychology, 50*, 1004–1012.

Hilgard, E. R. (1963). Ability to resist suggestions within the hypnotic state: Responsiveness to conflicting communications. *Psychological Reports, 12*, 3–13.

Hilgard, E. R. (1986). *Divided consciousness: Multiple controls in human thought and action* (expanded ed.). New York: Wiley.

Kirmayer, L. J. (1988). Word magic and the rhetoric of common sense: Erikson's metaphors for mind. *International Journal of Clinical and Experimental Hypnosis, 36*, 157–172.

Kirsch, I., Mobayed, C., Council, J., & Kenny, L. (1991). *Expert judgments of hypnosis from subjective state reports: New data on the altered state controversy*. Manuscript submitted for publication.

Kuhn, T. S. (1962). *The structure of scientific revolutions*. Chicago: University of Chicago Press.

Perry, C., Gelfand, R., & Marcovitch, R. (1979). The relevance of hypnotic susceptibility in the clinical context. *Journal of Abnormal Psychology, 88*, 592–603.

Piccione, C., Hilgard, E. R., & Zimbardo, P. G. (1989). On the stability of measured hypnotizability over a 25 year period. *Journal of Personality and Social Psychology, 56*, 289–295.

Sarbin, T. R. (1950). Contributions to role theory: 1. Hypnotic behavior. *Psychological Review, 57*, 255–270.

Sheehan, P. W. (1970). Analysis of the treatment effects of simulation instructions in the application of the real–simulator model of hypnosis. *Journal of Abnormal Psychology*, 75, 98–103.

Sheehan, P. W., & McConkey, K. (1982). *Hypnosis and experience: The exploration of phenomena and process*. Hillsdale, NJ: Erlbaum.

Spanos, N. P. (1986). Hypnotic behavior: A social psychological interpretation of amnesia, analgesia, and "trance logic." *Behavioral and Brain Sciences*, 9, 449–502.

Spanos, N. P., & Chaves, J. F. (Eds.). (1989). *Hypnosis: The cognitive–behavioral perspective*. Buffalo, NY: Prometheus Books.

Spanos, N. P., Cross, W. P., Menary, E. P., & Smith, J. (1988). Long term effects of cognitive skill training for the enhancement of hypnotic susceptibility. *British Journal of Experimental and Clinical Hypnosis*, 5, 73–78.

Spanos, N. P., & Flynn, D. M. (1989). Simulation, compliance, and skills training in the enhancement of hypnotizability. *British Journal of Experimental and Clinical Hypnosis*, 6, 1–8.

Spanos, N. P., Lush, N. I., & Gwynn, M. I. (1989). Cognitive skill-training enhancement of hypnotizability: Generalization effects and trance logic responding. *Journal of Personality and Social Psychology*, 56, 795–804.

Spanos, N. P., Robertson, L. A., Menary, E. P., & Brett, P. J. (1986). A component analysis of cognitive skill-training for the enhancement of hypnotic susceptibility. *Journal of Abnormal Psychology*, 95, 350–357.

Stam, H. J. (1989). From symptom relief to cure: Hypnotic interventions in cancer. In N. P. Spanos & J. F. Chaves (Eds.), *Hypnosis: The cognitive–behavioral perspective*. Buffalo, NY: Prometheus Books.

Stanley, S. M., Lynn, S. J., & Nash, M. R. (1986). Trance logic, susceptibility screening and transparency response. *Journal of Personality and Social Psychology*, 50, 447– 454.

Wadden, T. A., & Anderson, C. H. (1982). The clinical uses of hypnosis. *Psychological Bulletin*, 91, 215–243.

Wagstaff, G. F., & Benson, D. (1987). Exploring hypnotic processes with the cognitive-simulator comparison group. *British Journal of Experimental and Clinical Hypnosis*, 4, 83–91.

Weitzenhoffer, A. M. (1974). When is an "instruction" an "instruction"? *International Journal of Clinical and Experimental Hypnosis*, 22, 258–269.

White, R. W. (1941). An analysis of motivation in hypnosis. *Journal of General Psychology*, 24, 145–162.

Woody, E. Z., Bowers, K. S., & Oakman, J. M. (1991). *A conceptual analysis of hypnotic responsiveness: Experience, individual differences, and context*. Unpublished manuscript, University of Waterloo, Waterloo, Ontario, Canada.

Index